BLOOD CELLS

A PRACTICAL GUIDE

BLOOD CELLS
A PRACTICAL GUIDE

Barbara J. Bain
MBBS FRACP MRCPath
Department of Haematology
St Mary's Hospital Medical School
London

SECOND EDITION

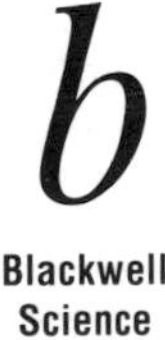

Blackwell
Science

Editorial Offices:
Osney Mead, Oxford OX2 0EL
25 John Street, London
WC1N 2BL
23 Ainslie Place, Edinburgh
EH3 6AJ
238 Main Street, Cambridge
Massachusetts 02142, USA
54 University Street, Carlton
Victoria 3053, Australia

Other Editorial Offices:
Arnette Blackwell SA
224, Boulevard Saint Germain
75007 Paris, France

Blackwell Wissenschafts-Verlag
GmbH
Kurfürstendamm 57
10707 Berlin, Germany

Zehetnergasse 6
A-1140 Wien
Austria

First published 1989
(Published by Gower Medical Publishing)
Second edition 1995
Reissued as paperback 1996

Set by Setrite Typesetters,
Hong Kong
Printed and bound in Italy
by G. Canale & C. S.p.A., Turin

Records for this title are available from the British Library and the Library of Congress

ISBN 0-86542-913-8 (hbk)
0-632-04155-2 (pbk)

DISTRIBUTORS

Marston Book Services Ltd
PO Box 269
Abingdon
Oxon OX14 4YN
(*Orders*: Tel: 01235 465500
Fax: 01235 465555)

USA
Blackwell Science, Inc.
238 Main Street
Cambridge, MA 02142
(*Orders*: Tel: 800 215–1000
617 876–7000
Fax: 617 492–5263)

Canada
Copp Clark, Ltd
2775 Matheson Blvd East
Mississauga, Ontario
Canada, L4W 4P7
(*Orders*: Tel: 800 263-4374
905 238-6074)

Australia
Blackwell Science Pty Ltd
54 University Street
Carlton, Victoria 3053
(*Orders*: Tel: 03 9347–0300
Fax: 03 9349–3016)

Contents

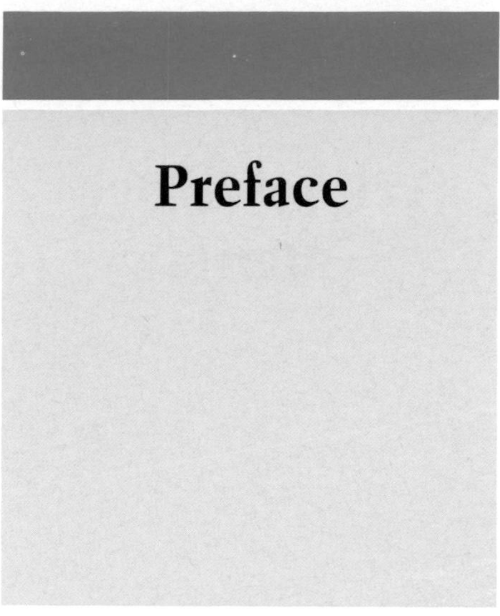

Preface

I have written this second edition of *Blood Cells* with both the practising haematologist and the trainee in mind. My aim has been to provide a guide for use in the diagnostic haematology laboratory, covering methods of collection of blood specimens, blood film preparation and staining, the principles of manual and automated blood counts and the assessment of the morphological features of blood cells. My objective has been that the practising haematologist should find this book sufficiently comprehensive to be a reference source while, at the same time, the trainee haematologist and laboratory scientist should find it a straight-forward and practical bench manual. I hope that the medically trained haematologist will gain a fuller understanding of the scientific basis of an important segment of laboratory haematology while the laboratory scientist will understand more of the purpose and clinical relevance of laboratory tests. I trust it is not too ambitious to hope to be 'all things to all men'. My overriding purpose has been to show that microscopy not only provides the essential basis of our haematological practice but can also lead to the excitement of discovery. If I succeed in sending the reader back to the microscope with renewed interest and enthusiasm I shall be well satisfied.

B.J.B.

Acknowledgements

I should like to thank Dr John Matthews and Mr Alan Dean who critically read the manuscript for the first edition of this book and Dr Kate Ozanne who did the same for the second edition. Many other colleagues and friends have reviewed sections of the manuscript and have given invaluable assistance by providing blood films or photographs. My thanks are also due to Mr Tony Macdonald, Mr Jim Griffiths and the manufacturers of the automated blood cell counters described for permitting me to observe various instruments in operation and for providing instrument printouts. Finally, I am grateful to those who have shared my pleasure in examining blood films over the last 25 years.

List of Abbreviations

ACTH	adrenocorticotrophic hormone
AIDS	acquired immune deficiency syndrome
ALL	acute lymphoblastic leukaemia
AML	acute myeloid leukaemia
ANAE	α-naphthyl acetate esterase
ANBE	α-naphthyl butyrate esterase
ATLL	adult T-cell leukaemia/lymphoma
ATP	adenosine triphosphate
CAE	chloroacetate esterase
CD	cluster of differentiation (immunophenotyping terminology)
CDA	congenital dyserythropoietic anaemia
CGL	chronic granulocytic leukaemia
CHCM	cellular haemoglobin concentration mean (Technicon H.1 series counters)
CLL	chronic lymphocytic leukaemia
CLL/PL	CLL, mixed cell type
CML	chronic myeloid leukaemia
CMML	chronic myelomonocytic leukaemia
CV	coefficient of variation
DNA	deoxyribonucleic acid
EBV	Epstein–Barr virus
EDTA	ethylene diamine tetra-acetic acid
ESR	erythrocyte sedimentation rate
FAB	French–American–British (classifications of haematological neoplasms)
FBC	full blood count
G6PD	glucose-6-phosphate dehydrogenase
G-CSF	granulocyte colony-stimulating factor
GM-CSF	granulocyte monocyte colony-stimulating factor
Hb	haemoglobin concentration
Hct	haematocrit
HDW	haemoglobin distribution width
HES	hypereosinophilic syndrome
HIV	human immune deficiency virus
HTLV-I	human T-cell lymphotropic virus I
ICSH	International Committee (now Council) for Standardization in Haematology
IL	interleukin
ITP	idiopathic (autoimmune) thrombocytopenic purpura
LCAT	lecithin–cholesterol acyl transferase
LI	lobularity index (H.1 series counters)
LUC	large unstained cells (H.1 series counters)
MCH	mean cell haemoglobin content
MCHC	mean cell haemoglobin concentration
MCV	mean cell volume
MDS	myelodysplastic syndrome(s)
MGG stain	May–Grünwald–Giemsa stain
MPO	myeloperoxidase
MPV	mean platelet volume

MPXI	mean peroxidase index (H.1 counter)
NAP	neutrophil alkaline phosphatase
NASA esterase	naphthol AS acetate esterase
NASDA esterase	naphthol AS-D acetate esterase
NRBC	nucleated red blood cell
PAS	periodic acid–Schiff
PCV	packed cell volume
PDW	platelet distribution width
PLL	prolymphocytic leukaemia
PNH	paroxysmal nocturnal haemoglobinuria
PRV	polycythaemia rubra vera
RBC	red cell count
RDW	red cell distribution width
RNA	ribonucleic acid
SBB	Sudan black B
SD	Standard deviation
SLVL	splenic lymphoma with villous lymphocytes
TNCC	total nucleated cell count
TRAP	tartrate-resistant acid phosphatase
TTP	thrombotic thrombocytopenic purpura
WBC	White cell count
WHO	World Health Organization
WIC	WBC in the impedance channel (Cell-Dyn instruments)
WOC	WBC in the optical channel (Cell-Dyn instruments)

Note to the reader

Unless otherwise stated, all photomicrographs have been stained with a May–Grünwald–Giemsa stain and have a final magnification of 912.

CHAPTER 1

Blood Sampling and Film Preparation

Obtaining a blood specimen

Performing an accurate blood count and correctly interpreting a blood film require that an appropriate sample from the patient, mixed with the correct amount of a suitable anticoagulant, is delivered to the laboratory without undue delay. No artefacts should be introduced during these procedures.

The identity of the patient requiring blood sampling should be carefully checked before performing a venepuncture. Patients should either sit or lie comfortably and should be reassured that the procedure causes only minimum discomfort; they should not be told that venepuncture is painless since this is not so. It is preferable for apprehensive patients to lie down. Chairs used for venepuncture should preferably have arm rests, both for convenience and to prevent a fainting patient falling from a chair. (I have personally observed one patient who sustained a skull fracture when he fainted at the end of a venepuncture and fell forward onto a hard floor, and two other patients, neither previously known to be epileptic, who suffered epileptiform convulsions during venepuncture. Such seizures may not be true epilepsy but consequent on hypoxia following brief vagal-induced cessation of heart beat [1].) If venepunctures are being performed on children or on patients unable to cooperate fully then the arm for venepuncture should be gently but firmly immobilized by an assistant. Gloves should be worn during venepuncture, for the protection of the person carrying out the procedure. The needle to enter the patient must not be touched so that it remains sterile.

Peripheral venous blood

In an adult, peripheral venous blood is most easily obtained from a vein in the antecubital fossa (Fig. 1.1) using a needle and either a syringe or an evacuated tube. Of the veins in the antecubital region the median cubital vein is preferred, since it is usually large and well anchored in tissues, but the cephalic and basilic veins are also often satisfactory. Other forearm veins can be used but they are often more mobile and therefore more difficult to penetrate. Veins on the dorsum of the wrist and hand often have a poorer flow and performing venepuncture at these sites is more likely to lead to bruising. This is also true of the anterior surface of the wrist where, in addition, venepuncture tends to be more painful.

When a vein is identified it is palpated to ensure it is patent. If a vein is not visible (in some dark-skinned or overweight people) it is identified by palpation after applying a tourniquet to achieve venous distention. If veins appear very small, warming of the arm to produce vasodilatation helps, as does tapping the vein and asking the patient to clench and unclench the fist several times.

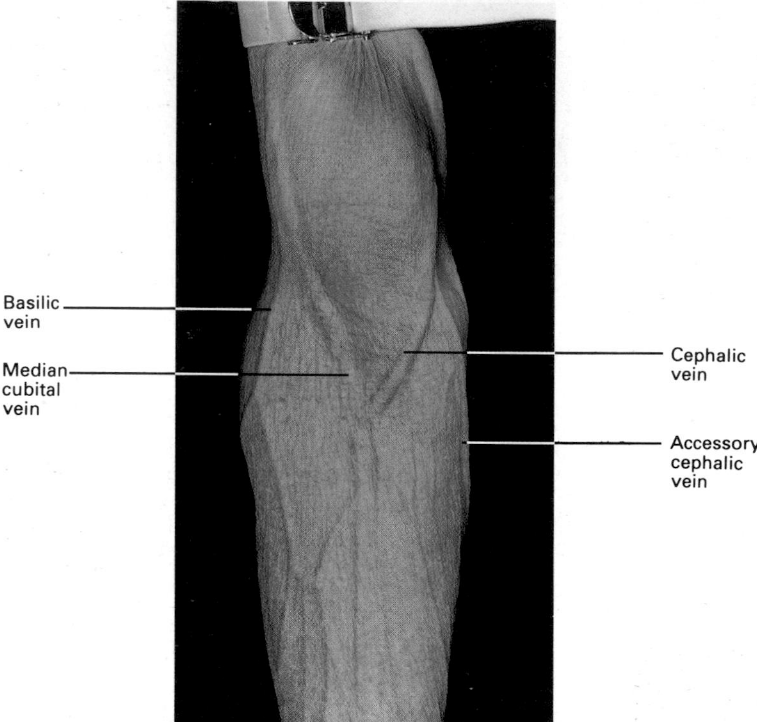

Fig. 1.1 Anterior surface of the left arm showing veins most suitable for venepuncture.

The arm should be positioned on the arm rest so that the vein identified is under some tension and its mobility is reduced. The skin should be cleaned with 70% ethanol or 0.5% chlorhexidine and allowed to dry. A tourniquet is applied to the arm, sufficiently tightly to distend the vein but not in such a manner as to cause discomfort. Alternatively, a sphygmomanometer cuff can be applied and inflated to diastolic pressure, but the use of a tourniquet is usually quicker and simpler. If it is particularly important to obtain a specimen without causing haemoconcentration, e.g., in a patient with suspected polycythaemia, the tourniquet should be left on the arm only long enough to allow penetration of the vein. Otherwise it can be left applied while blood is being obtained, to ensure a continuing adequate flow of blood. It is preferable that the tourniquet is applied for no more than a minute but the degree of haemoconcentration is not great, even after 10 minutes application. The increase of haemoglobin concentration and of red cell count is about 2% at 2 and at 10 minutes [2].

A 19 or 20 gauge needle is suitable for an adult and a 21 or 23 gauge for a child or an adult with small veins. The needle is attached to the syringe, which should have a side port rather than a central port, and the guard is removed. It is then inserted into the vein with the bevel upwards (Fig. 1.2). This may be done in a single movement or in two separate movements for the skin and the vein, depending on personal preference and on how superficial the vein is. With one hand steadying the barrel of the syringe so that the needle is not accidentally withdrawn from the vein, blood is withdrawn into the syringe using minimal negative pressure. Care should be taken not to aspirate more rapidly than blood is entering the vein, or the wall of the vein may be drawn against the bevel of the needle and cut off the flow of blood. If the tourniquet has not already been released this must be done before withdraw-

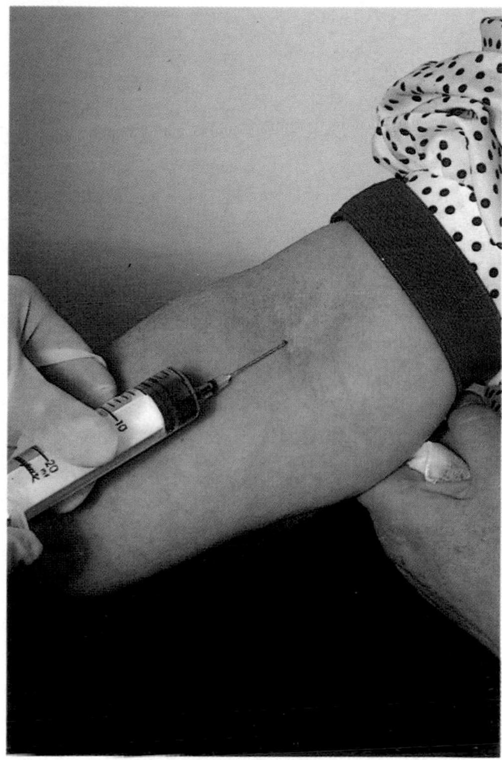

Fig. 1.2 Venepuncture technique using needle and syringe.

ing the needle. Following removal of the needle, direct pressure is applied to the puncture site with cotton wool or a sterile gauze square, the arm being kept straight and, if preferred, somewhat elevated. Adhesive plaster should not be applied until pressure has been sustained for long enough for bleeding from the puncture site to have stopped.

The needle should be removed from the syringe before expelling the blood into the specimen container, great care being taken to avoid self-injury with the needle. The needle should be put directly into a special receptacle for sharp objects without resheathing it. The blood specimen is expelled gently into a bottle containing anticoagulant and is mixed gently by inverting the container four or five times. Forceful ejection of the blood can cause lysis. Shaking should also be avoided. The specimen container is then labelled with the patient's name and identifying details and, depending on hospital procedure, possibly also with a bar-code label which is also applied to the request form and subsequently to the blood film. The time of venepuncture should also be recorded on the bottle. Bottles should not be labelled in advance away from the patient's bedside as this increases the chances of putting a blood sample into a mislabelled bottle. Recording the time of

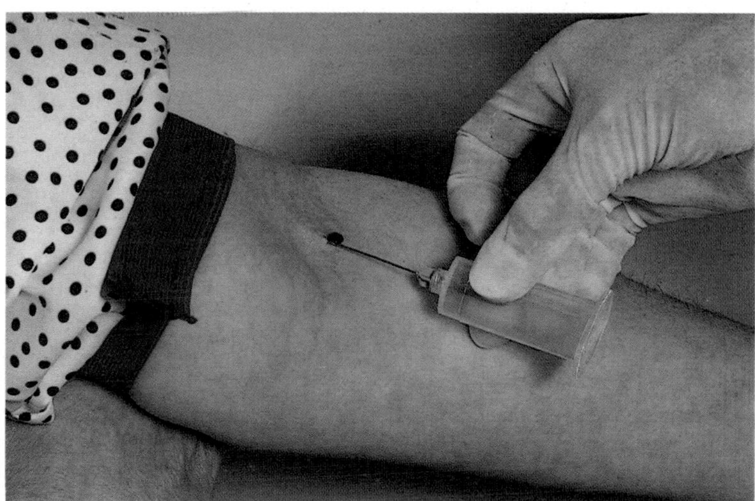

Fig. 1.3 Venepuncture technique using an evacuated container; the distal end of the needle has been screwed into the holder and the proximal needle has then been unsheathed and inserted into a suitable vein.

venepuncture is important both to allow the clinician to relate the laboratory result to the condition of the patient at the time and also to allow the laboratory to check that there has been no undue delay between venepuncture and performing the test.

When blood is taken into an evacuated tube the technique of venepuncture is basically similar. A double-ended needle is screwed into a holder which allows it to be manipulated for venepuncture (Fig. 1.3). Once the vein has been entered an evacuated tube is inserted into the holder and is pushed firmly so that its rubber cap is penetrated by the needle, breaking the vacuum and causing blood to be aspirated into the tube (Fig. 1.4). Evacuated tubes are very convenient if multiple specimens are to be taken, since several evacuated tubes can be applied in turn. Only sterile vacuum tubes should be used for obtaining blood specimens. In children and others with very small veins an appropriately small vacuum tube should be used so that excessive pressure does not cause the vein to collapse. Once all necessary specimen tubes have been filled, the needle is withdrawn from the vein, still attached to the holder. To reduce the possibility of a needle-prick injury it is necessary either to remove the needle from the holder with a specially designed safe device or to throw away the holder with the needle.

If a large specimen or a large number of specimens is required and an evacuated tube system is not in use, blood can be collected through a 'butterfly', that is through a needle fused to a small flexible tube. The tubing can easily be pinched off to allow several syringes in turn to be attached. This technique is also useful in children and when small veins make venepuncture difficult.

A blood specimen should not be taken from a vein above the site of an intravenous infusion since dilution can occur. However, venepuncture below the site of an infusion is not associated with clinically significant inaccuracy.

Anticoagulant and specimen container

The anticoagulant of choice for blood count specimens is one of the salts of ethylene diamine tetra-acetic acid (EDTA). K_2EDTA, K_3EDTA and Na_2EDTA have all been used. The preferred anticoagulant, recommended by the International Committee for Standardization in Haematology (ICSH), is K_2EDTA in a final concentration of 1.5–2.2 mg/ml [3]. Both dry EDTA and EDTA in solution are in use. A solution has the advantage that mixing of blood specimens is easier so clotted specimens are less common. However, it should be noted that some parameters are altered by dilution, and if too little blood is taken into a tube dilution may be appreciable. Excess EDTA

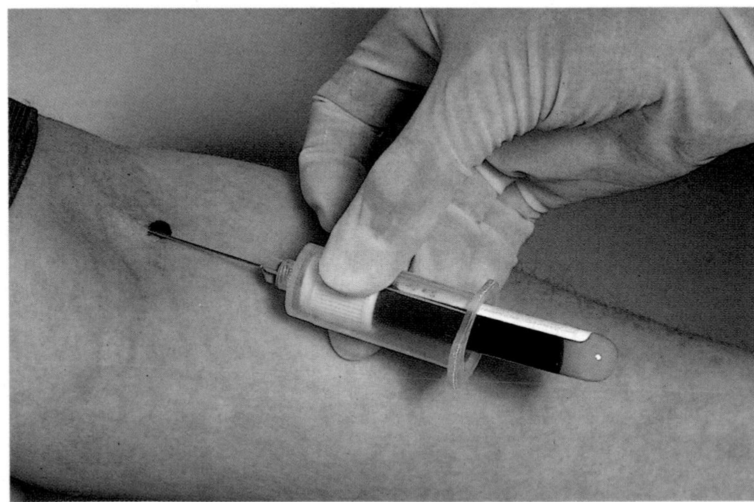

Fig. 1.4 Venepuncture technique using an evacuated container; the evacuated container has been inserted into the holder and forced onto the sharp end of the needle.

also has deleterious effects on cell morphology in stained blood films. Na_2EDTA is less soluble than the potassium salts. K_3EDTA causes undesirable cell shrinkage which is reflected in a lower microhaematocrit (see p. 19).

Many laboratories use automated blood counting instruments with a sampling device which is able to perforate the rubber cap of a blood specimen container and thus reduces unnecessary handling of blood. To take advantage of this it is necessary that not only evacuated tubes but also all blood containers have rubber caps which can be penetrated and resealed without permitting leakage.

Needle-prick injury

Precautions should be taken to avoid needle-prick (needle-stick) injuries. Hepatitis B can be readily transmitted by such injury, particularly when the patient is HB_e antigen positive. Overall transmission rates of 7–30% have been reported following needle-prick injuries involving infected patients. If the patient is HB_e antigen positive the rate of transmission is of the order of 20% if hepatitis B immune globulin is given after the injury [4] and about 30–40% if it is not given [5]. When sensitive techniques are used, the transmission of hepatitis C is found to be about 10% [6]. Human immune deficiency virus (HIV) is much less readily transmitted than hepatitis B or C but a risk does exist. In 3430 needle-prick injuries reported up to 1993 the overall transmission rate was 0.46% [7]. Other infections which have been occasionally transmitted by needle-prick injury include malaria, cryptococcosis and tuberculosis [8–10].

Because it has proved impossible to eliminate needle-stick injuries totally, staff who are performing venepunctures should be offered vaccination against hepatitis B and any who have not been vaccinated should be offered hepatitis B immune globulin after needle-prick injury involving an infected patient. Whether antiviral chemotherapy is useful after needle-prick injury involving an HIV-positive patient is unknown but it is clear that infection can be established despite zidovudine prophylaxis. Occupational health services should consider offering storage of serum samples from new staff so that baseline HIV testing is possible in the event of a subsequent needle-prick injury.

'Capillary blood'

It is often necessary to obtain blood by skin puncture in babies and infants and in adults with poor veins. 'Capillary' or, more probably, arteriolar blood may be obtained from a freely flowing stab wound made with a sterile lancet on the plantar surface of a warmed and cleansed heel (babies less than 3 months of age and infants), the plantar aspect of the big toe (infants) or a finger, thumb or ear lobe (older children and adults). The correct site for puncture of the heel is shown in Fig. 1.5. The lateral or posterior aspect of the heel should not be used in a baby as the underlying bone is much closer to the skin surface than it is on the plantar aspect. In older patients a finger (excluding the fifth finger) or the thumb is preferred to an ear lobe since bleeding from the ear lobe may be prolonged in a patient with a haemostatic defect and pressure is difficult to apply. The palmar surface of the distal phalanx is the preferred site on a digit since the underlying bone is closer to the skin surface on other aspects. Skin

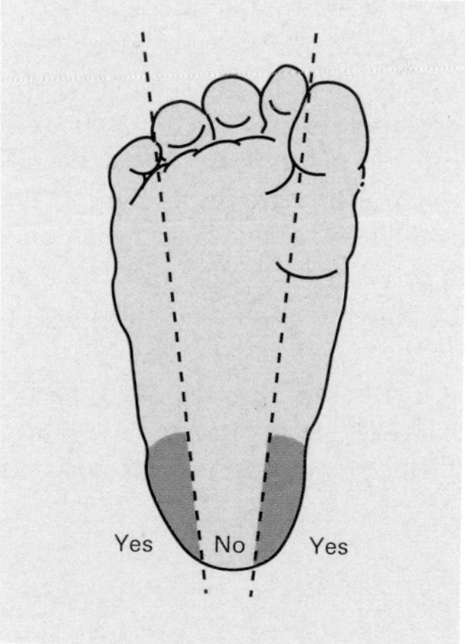

Fig. 1.5 The areas of the foot of a baby or infant which are suitable for obtaining capillary blood.

punctures should ideally be more than 1.5 mm deep in order that the lancet passes through the dermal–subcutaneous junction where the concentration of blood vessels is greatest, permitting a free flow of blood. Lancets used for heel puncture in babies must not exceed 2.4 mm in length since this is the depth below the skin of the calcaneal bone. Osteomyelitis of the calcaneal bone has resulted from inadvertent puncture of the bone [11]. Previous puncture sites should be avoided to reduce the risk of infection.

Capillary samples should be obtained from warm tissues so that a free flow of blood is more readily obtained. If the area is cool then it should be warmed with a wet cloth no hotter than 42°C. The skin should then be cleansed with 70% isopropanol and dried with a sterile gauze square (since traces of alcohol may lead to haemolysis of the specimen). The first drop of blood may be diluted with tissue fluid and should be wiped away with a sterile gauze square. Flow of blood may be promoted by gentle pressure, but a massaging or pumping action should not be employed since this may lead to tissue fluid being mixed with blood.

Capillary blood can be collected into re-usable glass pipettes or into glass capillary tubes. Capillary tubes containing EDTA may be used but tubes containing heparin are not suitable for full blood count (FBC) specimens since cellular morphology and staining characteristics are altered. Disposable pipettes complete with diluent, suitable for both automated and manual counts, are commercially available. Caution should be employed in the use of spring-loaded skin-prick devices since transmission of hepatitis B has occurred when there has been failure to change the platform as well as the lancet between patients [12].

Platelet counts performed on capillary blood are often lower than those on venous blood [13] and other parameters may also vary (see Chapter 5).

Cord blood

Blood samples can be obtained from the umbilical cord immediately after birth. Cord blood is best obtained with a syringe and needle. Expressing blood from the cut end of the cord can introduce Wharton's jelly into the blood sample with subsequent red cell agglutination. Haematological parameters on cord blood are not necessarily the same as those obtained from capillary or venous specimens from the neonate.

Other sites

It may sometimes be necessary to obtain blood from ankle veins, from the femoral vein or from indwelling cannulae in various sites. When blood is obtained from a cannula the first blood obtained may be diluted by infusion fluid or contaminated with heparin and should be discarded. In infants, blood can be obtained from scalp veins or jugular veins.

Making a blood film

A blood film may be made from non-anticoagulated (native) blood, obtained either from a vein or a capillary, or from EDTA-anticoagulated blood. Chelation of calcium by EDTA hinders platelet aggregation so that platelets are evenly spread and their numbers can be assessed more easily (Fig. 1.6). Films prepared from capillary blood usually show prominent platelet aggregation (Fig. 1.7) and films from native venous blood often show small aggregates (Fig. 1.8). Films prepared from native venous or capillary blood are free of artefacts due to storage or the effects of the anticoagulant. A few laboratories still use such films as a matter of routine, but otherwise their use is obligatory for investigating abnormalities such as red cell crenation or white cell or platelet aggregation which may be induced by storage or EDTA. Conversely, making a blood film from EDTA-anticoagulated blood after arrival of the blood specimen in the laboratory has the advantage that some of the artefacts which may influence the validity of results obtained from automated instruments are more likely to be detected, e.g., the formation of fibrin strands, aggregation of platelets or agglutination of red cells induced by cold agglutinins.

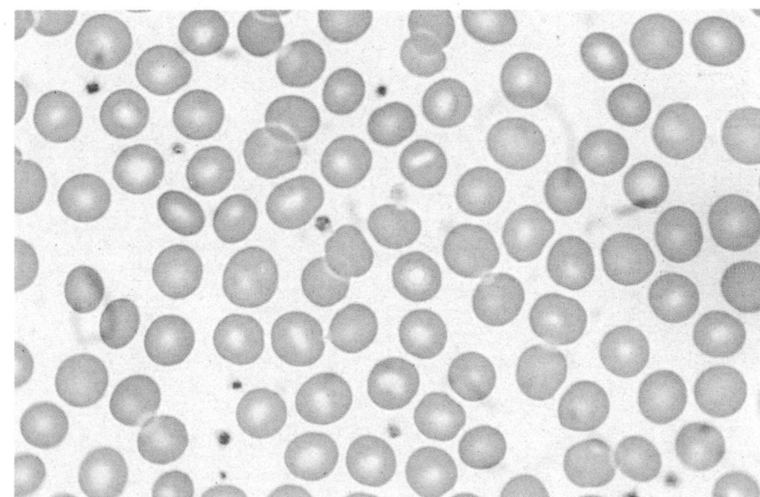

Fig. 1.6 A blood film from EDTA-anticoagulated blood showing an even distribution of platelets.

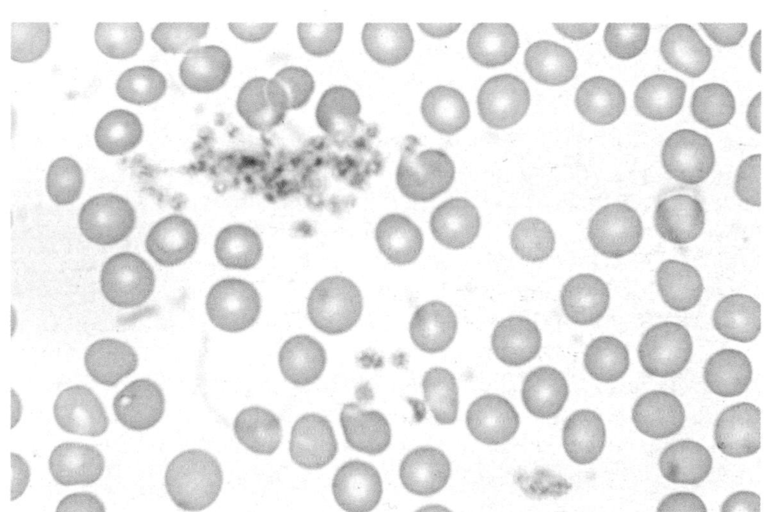

Fig. 1.7 A blood film from non-anticoagulated capillary blood showing the aggregation of platelets which usually occurs.

Manual spreading of a blood film on a glass slide (wedge-spread film)

Glass slides must be clean and free of grease. A spreader is also required and must be narrower than the slide. If a coverslip is to be applied it must also be narrower than the coverslip so that cells which are at the edge of the blood film are covered by the coverslip and can be easily examined microscopically. A spreader can be readily prepared by breaking the corner off a glass slide after incising it with a diamond pen; this provides a smooth-edged spreader which is large enough to be manipulated easily. Spreaders made by cutting transverse pieces from a slide are inferior since they are more difficult to handle and have at least one rough edge which may damage gloves or fingers.

The laboratory worker spreading blood films should wear gloves. A drop of blood (either native or anticoagulated) is placed near one end of the slide. Anticoagulated blood from screw-top con-

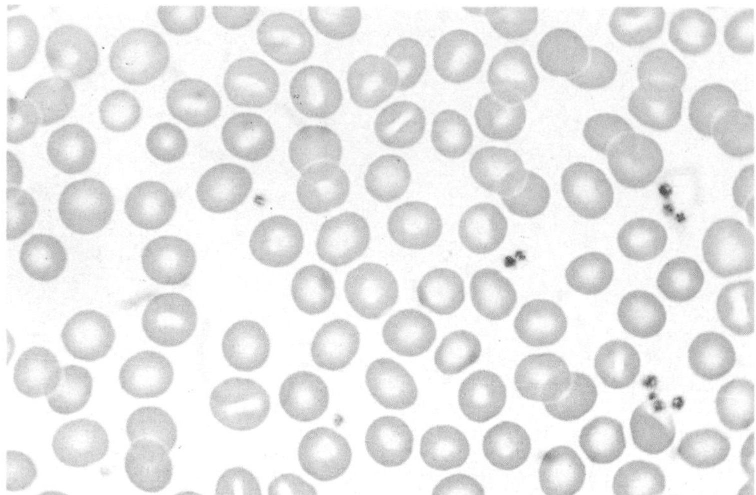

Fig. 1.8 A blood film from non-anticoagulated venous blood showing the minor degree of platelet aggregation which usually occurs.

tainers can be applied to the slide using a capillary tube which is then discarded. A drop of blood from specimen containers with penetrable lids can be applied to the slide by means of a special device which perforates the lid. The spreader is applied at an angle of 25–30°, in front of the drop of blood and is drawn back into it (Fig. 1.9). Once the blood has run along its back edge the spreader is advanced with a smooth steady motion so that a thin film of blood is spread over the slide. If the angle of the spreader is too obtuse or the speed of spreading is too fast, the film will be too short. An experienced operator learns to recognize blood with a higher than normal haematocrit (Hct), which is more viscous and requires a more acute angle to make a satisfactory film and, conversely, blood with a lower than normal Hct, which requires a more obtuse angle. It is important that the spreader is wiped clean with a dry tissue or gauze square after each use since it is otherwise possible to transfer abnormal cells from one blood film to another (Fig. 1.10).

As soon as slides are made they should be labelled with the patient's name and the date or with an identifying number. Small numbers of slides can be labelled with a diamond marker or by writing details on the thick part of the film. The fastest way to label large numbers of slides is with a methanol-resistant pen or by writing in pencil on the frosted end of a slide. Slides which are frosted at one end on *both* sides are useful because they avoid waste of staff time ensuring that the slide is the right way up. Slides should be dried rapidly. A fan to increase air circulation can be useful.

Figure 1.11 shows a well-spread film in comparison with examples of poor films resulting from faulty technique.

Unless otherwise stated, this book deals with morphology as observed in wedge-spread films. Most of the photographs are of manually spread films which have been prepared from recently collected EDTA-anticoagulated blood.

Other methods of spreading thin films

Automated spreading of blood films

Wedge-spread films can be prepared by mechanical spreaders which can be integrated with staining machines and automated full blood counters. A film of blood one cell thick can also be spread on a glass slide by centrifugation in a specially designed centrifuge but this method is losing popularity.

Films from blood with a very high Hct

If blood has a very high Hct, e.g., haemoglobin concentration (Hb) > 20 g/dl, it can be impossible

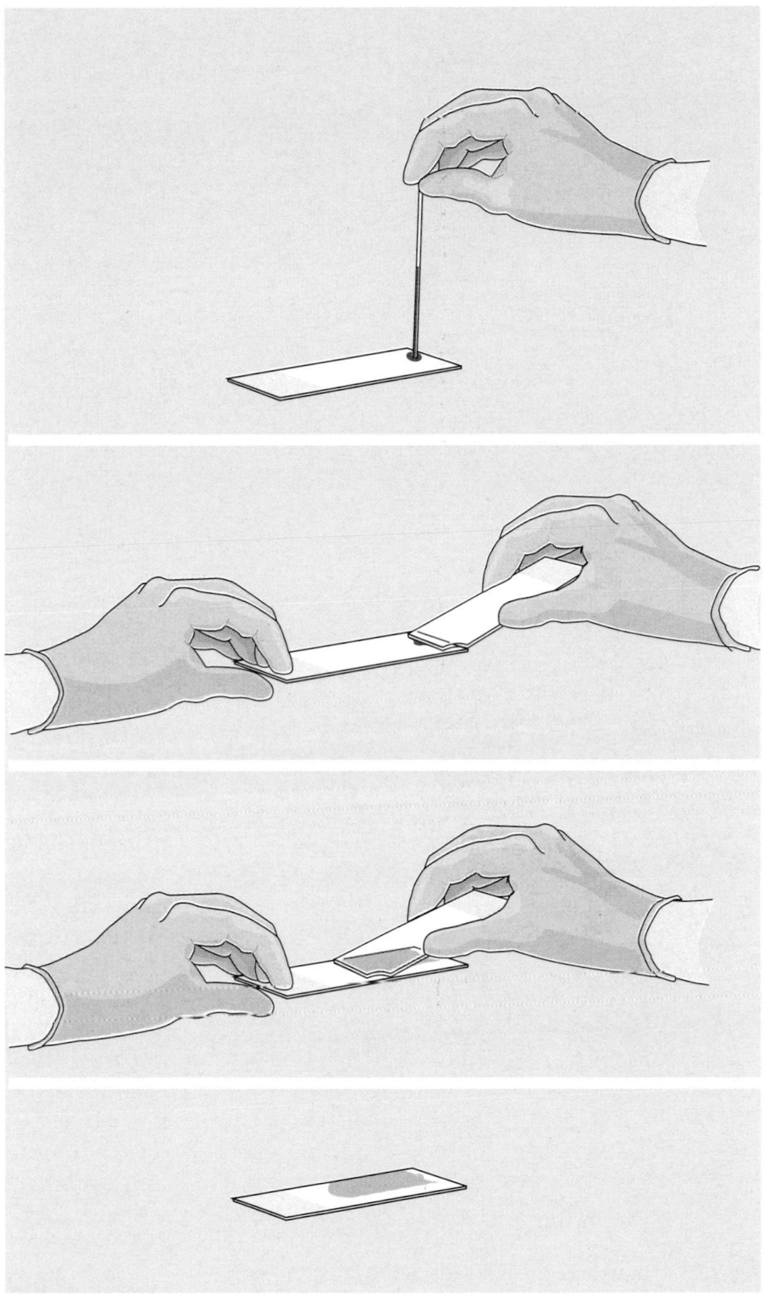

Fig. 1.9 The method of spreading a blood film.

to make a good blood film, even if the angle and the speed of spreading are adjusted. Mixing a drop of blood and a drop of saline or AB plasma reduces viscosity so that a film can be made in which details of red cell morphology can be appreciated.

Buffy coat films

Buffy coat films are useful to concentrate nucleated cells e.g., to look for low-frequency abnormal cells or bacteria. A tube of anticoagu-

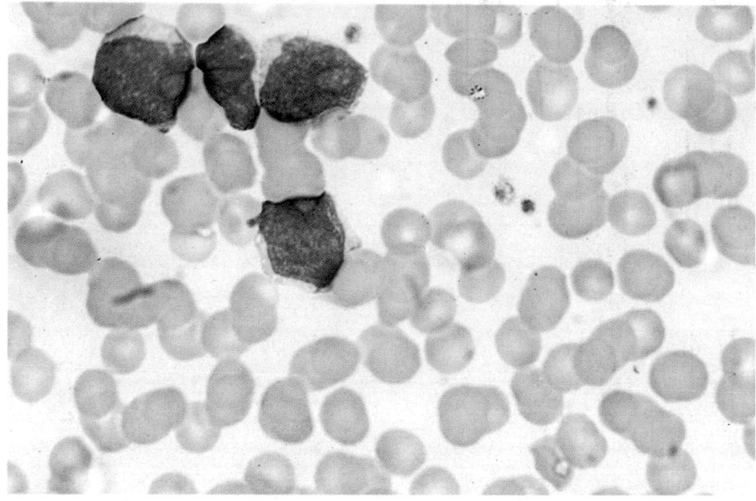

Fig. 1.10 Blast cells from a patient with acute leukaemia which have been inadvertently transferred to the blood film of another patient by the use of an inadequately cleaned spreader.

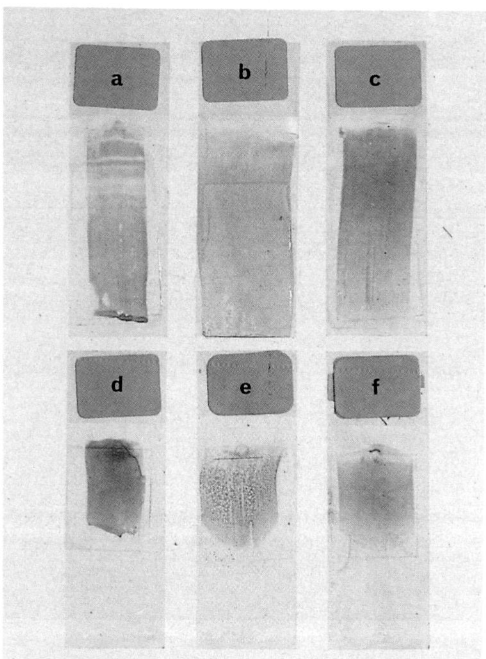

Fig. 1.11 Unsatisfactory and satisfactory blood films: (a) uneven pressure has produced ridges; (b) too broad and too long – the edges and the tail of the film cannot be examined adequately; (c) too long and streaked by an uneven spreader; (d) too thick and short due to the wrong angle or speed of spreading; (e) even distribution of blood cells has been interrupted because the slide was greasy; and (f) satisfactory.

lated blood is centrifuged and a drop of the buffy coat is mixed with a drop of autologous EDTA–plasma and spread in the normal manner.

Thick films

Thick films are required for examination for malarial parasites and certain other parasites, the red cells being lysed before the film is examined. Parasites are much more concentrated in a thick film so that searching for them requires less time. To make a thick film several drops of native or EDTA-anticoagulated blood are placed in the centre of a slide and stirred with a capillary tube or an orange stick into a pool of blood of such a thickness that typescript or a watch face can be read through the blood (Fig. 1.12). The blood film is not fixed but, after drying, is placed directly into an aqueous Giemsa stain so that lysis of red cells occurs; this allows the organisms to be seen more clearly.

Unstained films

Unstained films are useful for searching for motile parasites such as microfilariae which can be seen agitating the red cells. A drop of anticoagulated blood is placed on a slide and covered with a coverslip.

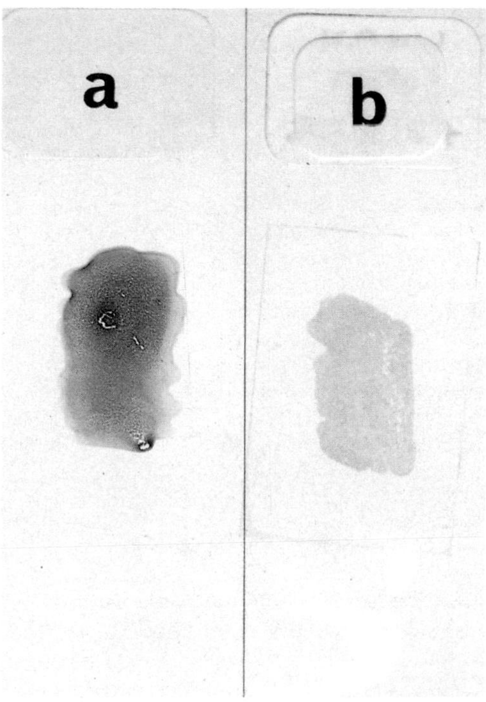

Fig. 1.12 Thick films for examination for malarial parasites: (a) unstained film showing the correct thickness of the film of blood; and (b) film stained without fixation, causing lysis of red cells.

Fixation, staining and mounting

Fixation

Following air drying, thin films are fixed in absolute methanol for 10–20 minutes. Poor fixation and characteristic artefactual changes occur if there is more than a few per cent of water in the methanol (Fig. 1.13); this renders interpretation of morphology, particularly red cell morphology, impossible. In warm, humid climates it may be necessary to change methanol solutions several times a day. Similar artefactual changes can be produced by condensation on slides. In humid climates slides should be fixed as soon as they are dry. A hot-air blower can be used to accelerate drying.

Staining

There is little consistency between laboratories in the precise stain used to prepare a blood film for microscopic examination, but the multiple stains in use are based on the Romanowsky stain, developed by the Russian protozoologist in the late nineteenth century [14]. Romanowsky used a mixture of old methylene blue and eosin to stain the nucleus of a malarial parasite purple and the

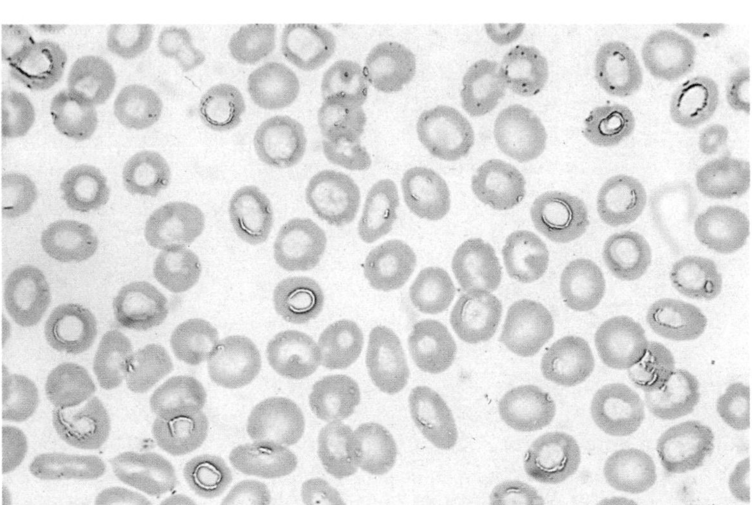

Fig. 1.13 Artefactual changes produced by 5% water in the methanol used for fixation.

cytoplasm blue. Subsequently, Giemsa modified the stain, combining methylene azure and eosin. The stain most commonly used in the UK is a combination of Giemsa's stain with May–Grünwald stain; it is therefore designated the May–Grünwald–Giemsa (MGG) stain. The stain most commonly used in North America is Wright's stain which contains methylene blue and eosin; the methylene blue has been heated, or 'polychromed', to produce analogues of methylene blue. It has been demonstrated by chromatography that dyes prepared by traditional organic chemistry methods are not pure, dyes sold under the same designation containing a variable mixture of five to 10 dyes [15]. Variation between different batches prepared by the same manufacturer also occurs.

The essential components of a Romanowsky-type stain are a basic or cationic dye, such as azure B, which conveys a blue–violet or blue colour to nucleic acids (DNA and RNA) and to nucleoprotein, to the granules of basophils and, weakly, to the granules of neutrophils; and an acidic or anionic dye, such as eosin, which conveys a red or orange colour to haemoglobin and the eosinophil granules. A stain containing azure B and eosin provides a satisfactory Romanowsky stain [14] as does a mixture of azure B, methylene blue and eosin [15]. The ICSH reference method for the Romanowsky stain [16] which uses pure azure B and eosin Y gives very satisfactory results but such pure dyes are expensive for routine use. Satisfactory and reasonably consistent staining can be achieved using good quality commercial stains and an automated staining machine. This method has been used for staining the majority of blood films photographed for this book.

Traditionally, cytoplasm which stains blue and granules which stain purple have both been designated 'basophilic' and granules which stain violet or pinkish-purple have been designated 'azurophilic'. In fact all these hues are achieved by the uptake of a single basic dye such as azure B or A. 'Acidophilic' and 'eosinophilic' both refer to uptake of the acidic dye, eosin, although 'acidophilic' has often been used to describe cell components staining pink and 'eosinophilic' to describe cell components staining orange. The range of colours which a Romanowsky stain should produce is shown in Table 1.1.

Table 1.1 Characteristic staining of different cell components with a Romanowsky stain

Cell component staining	Colour
Chromatin (including Howell–Jolly bodies)	Purple
Promyelocyte granules and Auer rods	Purplish-red
Cytoplasm of lymphocytes	Blue
Cytoplasm of monocytes	Blue–grey
Cytoplasm rich in RNA (i.e., 'basophilic cytoplasm')	Deep blue
Döhle bodies	Blue–grey
Specific granules of neutrophils, granules of lymphocytes, granulomere of platelets	Light purple or pink
Specific granules of basophils	Deep purple
Specific granules of eosinophils	Orange
Red cells	Pink

Staining must be performed at the correct pH. If the pH is too low, basophilic components do not stain well. Leucocytes are generally pale with eosinophil granules a brilliant vermillion. If the pH is too high, uptake of the basic dye may be excessive so that there is general overstaining, it becomes difficult to distinguish between normal and polychromatic red cells, eosinophil granules are deep blue or dark grey, and the granules of normal neutrophils are heavily stained, simulating toxic granulation.

Destaining an MGG-stained blood film can be done by flooding the slide with methanol, washing in water and then repeating the sequence until all the stain has gone. This can be useful if only a single blood film is available and a further stain, for example, an iron stain, is required.

Staining for malarial parasites

The detection and identification of malarial parasites is facilitated if blood films are stained with a Giemsa stain at pH 7.2. At this pH cells which have been parasitized by either *Plasmodium vivax* or *Plasmodium ovale* have different tinctorial qualities from non-parasitized cells and are easily identified. The inclusions in parasitized cells are also evident (see p. 116).

Mounting

If films are to be stored, mounting gives them protection against scratching and gathering of dust. As stated above, the coverslip should be sufficiently wide to cover the edges of the blood film. A neutral mountant which is miscible with xylene is required.

As an alternative to mounting, blood films can be sprayed with a polystyrene or acrylic resin.

If films are not to be stored a thin film of oil can be smeared on the stained slide to permit microscopic examination at low power before adding a drop of oil to permit examination with the oil immersion lens.

Storage of slides

Ideal patient care and continuing education of haematology staff dictate that blood films should be stored as long as possible, preferably for some years. Unfortunately, the very large numbers of blood specimens now being processed daily by many haematology laboratories means that this is often difficult. The most economical way to store slides is in metal racks in stacking drawers. Labels showing the patient's name, the date and the laboratory number should be applied in such a way that they can be read when the slides are in storage. Slides which have been freshly mounted should be stored in cardboard trays or stacked in racks separated from each other by wire loops until the mountant has hardened and dried. When the mountant is no longer sticky, slides can be stored stacked closely together for maximum economy of space. Glass slides are heavy and if large numbers are to be stored the floor of the room may need to be strengthened.

When a patient has a bone marrow aspiration performed a blood film should always be stored permanently with bone marrow films so that when it is necessary to throw out old peripheral blood films to make room for new ones at least this film is available for review. A laboratory should also separately file teaching slides which should include examples of rare conditions and typical examples of common conditions.

References

1 Roddy SM, Ashwal S, Schneider S. Venipuncture fits: a form of reflex anoxic seizure. *Pediatrics* 1983; 72: 715–17.

2 Mull JD, Murphy WR. Effects of tourniquet-induced stasis on blood determinations. *Am J Clin Pathol* 1993; 39: 134–6.

3 ICSH Expert Panel on Cytometry. Recommendations of the International Council for Standardization in Haematology for Ethylenediaminetetraacetic acid anticoagulation of blood for blood cell counting and sizing. *Am J Clin Pathol* 1993; 100: 371–2.

4 Masuko K, Mitsui T, Iwano K, Yamazaki C, Aikara S, Baba K, Takai E, Tsuda F *et al.* Factors influencing postexposure immunoprophylaxis of hepatitis B viral infection with hepatitis B immune globulin. High deoxyribonucleic acid polymerase activity in the inocula of unsuccessful cases. *Gastroenterology* 1985; 88: 151–5.

5 Seeff LB, Wright EC, Zimmerman HJ, Alter HJ, Dietz AA, Felsher BF, Finkelstein JD, Garcia-Pont P *et al.* Type B hepatitis after needle-stick exposure: prevention with hepatitis B immune globulin. A final report of the Veterans Administration Co-operative study. *Ann Intern Med* 1978; 88: 285–93.

6 Mitsui T, Iwano K, Masuko K, Yamazaki C, Okamoto H, Tsuda F, Tanaka T, Mishiro S. Hepatitis C virus infection in medical personnel after needle-stick accident. *Hepatology* 1992; 126: 1109–14.

7 Heptonstall J, Gill ON, Porter K, Black MB, Gilbart VL. Health care workers and HIV: surveillance of occupationally acquired infection in the United Kingdom. *Communicable Disease Report* 1993; 3: 147–53.

8 Bending MR, Maurice PD. Malaria: a laboratory risk. *Postgrad Med J* 1980; 56: 344–5.

9 Glaser JB, Garden A. Inoculation of cryptococcosis without transmission of the acquired immunodeficiency syndrome. *N Engl J Med* 1985; 312: 266.

10 Kramer F, Sasse SA, Simms JC, Leedom JM. Primary cutaneous tuberculosis after a needlestick injury from a patient with AIDS and undiagnosed tuberculosis. *Ann Intern Med* 1993; 119: 594–5.

11 Hammond KB. Blood specimen collection from infants by skin puncture. *Lab Med* 1980; 11: 9–12.

12 Polish LB, Shapiro CN, Bauer F, Klotz P, Ginier P, Roberto RR, Margolis HS, Alter MJ. Nosocomial transmission of hepatitis B virus associated with the use of a spring-loaded finger-stick device. *N Engl J Med* 1992; 326: 721–5.

13 Brecher G, Schneiderman M, Cronkite EP. The reproducibility and constancy of the platelet count. *Am J Clin Pathol* 1953; 23: 15–26.

14 Wittekind D. On the nature of the Romanowsky dyes and the Romanowsky–Giemsa effect. *Clin Lab Haematol* 1979; 1: 247–62.
15 Marshall PN, Bentley SA, Lewis SM. A standardized Romanowsky stain prepared from purified dyes. *J Clin Pathol* 1975; 28: 920–3.
16 ICSH. ICSH reference method for staining blood and bone marrow films by azure B and eosin Y (Romanowsky stain). *Br J Haematol* 1984; 57: 707–10.

CHAPTER 2

Performing a Blood Count

In the past, blood counts were performed by slow and labour-intensive manual techniques using counting chambers, microscopes, glass tubes, colorimeters, centrifuges and a few simple reagents. The only tests done with any frequency were estimations of Hb, packed cell volume (PCV) and white cell count (WBC). Hb was estimated by a method depending on optical density and was expressed as mass/volume or even as a percentage in relation to a rather arbitrary 'normal' which represented 100%. PCV was a measurement of the proportion of a column of centrifuged blood which was occupied by red cells. Now expressed as a decimal fraction representing volume/volume, it was initially expressed as a percentage. White cells were counted microscopically in a diluted blood sample in a haemocytometer, a counting chamber of known volume. All cell counts were expressed as the number of cells in a unit volume. The red cell count (RBC) was performed occasionally, mainly when there was a need to make an estimate of red cell size. Platelets were counted, by light or phase-contrast microscopy, only when there was a clear clinical need. From the primary measurements relating to red cells other values were derived: the mean cell volume (MCV), mean cell haemoglobin (MCH) and mean cell haemoglobin concentration (MCHC). The formulae for these derived measurements are as follows:

$$\text{MCV (fl)} = \frac{\text{PCV (l/l)} \times 1000}{\text{RBC (cells/l)} \times 10^{-12}}$$

$$\text{MCH (pg)} = \frac{\text{Hb (g/dl)} \times 10}{\text{RBC (cells/l)} \times 10^{-12}}$$

$$\text{MCHC (g/dl)} = \frac{\text{Hb (g/dl)}}{\text{PCV (l/l)}}$$

These and many other measurements are now made on automated and semi-automated instruments within minutes using either modifications of the manual techniques or totally new technologies. Measurements are precise, i.e., repeated measurements on the same sample give very similar results. As long as the instruments are carefully standardized and the blood has no unusual characteristics, measurements are also accurate, i.e., they give results which are very close to 'truth'. However, despite the widespread use of automated instruments, the manual techniques remain important both as reference methods and in the investigation of blood samples which appear to give anomalous test results on automated instruments. They also illustrate the principles which underlie various measurements.

Basic techniques

Haemoglobin concentration (Hb)

To measure Hb, a known volume of carefully

mixed whole blood is added to a diluent which lyses red cells to produce a haemoglobin solution; lysis occurs because of the hypotonicity of the diluent, but may be accelerated by the inclusion in the diluent of a non-ionic detergent to act as a lytic agent. The Hb is then determined from the light absorbance (optical density) of the solution of haemoglobin or its derivative at a selected wavelength.

Cyanmethaemoglobin method

The ICSH has recommended a reference method in which haemoglobin is converted to cyanmethaemoglobin (haemiglobincyanide) [1]. This method has three significant advantages. (i) Haemoglobin, methaemoglobin and carboxyhaemoglobin are all converted to cyanmethaemoglobin and are therefore included in the measurement. Of the forms of haemoglobin likely to be present in blood, only sulphaemoglobin — usually present in negligible amounts — is not converted to cyanmethaemoglobin, although carboxyhaemoglobin is more slowly converted than the other forms. (ii) Stable secondary standards which have been compared with the World Health Organization (WHO) international standard are readily available for calibration. (iii) Cyanmethaemoglobin has an absorbance band at 540 nm which is broad and relatively flat (Fig. 2.1), and thus measurements can be made either on a narrow-band spectrophotometer or on a filter photometer or colorimeter which reads over a wide band of wavelengths.

The reference method requires the addition of a diluent which contains: (i) potassium cyanide and potassium ferricyanide, to effect the conversion to methaemoglobin; (ii) dihydrogen potassium phosphate to lower the pH, accelerate the reaction, and allow the reading of light absorbance at 3 minutes rather than 10–15 minutes; and (iii) a non-ionic detergent, to accelerate cell lysis and reduce the turbidity due to precipitation of lipoproteins (and to a lesser extent red cell stroma) which is otherwise a consequence of the lower pH achieved by the dihydrogen potassium phosphate [2]. The absorbance of light by the solution is measured at 540 nm in a spectrophotometer. At this wavelength the light absorbance of the diluent is zero; either water or, preferably, the diluent can be used as the blank. No standard is required since the haemoglobin concentration can be calculated from the absorbance, given that the molecular weight and the millimolar extinction

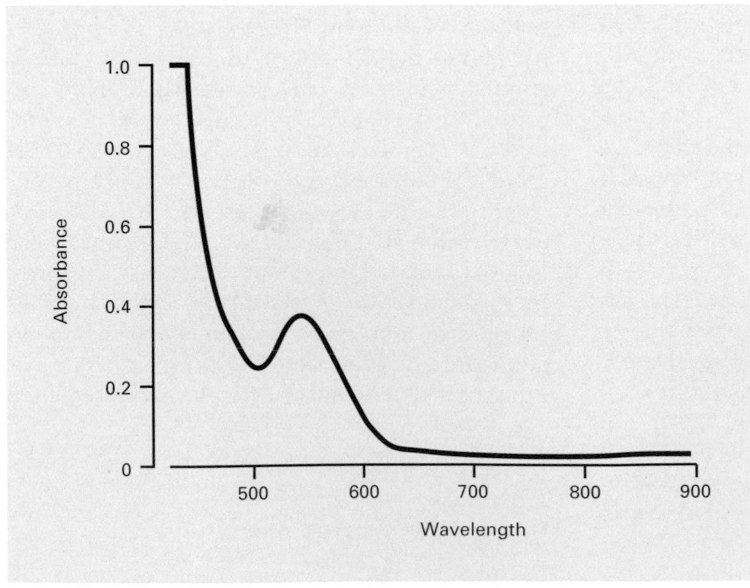

Fig. 2.1 Absorbance spectrum of cyanmethaemoglobin.

coefficient of haemoglobin are known. However, the wavelength of light produced by the instrument must be verified and the absorbance scale calibrated. A reference solution of cyanmethaemoglobin can be used for calibration.

In routine practice, Hb is usually measured by means of a photometer or colorimeter in which light of approximately 540 nm is produced by use of a yellow–green filter such as the Ilford 625. The light passing through the solution is detected by a photoelectric cell and the instrument scale shows either light absorbance or transmittance. Comparison of the instrument reading with that for a reference solution allows calculation of the Hb; this is most conveniently performed using a standard curve or a conversion table. Alternatively, the photometer can be calibrated to produce a direct readout of Hb; a reference cyanmethaemoglobin solution is suitable for verifying the accuracy of instruments of this type.

Certain characteristics of pathological blood samples may lead to inaccuracy in a cyanmethaemoglobin estimation of Hb. The presence of sulphaemoglobin will lead to slight underestimation of total haemoglobin: a concentration of 15 g/dl will be measured as 14.8 g/dl if 5% of haemoglobin is present as sulphaemoglobin [2]. The slow conversion of carboxyhaemoglobin to methaemoglobin leads to overestimation of the Hb if the test is read at 3 minutes, since carboxyhaemoglobin absorbs more light at 540 nm than does cyanmethaemoglobin. The maximum possible error which could be caused if 20% of the haemoglobin were in the form of carboxyhaemoglobin, a degree of abnormality which may be found in heavy smokers, would be 6% [2].

Spectrophotometers and photometers are both sensitive to the effect of turbidity, which may be caused by a high WBC, high concentrations of lipids or plasma proteins, or non-lysed red cells. Increased turbidity causes a factitiously elevated estimate of Hb. When the WBC is high, turbidity effects are circumvented by centrifugation or filtration of the solution prior to reading the absorbance. When turbidity is due to a high level of plasma protein (either when a paraprotein is present or when there is severe chronic infection or inflammation), it can be cleared by the addition of either potassium carbonate or a drop of 25% ammonia solution. When turbidity is due to hyperlipidaemia, a blank can be prepared from the diluent and the patient's plasma or the lipid can be removed by diethyl ether extraction and centrifugation. The target cells of liver disease or red cells containing haemoglobin S or C may fail to lyse in the diluent and, again, increased turbidity produces a factitiously high reading of Hb. Occasionally, this phenomenon is observed without any identifiable abnormality in the red cells to account for it. Making a 1 : 1 dilution in distilled water ensures complete lysis of osmotically resistant cells.

The cyanmethaemoglobin method has been modified for application in automated instruments by the use of various lytic agents and by reading absorbance after a shorter time or at a different wavelength.

Other methods

Alternative methods of measuring Hb are not widely used except when they have been incorporated into haemoglobinometers. Such methods usually require standardization by reference back to a cyanmethaemoglobin standard but they otherwise avoid the use of cyanide which is potentially toxic if released into the environment in large quantities.

Haemoglobin can be converted into a sulphated derivative with maximum absorbance at 534 nm by addition of sodium lauryl sulphate [3]. Conversion is instantaneous and methaemoglobin, but not sulphaemoglobin, is converted. The method correlates well with the reference method which is employed for calibration. This method is suitable for use with a spectrophotometer and has also been incorporated into several automated instruments.

Hb can also be measured following conversion to azidmethaemoglobin by the addition of sodium nitrate and sodium azide. This is the method employed by one portable haemoglobinometer (HemoCue, Clandon Scientific Ltd).

Hb can be measured as oxyhaemoglobin, in which case concentration of carboxyhaemoglobin, sulphaemoglobin and methaemoglobin will not be measured accurately. An artificial or secondary standard is needed. This method has been incorporated into directly reading haemoglobinometers which are standardized to give the same result as a cyanmethaemoglobin method.

Hb can be measured as haematin produced under alkaline conditions. The alkaline–haematin method measures carboxyhaemoglobin, sulphaemoglobin and methaemoglobin although it does not adequately measure haemoglobin F or haemoglobin Bart's which are resistant to alkaline denaturation. An artificial standard is required. The acid–haematin method is less reliable and is not recommended.

Hb can be estimated without chemical conversion by measuring absorbance at 548.5 nm, at which wavelength deoxyhaemoglobin and oxyhaemoglobin both have the same optical density and that of carboxyhaemoglobin is not much less. Hb is calculated by comparison of absorbance with that of an artificial standard. Absorbance can also be integrated between 500 and 600 nm, the integral absorbance of oxyhaemoglobin, deoxyhaemoglobin and carboxyhaemoglobin being similar over this waveband.

Recommended units

The ICSH has recommended that Hb be expressed as g/l (mass concentration), or as mmol/l (molar concentration) in terms of concentration of the haemoglobin monomer. The conversion factor is 0.06206, i.e., an Hb of 120 g/l = 120 × 0.06206 mmol/l = 7.45 mmol/l. If Hb is expressed in molar concentration then MCH and MCHC should also be expressed in this manner. There are no clear practical advantages in expressing Hb as molar concentration and the potential for confusion and risk to patients if conversion to these units were to be attempted might be considerable. Despite the advice of the ICSH many laboratories, preferring familiarity to correctness, continue to express Hb as g/dl.

Packed cell volume (PCV)

The PCV is the proportion of a column of centrifuged blood which is occupied by red cells. Some of the measured column of red cells represents plasma which is trapped between red cells. The PCV is expressed as a decimal fraction representing l/l (litres/litre). The terms packed cell volume and haematocrit (Hct) were initially synonymous and were used interchangeably but the ICSH has now recommended that PCV be reserved for estimates made by the traditional technique of centrifugation and Hct for estimates derived by other methods on automated instruments. The original method of measuring the PCV, as devised by Maxwell Wintrobe, required 1 ml of blood and prolonged (30 minutes to 1 hour) centrifugation in graduated glass tubes with a constant internal bore. This method, sometimes referred to as the macrohaematocrit, is the basis of the reference method [4] but for routine use it is cumbersome and slow. Since, for these reasons, it is no longer used in the diagnostic laboratory it will not be discussed further. It has been replaced by the microhaematocrit which has clinical usefulness by itself, can be combined with the Hb to derive an estimate of the MCHC and can be used to calibrate automated counters.

Microhaematocrit

A small volume of blood is taken by capillarity into an ungraduated capillary tube (usually 75 mm long with an internal diameter of 1.2 mm) leaving about 15 mm unfilled. The end of the tube distant from the column of blood is sealed by heat or by modelling clay or a similar product. It is then centrifuged for 5 or 10 minutes, at a high **g** value (for example 10 000–15 000 **g**) in a small, specially designed centrifuge, to separate the column of blood into red cells, buffy coat and plasma (Fig. 2.2). The PCV is read visually on a scale, the buffy coat of white cells and platelets being excluded from the measurement. The ICSH has published a selected method which employs 5 minutes centrifugation [5]. A further 3 minutes centrifugation is advisable if the sample is polycythaemic [6]. The microhaematocrit is usually measured on EDTA-anticoagulated venous blood but it can also be performed on capillary blood if the sample is taken into a microhaematocrit tube the interior of which is coated with heparin (2 IU).

The microhaematocrit has several sources of imprecision and inaccuracy. Because of the smallness of the tube, reading the level correctly can be difficult. Tubes may taper or be of an uneven

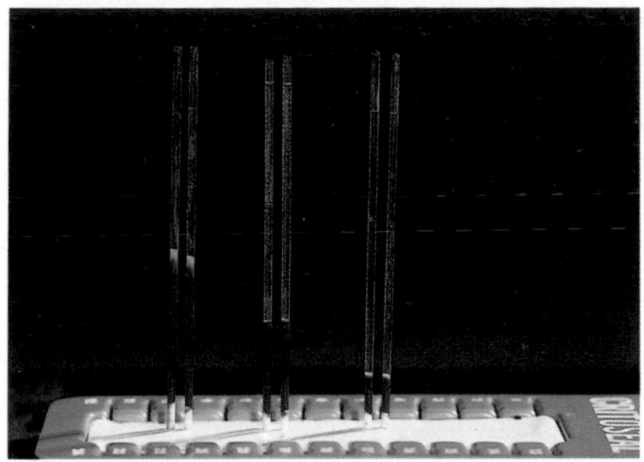

Fig. 2.2 Measurements of PCV by the microhaematocrit technique; paired tests from three patients are shown.

bore. The seal is not flat, tending to be convex if modelling clay is used and concave if heat sealing is employed, although the error introduced by the type of seal is usually minor [7]. The amount of plasma trapping is usually around 1–3% but is variable. It is less with longer periods of centrifugation and higher **g** values but is also affected by other technical factors and by the characteristics of the blood sample (Table 2.1). It should be noted that in the USA blood is usually taken into K_3EDTA and in the UK it is more usually taken into K_2EDTA; because of the cell shrinkage which occurs, the microhaematocrit with K_3EDTA is about 3% lower than with K_2EDTA [11]. The precision of the microhaematocrit can be improved by making at least three replicate measurements and taking the average; this is necessary when a manual PCV is used to calibrate an automated instrument.

Attempts have been made to make the microhaematocrit more accurate by 'correcting' the PCV for plasma trapping. A more accurate PCV means that an estimated MCV is also more accurate. In experimental conditions this can be done by labelling plasma proteins with ^{131}I and determining the amount of radioactive isotope which is trapped in the red cell column. The correction may itself be inaccurate since estimates of plasma trapping are lower when ^{131}I-labelled

Table 2.1 Some factors affecting the microhaematocrit

	Factors decreasing the microhaematocrit	Factors increasing the microhaematocrit
Consequent on dilution	Use of EDTA solution rather than dry EDTA	
Consequent on an alteration in the amount of trapped plasma	Longer period of centrifugation Increased centrifugal force (e.g., increased radius of centrifuge or increased speed of centrifugation) Elevated ESR	Shorter period of centrifugation Decreased centrifugal force Microcytosis (e.g., iron deficiency or thalassaemia trait) Sickle cell trait or sickle cell disease Spherocytosis Reduced flexibility of red cells on prolonged storage at room temperature
Consequent on red cell shrinkage	Excess EDTA [8,9] K_3EDTA rather than K_2EDTA or Na_2EDTA [7] Narrower tubes than recommended [10] Soda lime tubes [10]	K_2EDTA or Na_2EDTA Borosilicate tubes

fibrinogen is used than when ^{131}I-labelled albumin is used [7]. Such correction is clearly impracticable in routine diagnostic practice and it has been suggested that instead an arbitrary plasma trapping correction should be applied, particularly when the estimated PCV is to be used for calibration. This procedure is not recommended since, although the correction to be applied is based on experimental evidence it is, nevertheless, arbitrary when applied to an individual blood sample and there is no agreement as to what percentage correction is appropriate. Different studies have produced estimates varying from 1.3 to 3.2% for mean plasma trapping. The ICSH Committee on Cytometry does not recommend a correction. It is important that a standard procedure be used and that if a laboratory chooses to use a plasma trapping correction in calibrating an instrument it applies this correction when determining the reference range and continues to apply it when testing patient or blood donor samples.

Minor alterations in technique such as using or not using a plasma trapping correction can alter the percentage of blood donors whose donations are deferred or the clinician's assessment of whether or not a polycythaemic patient requires venesection. A similar variation of a few per cent in the MCV can be diagnostically important in screening for thalassaemia trait and can render nomograms devised for this purpose invalid. There is a similar effect on the use of MCV as a screening tool unless precisely the same technique is used in calibrating the instrument when the reference range is devised and when the patient samples are studied.

One circumstance in which a plasma trapping correction is considered appropriate is when a microhaematocrit is being used for estimation of total red cell mass. Allowance should be made for the greater degree of plasma trapping of polycythaemic blood. It is suggested that if the PCV is less than 0.50 after centrifugation for 5 minutes, 2% correction should be applied; if it is greater than 0.50, a further 5 minutes centrifugation should be carried out and the correction should be 3% [12].

With automated instruments in current use, Hct is computed from the number and size of electrical impulses generated by red cells passing through a sensor (see pp. 30 and 34).

The red cell count (RBC)

The RBC was initially performed by counting red cells microscopically in a carefully diluted sample of blood contained in a counting chamber (haemocytometer) with chambers of known volume [13]. Although this method was capable of producing satisfactory results if great care was exercised, it proved very unreliable in routine use because of a high degree of imprecision and it was also very time-consuming. For this reason the RBC and the parameters derived from it were measured or calculated on only a minority of blood specimens.

More precise and therefore more clinically useful RBCs can be performed on single-channel semi-automated impedance counters (see p. 28), such as the Coulter Counter model ZM, which count cells in an accurately fixed and known volume of diluted blood as they pass through an aperture. Although accurate setting of thresholds is needed, the instruments do not require calibration. The raw instrument cell counts produced are non-linear with increasing cell concentration because of the greater likelihood of two cells passing through the aperture simultaneously (coincidence); depending on the instrument, coincidence correction may be an automatic function of the instrument or may be carried out by the user by reference to a table. White cells are also included in the RBC. Because red cells are normally at least a 100-fold more numerous than white cells the inaccuracy introduced by this is usually not great. RBCs determined on single-channel impedence counters are much more precise than those produced in counting chambers and they can also be produced with much less labour. They are therefore more clinically useful. They can be used with a manual Hb and PCV to calculate MCV and MCH which are also much more precise than those derived from manual RBCs.

RBCs from single-channel semi-automated impedance counters can also be used to calibrate fully automated blood cell counters which count electrical impulses generated by red cells passing through a sensor (see p. 28). Automated instruments count of the order of 20 000–50 000 cells, so that precision is again much greater than that of a haemocytometer count based on 500–1000 cells.

Derived red cell variables

Given the three measured variables (Hb, PCV and RBC) MCV, MCH and MCHC can be derived. When no plasma trapping correction is used the MCV derived from a microhaematocrit will be an overestimate of the true value and the MCHC will be an underestimate. This is of no clinical consequence since reference ranges will be derived in the same manner. The measured and derived variables which describe the characteristics of red cells are often referred to collectively as the red cell indices.

The white cell count (WBC)

A manual WBC is performed after diluting an aliquot of blood in a diluent which lyses red cells and stains the nuclei of the white cells [13]. White cells are counted microscopically in a haemocytometer with chambers of known volume. Nucleated red blood cells (NRBC) cannot be readily distinguished from white cells in a counting chamber. If NRBC are present their percentage should be counted on a stained blood film and the total nucleated cell count (TNCC) should be corrected accordingly. The manual WBC is imprecise but this is of less practical importance than the imprecision of the RBC since clinically important changes in WBC are usually of sufficient magnitude to be detected even with an imprecise method.

White cells can also be counted in diluted whole blood following red cell lysis using a single-channel semi-automated impedance counter. In fully automated counters white cells are counted by impedance technology or light scattering.

Platelet count

Platelets can be counted in a haemocytometer using either diluted whole blood (in which red cells can be either left intact or lysed) or platelet-rich plasma (prepared by sedimentation or centrifugation). If very large platelets are present, a whole-blood method is preferred to the use of platelet-rich plasma to avoid the risk of large heavy platelets being lost during preparative procedures. Platelet-rich plasma may be preferred if the platelet count is low. When the method leaves platelets intact, large platelets can be distinguished from small red cells by the platelet's shape, which may be oval rather than round, and by its irregular outline, with fine projections sometimes being visible. Use of ammonium oxalate, which lyses red cells, as a diluent produces a higher and more accurate count than use of formol-citrate, which leaves red cells intact [14]. Platelet counts are best performed on anticoagulated venous blood obtained by a clean venepuncture. Counts on blood obtained by finger-prick tend to be lower.

Platelets can be visualized in the counting chamber by light or phase-contrast microscopy. When using light microscopy, brilliant cresyl blue can be added to the diluent. This stains platelets light blue and facilitates their identification. On light microscopy, platelet identification is aided by their refractility. It is easier to identify platelets by phase-contrast microscopy and such counts are therefore generally more precise.

Manual platelet counts are generally imprecise, particularly when the count is low. They are also very laborious so that when this was the only technique available counts were performed only when there was a clear clinical indication.

Platelets can be counted by semi-automated methods using impedance counters following the preparation of platelet-rich plasma. Coincidence correction and the use of two thresholds to exclude both debris and contaminating red cells and white cells is necessary. These techniques are also laborious and the several steps involved make them prone to error.

The only satisfactory way to perform the number of platelet counts required by modern medical practice is with fully automated full blood counters. Such instruments count platelets by either impedance or light-scattering technology. Counts are generally precise, even at low levels, but unusual characteristics of the blood sample can cause inaccuracy (see p. 138). Manual haemocytometer counts are necessary in some patients with giant platelets which with automated counters cannot be distinguished from red cells.

Differential white cell count

A differential white cell count is the assigning of leucocytes to their individual categories, this categorization being expressed as a percentage or, when the WBC is available, as an absolute count. A differential count carried out by a human observer using a microscope is referred to as a manual differential count. It is usually performed on a wedge-spread film, prepared either manually or with a mechanical film spreader. Automated differential counts are now generally performed by flow cytometry as part of an FBC, differentiation between categories being based on the physical characteristics of the cells and sometimes on their biochemical characteristics.

Cells which are normally present in the peripheral blood can be assigned to five or six categories, depending on whether segmented neutrophils are separated from non-segmented or band forms (see p. 67) or are counted with them. The differential count also includes any abnormal cells which may be present. NRBC can be included as a separate category in the differential count or, alternatively, their number can be expressed per 100 white cells. In the latter case the TNCC is corrected to a WBC by subtracting the number of NRBC. In the former case the uncorrected count is designated the TNCC rather than the WBC. Laboratories should consistently follow one or other convention of expressing counts.

Differential white cell counts, like all laboratory tests, are subject to both inaccuracy and imprecision. Manual differential counts are generally fairly accurate but their precision is poor, whereas automated counts are generally fairly precise but are sometimes inaccurate.

Inaccuracy

With a manual differential count, inaccuracy or deviation from the true count results both from maldistribution and from misidentification of cells.

Maldistribution of cells

The different types of white cells are not distributed evenly over a slide. The tail of the film contains more neutrophils and fewer lymphocytes whereas monocytes are fairly evenly distributed along the length of the film [15]. When large immature cells (blasts, promyelocytes and myelocytes) are present they are preferentially distributed at the edges of the film rather than in the centre and distally rather than proximally, in relation to lymphocytes, basophils, neutrophils and metamyelocytes [16]. The maldistribution of cells is aggravated if a film is too thin or if a spreader with a rough edge has been used. Various methods of tracking over a slide have been proposed to attempt to overcome errors due to maldistribution (Fig. 2.3). The method shown in Fig. 2.3a compensates for maldistribution between the body and the tail but not for maldistribution between the centre and the edge, whereas the 'battlement' method shown in Fig. 2.3b tends to do the reverse, since the customary 100-cell differential count will not cover a very large proportion of the length of the blood film. A modified battlement track (Fig. 2.3c) is a compromise between the two methods. In practice, the imprecision of a manual count is so great that a small degree of inaccuracy caused by maldistribution of cells is not of any great consequence. If there is white cell aggregation, the maldistribution of cells is so great that an accurate differential count is impossible.

Misidentification

Inaccuracy due to misidentification of cells is usually not great when differential counts are performed by experienced laboratory workers on high quality blood films. An exception to this is the differentiation between band forms and segmented neutrophils. Criteria for making this distinction differ between laboratories and there is also inconsistency in the application of the criteria within a laboratory because of an element of subjectivity. Occasionally, it is also difficult to distinguish a monocyte from a large lymphocyte or a degranulated basophil from a neutrophil. Marked storage artefact renders a differential

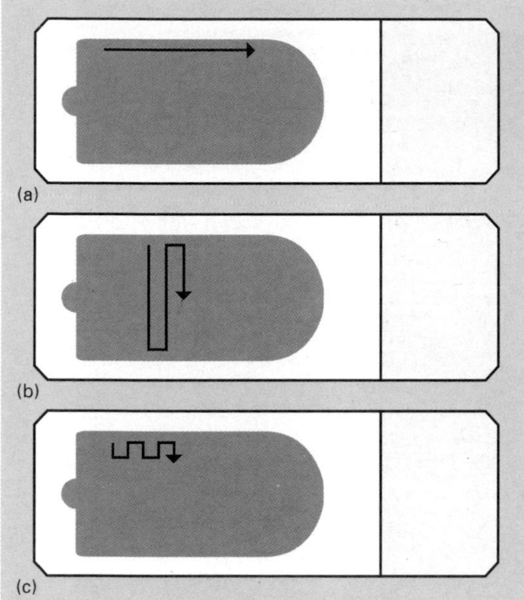

Fig. 2.3 Diagrams of blood films showing tracking patterns employed in differential WBC: (a) tracking along the length of the film; (b) battlement method; and (c) modified battlement method; two fields are counted close to the edge parallel to the edge of the film, then four fields at right angles, then two fields parallel to the edge and so on.

count very inaccurate; specifically, degenerating neutrophils may be misclassified as NRBC and preferential disintegration of neutrophils can cause a factitious elevation of the lymphocyte count. Inaccuracy can also be introduced into a count if many smear cells (see p. 97) are present and not included in the count. If the smear cells are, for example, lymphocytes then the percentage and absolute number of lymphocytes will be falsely low and the percentage and absolute number of all other cell types will be falsely high. Smear cells whose nature can be determined should be counted with the category to which they belong. Smear cells, the nature of which is not clear, should be counted as a separate category or the percentage and absolute number of cells of all categories will be falsely elevated.

Imprecision

The imprecision or lack of reproducibility of a count can be expressed as either the standard deviation (SD) or the coefficient of variation (CV) of replicate counts. The small number of cells conventionally counted in a manual differential count leads to poor precision [17]. When replicate counts are made of the percentage of cells of a given type among randomly distributed cells the SD of the count is related to the square root of the number of cells counted. Specifically, the SD of the proportion, θ, is equal to [18]:

$$\sqrt{\frac{\theta\,(1-\theta)}{n}}$$

The 95% confidence limits of the proportion, i.e., the limits within which 95% of replicate counts would be expected to fall, are equal to $\theta \pm 1.96$ SD. The confidence limits of a given percentage of cells when 100 or more cells are counted is shown in Table 2.2. It will be seen that the confidence limits are wide. For example, the confidence limits of a 10% eosinophil count on a 100-cell differential count are 4–18%. The precision of the absolute count of any given cell count cannot be any better than the precision of the percentage but, if it is calculated from an automated WBC which itself is quite a precise measurement, it is not a great deal worse. The imprecision of a manual differential count is greatest for those cells which are present in the smallest numbers, particularly the basophils. If it is diagnostically important to know whether or not there is basophilia then it is necessary to improve precision, either by performing an absolute basophil count in a haemocytometer or by counting many more than the usual 100 cells (e.g., 200 or 500 cells). Similarly, if neutrophils constitute only a small proportion of cells (e.g., in chronic lymphocytic leukaemia, CLL) it is again necessary to count a larger number of cells to improve precision and determine whether there is neutropenia. Although the precision of a manual count could be improved by routinely counting more cells, it is not feasible in a diagnostic laboratory to routinely count more than 100 or, at the most, 200 cells. The poor precision of the count of cells present in the smallest numbers means that the reference limits

Table 2.2 Precision achieved with differential counts of various numbers of leucocytes

Observed percentage of cells	Total number of cells counted (n)				
	100	200	500	1000	10 000
0	0–4	0–2	0–1	0–1	0–0.04
1	0–6	0–4	0–3	0–2	0.8–1.2
2	0–8	0–6	0–4	1–4	1.7–2.3
3	0–9	1–7	1–5	2–5	2.7–3.3
4	1–10	1–8	2–7	2–6	3.6–4.4
5	1–12	2–10	3–8	3–7	4.6–5.4
6	2–13	3–11	4–9	4–8	5.5–6.5
7	2–14	3–12	4–10	5–9	6.5–7.5
8	3–16	4–13	5–11	6–10	7.4–8.6
9	4–17	5–15	6–12	7–11	8.4–9.6
10	4–18	6–16	7–14	8–13	9.4–10.6
15	8–24	10–21	12–19	12–18	14.6–15.4
20	12–30	14–27	16–24	17–23	19.6–20.4
25	16–35	19–32	21–30	22–28	24.6–25.4
30	21–40	23–37	26–35	27–33	29.5–30.5
35	25–46	28–43	30–40	32–39	34.5–35.5
40	30–51	33–48	35–45	36–44	39.5–40.5
45	35–56	38–53	40–50	41–49	44.5–45.5
50	39–61	42–58	45–55	46–54	49.5–50.5

Confidence limits of 95% of the observed percentage of cells when the total number of cells counted (n) varies from 100 to 10 000. Ranges for $n = 100–1000$ are derived from Rümke [17].

for manual basophil and eosinophil counts include zero. It is therefore impossible on the basis of a manual count to say that a patient has basopenia or eosinopenia.

There is no internationally agreed reference method for the manual differential count though the USA National Committee for Clinical Laboratory Standards has established a reference method [19]. It uses a manually wedge-spread, Romanowsky-stained film. Two-hundred cells are counted by each of four trained observers using a 'battlement' track (see Fig. 2.3b). The results are averaged to produce an 800-cell differential count.

Reticulocyte count

Reticulocytes are young red cells, newly released from the bone marrow, which still contain ribosomal RNA. On exposure of unfixed cells to certain dyes, such as brilliant cresyl blue or new methylene blue, the ribosomes are precipitated and stained by the dye, to appear as a reticular network; as the cells are still living when exposed to the dye this is referred to as supravital staining. With new methylene blue, red cells stain a pale greenish-blue while the reticulum stains bluish-purple.

The amount of reticulum in a reticulocyte varies from a large clump in the most immature cells (group I reticulocytes) to a few granules in the most mature forms (group IV reticulocytes) (Fig. 2.4). The difficulty in determining whether one or two dots of appropriately stained material represent RNA has led to various definitions of a reticulocyte being proposed. The minimum requirement varies from a single dot, through two or three dots to a minimum network. Since the majority of reticulocytes in the peripheral blood are group IV, the precise definition of a reticulocyte which is employed will have an appreciable effect on the reticulocyte count. The USA National Committee for Clinical Laboratory Standards

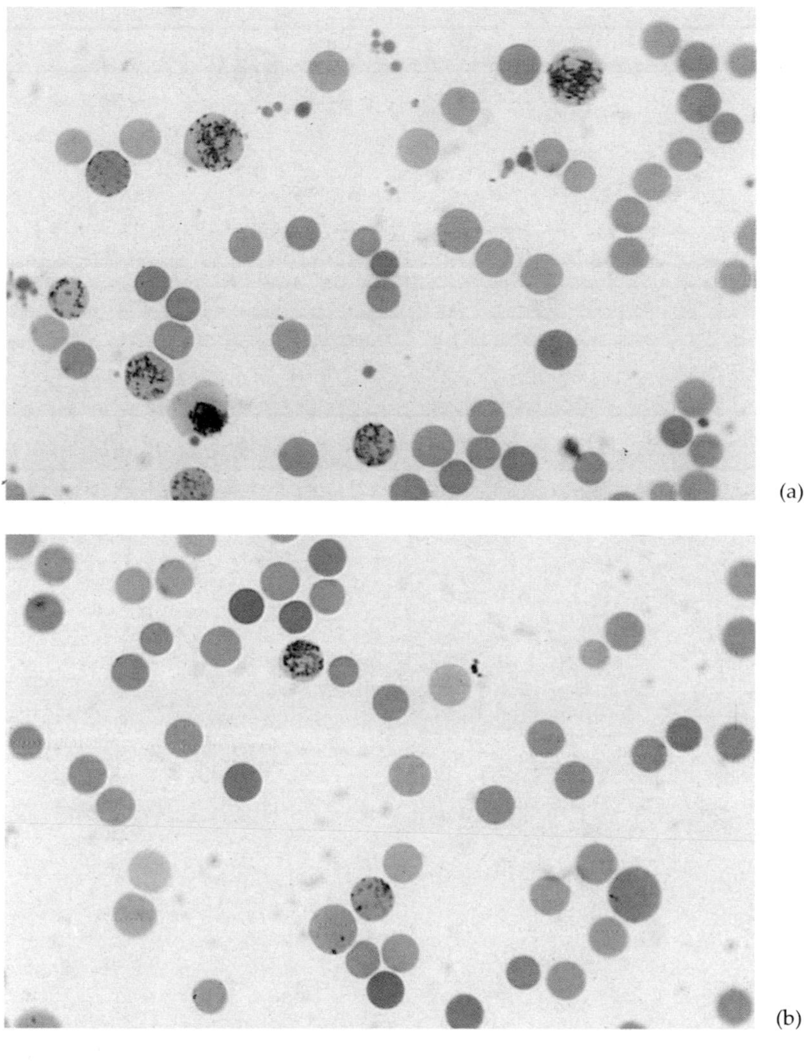

(a)

(b)

Fig. 2.4 Reticulocytes stained with new methylene blue. (a) A group I reticulocyte with a dense clump of reticulum, several group II reticulocytes with a wreath or network of reticulum and several group III reticulocytes with a disintegrated wreath of reticulum. (b) Group II, III and IV reticulocytes: the group IV reticulocyte has two granules of reticulum. There is also a cell with a single dot of reticulum. By some criteria this would also be classified as a reticulocyte. (c) Three reticulocytes and a Howell–Jolly body.

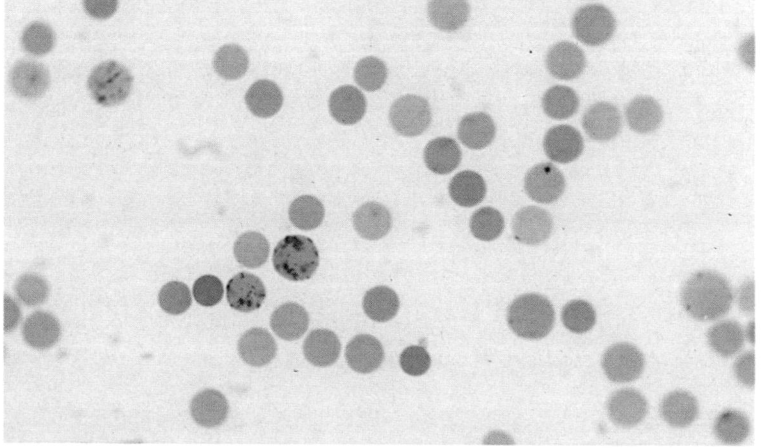

(c)

classifies as a reticulocyte 'any non-nucleated red cell containing two or more particles of blue-stained material corresponding to ribosomal RNA' [20]. This definition is also accepted by the ICSH [21].

The RNA which is responsible for forming the reticulum following supravital staining gives rise, on Romanowsky-stained films, to diffuse cytoplasmic basophilia. The combination of cytoplasmic basophilia with the acidophilia of haemoglobin produces staining characteristics known as polychromasia. Not all reticulocytes contain enough RNA to cause polychromasia on a Romanowsky-stained film but whether polychromatic cells correspond only to the least mature reticulocytes (equivalent to the group I reticulocytes) [22] or to all but the most mature reticulocytes (group I, II and III reticulocytes) [23] is not certain.

There are certain other inclusions which can be confused with the reticulum of reticulocytes. Methods of making the distinction are given in Table 2.3 and these other inclusions are discussed in more detail in Chapter 7. Cells containing Pappenheimer bodies, in particular, can sometimes be difficult to distinguish from late reticulocytes with only a few granules of reticulofilamentous material. If necessary, a reticulocyte preparation can be counterstained with a Perls' stain (see p. 186) to identify Pappenheimer bodies, or by a Romanowsky stain to identify Howell–Jolly bodies. When a reticulocyte preparation is fixed in methanol and counterstained with a Romanowsky stain the vital dye, e.g., the new methylene blue, is washed out during the methanol fixation. The reticulum is then stained by the basic component of the Romanowsky stain [24].

Reticulocytes are usually counted as a percentage of red blood cells. The use of an eyepiece containing a Miller ocular micrometer disc (Fig. 2.5) facilitates counting; reticulocytes are counted in the large squares and the total red cells in the small squares, which are one-ninth of the size of the large cells. If 20 fields are counted, the reticulocytes among about 2000 cells are counted and the reticulocyte percentage is equal to:

$$\frac{\text{reticulocytes in 20 large squares} \times 100}{\text{erythrocytes in 20 small cells} \times 9}$$

This method gives superior precision to counting the proportion of reticulocytes without an ocular insert [25]. Consecutive rather than random fields should be counted since there is otherwise a tendency to subconsciously select fields with more reticulocytes [25]. The number of cells to be

Table 2.3 The characteristic appearance of various red cell inclusions on a new methylene blue reticulocyte preparation

Reticulum	Ribosomal RNA	Reticulofilamentous material or scanty small granules
Pappenheimer bodies	Iron-containing inclusions	One or more granules towards the periphery of the cell, may stain a deeper blue than reticulum
Heinz bodies	Denatured haemoglobin	Larger than Pappenheimer bodies, irregular in shape, usually attached to the cell membrane and may protrude through it, pale blue
Howell–Jolly bodies	DNA	Larger than Pappenheimer bodies, regular in shape, distant from the cell membrane, pale blue
Haemoglobin H inclusions	Denatured haemoglobin H	Usually do not form with short incubation periods; if present they are multiple and spherical giving a 'golf-ball' appearance; pale greenish-blue

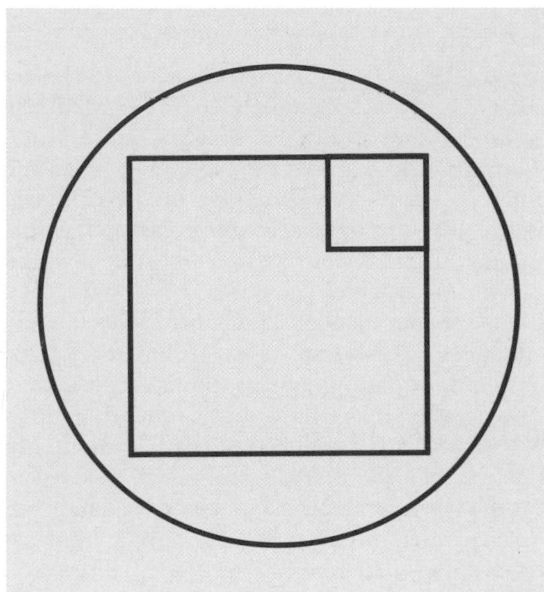

Fig. 2.5 The appearance of a Miller ocular micrometer for use in counting reticulocytes.

counted to achieve an acceptable degree of reproducibility increases as the percentage of reticulocytes falls. If a Miller graticule is used, the number of cells which should be counted to achieve a CV of about 10% is shown in Table 2.4 [21].

Reticulocyte counts have traditionally been expressed as a percentage. If an RBC is available an absolute reticulocyte count, which gives a more accurate impression of bone marrow output, can be calculated. As an alternative, a result which is more meaningful than a percentage can be produced by correcting for the degree of anaemia as follows:

$$\text{reticulocyte index} = \frac{\text{reticulocyte percentage} \times \text{observed PCV}}{\text{normal PCV}}$$

for example,

$$\text{reticulocyte index} = \frac{1.2 \times 0.29}{0.45} = 0.77$$

This example shows that an apparently normal reticulocyte count can be demonstrated to be low if allowance is made for the presence of anaemia. This procedure and the use of an absolute reticulocyte count give similar information. A more complex correction [26] can be made which allows for the fact that in anaemic persons, under the influence of an increased concentration of erythropoietin, reticulocytes are released prematurely from the bone marrow and spend longer in the blood before becoming mature red cells. The reticulocyte index and the absolute reticulocyte count both give a somewhat false impression of marrow output in this circumstance. The reticulocyte production index [26] is calculated by dividing the reticulocyte index by the average maturation time of a reticulocyte in the peripheral blood at any degree of anaemia. Although the reticulocyte index and the reticulocyte production index have not found general acceptance the concepts embodied in them should be borne in mind when reticulocyte counts are being interpreted.

Although the absolute reticulocyte count or one of the reticulocyte indices is to be preferred as an indicator of bone marrow output, the reticulocyte percentage has the advantage that it gives an indication of red cell lifespan. If a patient with a stable haemolytic anaemia has a reticulocyte count of 10% it is apparent that one cell in 10 is less than 1–3 days old.

The reticulocyte count is stable with storage of EDTA-anticoagulated blood for up to 24 hours at room temperature [27] and for several days at 4°C [21].

Table 2.4 Cells to be counted to achieve a reasonably precise reticulocyte count

Reticulocyte count (%)	Approximate number of cells to be counted in small squares for CV of 10%	Equivalent to total count of
1–2	1000	9000
3–5	500	4500
6–10	200	1800
20–25	100	900

The number of cells to be counted in the small square of a Miller graticule to achieve an acceptable degree of precision for the reticulocyte count. From ICSH [21].

Principles of operation of automated haematology counters

The latest fully automated blood cell counters aspirate and dilute a blood sample and determine 8–23 variables relating to red cells, white cells and platelets. Many counters are also capable of identifying a blood specimen (e.g., by bar-code reading), mixing it, transporting it to the sampling tube and checking it for adequacy of volume and absence of clots. To avoid any unnecessary handling of blood specimens by instrument operators, sampling is usually by piercing a cap. Apart from the measurement of Hb, all variables depend on counting and sizing of particles, whether red cells, white cells or platelets. Particles can be counted and sized either by electrical impedance or by light scattering. Automated instruments have at least two channels. In one channel a diluent is added and red cells are counted and sized. In another channel a lytic agent is added, together with diluent, to reduce red cells to stroma, leaving the white cells intact for counting and also producing a solution in which Hb can be measured. Further channels are required for a differential WBC which is often dependent on study of cells by a number of modalities, e.g., impedance technology with current of various frequencies, light scattering and light absorbance. A separate channel or an independent instrument may be required for a reticulocyte count.

Automated instruments cannot recognize all the significant abnormalities which can be recognized by a human observer. They are therefore designed to produce accurate and precise blood counts on specimens which are either normal or show only numerical abnormalities, and to alert the instrument operator when the specimen has unusual characteristics which could either lead to an inaccurate measurement or which require review of a blood film. This is often referred to as 'flagging'. Results should be flagged: (i) when the blood sample contains blast cells, immature granulocytes, NRBC or atypical lymphocytes; (ii) when there are giant or aggregated platelets or for any reason red cell and platelet populations cannot be separated; and (iii) when there is an abnormality likely to be associated with factitious results.

Coulter counters and other impedance counters

Blood cells are extremely poor conductors of electricity. When a stream of cells in a conducting medium flows through a small aperture across which an electric current is applied (Fig. 2.6) there is a measurable increase in the electrical impedance across the aperture as each cell passes through, this increase being proportional to the volume of conducting material displaced. The change in impedance is proportional to the cell volume. Cells can thus be both counted and sized from the electrical impulses which they generate. This is the principle of impedance counting which was devised and developed by Wallace Coulter in the late 1940s and 1950s and which ushered in the modern era of automated blood cell counting.

Aperture impedance is determined by capacitance and inductance as well as by resistance. Various factors apart from cell volume influence the amplitude, duration and form of the pulse, these being related to the disturbance of electrical lines of force as well as to the displacement of the conducting medium. Cell shape is relevant, as well as cell volume, so that cells of increased deformability which can elongate in response to shear forces as they pass through the aperture appear smaller than their actual size and rigid cells appear larger [28]. Furthermore, cells which pass through the aperture off centre produce aberrant impulses and appear larger than their actual size. Cells which recirculate through the edge of an electrical field produce an aberrant impulse which is smaller than that produced by a similar cell passing through the aperture; a recirculating red cell can produce an impulse similar to that of a platelet passing through the aperture. Cells which pass through the aperture simultaneously, or almost so, are counted and sized as a single cell; the inaccuracy introduced requires correction known as coincidence correction. Aberrant impulses can be edited out electronically. Sheathed flow or hydrodynamic focusing can direct cells to the centre of the aperture to reduce the problems caused both by coincidence and by aberrant impulses. Both sheathed flow and sweep flow behind an aperture can prevent recirculation of cells.

Impedance counters generally produce very

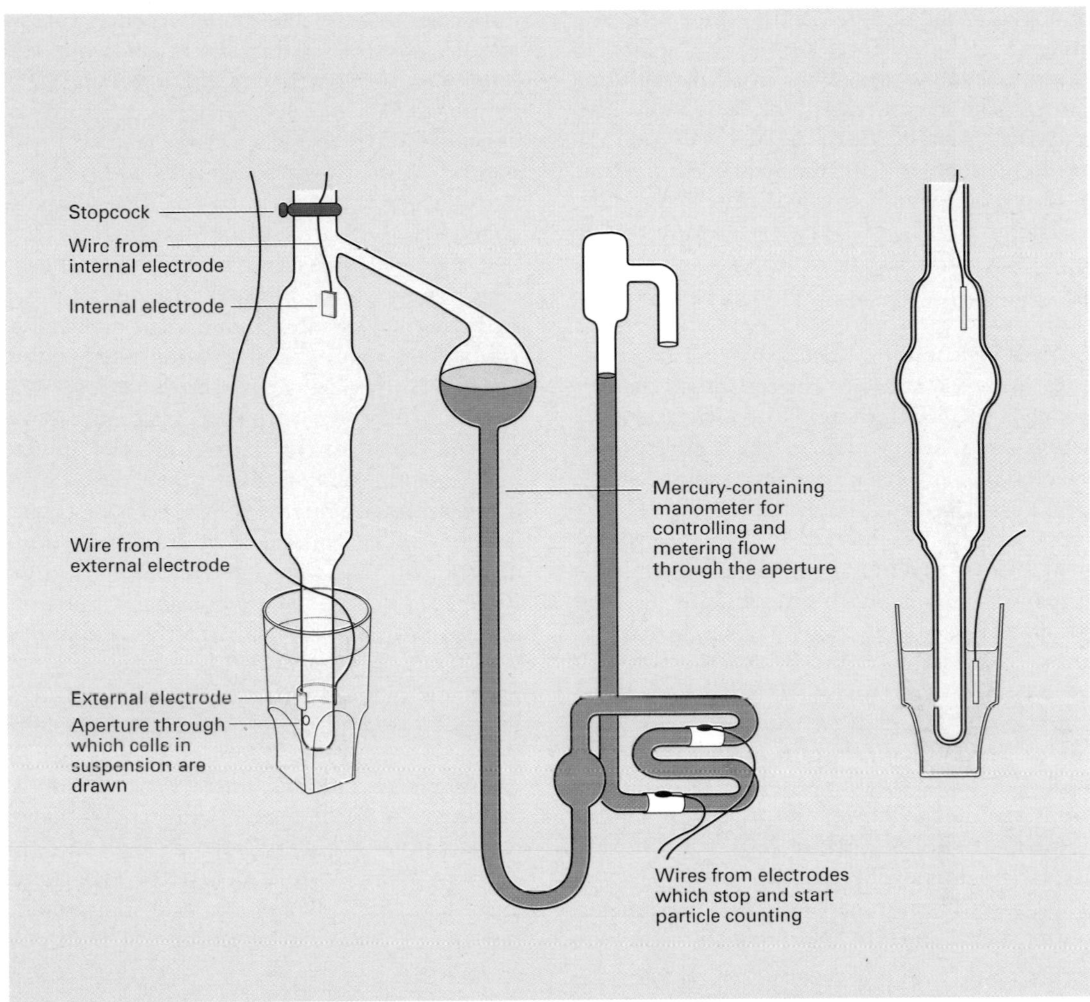

Fig. 2.6 Semi-diagrammatic representation of part of Coulter Counter, model FN showing the aperture tube and the manometer used for metering the volume of cell suspension counted. Right: diagrammatic representation of the cross-section of the aperture tube of an impedance counter.

precise measurements of cell volume and haemoglobin content and concentration. However, there are some inaccuracies inherent in the method which are greater when cells are abnormal. The voltage pulse produced by a cell passing through the sensing zone can be regarded as the cell's electrical shadow, which suggests a particle of a certain size and shape. A normal red cell probably passes through the aperture in a fusiform or cigar shape [28] producing an electrical shadow similar to its actual volume, whereas a sphere produces an electrical shadow 1.5 times its actual volume [28]. A fixed rigid cell will appear larger than its actual volume. Furthermore, cell deformability is a function of haemoglobin concentration within an individual cell.

Coulter counters

Coulter counters measure Hb by a modified cyanmethaemoglobin method. For example, with the Coulter Counter S Plus IV Hb is derived from the optical density at approximately 525 nm after a reaction time of 20–25 seconds. Coulter instruments count and size red cells, white cells and platelets by impedance technology. Platelets and red cells are counted and sized in the same channel. The measurement of MCV and RBC allow the Hct (PCV) to be derived and the measurement of MPV and the platelet count allow the derivation of an equivalent platelet variable, the plateletcrit. The MCH is derived from the Hb and the RBC. The MCHC is derived from the Hb, RBC and MCV. The variation in size of red cells is indicated by the red cell distribution width (RDW), which is the SD of individual measurements of red cell volume. The equivalent platelet variable is the platelet distribution width (PDW). There is often some overlap in size between small red cells and large platelets. Depending on the model of instrument, platelets and red cells may be separated from each other by a fixed threshold, e.g., at 20 fl, or by a moving threshold, or the data from counts between two thresholds, e.g., 2 and 20 fl, may be used to fit a curve which is extrapolated so that platelets falling beyond these thresholds, e.g., between 0 and 70 fl, are also included in the count. White cells are counted in a separate channel, the Hb channel, following red cell lysis. Some, but not necessarily all, of any NRBC present are included in the 'WBC'. Histograms of volume distribution of white cells, red cells and platelets are provided (Fig. 2.7).

The latest fully automated Coulter instruments (Coulter STKS and MAXM) produce a five-part differential white cell count which is based on various physical characteristics of white cells, following partial stripping of cytoplasm (Fig. 2.8 & Table 2.5). Three simultaneous measurements are made on each cell: (i) impedance measurements with low-frequency electromagnetic current, dependent mainly on cell volume; (ii) conductivity measurements with high-frequency (radiofrequency) electromagnetic current, dependent mainly on the internal structure of the cell including nucleocytoplasmic ratio, nuclear density and granularity; (iii) forward light scattering at 10–70° when cells pass through a laser beam, determined by structure, shape and reflectivity of the cell. Five cell populations are discriminated by three-dimensional cluster analysis. Clusters are represented graphically by plots of cell volume (determined by impedance analysis) against three discriminant functions derived from the data. Plots of size against discriminant function 1 (mainly derived from light scatter) separate cells into four clusters: neutrophils, eosinophils, monocytes and lymphocytes plus basophils (Fig. 2.8a). Basophils are in the upper right hand quadrant of the lymphocyte box. Plots of size against discriminant function 2 (mainly based on conductivity measurements with high-frequency electromagnetic current) separate cells into three clusters, lymphocytes, monocytes and granulocytes (Fig. 2.8b). A plot of size against discriminant function 3, obtained by gating out neutrophils

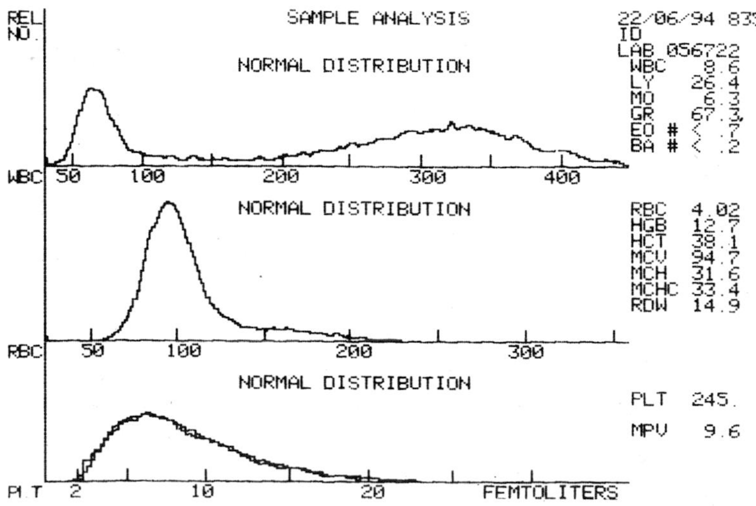

Fig. 2.7 Histograms produced by a Coulter S Plus IV automated counter showing volume distribution of white cells, red cells and platelets.

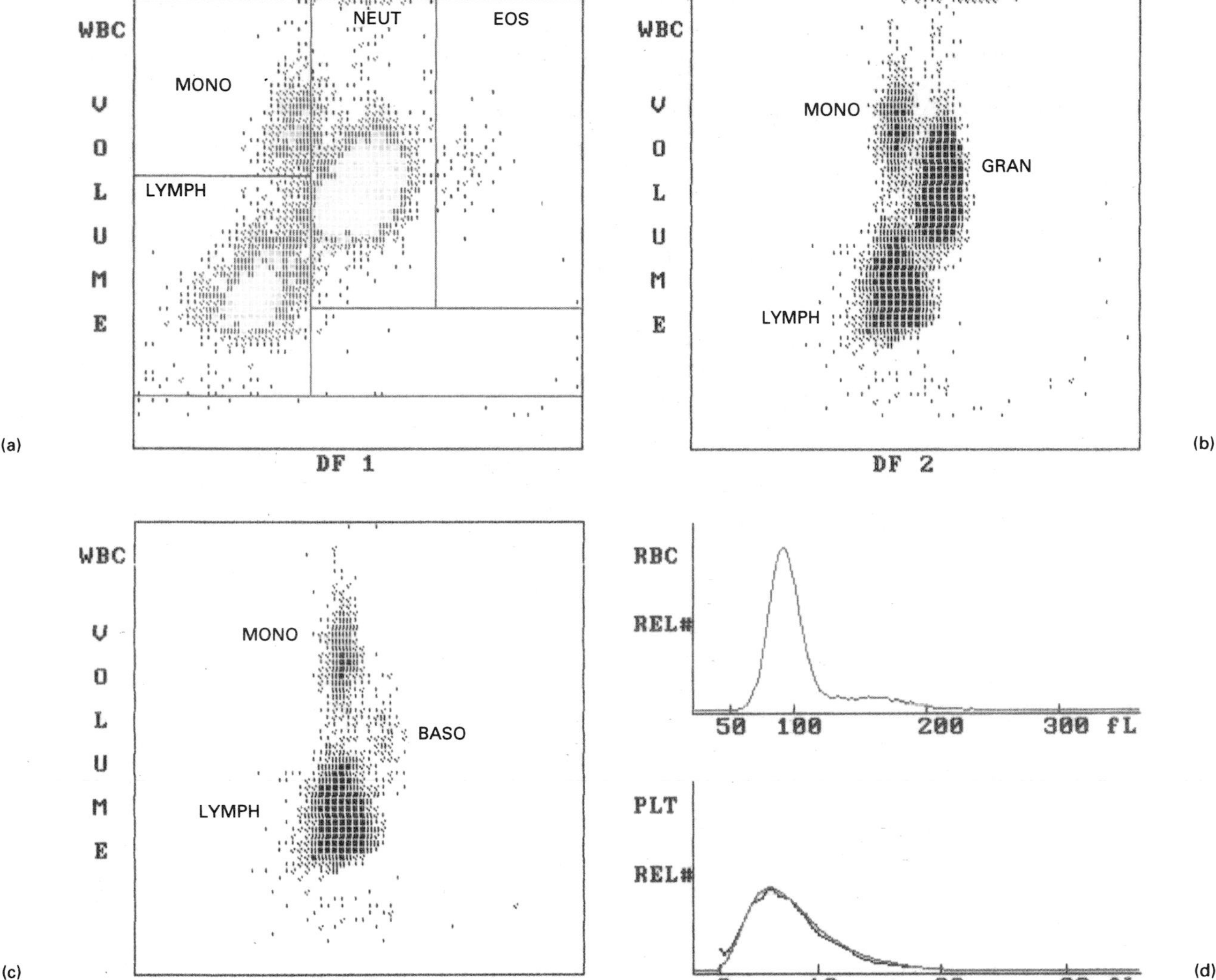

Fig. 2.8 Printouts of Coulter STKS automated counter. (a) Scatter plot of white cell volume against discriminant function 1. There are four white cell populations: NEUT, neutrophils; EOS, eosinophils; MONO, monocytes; and LYMPH, lymphocytes. (b) Scatter plots of white cell volume against discriminant function 2 showing three white cell populations: GRAN, neutrophils, eosinophils and basophils; MONO, monocytes; and LYMPH, lymphocytes. (c) Scatter plots of white cell volume against discriminant function 3 showing three white cell populations; BASO, basophils; MONO, monocytes; and LYMPH, lymphocytes. (d) Histogram showing size distribution of red cells and platelets.

and eosinophils, shows basophils as a cluster separate from lymphocytes and monocytes (Fig. 2.8c).

Earlier Coulter instruments (the S Plus series and the STKR) produce a three-part differential count based solely on impedance sizing following partial stripping of cytoplasm, the categories of white cell being granulocyte, lymphocyte and mononuclear cell.

Table 2.5 Technology employed in automated full blood counters performing five- to seven-part differential counts

Instrument	Technology
Coulter STKS (Coulter Electronics Ltd)	Impedance with low-frequency electromagnetic current Conductivity with high-frequency electromagnetic current Laser light scattering
Sysmex SE-9000 (Toa Medical Electronic)	Impedance with direct current Capacitance with high-frequency current Impedance with direct current at low and high pH
H.1 series (Technicon Division of Bayer)	Light scattering following peroxidase reaction Light absorbance following peroxidase reaction Light scattering following stripping of cytoplasm from cells other than basophils by a lytic agent at low pH
Cell-Dyn 3500 (Abbott Diagnostics)	Forward light scatter Narrow-angle light scatter Orthogonal light scatter Polarized orthogonal light scatter
Cobas Argos 5000 (Roche Products Ltd)	Impedance Light absorbance following staining of eosinophils Impedance following preferential stripping of cytoplasm from basophils at low pH

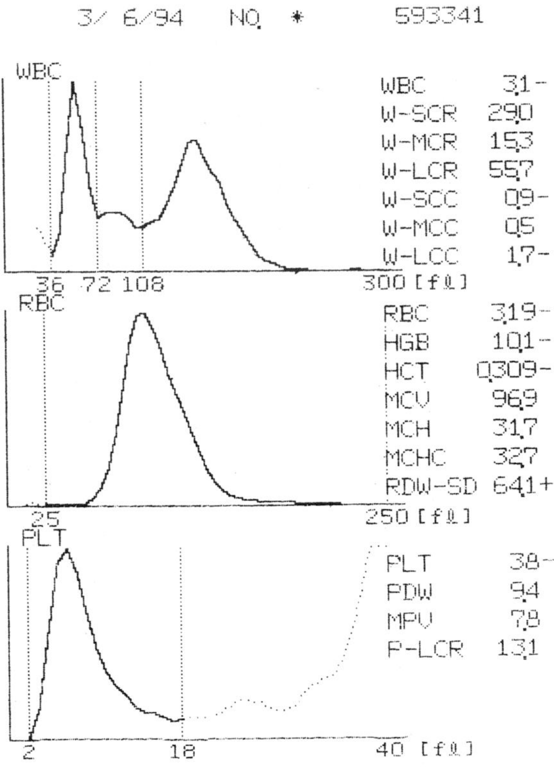

Fig. 2.9 Numerical printout and histograms of white blood cell (WBC), red blood cell (RBC) and platelet (PLT) volume produced by a Toa-Sysmex E 5000 automated haematology analyser. White cells are classified into small cells (W-SC) which are mainly lymphocytes, intermediate sized cells (W-MC) which are mainly monocytes and large cells (W-LC) which are mainly neutrophils.

Toa-Sysmex and other impedance counters

After the expiry of the initial patent of Coulter Electronics, impedance counters were introduced by a number of other manufacturers. These operate according to similar principles to those of Coulter instruments. Some instruments integrate the pulse heights from the red cell channel to produce Hct and derive the MCV from the RBC and Hct while others do the reverse. Parameters produced are similar to those of Coulter analysers, often including a three-part differential count (Fig. 2.9). Platelets may be separated from red cells by fixed thresholds or moving thresholds. The RDW on most instruments represents the SD of cell size measurements. Toa-Sysmex instruments give the option of CV as an index of RDW. Most impedance counters measure Hb by a modified cyanmethaemoglobin method. An exception is found with Toa-Sysmex instruments which are progressively introducing a lauryl sulphate method.

The latest Toa-Sysmex instrument, the SE-9000, has an Hb channel which is separate from the WBC channel. This permits the use of a strong lytic agent so that high WBCs are unlikely to interfere with Hb estimates. Hb estimation is by a lauryl sulphate method. There are moving thresh-

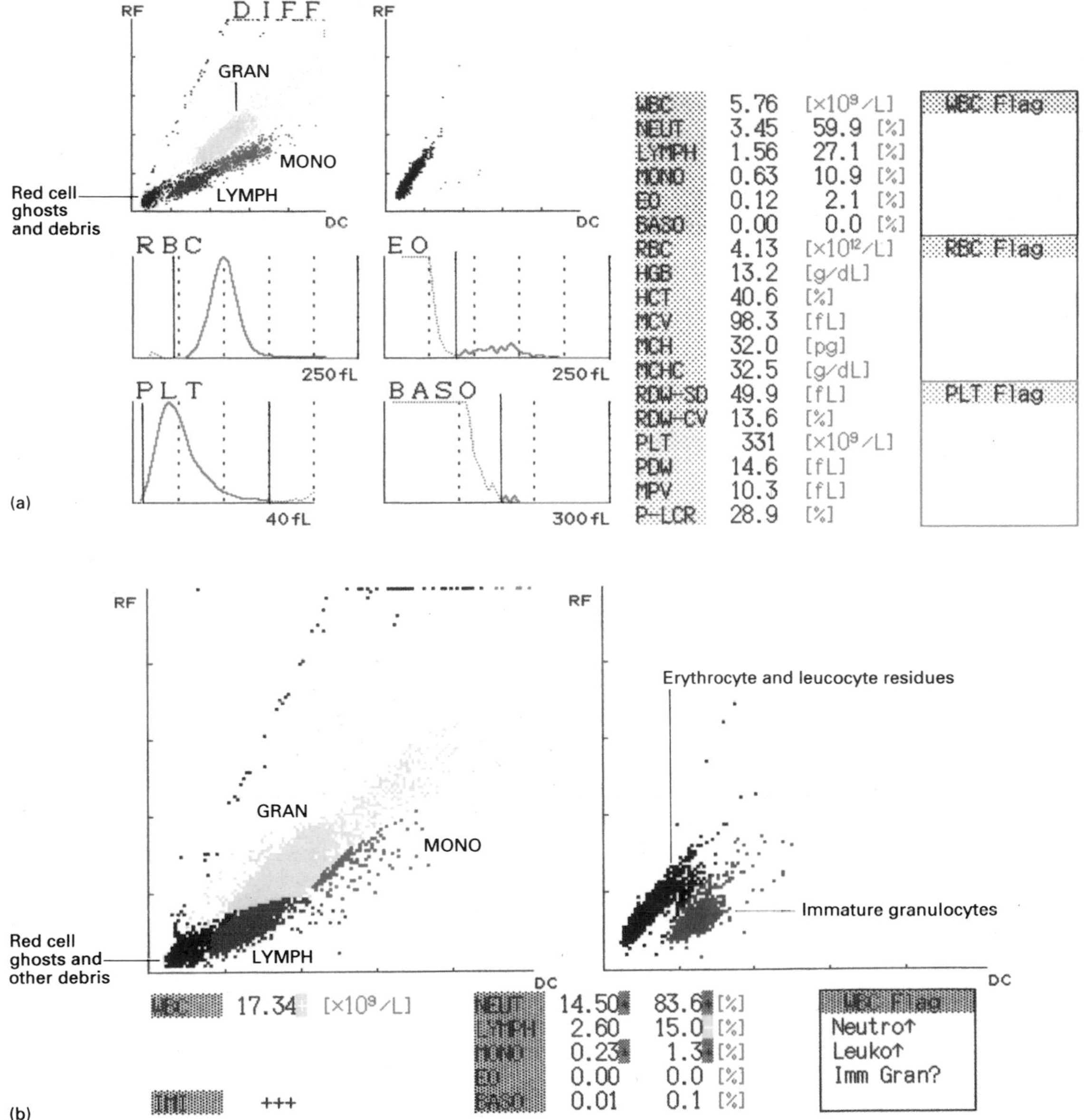

Fig. 2.10 Graphic output of Toa-Sysmex SE-9000 automated haematology analyser. (a) White cell scatter plots and red cell, platelet, eosinophil and basophil volume histograms on a normal sample. (b) White cell scatter plots — radiofrequency (RF) against direct current (DC) — of an abnormal sample with an increase of immature granulocytes. White cell populations shown are: GRAN, granulocytes; LYMPH, lymphocytes; MONO, monocytes (left); and immature granulocytes in a separate cluster from erythrocytes and residues of other leucocytes (right).

olds for both red cells and platelets. As with earlier instruments, histograms of red cell, white cell and platelet volume distribution are provided (Fig. 2.10a). A five-part differential count is produced by combining data from three channels (see Table 2.5). In the granulocyte–lymphocyte–monocyte channel leucocytes are separated from red cell ghosts and platelet clumps and are divided into three major clusters (Fig. 2.10) by a plot of radiofrequency capacitance measurements against direct current impedance measurements. Radiofrequency measurements depend on internal cellular structure — nucleocytoplasmic ratio, chromatin structure and cytoplasmic granularity — while direct current measurements depend on cell size. Eosinophils are detected by direct current measurements of cell size following exposure to a lytic agent at alkaline pH. Basophils are detected by direct current measurements of cell size following exposure to a lytic agent at acid pH. The neutrophil count is determined by subtracting basophil and eosinophil counts from the granulocyte count. Immature granulocytes can be separated from erythrocytes and the residues of other leucocytes in the immature myeloid information (IMI) channel (Fig. 2.10b, right). Any abnormalities can thus be flagged as: ?left shift, ?immature granulocytes or ?blasts.

Technicon instruments and other light-scattering or light-scattering/impedance instruments.

A cell passing through a focused beam of light scatters the light which may then be detected by photo-optical detectors placed lateral to the light beam. The degree of scatter is related to the cell size so that the cell can be both counted and sized. By placing a detector in the line of the light beam it is also possible to measure light absorbance. The light beam can be either white light or a high-intensity, coherent laser which has superior optical qualities. The light detector can be either a photomultiplier or a photodiode which converts light to electrical impulses which can be accumulated and counted.

Technicon instruments

The latest Technicon instruments (Bayer Diagnostics) — the H.1, H.2 and H.3 — count and size cells by light scattering, using white light for counting and sizing leucocytes and a laser for counting and sizing red cells and platelets. The red cells are isovolumetrically sphered so that light scatter is not dependent on cell shape and can be predicted from the laws of physics. Cells move through a laser beam and light scattered forward is measured at a narrow (2–3°) and a wider (5–15°) angle. A comparison of the two allows the computation of the size and haemoglobin concentration of individual red cells. Histograms showing the distribution of red cell volume and haemoglobin concentration are provided, together with a plot of volume against haemoglobin concentration (Fig. 2.11). The histogram of the cell volumes permits the derivation of the MCV, RDW and Hct (PCV).

Similarly, the histogram of haemoglobin concentrations permits the derivation of the cellular haemoglobin concentration mean (CHCM) and the haemoglobin distribution width (HDW), the latter being indicative of the variation in haemoglobin concentration between individual cells. Technicon instruments measure Hb by a modification of conventional cyanmethaemoglobin methodology, and the MCH and MCHC are computed from the Hb, RBC and MCV. An optional lauryl sulphate method for Hb estimation is also available. The MCHC and CHCM are independently derived measurements, both representing the average haemoglobin concentration in a cell. They should give essentially the same result. This acts as an internal quality control mechanism since errors in the estimation of Hb, e.g., consequent on a very high WBC, cause a discrepancy between these two measurements. It would be theoretically possible to omit the haemoglobin channel and compute Hb from the CHCM, RBC and MCV derived from light-scattering measurements.

The technology of the H.1 series of instruments appears to produce accurate estimations of MCV, PCV and MCHC which agree well with reference methods [29,30]. It has been possible to avoid the inaccuracies of earlier light-scattering instruments (in which light scattering was influenced by cellular haemoglobin concentration as well as cell size) and the inaccuracies inherent in impedance counters (in which the electrical shadow is influenced by cellular deformability as well as cell size). Cells which cannot be isovolumetrically sphered, e.g., irreversibly sickled cells, will not be sized accurately. Similar measurements of two-angle light scatter permit platelets to be counted and sized (platelet count and MPV). A plateletcrit and PDW, a measure of platelet anisocytosis, are also computed.

The differential count of the H.1 series is

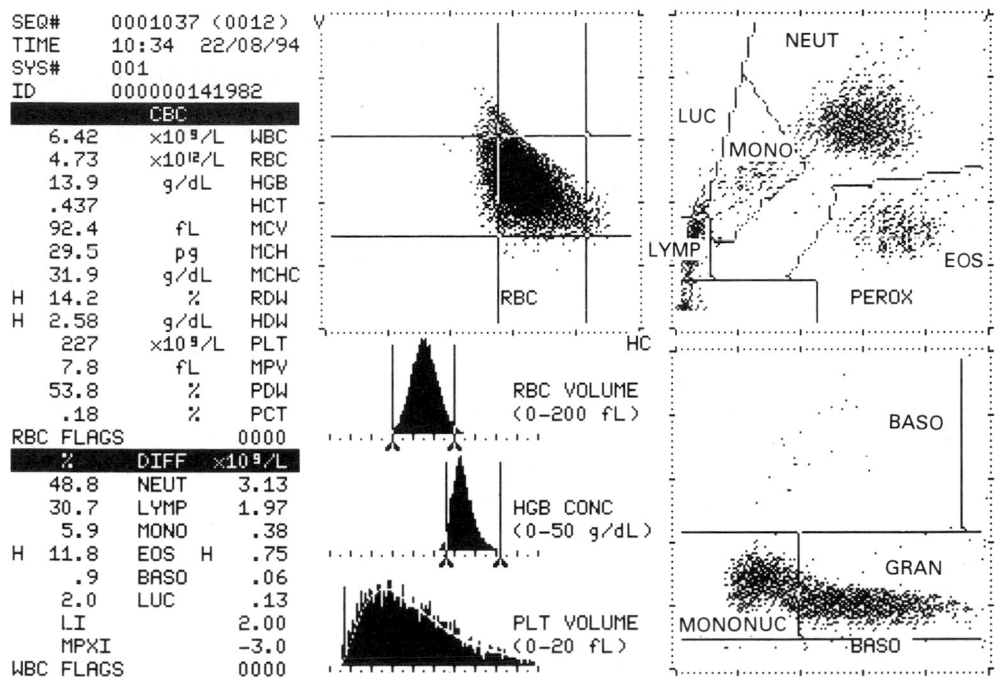

Fig. 2.11 Histograms and scatter plots of red cell volume and red cell haemoglobin concentration and white cell scatter plots produced by a Technicon H.2 counter. In the peroxidase channel forward light scatter, largely determined by cell volume is plotted against light absorbance, largely determined by the intensity of the peroxidase reaction. There are five white cell populations: NEUT, neutrophils; MONO, monocytes; LYMPH, lymphocytes; EOS, eosinophils; and LUC, large unstained cells, which are large, peroxidase-negative cells. In the basophil/lobularity channel forward light scatter, representing cell volume following differential cytoplasmic stripping is plotted against high-angle light scatter which is determined largely by cellular structure. There are three cell clusters, two of which overlap: BASO, basophils; MONONUC, mononuclear cells (lymphocytes and monocytes); and GRAN, granulocytes (neutrophils and eosinophils).

derived from two channels (see Table 2.5). The peroxidase channel uses white light and incorporates a cytochemical reaction in which the peroxidase of neutrophils, eosinophils and monocytes acts on a substrate, 4-chloro-1-naphthol, to produce a black reaction product which absorbs light. Light scatter, which is proportional to cell size, is then plotted against light absorbance, which is proportional to the intensity of the peroxidase reaction (see Fig. 2.11). Neutrophils, eosinophils, monocytes and lymphocytes fall into four clusters which are separated from each other and from cellular debris by a mixture of moving and fixed thresholds. A further cluster of cells which are peroxidase-negative and larger than most lymphocytes are designated large unstained cells (LUC). In healthy subjects, LUC are mainly large lymphocytes but abnormal cells such as blast cells and atypical lymphocytes can fall into this category. In the peroxidase channel, basophils fall in the lymphocyte category. They are separated from all other leucocytes in an independent basophil/lobularity channel, on the basis of their resistance to stripping of cytoplasm by a lytic agent in acid conditions. Basophils, sized by forward light scatter, are larger than the stripped residues of other cells (see Fig. 2.11). The basophil/lobularity channel is also used to detect the presence of blasts. Forward light scatter, which is proportional to cell size, is plotted against high-angle light scatter which is a measure of increasing nuclear density and lobulation. Blasts are detected as a population with an abnormally low nuclear density. In addition, the 'lobularity index' (LI) is a measure of the ratio of the number of cells producing a lot of high-angle light scatter (lobulated neutrophils) to cells producing less high-angle light scatter (mononuclear cells, immature granulocytes and blasts).

Instruments of the H.1 series, in addition to 'flagging' the presence of blasts, atypical lymphocytes, immature granulocytes and NRBC, produce two new white cell parameters — LI (described above) and the mean peroxidase index (MPXI). This latter is a measure of average peroxidase activity and is decreased in inherited peroxidase deficiency and also in acquired deficiency, as occurs in some myelodysplastic syndromes and myeloid leukaemias. MPXI is increased in infection, in some myeloid leukaemias and myelodysplastic syndromes, in acquired immune deficiency syndrome (AIDS) and in megaloblastic anaemia.

Cell-Dyn instruments

The Cell-Dyn 3500 (Abbott Diagnostics) is a multichannel automated instrument incorporating both laser light-scattering and impedance technology. Hb is measured as cyanmethaemoglobin. Red cells, white cells and platelets are counted and sized by impedance technology following cytoplasmic stripping of white cells. Histograms of size distribution are provided (Fig. 2.12).

The WBC is also estimated in a light-scattering (laser) channel which provides, in addition, an automated five-part differential count [31] (see Table 2.5). White cells mainly maintain their integrity and are hydrodynamically focused to pass in single file through the laser beam. In this channel red cells are rendered transparent because their refractive index is the same as that of the sheath reagent. Four light-scattering parameters are measured: (i) forward light scatter at 1–3° (referred to as 0° scatter) which is mainly dependent on cell size; (ii) narrow-angle light scatter at 7–11° (referred to as 10° scatter) which is dependent on cell structure and complexity; (iii) total polarized orthogonal light scatter at 70–100° (referred to as 90° scatter); and (iv) depolarized orthogonal light scatter at 70–100° (referred to as 90°D scatter). Scatter plots of white cell populations are provided (Fig. 2.13). Cells are first separated into granulocytes and mononuclear cells (Fig. 2.13a) on the basis of their lobularity and complexity. Next, granulocytes are separated into eosinophils and neutrophils on the basis of the unique ability of eosinophils to depolarize light (Fig. 2.13b). Next, the mononuclear cells are separated into monocytes, lymphocytes and degranulated basophils (basophil granules being soluble in the sheath reagent) on the basis of cell size and complexity (Fig. 2.13c). Finally, all five populations are indicated (colour coded) on a plot of lobularity against size (Fig. 2.13d). The identification of cell clusters with anomalous characteristics permits blasts, atypical lymphocytes, NRBC and immature granulocytes to be flagged.

The measurement of WBC by two technologies provides an internal quality control mechanism.

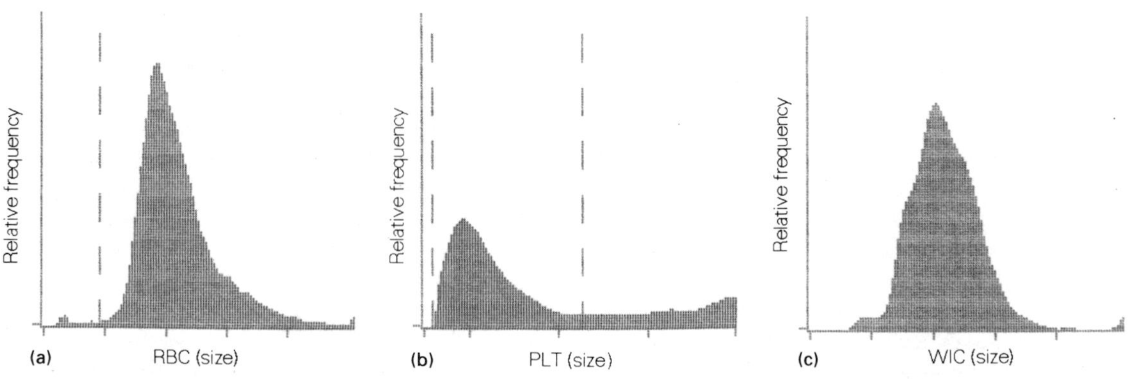

Fig. 2.12 Graphic output of Cell-Dyn 3500 automated counter showing histograms of volume distribution of RBC, platelets (PLT) and WIC derived from the impedance channel.

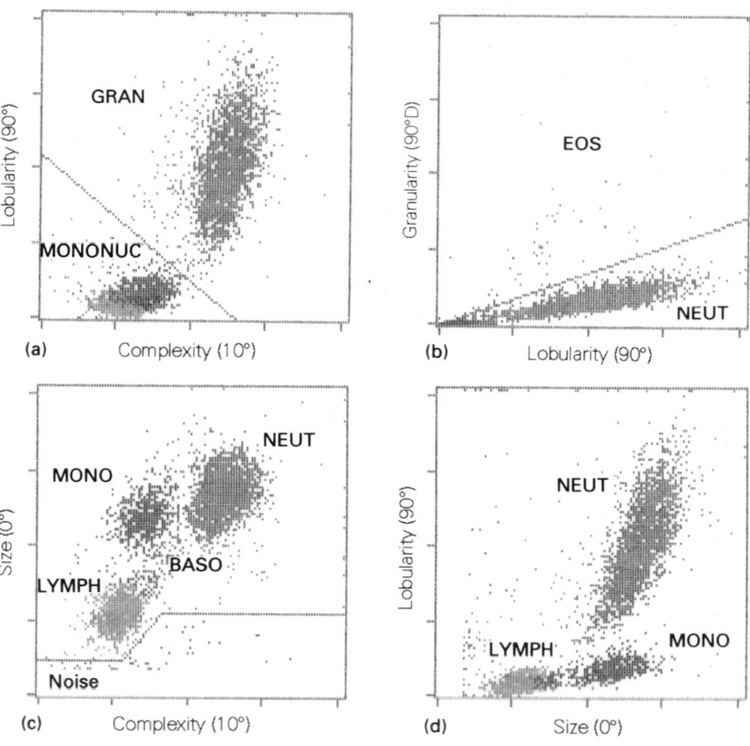

Fig. 2.13 Graphic output of a Cell-Dyn 3500 counter showing white cell scatter plots derived from the white cell optical channel. (a) A plot of 90° scatter (indicating lobularity) against 10° scatter (indicating complexity) separates a granulocyte cluster from a mononuclear cluster. (b) 90°D (depolarized) scatter against 90° scatter separates the granulocyte cluster into eosinophils (which depolarize light) and neutrophils (which do not). (c) 0° scatter (related to size) against 10° scatter (related to complexity) separates the mononuclear cell cluster into lymphocytes, monocytes and degranulated basophils. (d) The five populations thus identified are shown on a plot of 90° scatter (related to lobularity) against 0° scatter (related to size).
GRAN, granulocytes; MONONUC, mononuclear cells; NEUT, neutrophils; MONO, monocytes; LYMPH, lymphocytes; and EOS, eosinophils.

The WBC in the impedance channel (WIC) is falsely elevated if NRBC are present whereas the WBC in the optical channel (WOC) excludes NRBC by means of a moving threshold. However, since the optical channel employs a less potent lytic agent, WOC may be falsely elevated when there are osmotically resistant red cells, as occurs with some neonatal blood samples. The likelihood of NRBC or osmotically resistant red cells is flagged and an algorithm selects the preferred result. If a suspicion of *both* NRBC and osmotically resistant cells is flagged an extended period of lysis can be used to produce an accurate WOC.

Cobas Argos instruments

Cobas Argos 5 Diff and Cobas Argos 5000 instruments (Roche Products Ltd) are multichannel automated instruments incorporating light absorbance measurements and impedance technology. Red cells, white cells and platelets are counted and sized by impedance technology and histograms of size distribution are provided. A six-part differential count, displayed graphically, is based on measurements of light absorbance and electrical impedance following staining of eosinophils so that they can be differentiated from other cells by their greater light absorbance (Fig. 2.14 and see Table 2.5). It includes 'large immature cells' (comprised of blasts and immature granulocytes) and 'atypical lymphocytes' (including small blasts). Basophils are differentiated from other white cells by impedance measurements following differential cytoplasmic stripping to provide a final seven-part differential count.

Automated reticulocyte counts

Most automated reticulocyte counts depend on the ability of various fluorochromes to combine with the RNA of reticulocytes. Fluorescent cells can then be counted in a flow cytometer. The

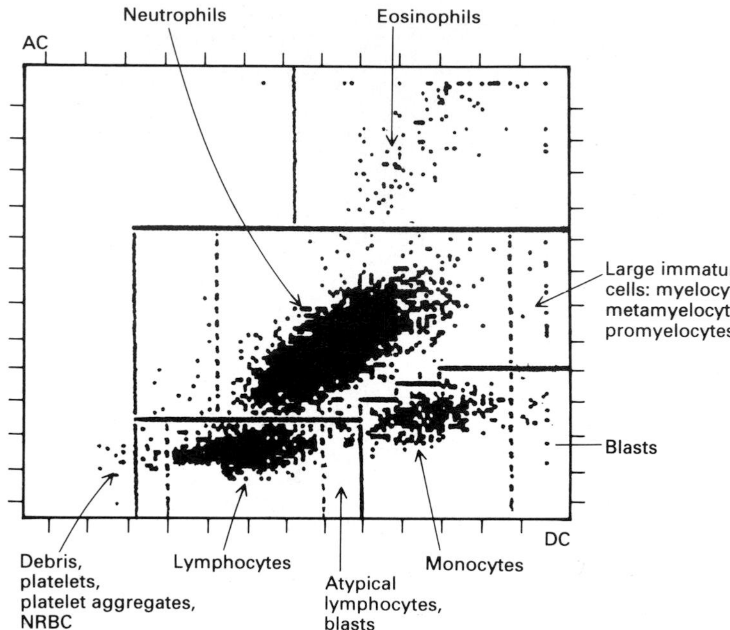

Fig. 2.14 Diagrammatic representation of the white cell scatter plot produced by a Cobas 5000 or Cobas Helios automated counter. Light absorbance (AC) is plotted against an impedance measurement of volume (DC).

fluorochromes also combine with DNA so that nucleated cells fluoresce. An alternative technology is based on staining of RNA by a non-fluorescent nucleic acid stain such as new methylene blue or oxazine 750. Reticulocytes are then detected by their light absorbance. White cells, nucleated red cells and platelets can usually be separated from reticulocytes on the basis of gating for size and either their light absorbance or the intensity of their fluorescence. Reticulocyte counts can be expressed as an absolute count or as a percentage of total red cells.

Because of the large number of cells counted, automated reticulocyte counts are much more precise than manual counts. It was hoped that they might also be more accurate, since the subjective element in recognizing late reticulocytes with only one or two granules of positively staining material is eliminated. However, the automated count is altered by (i) the choice of fluorochrome; (ii) the duration of exposure of the blood to the fluorochrome; (iii) the temperature at which the sample is kept after mixing; and (iv) the setting of thresholds — the upper threshold to exclude fluorescing nucleated cells and the lower threshold to exclude background autofluorescence.

Similar considerations apply to automated reticulocyte counts using non-fluorescent nucleic acid stains. A reference range for an automated reticulocyte count is therefore specific to an instrument and method. Reference ranges which have been established show considerable variation. It is still necessary to consider the manual count to decide whether a range represents 'truth'. Ideally, automated and manual counts should show a close correlation; mean counts should be similar and the intercept on the *y*-axis of the regression line of automated counts on manual counts should be small.

Automated reticulocyte counts can be performed on general purpose flow cytometers, such as the Becton Dickinson FACScan or the Coulter EPICS XL, or on a dedicated reticulocyte counter, such as the Sysmex-Toa R-1000 or R-3000 (Fig. 2.15). An automated reticulocyte counting capacity can also be incorporated into an automated full blood counter as in the Technicon H.3 (Figs 2.16 & 2.17) and the latest versions of the Coulter STKS and MAXM (Fig. 2.18).

Automated reticulocyte counters can also provide an index of reticulocyte immaturity since intensity of fluorescence or uptake of the nucleic

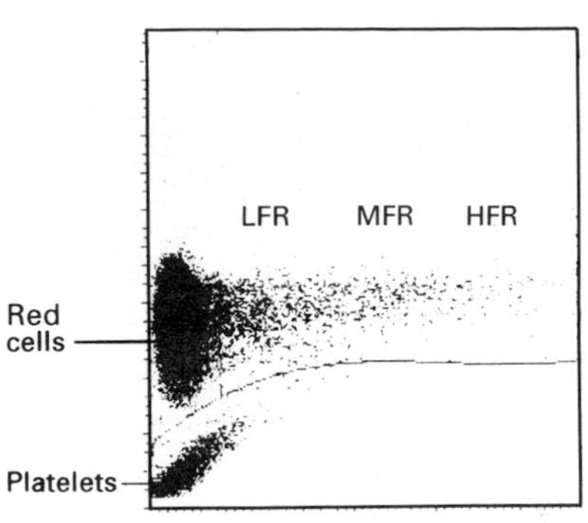

15 : 46
NO. 596925

+RET %	11.52 [%]
+RET #	299.5 [x10^9/ℓ]
-RBC	2.60 [x10^{12}/ℓ]
-LFR	66.0 [%]
+MFR	25.7 [%]
+HFR	8.3 [%]

PLT DISCRIMINATION ERROR

Fig. 2.15 Scatter plot of the reticulocyte count of the Sysmex R.3000. Cell volume is plotted against fluorescence intensity. A threshold separates red cells from platelets. Reticulocytes are divided into high fluorescence (HFR) representing the most immature reticulocytes, intermediate fluorescence (MFR) and low fluorescence (LFR) representing late reticulocytes.

RETICULOCYTE	%
RETIC	1.8

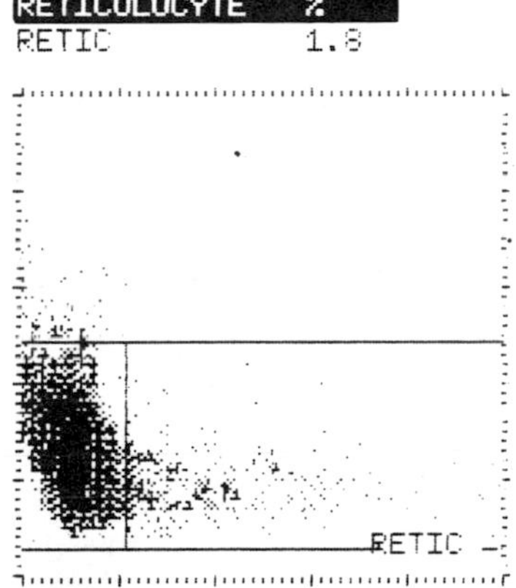

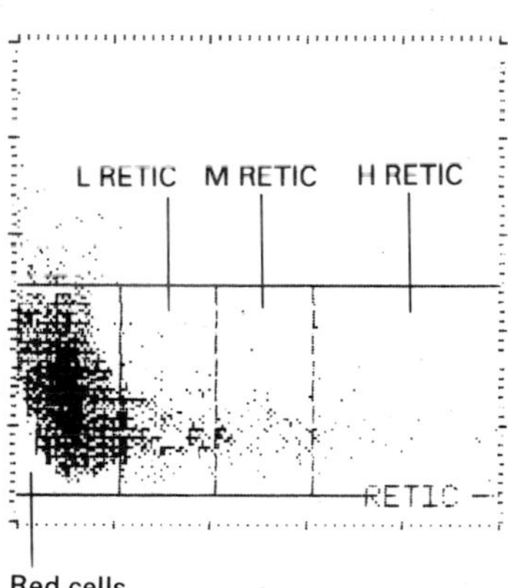

RETICULOCYTE CELLS	%	#
NEG RBC	98.2	19169
RETIC	1.8	351
L RETIC	67.0	235
M RETIC	23.4	82
H RETIC	9.7	34
CELLS ACQUIRED		19693
CELLS ANALYZED		19582
GATED CELLS		19520
MEAN ABSORPTION		10.70
CAL FACT USED		1.00

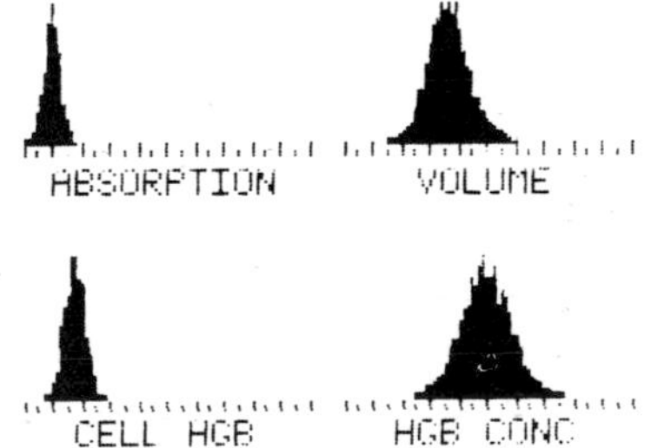

RETICULOCYTE INDICES	RETIC CELLS	GATED CELLS	
MCVr	106.3	74.4	fL
CHCMr	17.4	25.1	g/dL
RDWr	24.1	21.4	%
HDWr	3.38	4.65	g/dL
CHr	17.8	17.9	pg
CHDWr	4.5	3.7	pg

Fig. 2.16 Printout of a Technicon H.3 counter showing the scatter plot of the reticulocyte counting channel. The volume and haemoglobin content of reticulocytes and other red cells is determined by high- and low-angle light scattering and light absorbance is measured following uptake of a nucleic acid dye, oxazine 750. Six parameters of potential clinical usefulness are measured for reticulocytes as well as for total red cells. They are MCV, CHCM (= MCHC), RDW, HDW (in g/dl), CH (= MCH) and CHDW (HDW in pg). Cell volume is plotted against light absorbance. Reticulocytes are divided into high absorbance. (H RETIC) representing early reticulocytes, intermediate absorbance (M RETIC) and low absorbance (L RETIC) representing late reticulocytes.

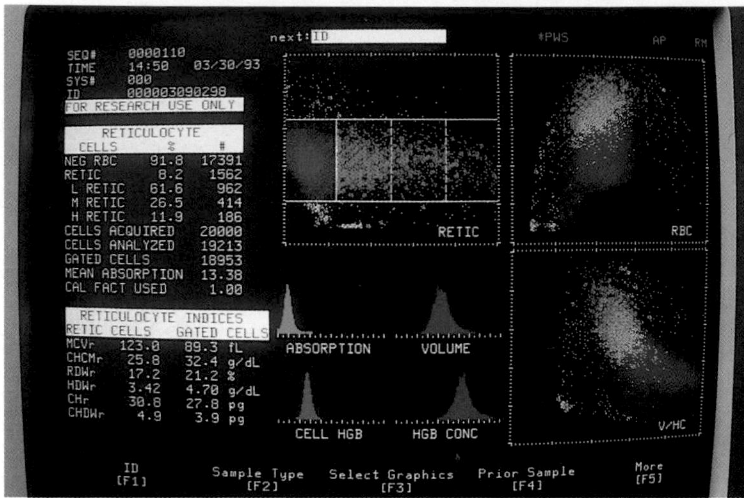

Fig. 2.17 Photograph of the colour monitor of a Technicon H.3 automated counter. The scattergram shows volume and haemoglobin content of reticulocytes (blue) in relation to size and haemoglobin content of other red cells (red) on both a Mie map and a red cell cytogram. This sample had a greatly increased reticulocyte count as a consequence of a haemolytic transfusion reaction.

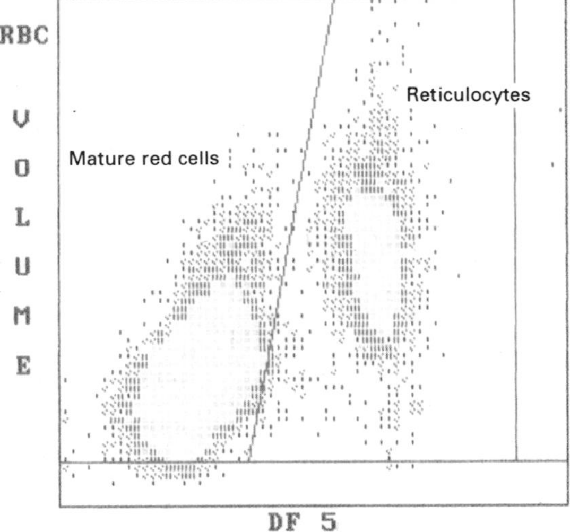

Fig. 2.18 Scatter plot of the reticulocyte channel of the Coulter Counter STKS showing clusters of mature red cells (left) and reticulocytes (right) following vital staining of reticulocytes by new methylene blue.

acid stain is proportional to the amount of RNA in the cell. Such measurements may be of clinical significance. In anaemia consequent on haemolysis or blood loss, the percentage of immature reticulocytes rises as the total reticulocyte count rises [32]. However, when there is dyserythropoiesis the percentage of immature reticulocytes may be elevated despite a normal or reduced total reticulocyte count. This has been observed, for example, in acute myeloid leukaemia (AML), the myelodysplastic syndromes (MDS), megaloblastic anaemia and aplastic anaemia [32,33]. A disproportionate increase in immature reticulocytes indicates abnormal maturation of reticulocytes [33]. In other anaemias with little dyserythropoiesis but with a poor reticulocyte response, e.g., iron-deficiency anaemia or the anaemia of chronic renal failure, the absolute reticulocyte count is reduced but the percentage of immature reticulocytes is normal.

References

1 International Committee for Standardization in Haematology. Recommendations for reference method for haemoglobinometry in human blood (ICSH Standard EP 6/2: 1977) and specifications for international haemiglobincyanide reference preparation (ICSH Standard EP 6/3: 1977). *J Clin Pathol* 1978; 31: 139–43.

2 van Kampen EJ, Zijlstra WG. Spectrophotometry of hemoglobin and hemoglobin derivatives. *Adv Clin Chem* 1983; 23: 199–257.

3 Lewis SM, Garvey B, Manning R, Sharp SA, Wardle J. Lauryl sulphate haemoglobin: a non-hazardous substitute for HiCN in haemoglobinometry. *Clin Lab Haematol* 1991; 13: 279–90.

4 International Committee for Standardization in Haematology Expert Panel on Blood Cell Sizing.

Recommendation for reference method for determination by centrifugation of packed cell volume of blood. *J Clin Pathol* 1980; 33: 1–2.

5 ICSH. Selected methods for the determination of the packed cell volume. In: van Assendelft OW & England JM, eds. *Advances in Hematological Methods: the blood count*. Boca Raton: CRC Press, 1982: 93–8.

6 Guthrie DL, Pearson TC. PCV measurement in the management of polycythaemic patients. *Clin Lab Haematol* 1982; 4: 257–65.

7 Crosland-Taylor PJ. The micro PCV. In: van Assendelft OW & England JM, eds. *Advances in Hematological Methods: the blood count*. Boca Raton: CRC Press, 1982: 85–92.

8 Lampasso JA. Error in hematocrit value produced by excessive ethylenediaminetetraacetate. *Am J Clin Pathol* 1965; 44: 109–10.

9 Pennock CA, Jones KW. Effects of ethylene-diamine-tetra-acetic acid (dipotassium salt) and heparin on the estimation of packed cell volume. *J Clin Pathol* 1966; 19: 196–9.

10 Karlow MA, Westengard JC, Bull BS. Does tube diameter influence the packed cell volume? *Clin Lab Haematol* 1989; 11: 375–83.

11 Lines RW, Grace E. Choice of anticoagulants for packed cell volume and mean cell volume determination. *Clin Lab Haematol* 1984; 6: 305–6.

12 International Committee for Standardization in Haematology. Recommended methods for measurement of red cell and plasma volume. *J Nucl Med* 1980; 21: 793–800.

13 Dacie JV, Lewis SM revised by Bain BJ. Basic haematological techniques. In: Dacie JV & Lewis SM, eds. *Practical Haematology*, 8th edn. Edinburgh: Churchill Livingstone, 1994: 48–82.

14 Lewis SM. Visual haemocytometry. In: van Assendelft OW & England JM, eds. *Advances in Hematological Methods: the blood count*. Boca Raton: CRC Press, 1982: 39–47.

15 Talstad I. Problems in microscopic and automatic cell differentiation of blood and cell suspensions. *Scand J Haematol* 1981; 26: 398–406.

16 Davidson E. The distribution of cells in peripheral blood smears. *J Clin Pathol* 1958; 11: 410–11.

17 Rümke CL. Variability of results in differential cell counts on blood smears. *Triangle* 1960; 4: 154–7.

18 England JM, Bain BJ. Total and differential leucocyte count. *Br J Haematol* 1976; 33: 1–7.

19 NCCLS. *Approved Standard H20-A. Leukocyte differential counting*. Villanova, Pennsylvania: USA National Committee for Clinical Laboratory Standards, 1992.

20 Koepke JF, Koepke JA. Reticulocytes. *Clin Lab Haematol* 1986; 8: 169–79.

21 The Expert Panel on Cytometry of the International Council for Standardization in Haematology. *ICSH Guidelines for Reticulocyte Counting by Microscopy of Supravitally Stained Preparations*. Geneva: World Health Organization, 1992.

22 Perrotta AL, Finch CA. The polychromatophilic erythrocyte. *Am J Clin Pathol* 1972; 57: 471–7.

23 Crouch JY, Kaplow LS. Relationship of reticulocyte age to polychromasia, shift cells, and shift reticulocytes. *Arch Pathol Lab Med* 1985; 109: 325–9.

24 Lowenstein ML. The mammalian reticulocyte. *Int Rev Cytol* 1959; 9: 135–74.

25 Brecher G, Schneiderman MR. A time-saving device for counting of reticulocytes. *Am J Clin Pathol* 1950; 20: 1079–83.

26 Hillman RS, Finch CA. The misused reticulocyte. *Br J Haematol* 1969; 17: 313–15.

27 Fannon M, Thomas R, Sawyer L. Effect of staining and storage times on reticulocyte counts. *Lab Med* 1982; 13: 431–3.

28 Rowan RM. *Blood Cell Volume Analysis*. London: Albert Clark, 1983.

29 Mohandas N, Kim YR, Tycko DH, Orlik J, Wyatt J, Groner W. Accurate and independent measurement of volume and hemoglobin concentration of individual red cells by laser light scattering. *Blood* 1986; 68: 506–13.

30 von Feltan U, Furlan M, Frey R, Bucher U. Test of a new method for hemoglobin determinations in automatic analysers. *Med Lab* 1978; 31: 223–31.

31 Cornbleet PJ, Myrick D, Judkins S, Levy R. Evaluation of the CELL-DYN 3000 differential. *Am J Clin Pathol* 1992; 98: 603–14.

32 Watanabe K, Kawai Y, Takeuchi K, Shimizu N, Iri H, Ikeda Y, Houwen B. Reticulocyte maturity as an indicator for estimating qualitative abnormality of erythropoiesis. *J Clin Pathol* 1994; 47: 736–9.

33 Daliphard S, Bizet M, Callat MP, Beufe S, Latouche JB, Soufiani H, Monconduit M. Evaluation of reticulocyte subtype distribution in myelodysplastic syndromes. *Am J Hematol* 1993; 44: 210–20.

CHAPTER 3

Morphology of Blood Cells

Examining the blood film

Blood films should be examined in a systematic manner, as follows.

1 Patient identification should be checked and confirmed and the microscope slide matched with the corresponding FBC report. The sex and age of the patient should be noted since the blood film cannot be interpreted without this information. In a multiracial community it is also helpful to know the ethnic origin of the patient.

2 The film should be examined macroscopically to confirm adequate spreading and to look for any unusual spreading or staining characteristics. The commonest such abnormality is an increased blue coloration caused by hypergammaglobulinaemia (Fig. 3.1) due either to a paraprotein, e.g., in multiple myeloma and related conditions, or to a reactive increase in immunoglobulins, e.g., in cirrhosis or rheumatoid arthritis. Abnormal staining characteristics are also caused by the presence of foreign substances such as heparin, which conveys a pink tinge, or the vehicles of certain intravenous drugs. Occasionally, macroscopic abnormalities are caused by precipitation of cryoglobulin, gross red cell agglutination, platelet clumping or the presence of clumps of tumour cells (Figs 3.2–3.4).

3 The film should be examined microscopically, using a microscope correctly set up to give optimal illumination [1]. Examination should take place first under a low power (for example with the ×10 or ×25 objective) and then with a higher power (×40 or ×50 objective) with an eyepiece magnification of ×10 or ×12. It is only necessary to use oil immersion and a ×100 objective when observation of fine detail is required or when searching for malarial parasites. Laboratories using unmounted films may find it useful to have a ×50 oil immersion objective in addition to a ×100. The use of a relatively low power is important since it allows rapid scanning of a large part of the film and facilitates the detection of abnormal cells when they are present at a low frequency. It is also useful in the appreciation of rouleaux and red cell and white cell agglutination. Examination of the blood film must also include examination of the edges and the tail since large abnormal cells and clumps of cells are often distributed preferentially in these areas. Platelet aggregates and fibrin strands, if present, are often found in the tail of the film.

On placing a film under the microscope the first decision to be made is whether or not it is suitable for further examination. Spreading, fixation and staining must be satisfactory and there should be no artefactual changes produced by excess EDTA or prolonged storage (see p. 43). It is unwise to give an opinion on an inadequate blood film. A well-spread film should have an appreciable area where cells are a monolayer, i.e., where they are touching but not overlapping.

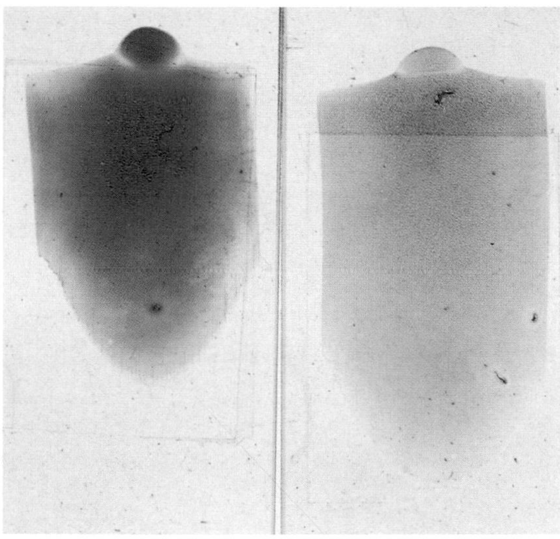

Fig. 3.1 Peripheral blood film of a patient with multiple myeloma (left) compared with another blood film stained in the same batch (right). The deeper blue staining occurs because the high concentration of immunoglobulin leads to increased uptake of the basic component of the stain.

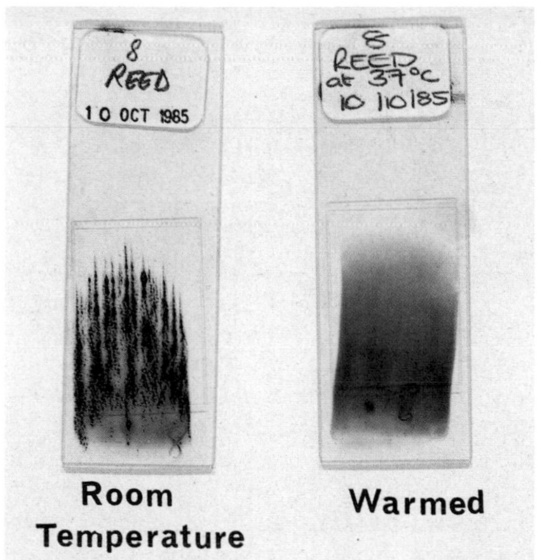

Fig. 3.2 Peripheral blood films from a patient with a potent cold agglutinin. The left hand film, which shows marked agglutination, was prepared from EDTA-anticoagulated blood which had been standing at room temperature. The right hand film, which shows no macroscopic agglutination, was prepared from blood warmed to 37°C.

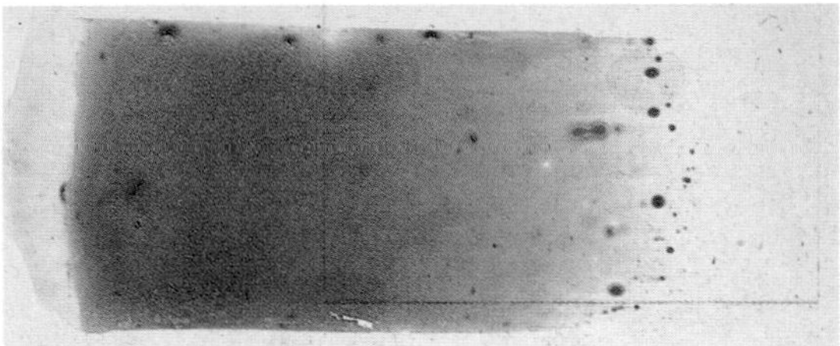

Fig. 3.3 Peripheral blood film from a patient with multiple myeloma showing cryoglobulin precipitates. Courtesy of Dr Sue Fairhead, London.

White cells should be distributed regularly without undue concentration along the edges or in the tail, such as occurs when the film is spread too thinly. Granulocytes are found preferentially along the edges and in the tail of a wedge-spread film and lymphocytes are preferentially in the centre but in a carefully spread film the difference is not great (see p. 22).

Blood films should be examined for platelet aggregates (Fig. 3.5), which may cause the platelet count to be falsely low, or fibrin strands (Fig. 3.6) which indicate partial clotting of the sample with the likelihood that the platelet count and possibly other variables are invalid. Platelets which have discharged their granules following aggregation may appear as pale blue masses not immediately identifiable as platelets.

Storage-induced artefacts

Blood films should be made without delay but laboratories which receive specimens by post or transported from a distance should be aware of the changes induced by storage. Prolonged storage of EDTA-anticoagulated blood causes crenation or echinocytic changes in red cells (Fig. 3.7), degeneration of neutrophils (Fig. 3.7) and lobulation of some lymphocyte nuclei (Fig. 3.8). Excess EDTA may itself cause crenation of red cells and also accelerates the development of storage changes. Degenerating neutrophils may have a similar appearance to necrobiotic neutrophils formed *in vivo* (see Fig. 3.67) or may be completely amorphous. If there has been prolonged delay in the blood specimen reaching the laboratory, e.g., 3 days or more, most of the neutrophils will have

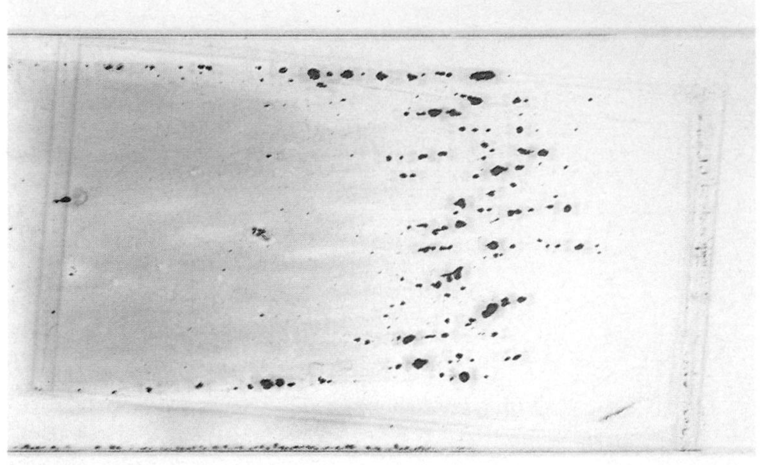

(a)

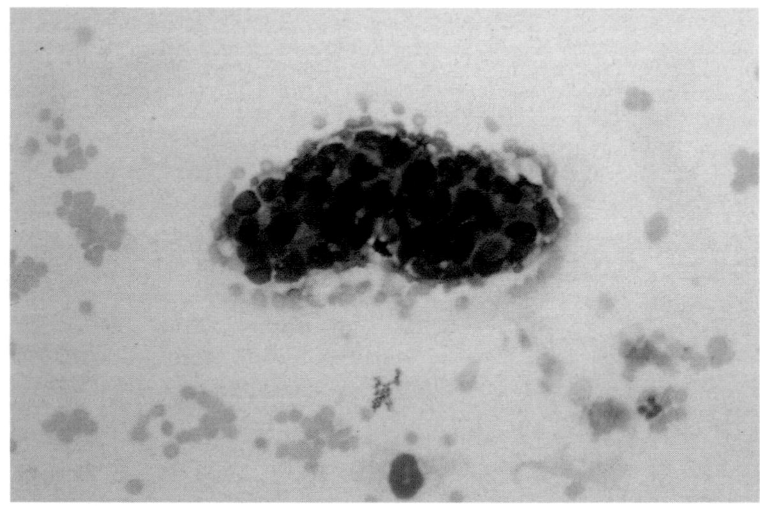

(b)

Fig. 3.4 Peripheral blood film showing visible aggregates of tumour cells. (a) Macroscopic photograph of slide. (b) Photomicrograph showing that the visible masses are clumps of tumour cells. Courtesy of Dr Sue Fairhead.

degenerated and the WBC will have fallen in consequence. If an inexperienced laboratory worker does not recognize the storage artefact and attempts to perform a differential count, a factitious neutropenia and lymphocytosis will be recorded. Inexperienced observers may also misclassify neutrophils with a single rounded nuclear mass as NRBC. Storage also leads to artefactual changes in automated blood counts.

Another unusual artefactal change is produced by accidentally heating samples, e.g., by transporting a blood specimen in a hot car [2]. This causes dramatic fragmentation of red cells (Fig. 3.9) which can be confused with hereditary pyropoikilocytosis.

If a blood film is regarded as suitable for further examination then all cell types and also the background staining should be evaluated systematically. The film appearances should be compared with the FBC and a judgement made as to whether the WBC, Hb, MCV and platelet count are consistent with the film, or whether there is some unusual feature which could invalidate them. If the FBC and the film are inconsistent with each

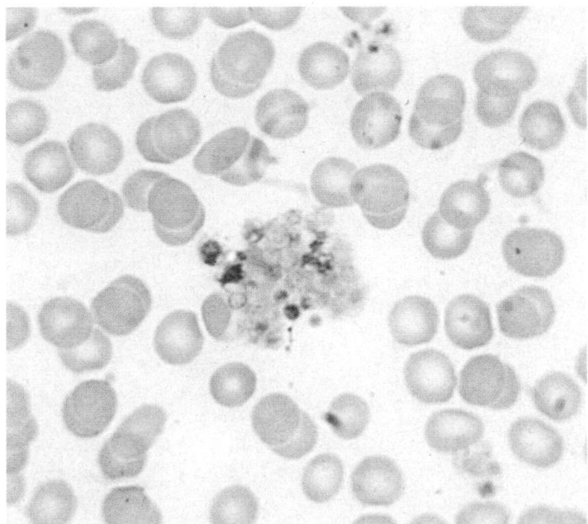

Fig. 3.5 Platelet aggregate in a peripheral blood film. The platelets have agglutinated and some have discharged their granule contents and thus appear grey.

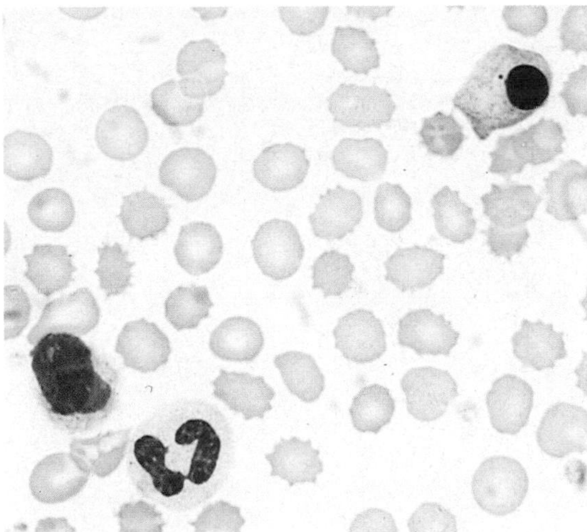

Fig. 3.7 Peripheral blood film showing storage artefact — crenation (echinocytosis), a disintegrated cell and a neutrophil with a rounded pyknotic nucleus.

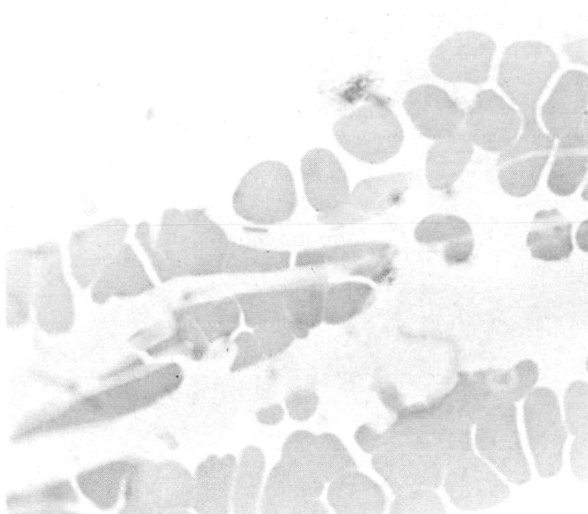

Fig. 3.6 Fibrin strands in a peripheral blood film from a patient with a hypercoagulable state. The fibrin strands are very weakly basophilic and cause deformation of the red cells between which they pass. Fibrin strands can also form when there has been partial clotting of a blood specimen because of difficulty in venepuncture.

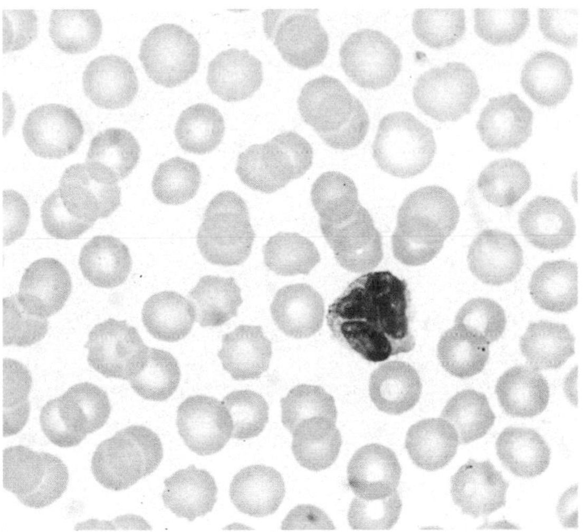

Fig. 3.8 Peripheral blood film showing storage artefact — mild crenation and lobulation of a lymphocyte nucleus.

other then the blood specimen should be inspected and the FBC — and if necessary the film — should be repeated. Such discrepancies may be due to: (i) a poorly mixed or partly clotted specimen; (ii) a specimen which is too small so that the instrument has aspirated an inadequate volume; or (iii) the blood film and FBC being derived from different blood specimens. If such technical errors are eliminated, discrepancy may be due to an abnormality in the specimen such as hyperlipidaemia

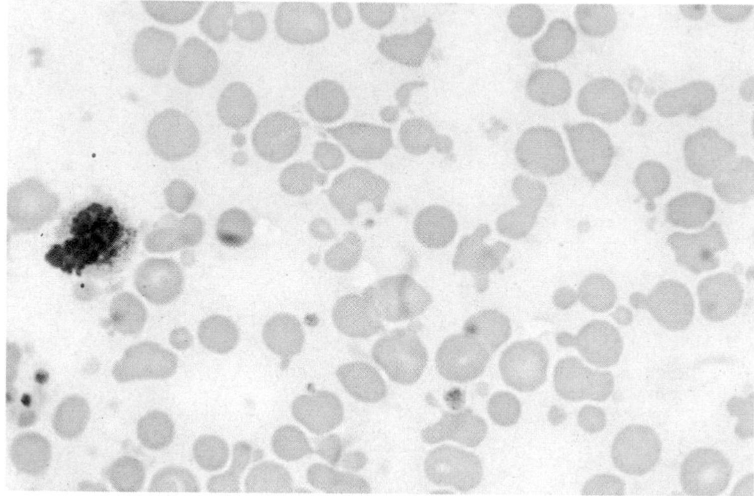

Fig. 3.9 Peripheral blood film from a blood specimen which has been transported in a hot motor vehicle showing red cell budding and fragmentation.

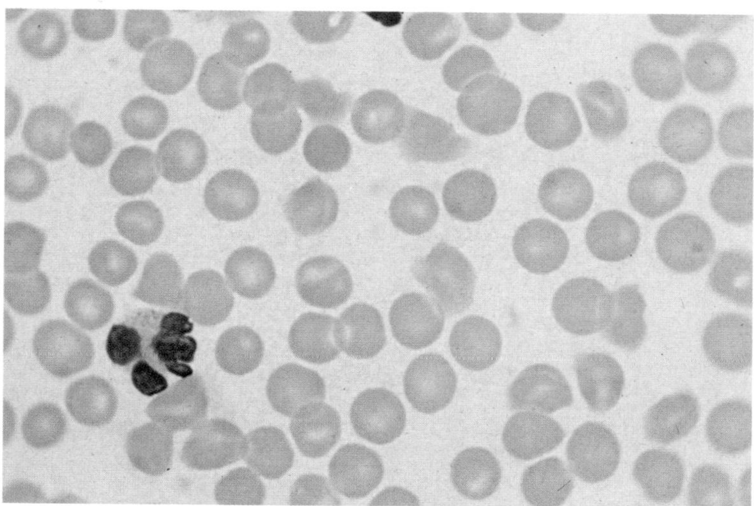

Fig. 3.10 Peripheral blood film from a patient with hyperlipidaemia showing misshapen red cells with fuzzy outlines and blurring of the outline of the lobes of a neutrophil consequent on the high concentration of lipids.

or the presence of a cold agglutinin. Hyperlipidaemia may be suspected when there are blurred red cell outlines (Fig. 3.10) and red cell agglutinates are often present in the film when there is a cold agglutinin (Fig. 3.11). The validation of the blood count by comparison with the blood film and by other means is dealt with in Chapter 4.

Erythrocytes

The majority of normal red cells or erythrocytes are disciform in shape (Fig. 3.12); a minority are bowl shaped. On a stained peripheral blood film they are approximately circular in outline and show only minor variations in shape and moderate variations in size (Fig. 3.13). The average diameter is about 7.5 μm. In the area of a film where cells form a monolayer a paler central area occupies approximately the middle third of the cell.

The normal shape and flexibility of a red cell are dependent on the integrity of the cytoskeleton to which the lipid membrane is bound. An abnormal shape can be caused by a primary defect of the cytoskeleton or membrane or be secondary

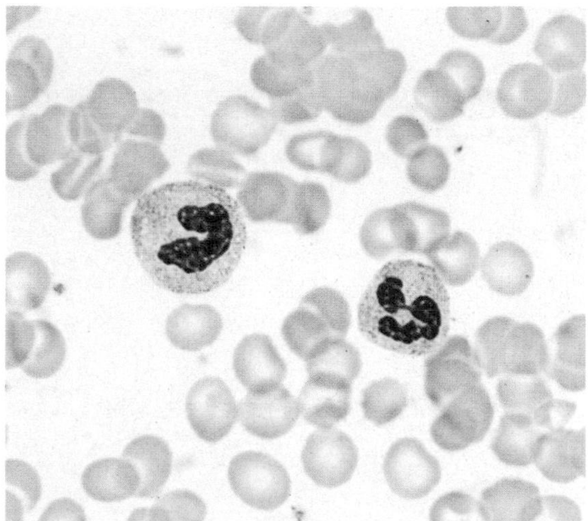

Fig. 3.11 Red cell agglutinates in peripheral blood film of a patient with a high titre cold agglutinin.

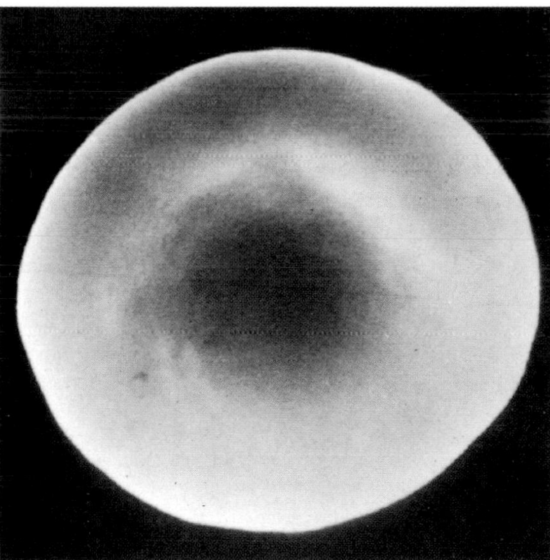

Fig. 3.12 Scanning electron micrograph of a normal red cell (discocyte). Courtesy of Professor A. Polliack, Jerusalem, from Hoffbrand and Pettit [187].

to red cell fragmentation or to polymerization, crystallization or precipitation of haemoglobin. The red cell membrane is a lipid bilayer crossed by several transmembrane proteins, most importantly protein 3 and the glycophorins. The principal

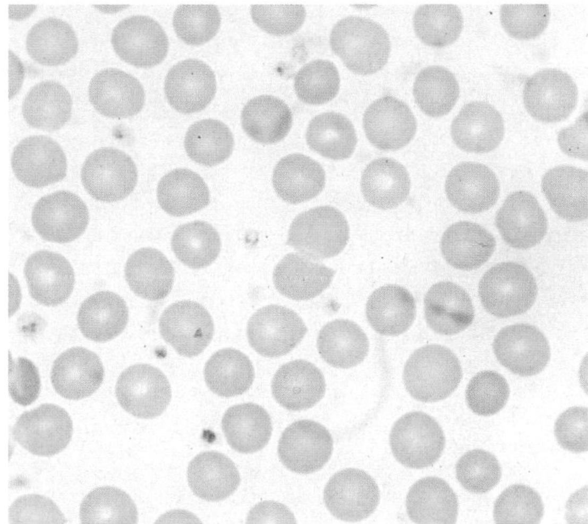

Fig. 3.13 Peripheral blood film of a healthy subject showing normal red cells and platelets. The red cells show little variation in size and shape. Some of the platelets show granules dispersed through the cytoplasm while others have a granulomere and a hyalomere.

protein of the cytoskeleton is spectrin; heterodimers composed of α- and β spectrin chains assemble into spectrin tetramers which are bound to other spectrin tetramers to form a complex network. The cytoskeletal network is bound to the lipid bilayer by interactions of spectrin β-chain with ankyrin and the transmembrane protein, protein 3, and interactions of spectrin α- and β-chains with actin, protein 4.1 and the transmembrane protein, glycophorin C.

Certain terms used to describe red cell morphology require definition. Two terms are used to describe cells of normal morphology: (i) normocytic, which means that the cells are of normal size; and (ii) normochromic, which means that the cells contain the normal amount of haemoglobin and therefore stain normally. Other descriptive terms imply that the morphology is abnormal and they should therefore not be used, when reporting blood films, to describe normal physiological variation. For example, the cells of a neonate should not be reported as 'macrocytic' since it is normal for the cells of a neonate to be larger than those of an adult. Similarly, the red cells of a healthy pregnant woman should not be reported as showing 'anisocytosis' or 'poikilocytosis' since no abnormality is present. Policy differs between laboratories as to whether every normal film is reported as being normocytic and normochromic or whether a comment on the red cell morphology is made only when it is abnormal or when it is particularly significant that it is normal. Either policy is acceptable as long as it is consistently applied and clinical staff are aware of it. If a patient is anaemic but the red cells are normocytic and normochromic it is useful to say so since this narrows the diagnostic possibilities.

Anisocytosis

Anisocytosis is an increase in the variability of erythrocyte size beyond that which is observed in a normal healthy subject. Anisocytosis is a common, non-specific abnormality in haematological disorders. In automated instrument counts an increase in RDW (see p. 30) is indicative of anisocytosis.

Microcytosis

Microcytosis is a decrease in the size of the erythrocytes. Microcytes are detected on a blood film by a reduction of red cell diameter to less than 7–7.2 μm (Fig. 3.14). The nucleus of a small lymphocyte which has a diameter of approximately 8.5 μm is a useful guide to the size of a red cell. Microcytosis may be general or there may be a population of small red cells. If all or most of the red cells are small there is a reduction in the MCV (see p. 15) but a small population of microcytes can be present without the MCV falling below the reference range. Some of the causes of microcytosis are listed in Table 3.1.

The red cells of healthy children are smaller than those of adults, so that cell size must be interpreted in the light of the age of the subject. As a group, black people have smaller red cells than white people; this is likely to be consequent on a high prevalence of α-thalassaemia trait, together with a lower prevalence of β-thalassaemia trait, haemoglobin C trait and other haemoglobinopathies which are associated with microcytosis, rather than to any intrinsic ethnic difference in red cell size.

Table 3.1 Some causes of microcytosis

Inherited
β-thalassaemia trait (heterozygosity) for β-thalassaemia)
β-thalassaemia major (homozygosity or compound heterozygosity for β-thalassaemia)
δβ- and γδβ-thalassaemia heterozygotes and homozygotes
Heterozygotes and homozygotes for haemoglobin Lepore
Homozygotes and some heterozygotes for hereditary persistence of fetal haemoglobin
α-thalassaemia trait (particularly α_1-thalassaemia trait and haemoglobin Constant Spring trait)
Haemoglobin H disease
Sickle cell trait [3,4]
Haemoglobin C heterozygotes [3,4] and homozygotes
Sickle cell/haemoglobin C disease [5]
Haemoglobin E heterozygotes [6] and homozygotes [7]
Haemoglobin $D^{\text{Los Angeles}}$ (D^{Punjab}) trait
Other rare abnormal haemoglobins producing thalassaemia-like conditions (haemoglobin Tak, haemoglobin Indianapolis)
Congenital sideroblastic anaemia
Atransferrinaemia
Ferrochelatase deficiency [8]
Acquired
Iron deficiency
Anaemia of chronic disease
Myelodysplastic syndromes, particularly but not only [9] caused by acquired haemoglobin H disease
Secondary acquired sideroblastic anaemia (e.g., caused by various drugs; some cases of lead poisoning and some cases of copper deficiency [10] or zinc excess with functional copper deficiency [11,12])
Hyperthyroidism [13]
Lead poisoning
Cadmium poisoning [14]
Aluminium poisoning
Antibody to erythroblast transferrin receptor [15]

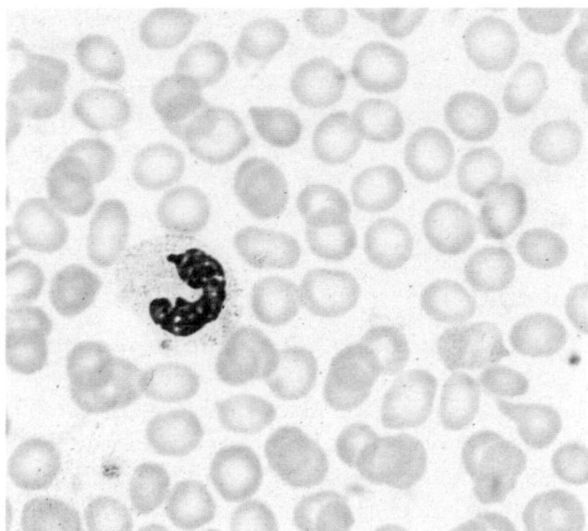

Fig. 3.14 Microcytosis in a patient with β-thalassaemia trait; MCV was 62 fl. The blood film also shows mild hypochromia, anisocytosis and poikilocytosis.

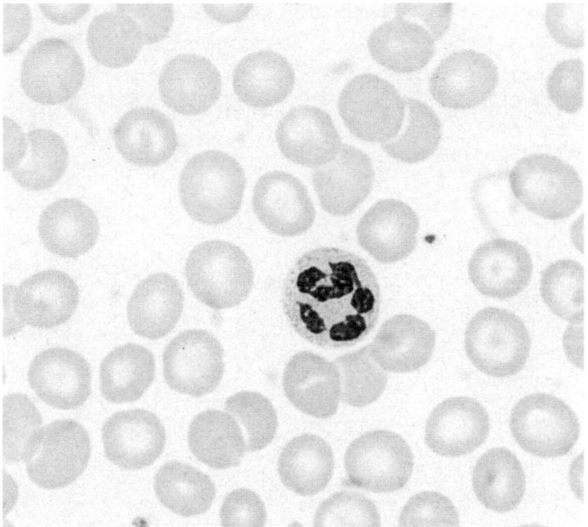

Fig. 3.15 Macrocytosis associated with liver disease; MCV was 105 fl. Several target cells are also present.

Macrocytosis

Macrocytosis is an increase in the size of erythrocytes. It is recognized on a blood film by an increase in cell diameter (Fig. 3.15). It may be a generalized change, in which case MCV (see p. 15) will be raised, or it may affect only a proportion of the red cells. Macrocytes may be round or oval in outline, the diagnostic significance being somewhat different. Some of the causes of macrocytosis are listed in Table 3.2.

The erythrocytes of neonates show a considerable degree of macrocytosis if they are assessed in relation to those of adults (see p. 104). Fetal red cells are also much larger than those of adults. A slight degree of macrocytosis is also seen as a physiological feature of pregnancy [19] and in older adults [17].

Hypochromia

Hypochromia is a reduction of the staining of the red cell (Fig. 3.16); there is an increase in central pallor which occupies more than the normal approximate third of the red cell diameter. Hypochromia may be general or there may be a population of hypochromic cells. Severe hypochromia may be reflected in a reduction in the MCHC but the sensitivity of this measurement to hypochromia depends on the method by which it is measured (see p. 138). Any of the conditions leading to microcytosis may also cause hypochromia, although in some subjects with α- or β-thalassaemia trait the blood film shows microcytosis without appreciable hypochromia and in rare patients with copper-deficiency hypochromia is associated with macrocytosis [16]. Red cells of healthy children are often hypochromic if assessed in relation to the appearance of the red cells of adults. Since the intensity of staining of the red cell is determined by the thickness of the cell as well as by the concentration of haemoglobin, hypochromia can also be noted in cells which are thinner than normal but have a normal volume and haemoglobin concentration; such cells are designated leptocytes.

Hyperchromia

The term hyperchromia is rarely used in describing blood films. It can be applied when cells are more intensely stained than normal but it is more useful to indicate why a cell is hyperchromic. Spherocytes (see p. 52) and irregularly contracted cells (see p. 54) stain more intensely than normal; the MCHC may be increased, indicating

Table 3.2 Some causes of macrocytosis

Associated with reticulocytosis
Haemolytic anaemia
Haemorrhage
Associated with megaloblastic erythropoiesis
Vitamin B_{12} deficiency and inactivation of vitamin B_{12} by chronic exposure to nitric oxide
Folic acid deficiency and antifolate drugs (including methotrexate, pentamidine, pyrimethamine and trimethoprin)
Scurvy
Drugs interfering with DNA synthesis — used as anti-cancer drugs, immunosuppressive agents and in the treatment of AIDS (including doxorubicin, daunorubicin, azathioprine, mercaptopurine, cyclophosphamide, cytosine arabinoside, fluorouracil, hydroxyurea, procarbazine, thioguanine and azidothymidine (zidovudine))
Rare inherited defects of DNA synthesis (including hereditary orotic aciduria, thiamine-responsive anaemia and the Lesch–Nyhan syndrome)
Associated with megaloblastic or macronormoblastic erythropoiesis
Myelodysplastic syndromes including primary acquired sideroblastic anaemia
Di Guglielmo's syndrome
Some acute myeloid leukaemias
Multiple myeloma
Ethanol intake
Liver disease
Phenytoin therapy
Some cases of copper deficiency [16]
Associated with macronormoblastic erythropoiesis
Some congenital dyserythropoietic anaemias, particularly CDA type I
Pure red cell aplasia of infancy (Blackfan–Diamond syndrome)
Aplastic anaemia
Uncertain mechanism
Cigarette smoking [17]
Down's syndrome [18]
Chronic obstructive airways disease

that the hyperchromia is related not only to a change in the shape of the cell but also to a true increase in the haemoglobin concentration. Some macrocytes are thicker than normal and this causes them to be hyperchromic without any increase in haemoglobin concentration; central pallor may be totally lacking.

Anisochromasia

Anisochromasia describes an increased variability in the degree of staining or haemoglobinization of the red cell (Fig. 3.16). In practice, it usually means that there is a spectrum of staining from hypochromic to normochromic. Anisochromasia commonly indicates a changing situation, such as iron deficiency developing or responding to treatment or anaemia of chronic disease developing or regressing. Anisochromasia is reflected in an elevated HDW measured by some automated instruments (see p. 34).

Dimorphism

Dimorphism indicates the presence of two distinct populations of red cells (Fig. 3.17). The term most often applies when there is one population of hypochromic, microcytic cells and another population of normochromic cells which are either normocytic or macrocytic. Since the term is a general one, it is necessary to describe the two populations. They may differ in their size, haemoglobin content or shape and this is relevant to the differential diagnosis. Automated counters may confirm the visual impression of dimorphism, although some instruments may be unable to distinguish between a difference in size and a difference in haemoglobin concentration (see p. 136). Causes of a dimorphic film included iron deficiency anaemia (following administration of iron or blood transfusion), sideroblastic anaemia, the heterozygous state for hereditary sideroblastic anaemia, macrocytic anaemia post-transfusion, double deficiency of iron and either vitamin B_{12} or folic acid, unmasking of iron deficiency following treatment of megaloblastic anaemia and delayed transfusion reactions. A recently described rare cause is mosaicism for β-thalassaemia trait associated with a constitutional chromosomal abnormality [20].

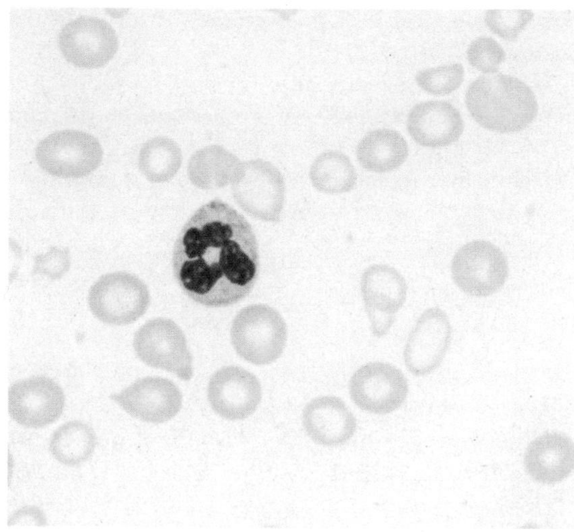

Fig. 3.16 Hypochromic red cells in a patient with iron deficiency anaemia. The film also shows anisochromasia.

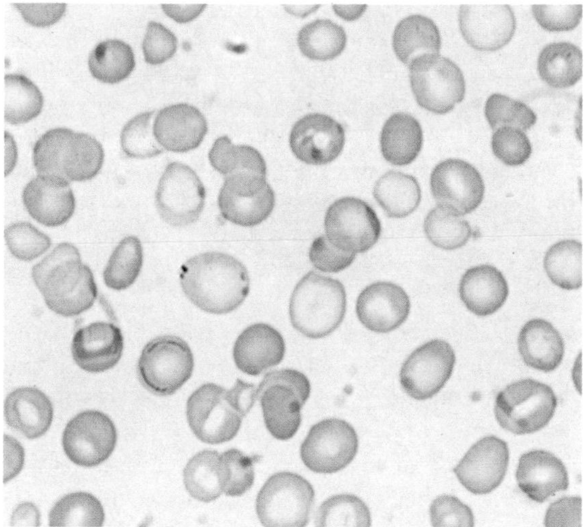

Fig. 3.17 A dimorphic peripheral blood film from a patient with sideroblastic anaemia as a consequence of a myelodysplastic syndrome. One population of cells is normocytic and normochromic while the other is microcytic and hypochromic. One of the poorly haemoglobinized red cells contains some Pappenheimer bodies.

Polychromasia

Polychromasia or polychromatophilia describes red cells which are pinkish-blue as a consequence of uptake both of eosin (by haemoglobin) and of basic dyes (by residual ribosomal RNA). Since reticulocytes (see p. 24) are cells in which ribosomal RNA takes up a vital dye to form a visible reticulum it will be seen that there is likely to be a relationship between reticulocytes and polychromatic cells. Both are immature red cells newly released from the bone marrow. However, the number of polychromatic cells in a normal blood film is usually less than 0.1% [21], considerably less than the normal reticulocyte count of around 1–2%. This is because only the most immature (grade I) reticulocytes are polychromatic. In conditions of transient or persistent haemopoietic stress, when erythropoietin levels are high, immature reticulocytes are released from the bone marrow. They are considerably larger than mature erythrocytes and, as a consequence of a reduced haemoglobin concentration, are less dense. On average their diameter is about 28% greater than that of a mature erythrocyte [21]. On scanning electron microscopy they have an irregular, multilobated surface (Fig. 3.18). They are readily recognized in MGG-stained films by their greater diameter, their lack of central pallor and their polychromatic qualities (Fig. 3.19). They are often referred to as 'polychromatic macrocytes'. Late reticulocytes, which are the only forms present in the blood of haematologically normal subjects, are cup-shaped and only slightly larger than mature erythrocytes. They are therefore difficult to recognize on an MGG-stained film.

The total number of reticulocytes, the proportion of early reticulocytes and the number of polychromatic macrocytes increase as a physiological response to increasing altitude or other hypoxic stimulus and as a normal response to anaemia when there are no factors limiting erythropoiesis. In severely anaemic patients, a lack of polychromasia is significant. It is absent in pure red cell aplasia and in aplastic anaemia and is inconspicuous in the anaemia of chronic disease and often in renal failure when the erythropoietin response is inadequate. The absence of polychromasia in a patient with sickle cell anaemia or other haemolytic anaemia is important since it may indicate complicating parvovirus-induced red cell aplasia.

Polychromatic erythrocytes are increased in myelofibrosis and in metastatic carcinoma of the

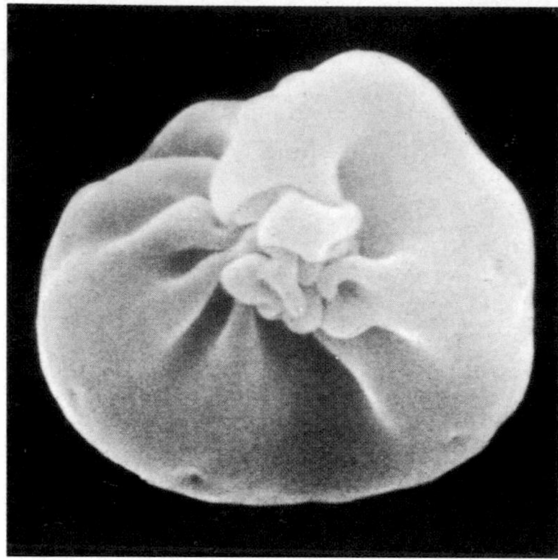

Fig. 3.18 Scanning electron microscopy of a reticulocyte. Courtesy of Professor A. Polliack, from Hoffbrand and Pettit [187].

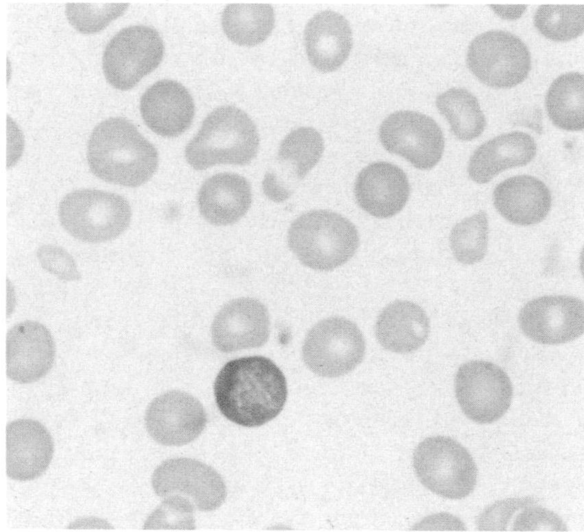

Fig. 3.19 A polychromatic cell which is also larger then a normal cell; it may be designated a polychromatic macrocyte. The film also shows anisocytosis and poikilocytosis.

bone marrow. In these conditions the number of polychromatic cells is greater than would be expected from the degree of anaemia and the polychromatic cells may be abnormal — more deeply basophilic than normal and not always increased in size [21].

When the reticulocyte count is increased, automated counters show an increased MCV and RDW. Technicon H.1 series counters show, in addition, an increased HDW and reticulocytes are seen as hypochromic macrocytes on the red cell cytogram (see Fig. 8.49).

Poikilocytosis

A cell of abnormal shape is a poikilocyte. Poikilocytosis is therefore a state in which there is an increased proportion of cells of abnormal shape. High altitude produces some degree of poikilocytosis in haematologically normal subjects [22]. Poikilocytosis is also a common, often non-specific abnormality in many haematological disorders. It may result from the production of abnormal cells by the bone marrow or from damage to normal cells after release into the blood stream. If poikilocytosis is very marked, diagnostic possibilities include myelofibrosis, congenital and acquired dyserythropoietic anaemias and hereditary pyropoikilocytosis. The presence of poikilocytes of certain specific shapes, e.g., spherocytes or elliptocytes, may have a particular significance (see below).

Spherocytosis

Spherocytes are cells which, rather than being disciform, are spherical or near spherical in shape (Fig. 3.20). They are cells which have lost membrane without equivalent loss of cytosol, as a consequence of an inherited or acquired abnormality of the red cell cytoskeleton and membrane. In a stained blood film, spherocytes lack the normal central pallor. The diameter of a sphere is less than that of a disc-shaped object of the same volume, and thus a spherocyte may appear smaller than a discocyte. It is preferable, however, to restrict the term 'microspherocyte' to cells of reduced volume rather than merely reduced diameter. In examining a blood film for the presence of spherocytes it is important to examine that part of the film where the cells are just touching, since normal cells may lack central pallor near the tail of the film. Spherocytes do not

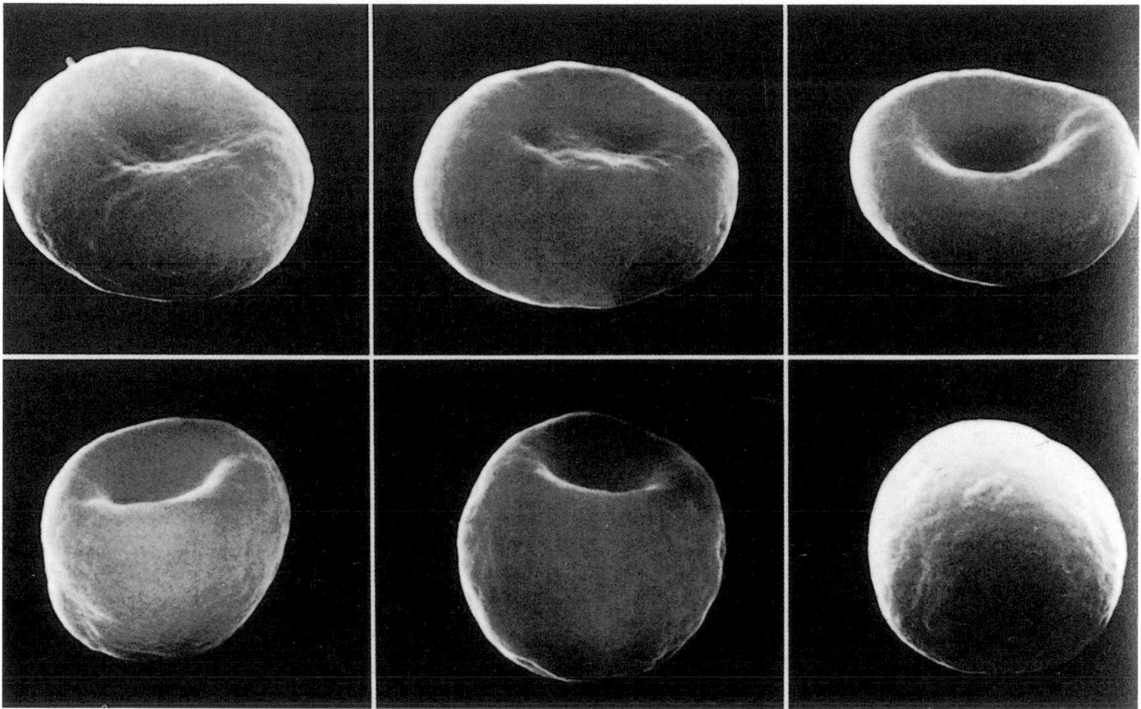

Fig. 3.20 Scanning electron micrography of spherocytes and forms intermediate between discocytes and spherocytes in a patient with hereditary spherocytosis. From Bessis [23].

stack well into rouleaux.

The distinction between spherocytes and irregularly contracted cells (see below) is important since the diagnostic significance is different.

Some of the causes of spherocytosis are shown in Table 3.3. There are a variety of underlying mechanisms responsible. In hereditary spherocytosis there is an abnormality of the cytoskeleton with a secondary destabilization and loss of membrane. In acquired conditions spherocytosis can result from direct damage to the red cell membrane, e.g., by heat (Fig. 3.21), clostridial toxins (Fig. 3.22) or snake venoms. Loss of membrane can follow antibody coating of the cell by alloantibodies (Fig. 3.23), autoantibodies or drug-induced antibodies; the macrophages of the reticuloendothelial system recognize immunoglobulin or complement on the surface of the cell and remove pieces of membrane. When red cells fragment those fragments with a relative lack of membrane form microspherocytes; this is the

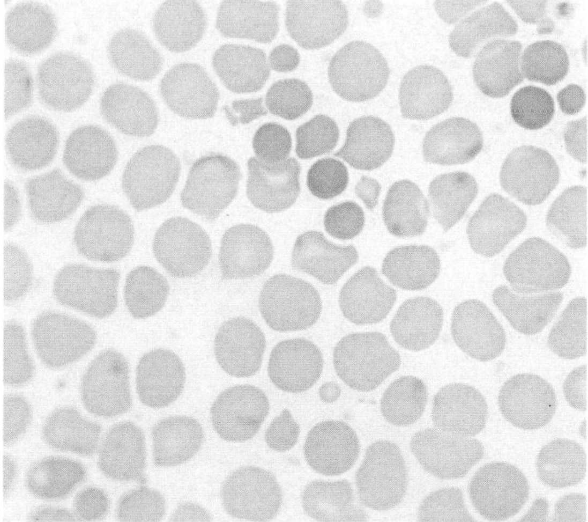

Fig. 3.21 Peripheral blood film of a patient with severe burns showing spherocytes, microspherocytes and red cells which appear to be budding off very small spherocytic fragments.

Table 3.3 Some causes of spherocytosis

Conditions which may be associated with numerous spherocytes
Hereditary spherocytosis
Warm autoimmune haemolytic anaemia
Delayed transfusion reactions
ABO haemolytic disease of the newborn
Clostridium welchii sepsis
Drug-induced immune haemolytic anaemia (innocent bystander mechanism)
Zieve's syndrome*
Low erythrocyte ATP caused by phosphate deficiency [24,25]
Snake-bite induced haemolysis
Bartonellosis (Oraya fever)
Fresh-water drowning or intravenous infusion of water
Conditions which may be associated with smaller numbers of spherocytes
As an isolated feature
Immediate transfusion reaction
Acute cold autoimmune haemolytic anaemia
Chronic cold haemagglutinin disease
Rhesus haemolytic disease of the newborn
Penicillin-induced haemolytic anaemia
Acute attacks of paroxysmal cold haemoglobinuria
Infusion of large amounts of intravenous lipid [26]
In association with other poikilocytes
Normal neonate
Hyposplenism
Sickle cell anaemia
Microangiopathic haemolytic anaemia
Mechanical haemolytic anaemia
Homozygous hereditary elliptocytosis and hereditary elliptocytosis with transient severe manifestations in infancy [27]
Hereditary pyropoikilocytosis
Rh null phenotype

* Irregularly contracted cells may be more characteristic

mechanism of formation of spherocytes in microangiopathic haemolytic anaemia, mechanical haemolytic anaemia and hereditary pyropoikilocytosis. Erythrocytes stored for transfusion become spheroechinocytes as the blood ages (see below). Rarely, marked spherocytosis has been described in hypophosphataemia, e.g., in liver disease [24] or in acute diabetic ketoacidosis [25]; the mechanism is likely to be adenosine triphosphate (ATP) depletion. In Heinz body haemolytic anaemias, although most abnormal cells are irregularly contracted cells (see below), there are usually also some spherocytes.

Irregularly contracted cells

Irregularly contracted cells lack central pallor and appear smaller and denser than normal erythrocytes without being as regular in shape as spherocytes (Fig. 3.24). Irregularly contracted cells are formed when there is oxidant damage to erythrocytes, or damage to red cell membranes by precipitation of unstable haemoglobin or free α- or β-chains. Blood films showing irregularly contracted cells often also show some spherocytes; these are formed when a red cell inclusion such as a Heinz body has been removed by the pitting action of splenic macrophages with associated loss of red cell membrane. Some causes of irregularly contracted cells are shown in Table 3.4.

Table 3.4 Some conditions which are associated with irregularly contracted cells

Conditions which may be associated with numerous irregularly contracted cells
Haemoglobin C disease
Haemoglobin C/β-thalassaemia
Sickle cell/haemoglobin C disease
Unstable haemoglobins
Acute haemolysis in G6PD deficiency or other abnormalities of the pentose shunt
Severe oxidant stress (drugs or chemicals) in patients without abnormalities of the pentose shunt
Zieve's syndrome
Conditions which may be associated with smaller numbers of irregularly contracted cells
Minor haemolytic episodes in G6PD deficiency
Moderate oxidant stress in patients without abnormalities of the pentose shunt
Haemoglobin C trait
Unstable haemoglobins
β-thalassaemia trait
Haemoglobin H disease
Haemoglobin E disease or trait
Hereditary xerocytosis (dehydrated variant of hereditary stomatocytosis)

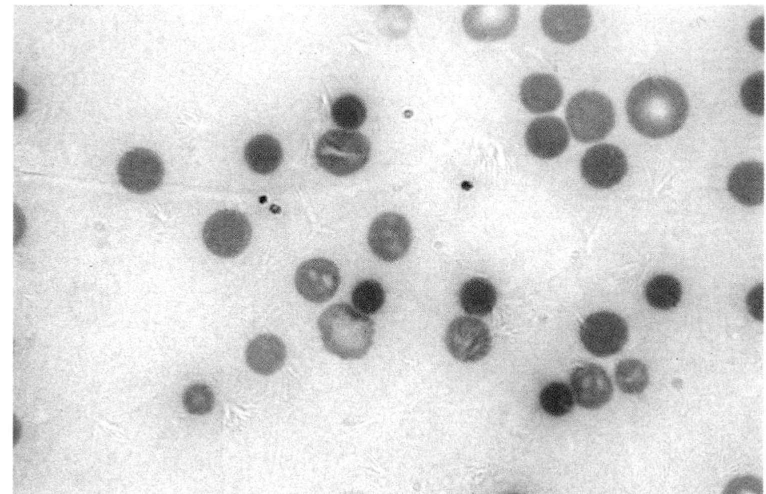

Fig. 3.22 Peripheral blood film of a patient with clostridial septicaemia showing many spherocytes. Courtesy of Professor H. Smith, Brisbane.

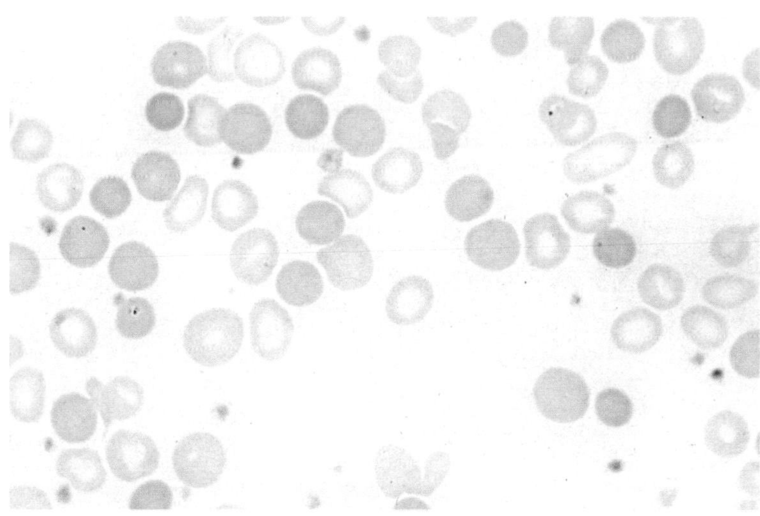

Fig. 3.23 Spherocytes in the peripheral blood film of an iron deficient patient who suffered a delayed transfusion reaction due to an anti-D antibody; the film is dimorphic showing a mixture of the recipient's hypochromic microcytic cells and the donor cells which have become spherocytic.

Elliptocytosis and ovalocytosis

Elliptocytosis indicates the presence of increased numbers of elliptocytes and ovalocytosis the presence of increased numbers of ovalocytes. These terms have not been used in any consistent manner but it has been suggested that a cell with a long axis more than twice its short axis should be designated an elliptocyte while cells with the long axis less than twice its short axis are designated ovalocytes [28]. When elliptocytes or ovalocytes are numerous (Fig. 3.25) and are the dominant abnormality it is likely that the patient has an inherited abnormality affecting the red cell cytoskeleton such as hereditary elliptocytosis (see p. 230). Smaller numbers of elliptocytes or ovalocytes may be seen in iron deficiency, in some patients with thalassaemia, megaloblastic anaemia, myelofibrosis and occasionally inherited red cell enzyme abnormalities. Macrocytic ovalocytes or oval macrocytes are characteristic of megaloblastic anaemia and South-East Asian

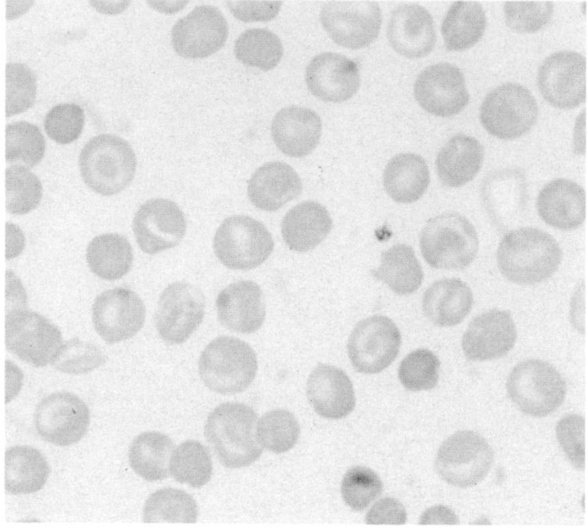

Fig. 3.24 Peripheral blood film of a patient with haemoglobin C disease showing irregularly contracted cells and several target cells.

ovalocytosis (see p. 233) and are also seen in dyserythropoiesis, e.g., in idiopathic myelofibrosis. Elliptocytes are biconcave and thus are capable of forming rouleaux.

Tear drop cells (dacrocytes)

Tear drop or pear-shaped cells (dacrocytes) (Fig. 3.26) occur when there is bone marrow fibrosis or severe dyserythropoiesis and also in some haemolytic anaemias. They are particularly characteristic of megaloblastic anaemia, thalassaemia major and myelofibrosis, either idiopathic myelofibrosis or myelofibrosis secondary to metastatic carcinoma or other bone marrow infiltration. In both thalassaemia major and idiopathic myelofibrosis the proportion of tear drop cells decreases following splenectomy suggesting either that they are the product of extramedullary haemopoiesis or that they are formed when the spleen causes further damage to abnormal red cells. Tear drop cells which are present in occasional cases of autoimmune haemolytic anaemia [29] and in Heinz body haemolytic anaemias are likely to be consequent on the action of splenic macrophages on abnormal erythrocytes.

Spiculated cells

The terminology applied to spiculated cells is confused. In particular, the term 'burr cell' has been used by different authors to describe different cells and therefore is better abandoned. The terminology of Bessis [23] is recommended since it is based on careful study of abnormal cells by scanning electron microscopy and is clear and relatively easy to apply. Bessis has divided spiculated cells into echinocytes, acanthocytes, keratocytes and schistocytes.

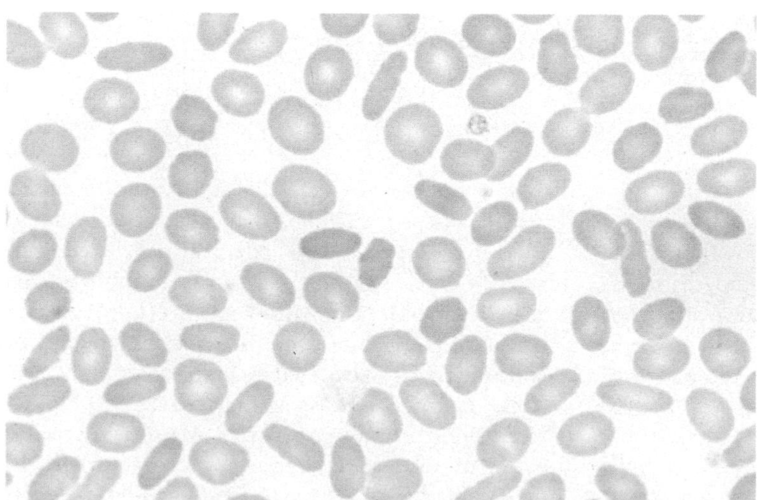

Fig. 3.25 Peripheral blood film of a patient with hereditary elliptocytosis showing elliptocytes and ovalocytes.

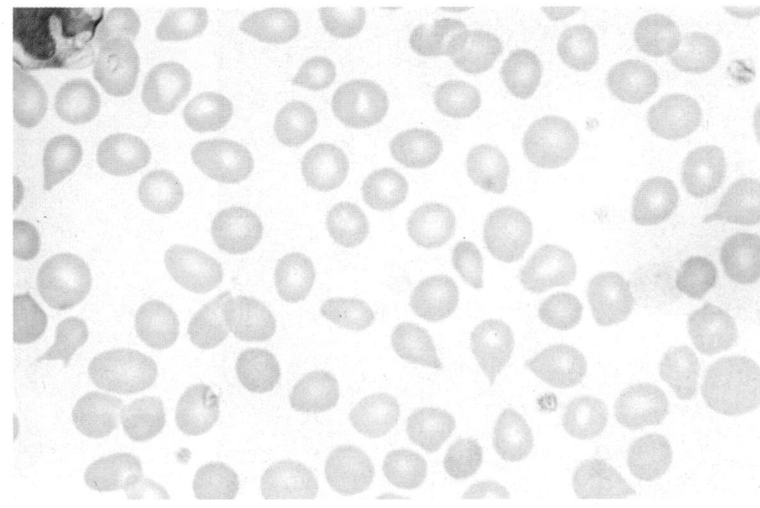

Fig. 3.26 Peripheral blood film of a patient with idiopathic myelofibrosis showing tear drop poikilocytes (dacrocytes).

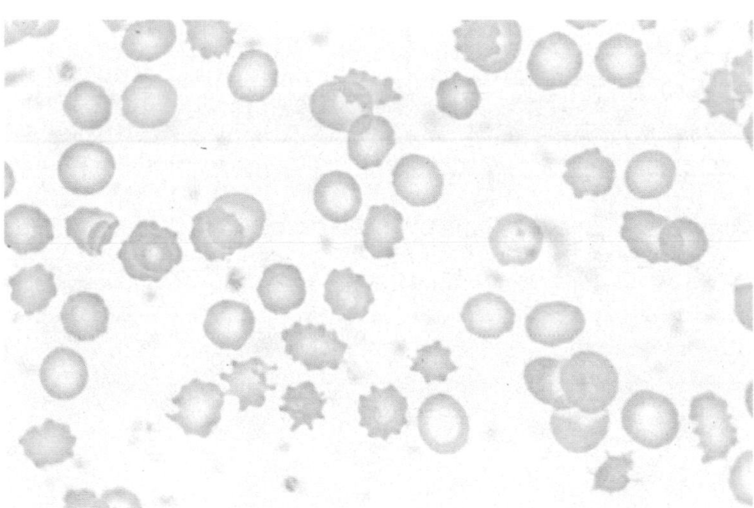

Fig. 3.27 Echinocytes in the peripheral blood film of a patient with chronic renal failure.

Echinocytes

Echinocytes are erythrocytes which have lost their disc shape and are covered with 10–30 short blunt spicules of fairly regular form (Figs 3.27 & 3.28). The main causes of echinocytosis are shown in Table 3.5. Echinocytes may be produced *in vitro* by exposure to fatty acids and certain drugs or simply by incubation. The end stage of a discocyte–echinocyte transformation is a spheroechinocyte. A spheroechinocyte is also formed when a spherocyte undergoes an echinocytic change and, similarly, other abnormally shaped cells, e.g., acanthocytes, can undergo an echinocytic change.

When donor blood is stored for transfusion cells become spheroechinocytes (Fig. 3.29) as lysolecithin is formed and as ATP concentration decreases; membrane lipid, both cholesterol and phospholipid, is then lost when microvesicles containing small amounts of haemoglobin are shed from the tips of the spicules. When blood is transfused and there is resynthesis of ATP many of the cells revert to cup-shaped stomatocytes

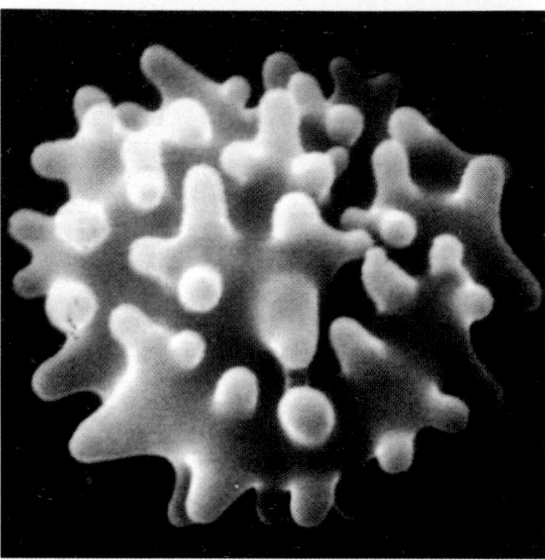

Fig. 3.28 Scanning electron micrograph of an echinocyte. Courtesy of Professor A. Polliak, from Hoffbrand and Pettit [187].

rather than to discocytes; those which have lost a lot of membrane remain spherocytic.

In vivo, echinocyte formation may be related to increased plasma fatty acids such as occurs during heparin therapy, ATP depletion and lysolecithin formation. During echinocyte formation there is entry of calcium into cells with polymerization

Table 3.5 Some causes of echinocytosis

Storage artefact
Liver disease, particularly with coexisting renal failure
Nutritional phosphate deficiency
Pyruvate kinase deficiency
Phosphoglycerate kinase deficiency
Aldolase deficiency [30]
Decompression phase of diving [31]
Haemolytic uraemic syndrome
Following burns
Following cardiopulmonary bypass
Post-transfusion (spheroechinocytes)

of spectrin. Echinocytosis is reversible *in vitro* and *in vivo*, e.g., by suspending cells in fresh plasma or by allowing ATP resynthesis.

In laboratories which make films from EDTA-anticoagulated blood rather than fresh blood by far the most common cause of echinocytosis is delay in making the blood film (see Fig. 3.7). This storage artefact, often referred to as 'crenation', is likely to be caused by a fall in ATP or by lysolecithin formation. Echinocytosis, other than as an artefactual change, is quite uncommon. The incidence is higher in neonates [32]. It can occur in liver disease [32] but acanthocytosis (see below) is commoner. It can occur in the early stages of the haemolytic uraemic syndrome but subsequently echinocytosis resolves leaving only the

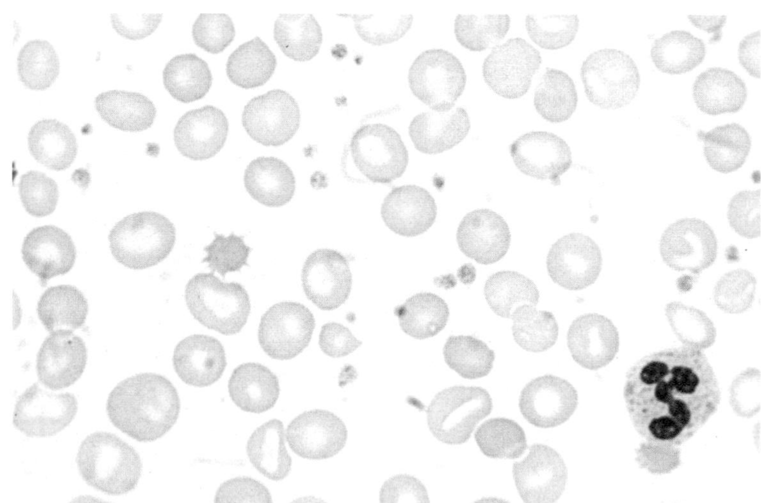

Fig. 3.29 Spheroechinocyte in a peripheral blood film made from blood taken shortly after a blood transfusion. The spheroechinocyte is a transfused cell.

features of microangiopathic haemolytic anaemia. Echinocytosis is probably most common in critically ill patients with multiorgan failure including both hepatic and renal failure.

Echinocytosis which has been observed following the development of hypophosphataemia in patients on parenteral feeding is attributable to a fall in ATP concentration and this may also be the mechanism operating when echinocytes develop in hereditary pyruvate kinase deficiency and in phosphoglycerate kinase deficiency. Echinocytosis occurring in hypothermic, heparinized patients on cardiopulmonary bypass has been attributed to a rise of free fatty acid concentration. The echinocytosis which has been noted as a delayed response in severely burned patients may be consequent on lipid abnormalities.

Acanthocytes

Acanthocytes are cells of approximately spherical shape bearing between two and 20 spicules which are of unequal length and distributed irregularly over the red cell surface (Figs 3.30–3.33). Some of the spicules have club-shaped rather than pointed ends. Causes of acanthocytosis are shown in Table 3.6. Acanthocyte formation probably results from a preferential expansion of the outer leaflet of the lipid bilayer which comprises the red cell membrane [35]. Acanthocytes cannot form rouleaux. Unlike echinocytosis, acanthocytosis is not reversible on suspending cells in fresh plasma. In acanthocytosis associated with abetalipoproteinaemia or liver disease the cholesterol/phospholipid ratio in the red cells is increased. This is in contrast to the target cells associated with liver disease in which the cholesterol and phospholipid concentrations rise in parallel.

Acanthocytosis as an inherited phenomenon is associated with a number of different syndromes and its presence may help in their diagnosis. It was first described in association with retinitis pigmentosa, degenerative neurological disease, fat malabsorption and abetalipoproteinaemia [36]. Subsequently, it was recognized in association with several rare degenerative neurological diseases with normal β-lipoproteins. In one syndrome found in white people and usually having an autosomal recessive inheritance there is choreoathetosis and acanthocytosis [37]. In another syndrome found in Japanese and probably also autosomal recessive there is tongue-biting, peripheral nerve degeneration and an elevated creatine phosphokinase [38]. Several inherited abnormalities of red cell antigens are characterized by acanthocytosis. In the In(Lu) phenotype in which there is suppression of Lu and several other blood group antigen systems there are no associated abnormalities [39] whereas some cases of the McLeod phenotype in which Kell antigens are

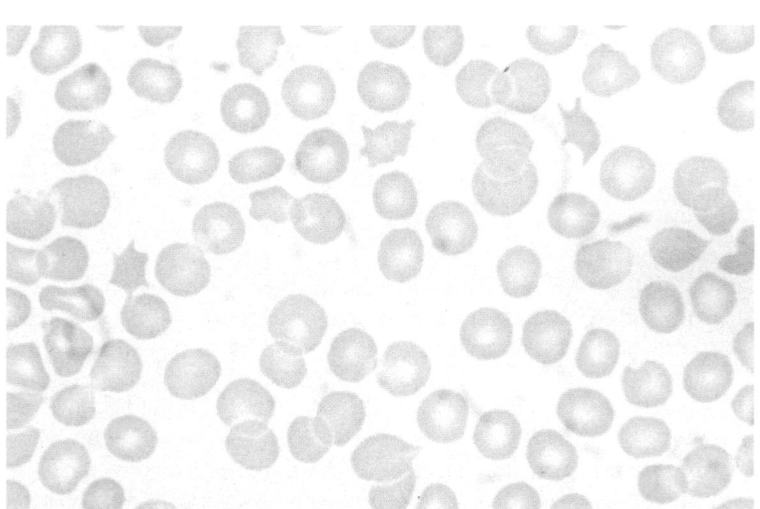

Fig. 3.30 Acanthocytes in a patient with anorexia nervosa.

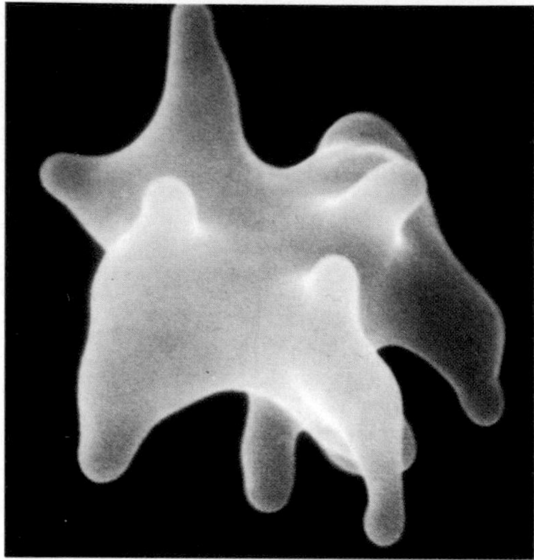

Fig. 3.31 Scanning electron micrograph of an acanthocyte. Courtesy of Professor A. Polliack, from Hoffbrand and Pettit [187].

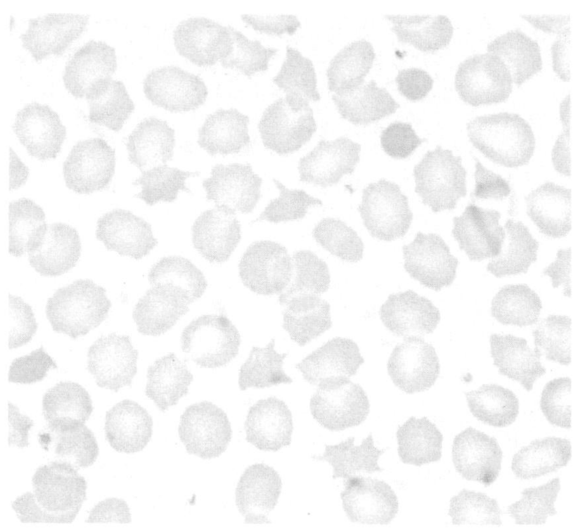

Fig. 3.32 Unusually numerous acanthocytes in the peripheral blood film of a haematologically normal subject who has had a splenectomy.

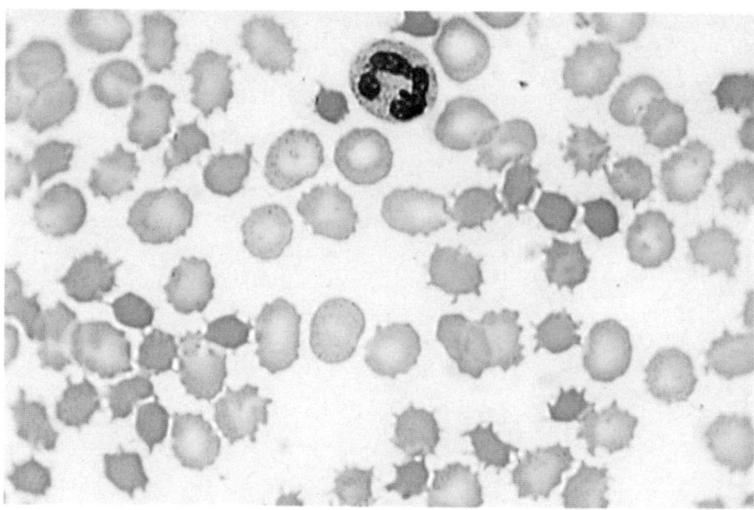

Fig. 3.33 Numerous acanthocytes in a patient with abetalipoproteinaemia.

lacking also have chronic granulomatous disease. Acanthocytosis has also been associated with a deficiency of band 3 protein [33].

Keratocytes

Keratocytes (or horned cells) (Fig. 3.34) are cells with pairs of spicules, usually two but sometimes four or six, which have been formed by the fusion of opposing membranes to form a pseudovacuole with subsequent rupture of the membrane at the cell surface. They are formed when there is mechanical damage to red cells, e.g., by fibrin strands or a malfunctioning cardiac prosthesis. They have been observed in microangiopathic haemolytic anaemia, in disseminated intravascular

Table 3.6 Some causes of acanthocytosis

Conditions associated with large numbers of acanthocytes
Inherited
Hereditary abetalipoproteinaemia
Hereditary hypobetalipoproteinaemia (some cases)
Associated with degenerative neurological disease but with normal lipoproteins
McLeod red cell phenotype
In (Lu) red cell phenotype
Associated with abnormal band 3 of red cell membrane [33]
Acquired
Hypobetalipoproteinaemia caused by malnutrition or lipid deprivation
'Spur cell' haemolytic anaemia associated with liver disease (usually associated with alcoholic cirrhosis but also occasionally with severe viral hepatitis, neonatal hepatitis, cardiac cirrhosis, haemochromatosis or Wilson's disease)
Infantile pyknocytosis
Vitamin E deficiency in premature neonates
Myelodysplastic syndrome [34]
Conditions associated with small numbers of acanthocytes
Inherited
Heterozygotes for the McLeod phenotype
Pyruvate kinase deficiency
Woronet's trait
Acquired
Post-splenectomy and hyposplenism
Anorexia nervosa and starvation
Myxoedema and panhypopituitarism

coagulation and in renal disease, e.g., glomerulonephritis, uraemia and post-transplantation.

Schistocytes

Schistocytes are fragments of red cells formed either by fragmentation of abnormal cells, e.g., in hereditary pyropoikilocytosis, or following mechanical, toxin or heat-induced damage of previously normal cells (Fig. 3.35). When consequent on mechanical damage, schistocytes often coexist with keratocytes. Many schistocytes are spiculated. Others have been left with too little membrane for their cytoplasmic volume and therefore have formed microspherocytes (spheroschistocytes). The commonest causes of schistocyte formation are microangiopathic and mechanical haemolytic anaemias.

Table 3.7 Some causes of target cell formation

Conditions which are often associated with large numbers of target cells
Obstructive jaundice
Hereditary LCAT deficiency
Haemoglobin C disease
Sickle cell anaemia
Compound heterozygosity for haemoglobin S and haemoglobin C
Haemoglobin D disease
Haemoglobin O-Arab homozygotes
Conditions which may be associated with moderate or small numbers of target cells
Parenchymal liver disease
Splenectomy and other hyposplenic states
Haemoglobin C trait
Haemoglobin S trait
Haemoglobin E trait and disease
Haemoglobin Lepore trait
β-thalassaemia trait and major
Haemoglobin H disease
Iron deficiency
Sideroblastic anaemia
Hereditary xerocytosis (dehydrated variant of hereditary stomatocytosis) [40]
Analphalipoproteinaemia [41] and hypoalphalipoproteinaemia [42]

Target cells

Target cells have an area of increased staining which appears in the middle of the area of central pallor (Figs 3.36 & 3.37). Target cells are formed as a consequence of there being redundant membrane in relation to the volume of the cytoplasm. They may also be thinner than normal cells. *In vivo* they are bell-shaped and this can be demonstrated on scanning electron microscopy. They flatten on spreading to form the characteristic cell seen on light microscopy. Target cells may be microcytic, normocytic or macrocytic, depending on the underlying abnormality and the mechanism of their formation. Some of the cause of target cell formation are shown in Table 3.7.

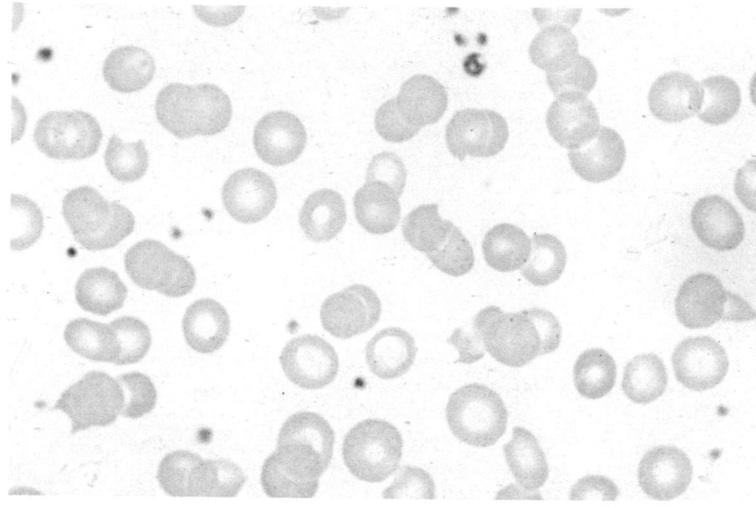

Fig. 3.34 Keratocytes in the peripheral blood film of a patient with microangiopathic haemolytic anaemia.

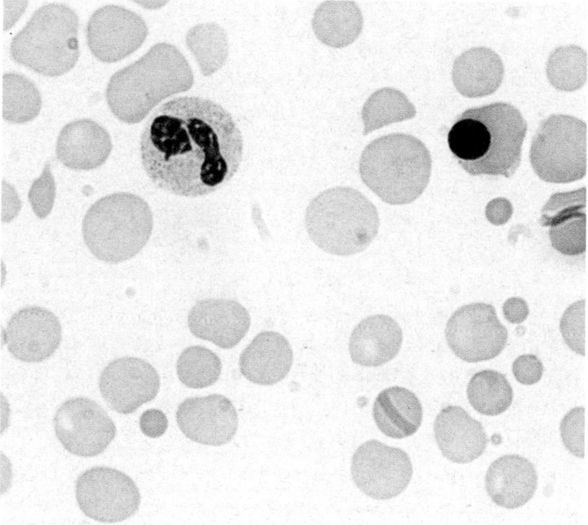

Fig. 3.35 Fragments including microspherocytes in the peripheral blood film of a patient with the haemolytic uraemic syndrome. The film also shows polychromasia and an NRBC.

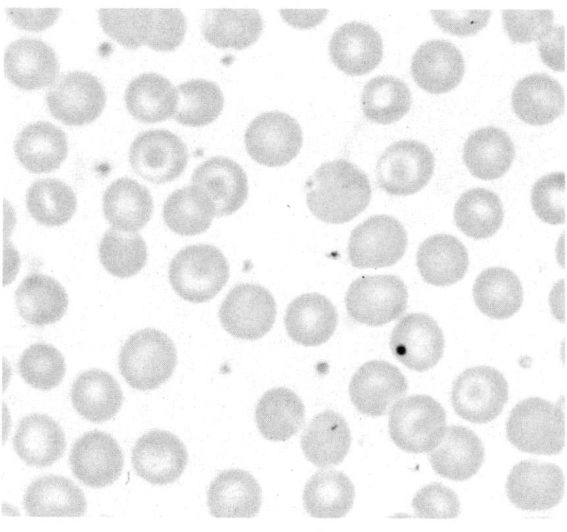

Fig. 3.36 Peripheral blood film of a haematologically normal patient who has had a splenectomy, showing target cells and a Howell–Jolly body.

Target cells may be formed because of an excess of red cell membrane as when there is excess membrane lipid. This is the mechanism of formation in obstructive jaundice, severe parenchymal liver disease and hereditary deficiency of lecithin–cholesterol acyl transferase (LCAT). The ratio of membrane cholesterol to cholesterol ester is increased. Red cells lack enzymes for the synthesis of cholesterol and phospholipid and for the esterification of cholesterol so that changes in the membrane lipids are passive, reflecting changes in plasma lipids. When LCAT activity is reduced the ratio of cholesterol to cholesterol ester in the red cell membrane increases. There may also be an increase in total membrane cholesterol, with a proportionate increase in lecithin and with a

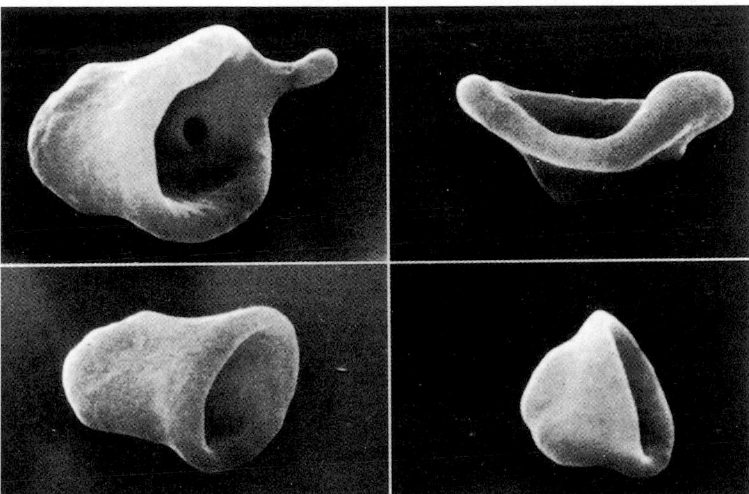

Fig. 3.37 Scanning electron micrographs of target cells. From Bessis [23].

decrease in ethanolamine. LCAT is synthesized in hepatocytes and so it may be reduced in liver disease. In obstructive jaundice very high levels of bile salts inhibit LCAT. This does not, however, appear to be the sole mechanism of target cell formation in obstructive jaundice since patients may have target cells without their plasma being able to inhibit the LCAT activity of normal plasma. When target cells are formed as a consequence of plasma lipid abnormalities they revert to a normal shape on being transfused into a subject with normal plasma lipids. If changes in membrane lipids which would normally cause target cell formation occur in patients with spherocytosis the cells become more disciform; this phenomenon may be observed when a patient with hereditary spherocytosis develops obstructive jaundice.

An alternative mechanism of target cell formation is a reduction of cytoplasmic content without a proportionate reduction in the quantity of membrane. This is the mechanism of target cell formation in a group of conditions such as iron deficiency, thalassaemias and haemoglobinopathies in which target cells are associated with hypochromia or microcytosis. Target cells are much less numerous in iron deficiency than in thalassaemias. The reason for this is not clear.

Stomatocytosis

Stomatocytes are cells which, on a stained blood film, have a central linear slit or stoma (Fig. 3.38). Occasionally such cells are seen in the blood films of healthy subjects. On scanning electron microscopy or in wet preparations with the cells suspended in plasma they are cup- or bowl-shaped (Fig. 3.39). Stomatocytes can be formed *in vitro*, e.g., in response to low pH or exposure to cationic lipid-soluble drugs such as chlorpromazine; the change in shape is reversible. The end stage of a discocyte–stomatocyte transformation is a spherostomatocyte. Stomatocytosis results from a variety of membrane abnormalities but probably essentially from expansion of the inner leaflet of the lipid bilayer which comprises the red cell membrane [35]. In liver disease their formation has been attributed to an increase of lysolecithin in the inner layer of the red cell membrane. In hereditary spherocytosis and autoimmune haemolytic anaemia progressive loss of membrane leads to formation of stomatocytes, spherostomatocytes and spherocytes.

Stomatocytes have been associated with a great variety of clinical conditions [43,44] but an aetiological connection has not always been established. The commonest cause of stomatocytosis is alcohol excess and alcoholic liver disease; in these cases there is often associated macrocytosis

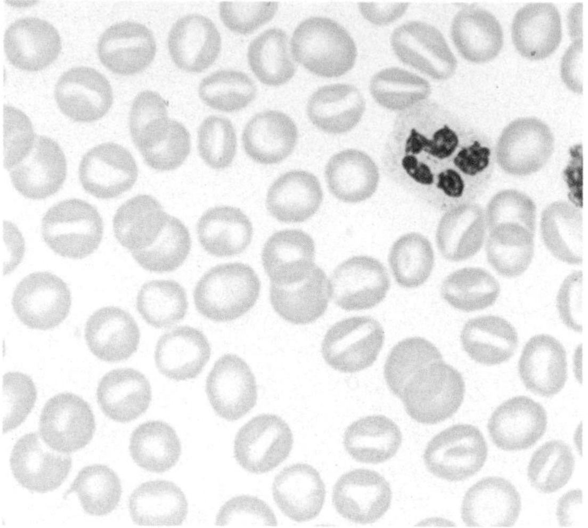

Fig. 3.38 Peripheral blood film showing stomatocytes.

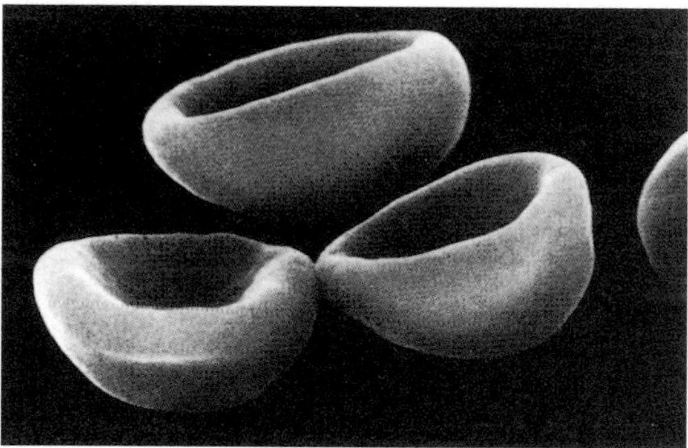

Fig. 3.39 Scanning electron micrograph of stomatocytes. From Bessis [23].

and in those with very advanced liver disease there may also be triconcave cells [45]. The combination of stomatocytosis and macrocytosis also seen in patients receiving hydroxyurea and occasionally in the myelodysplastic syndromes. It is possible that chlorpromazine exposure can cause stomatocytosis *in vivo* as well as *in vitro* since an association has been observed [44]. Certain inherited erythrocyte membrane abnormalities are characterized by stomatocytes either alone — in hereditary stomatocytosis and hereditary xerocytosis — or in association with other abnormalities in Rh_{null} or Rh_{MOD} syndromes [46] and South-East Asian ovalocytosis. Analphalipoproteinaemia [41] and hypoalphalipoproteinaemia [42] are associated with stomatocytosis. LCAT deficiency shows both target cells and stomatocytes. An increased incidence of stomatocytosis has been reported in healthy Mediterranean (Greek and Italian) subjects in Australia [47].

Inclusions in erythrocytes

Howell–Jolly bodies

Howell–Jolly bodies (see Fig. 3.36) are medium sized, round, cytoplasmic red cell inclusions which have the same staining characteristics as the nucleus and can be demonstrated to be composed of DNA. A Howell–Jolly body is a fragment of nuclear material. It can arise by karyorrhexis (the breaking up of a nucleus) or by incomplete nuclear expulsion, or can represent chromosomes which have separated from the mitotic spindle during abnormal mitosis. Some Howell–Jolly bodies are found in erythrocytes within the bone marrow in haematologically normal subjects but, as they are removed by the spleen, they are not seen in the peripheral blood. They appear in the blood following splenectomy and are also present in other hyposplenic states. They are a normal finding in neonates (in whom the spleen is functionally immature). The rate of formation of Howell–Jolly bodies is increased in megaloblastic anaemias and, if the patient is also hyposplenic, large numbers of Howell–Jolly bodies will be seen in the peripheral blood.

Basophilic stippling

Basophilic stippling (Fig. 3.40) or punctate basophilia describes the presence in erythrocytes of considerable numbers of small basophilic inclusions which are dispersed through the erythrocyte cytoplasm and can be demonstrated to be RNA. They are composed of aggregates of ribosomes; degenerating mitochondria and siderosomes may be included in the aggregates but most such inclusions are negative with Perls' acid ferrocyanide stain for iron. Very occasional cells with basophilic stippling can be seen in normal subjects. Increased numbers are seen in

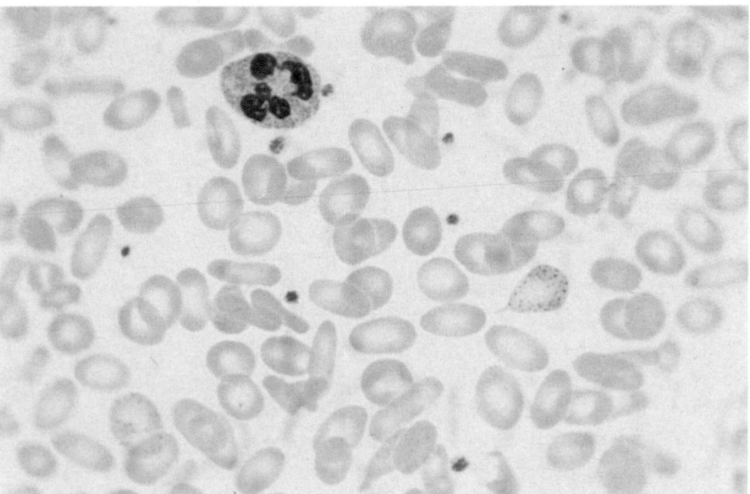

Fig. 3.40 Prominent basophilic stippling in the peripheral blood film of a patient who has inherited both β-thalassaemia trait and hereditary elliptocytosis. The film also shows microcytosis and numerous elliptocytes and ovalocytes. One of the heavily stippled cells is a tear drop poikilocyte. Courtesy of Dr F. Toolis, Dumfries.

the presence of thalassaemia trait (particularly β-thalassaemia trait and with haemoglobin Constant Spring), thalassaemia major, megaloblastic anaemia, unstable haemoglobins, haemolytic anaemia, dyserythropoietic states in general (including sideroblastic anaemia, erythroleukaemia and idiopathic myelofibrosis), liver disease and poisoning by heavy metals such as lead, arsenic, bismuth, zinc, silver and mercury. Basophilic stippling is a prominent feature of hereditary deficiency of pyrimidine 5′ nucleotidase [48], an enzyme which is required for RNA degradation. Inhibition of this enzyme may also be responsible for the prominent basophilic stippling in some patients with lead poisoning.

Pappenheimer bodies

Pappenheimer bodies (see Fig. 3.17) are basophilic inclusions which may be present in small numbers in erythrocytes; they often occur in small clusters towards the periphery of the cell and can be demonstrated to contain iron. They are composed of ferritin aggregates, or mitochondria or phagosomes containing aggregated ferritin. They stain on a Romanowsky stain because clumps of ribosomes are coprecipitated with the iron-containing organelles. A cell containing Pappenheimer bodies is a siderocyte. Reticulocytes often contain Pappenheimer bodies. Following splenectomy in a haematologically normal subject, small numbers of Pappenheimer bodies appear, these being ferritin aggregates. In pathological conditions, such as lead poisoning or sideroblastic anaemia, Pappenheimer bodies can also represent iron-laden mitochondria or phagosomes. If the patient has also had a splenectomy they will be present in much larger numbers.

Microorganisms in erythrocytes

Both protozoan parasites (see pp. 111–13) and other microorganisms (see p. 108) can be seen within red cells.

Circulating nucleated red cells

Except in the neonatal period and occasionally in pregnancy the presence of NRBC (see Fig. 3.35) in the peripheral blood is abnormal, generally indicating hyperplastic erythropoiesis or bone marrow infiltration. If granulocyte precursors are also present the film is described as leucoerythroblastic (see p. 171). NRBC in the peripheral blood may be morphologically abnormal; e.g., they may be megaloblastic or show the features of iron deficient or sideroblastic erythropoiesis. An increased frequency of karyorrhexis in circulating NRBC may be seen in arsenic and lead poisoning [49] and in certain dyserythropoietic states such as erythroleukaemia and severe iron-deficiency anaemia. Examination of a buffy coat film is helpful if assessment of morphological abnormalities in NRBC is required.

Red cell agglutination and rouleaux formation

Red cell agglutinates (see Fig. 3.11) are irregular clumps of cells whereas rouleaux (Fig. 3.41) are stacks of erythrocytes resembling a pile of coins.

Reticulocytes may form agglutinates when their numbers are increased; this is a normal phenomenon. Mature red cells agglutinate when they are antibody-coated. Small agglutinates may be seen in warm autoimmune haemolytic anaemia whereas the presence of cold agglutinates may cause massive agglutination (see Fig. 3.2).

Rouleaux formation is increased when there is an increased plasma concentration of proteins of high molecular weight. The most common causes are pregnancy (in which fibrinogen concentration is increased), inflammatory conditions (in which polyclonal immunoglobulins, α_2-macroglobulin and fibrinogen are increased) and plasma cell dyscrasias such as multiple myeloma (in which increased immunoglobulin concentration is caused by the presence of a monoclonal paraprotein). Rouleaux formation may be artefactually increased if a drop of blood is left standing for too long on a microscope slide before the blood is spread.

Abnormal clumping of red cells can also occur in patients receiving certain intravenous drugs which use polyethoxylated castor oils as a carrier (for example miconazole, phytomenadione and cyclosporin).

Leucocytes

Normal peripheral blood leucocytes are classified as polymorphonuclear leucocytes or mononuclear cells, the latter term indicating lymphocytes and monocytes. Polymorphonuclear leucocytes are also referred to as polymorphonuclear granulocytes, polymorphs or granulocytes. The term granulocyte has also been used to refer more generally to both the mature polymorphonuclear leucocytes usually seen in the peripheral blood and their granulated precursors. Polymorphs have lobulated nuclei which are very variable in shape, hence 'polymorphic', and prominent cytoplasmic granules which differ in staining characteristics between the three classes — neutrophil, eosinophil and basophil. Mononuclear cells may also have granules; in the case of the monocyte they are inconspicuous, whereas in the lymphocyte they are sometimes prominent but are not numerous. In pathological conditions and in certain physiological conditions, such as pregnancy and during the neonatal period, precursors of polymorphs may appear in the peripheral blood. A variety of abnormal leucocytes may also be seen in certain disease states.

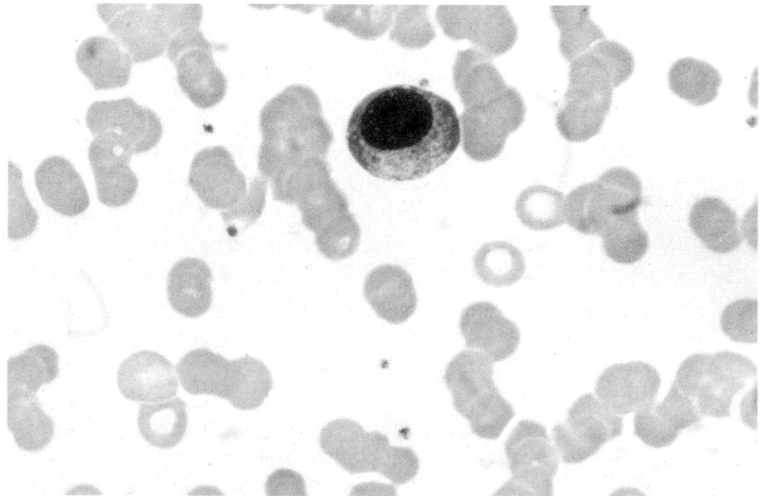

Fig. 3.41 Peripheral blood film of a patient with multiple myeloma showing increased rouleaux formation consequent on the presence of a paraprotein; the film also shows increased background staining and a circulating myeloma cell.

The neutrophil

The mature neutrophil measures 12–15 μm in diameter. The cytoplasm is acidophilic with many fine granules. The nucleus has clumped chromatin and is divided into two to five distinct lobes by filaments which are narrow strands of dense heterochromatin bordered by nuclear membrane (Fig. 3.42). The nucleus tends to follow an approximately circular form since in the living cell the nuclear lobes are arranged in a circle around the centrosome. In normal females a 'drumstick' may be seen protruding from the nucleus of a proportion of cells (Fig. 3.43). A normal neutrophil has granules spread evenly through the cytoplasm but there may be some agranular cytoplasm protruding at one margin of the cell. This may represent the advancing edge of a cell in active locomotion.

Characteristics of the nucleus

The neutrophil band form and left shift

A cell which otherwise resembles a mature neutrophil but which lacks nuclear lobes (Fig. 3.44) is referred to as a neutrophil band form or a 'stab' form (from the German *stabzelle* referring to a shepherd's staff or crook). The Committee for the Clarification of Nomenclature of Cells and Diseases of the Blood Forming Organs has defined a band cell as 'any cell of the granulocyte series which has a nucleus which could be described as a curved or coiled band, no matter how marked the indentation, if it does not completely segment the nucleus into lobes separated by a filament'. A filament is a thread-like connection with 'no significant nuclear material' [50]. A band is differentiated from a metamyelocyte (see below) by having an appreciable amount of nucleus with parallel sides. Small numbers of band cells are seen in healthy subjects. An increase in the number of band cells in relation to normal neutrophils is known as a left shift. When a left shift occurs, neutrophil precursors more immature than band forms (metamyelocytes, myelocytes, promyelocytes and blast cells) may also be released into the blood. A left shift is a physiological occurrence in pregnancy. In the non-pregnant patient it commonly indicates response to infection or inflammation, or some other stimulus to the bone marrow. A left shift, including even a few blast cells, is produced by the administration of cytokines such as granulocyte colony-stimulating factor (G-CSF) and granulocyte macrophage colony-stimulating factor (GM-CSF).

The actual percentage or absolute number of band forms or the ratio of band forms to neutrophils which is regarded as normal is dependent on the precise definition of band form used and how the definition is applied in practice. Inconsistency between laboratories with regard to definition

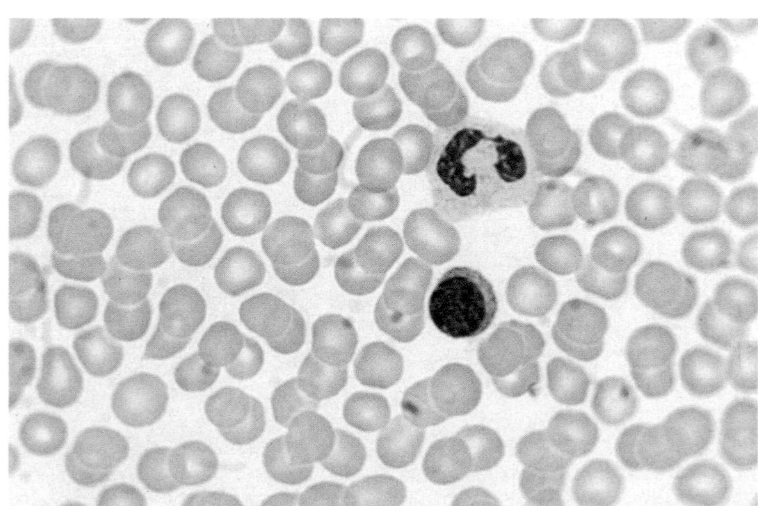

Fig. 3.42 Peripheral blood film of a healthy subject showing a normal polymorphonuclear neutrophil and normal small lymphocyte. The disposition of the nuclear lobes around the circumference of a circle is apparent.

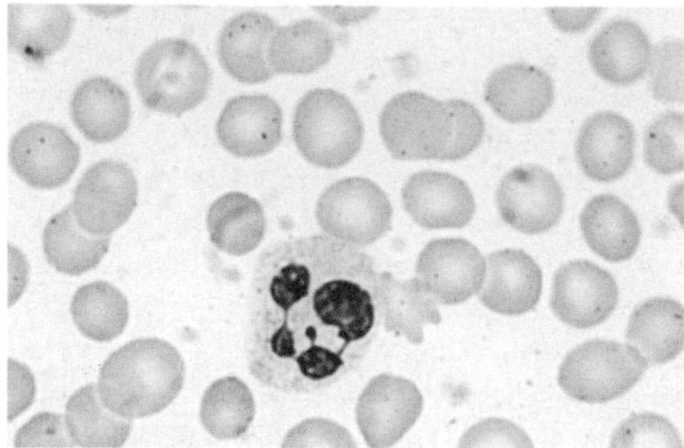

Fig. 3.43 Peripheral blood film of a healthy female showing a normal neutrophil with a drumstick.

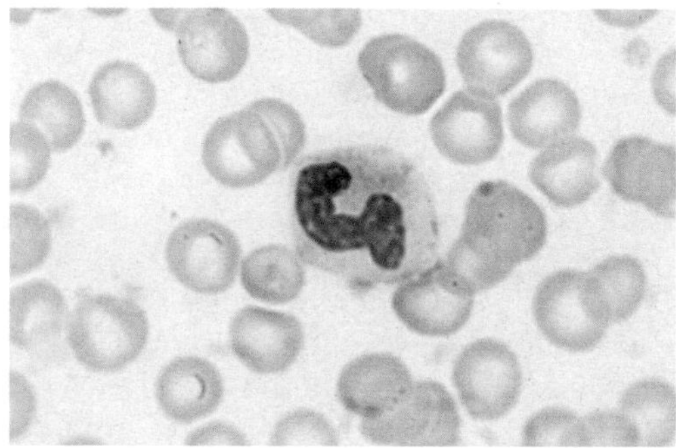

Fig. 3.44 A neutrophil band form. The nucleus is non-segmented and also has chromatin which is less condensed than that of the majority of segmented neutrophils.

is common, as is variation between and within laboratories as to how definitions are applied.

Band cell counts have been employed in the detection of infection in neonates, but again various definitions have been applied [51,52]. For example, Akenzua *et al.* [51] defined a (segmented) neutrophil as a cell with lobes separated by a thin filament whose width is less than one-third the maximum diameter of the lobes whereas Christensen *et al.* [53] required the lobes to be separated by a definite nuclear filament.

The neutrophil lobe count and right shift

In normal blood, most neutrophils have one to five lobes. Six-lobed neutrophils are rare. A right shift is said to be present if the average lobe count is increased or if there is an increased percentage of neutrophils with five or six lobes. The average lobe count of normal neutrophils varies between observers, with values of 2.5–3.3 obtained in different studies [54]. In practice, a formal lobe count is time-consuming and the presence of more than 3% of neutrophils with five lobes or more (Fig. 3.45) is a more practical indicator of right shift. This is also a more sensitive index of neutrophil hypersegmentation than the average lobe count and allows hypersegmentation to be detected in patients in whom a simultaneous increase in band forms means that the average lobe count is normal. A further index of right shift which has been found to be more sensitive than either of the above (see p. 224) is the segmentation index:

$$\frac{\text{number of neutrophils with five lobes or more} \times 100}{\text{number of neutrophils with four lobes}}$$

Values of greater than 16.9 are abnormal [55].

A right shift or neutrophil hypersegmentation is seen in megaloblastic anaemia and in occasional patients with iron deficiency, infection or uraemia. It also occurs as a rare hereditary characteristic with an autosomal dominant inheritance [56]. In the inherited condition known as myelokathexis there is neutropenia in association with a defect of neutrophil lobulation [57]. Neutrophils are hypersegmented with long chromatin filaments separating the lobes. Rarely, a similar anomaly is seen in the myelodysplastic syndromes but at least some of these cases differ from the inherited condition in that the hypersegmented neutrophils are tetraploid (Fig. 3.46).

The presence of macropolycytes with more than five lobes (see p. 80) is not an indication of right shift since the increased number of lobes is consequent on an increased DNA content rather than on any abnormality of nuclear segmentation.

The neutrophil drumstick, sessile nodules and other nuclear projections

Some neutrophils in normal females have a drumstick-shaped nuclear appendage about 1.5 μm in diameter which is linked to the rest of the

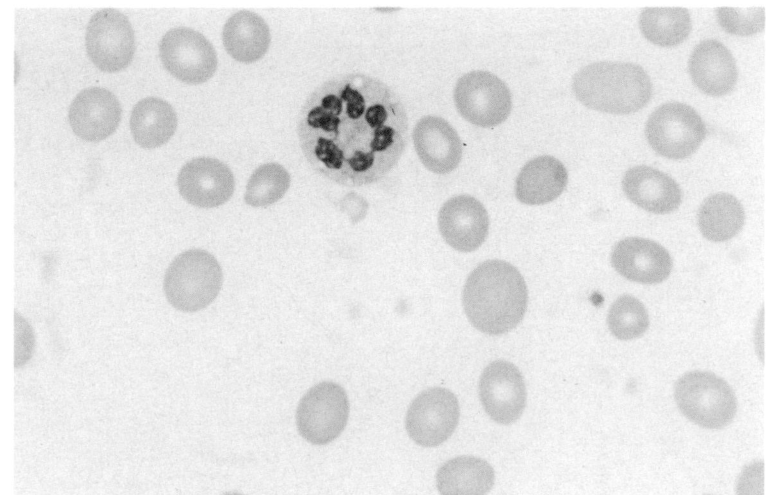

Fig. 3.45 A hypersegmented neutrophil showing seven nuclear lobes. The film also shows anisocytosis with both microcytes and macrocytes.

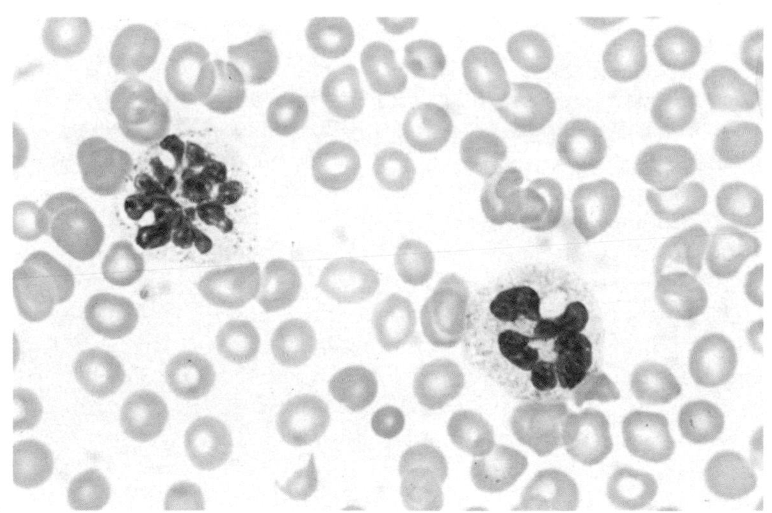

Fig. 3.46 Peripheral blood film of a patient with a myelodysplastic syndrome showing two neutrophils. Both are macropolycytes (tetraploid neutrophils) and one shows a defect of nuclear segmentation resembling myelokathexis.

nucleus by a filament [58] (see Fig. 3.43). These drumsticks represent the inactive X chromosome of the female. Similar projections with central pallor (racquet forms) are not drumsticks and do not have the same significance. In cells without drumsticks the inactive X chromosome may be condensed beneath the nuclear membrane, where it can be detected in some neutrophil band forms [59], or it may protrude from the nucleus as a sessile nodule (Fig. 3.47). Like drumsticks, sessile nodules are usually only found in females. In one study the frequency of drumsticks was found to vary from one in 38 to one in 200 neutrophils, and to be characteristic of the individual but also proportional to the lobe count [58,60]. If a left shift occurs, the proportion of cells with drumsticks reduces, whereas in macropolycytes (see p. 80), and when there is right shift due to megaloblastic anaemia or hereditary hypersegmentation of neutrophils, the frequency of drumsticks is increased.

The presence and frequency of drumsticks is related to the number of X chromosomes, They do not occur in normal males, in individuals with

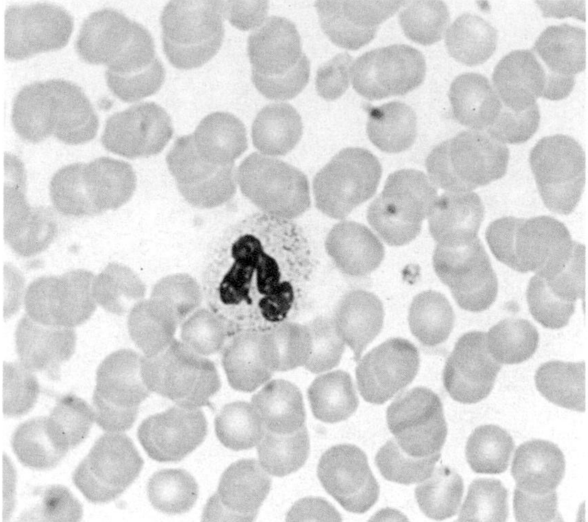

Fig. 3.47 Peripheral blood film of a healthy female showing a band neutrophil with a sessile nodule.

the testicular feminization syndrome who are phenotypically female but genetically (XY) male, or in Turner's syndrome (XO) females. In males with Klinefelter's syndrome (XXY) drumsticks are found but in lower numbers than in females. Paradoxically, XXX females rarely have cells with double drumsticks and on average their lobe count and frequency of drumsticks are lower than those of normal females; they have an increased incidence of sessile nodules and it has been suggested that the presence of an extra X chromosome inhibits nuclear segmentation [61]. Females with an isochromosome of the long arms of the X chromosome have larger and more frequent drumsticks, whereas females with deletions from the X chromosome have smaller drumsticks [56]. Natural human chimaeras whose cells are a mixture of cells of male and female origin have a drumstick frequency consistent with a male/female mixture of neutrophils [60] and similarly, an alteration of the drumstick count may be seen after bone marrow transplantation when bone marrow from a female has been transplanted into a male or vice versa.

The proportion of neutrophils with drumsticks and sessile nodules is reduced in women with chronic granulocytic leukaemia but returns to normal when the WBC falls on treatment [62].

The drumstick count (and the average lobe count) are reduced in Down's syndrome [63].

In addition to drumsticks and sessile nodules, neutrophil nuclei may have other projections which can have the shape of clubs, hooks or tags. These projections can also be seen in the neutrophils of males. Increased nuclear projections are a relatively uncommon feature of the myelodysplastic syndromes (Fig. 3.48).

Other abnormalities of neutrophil nuclei (Table 3.8)

Reduced neutrophil segmentation which is not consequent on temporary bone marrow stimulation with release of immature cells is seen as an inherited anomaly (the Pelger–Hüet anomaly) or as an acquired anomaly (the pseudo- or acquired Pelger–Hüet anomaly). The Pelger–Hüet anomaly was first described by Pelger in 1928 and its familial nature was recognized by Hüet in 1931 [78]. It is inherited as an autosomal dominant characteristic with a prevalence between one in 100 and one in 10 000 in different communities [79]. It has been recognized in many ethnic groups including white and black people, Chinese, Japanese and Indonesians. The abnormality is distinctive. The majority of neutrophils have bilobed nuclei (Fig. 3.49a), the lobes being rounder than normal and the chromatin more condensed; a characteristic spectacle or *pince-nez* shape is common. Other nuclei are shaped like dumbells or peanuts (Fig. 3.49b). A small proportion of neutrophils, usually not more than 4%, have non-lobed nuclei (Fig. 3.49c); they are distinguished from myelocytes by a lower nucleocytoplasmic ratio, the condensation of nuclear chromatin and the maturity of the cytoplasm. In rare homozygotes with the Pelger–Hüet anomaly all the neutrophils have round or oval nuclei. The distinction between the Pelger–Hüet anomaly and a left shift is important since the inherited condition is of no clinical significance. If a left shift occurs in a patient with the Pelger–Hüet anomaly the proportion of non-lobed neutrophils is further increased. If a subject with the Pelger–Hüet anomaly develops megaloblastic erythropoiesis, a right shift occurs and neutrophils with three, four or even five lobes are seen [80]; megaloblastosis

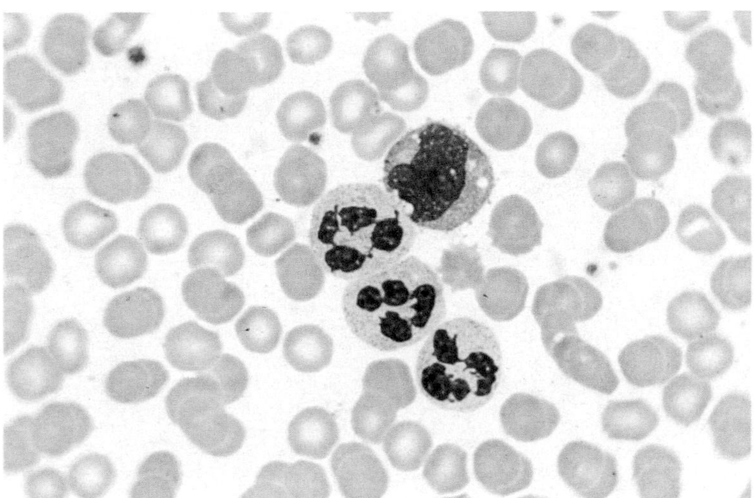

Fig. 3.48 Peripheral blood film of a patient with chronic myelomonocytic leukaemia showing neutrophils with abnormal nuclear projections.

also causes loss of the characteristic dense clumping of the nuclear chromatin and drumsticks may become identifiable. Subjects with the Pelger–Hüet anomaly also show reduced lobulation of eosinophils and basophils [81].

In another congenital anomaly, sometimes designated lactoferrin deficiency, neutrophils with a marked reduction in the numbers of specific granules also have bilobed nuclei [64,82].

A single patient has been described in whom non-lobed neutrophils were associated with skeletal malformations, microthalmia and mental retardation [65].

The acquired Pelger–Hüet anomaly (Fig. 3.50) is common in myelodysplastic syndromes and in acute myeloid leukaemias. It occurs occasionally in other haematological neoplasms, particularly idiopathic myelofibrosis and during the evolution of chronic granulocytic leukaemia (CGL). Features which help in making the distinction from the inherited Pelger–Hüet anomaly are that the percentage of affected neutrophils is usually less and there is commonly an association with neutropenia, hypogranularity of neutrophils, Döhle bodies (see p. 76) or dysplastic features in other lineages.

Reduced neutrophil lobulation is rarely seen in other circumstances but has been described in association with therapy with colchicine, ibuprofen and other drugs, and in infectious mononucleosis, malaria, myxoedema, metastatic carcinoma of the bone marrow, CLL and acute enteritis [56,83].

Neutrophils with ring or doughnut nuclei (Fig. 3.51) are seen occasionally in normal subjects. Their frequency is increased in CGL, in chronic neutrophilic leukaemia and probably in the myelodysplastic syndromes [71]; occasionally they are prominent in AML [72].

Another acquired defect of the neutrophil nucleus is radial segmentation to form a 'botryoid' nucleus, i.e., a nucleus with a shape resembling a bunch of grapes. The change is consequent on contraction of microfilaments radiating from the centriole. It has been demonstrated in heat stroke [75] and in hyperthermia arising from brain stem haemorrhage [76].

Excessive clumping of the neutrophil nuclear chromatin is observed sometimes in the myelodysplastic syndromes and in AML.

Rarely, neutrophils have detached nuclear fragments (Fig. 3.52) equivalent to the Howell–Jolly bodies of erythrocytes; their nature can be confirmed by a Feulgen stain for DNA. Such inclusions are indicative of dysgranulopoiesis. They are seen mainly in patients on anti-cancer chemotherapeutic agents or azathioprine, and in patients infected with HIV, the latter in the absence of any drug therapy.

The administration of G-CSF and GM-CSF can

(a) 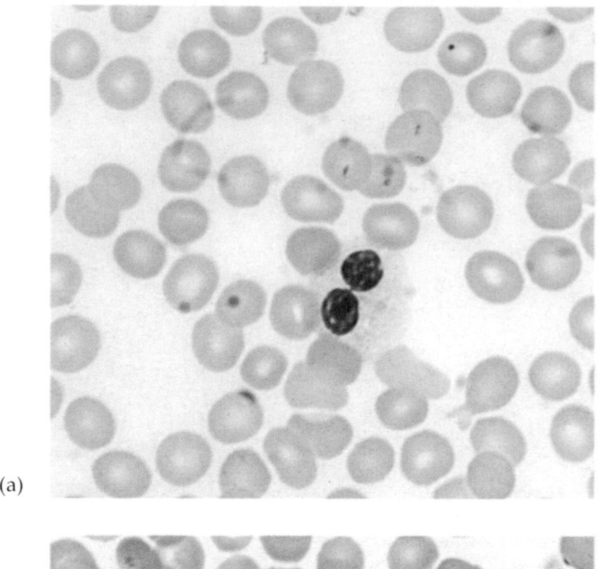

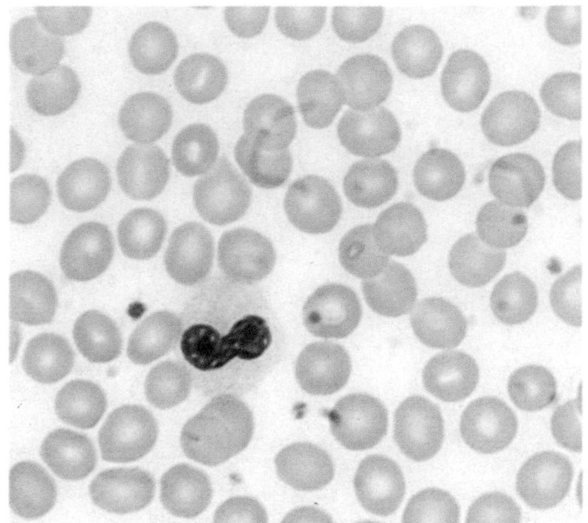 (b)

(c) 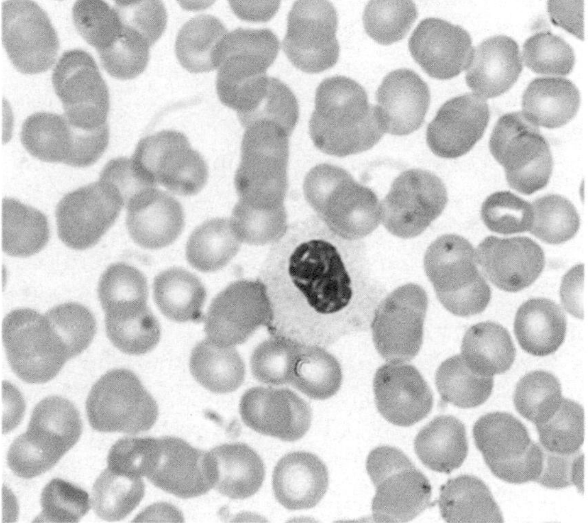

Fig. 3.49 Peripheral blood film of a patient with the inherited Pelger–Hüet anomaly showing three neutrophils with (a) bilobed nucleus, (b) peanut-shaped nucleus, and (c) non-lobed nucleus.

be associated with the appearance of a proportion of neutrophils with hypersegmented, hyposegmented and ring nuclei [84].

Abnormalities of neutrophil cytoplasm (Table 3.9)

Reduced granulation

Reduced granulation of neutrophils occurs as a congenital anomaly, e.g., in lactoferrin deficiency, but this is rare. It is usually an acquired abnormality, most often as a feature of one of the myelodysplastic syndromes (Fig. 3.53). In HIV infection some neutrophils may show reduced granulation but this is not as marked as in the myelodysplastic syndromes.

Increased granulation

Increased granulation of neutrophils with granules appearing both larger and more basophilic than normal, is designated as toxic granulation (Fig. 3.54). When neutrophil maturation is normal the azurophilic or primary granules become less strongly azurophilic as the cell matures so that,

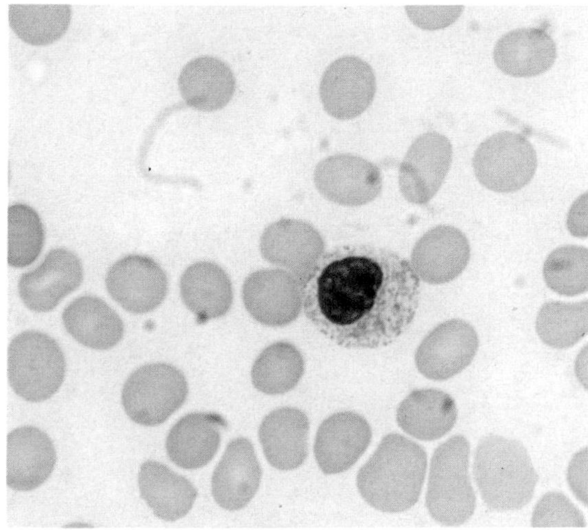

(a)

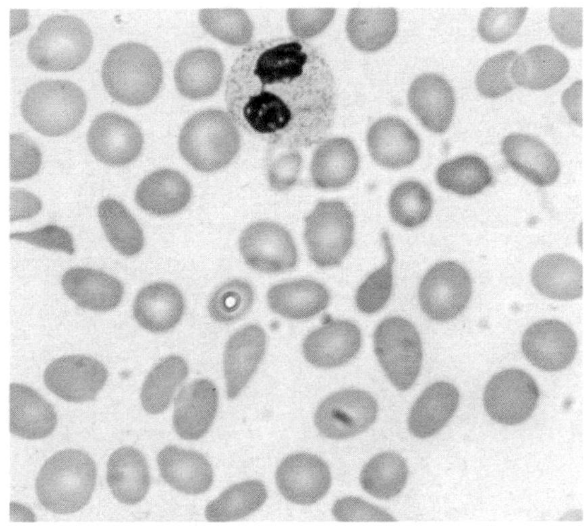

(b)

Fig. 3.50 Peripheral blood film of a patient with the acquired Pelger–Hüet anomaly as part of a post-chemotherapy myelodysplastic syndrome showing (a) neutrophil with non-lobed nucleus, and (b) anisocytosis, poikilocytosis and neutrophil with bilobed nucleus.

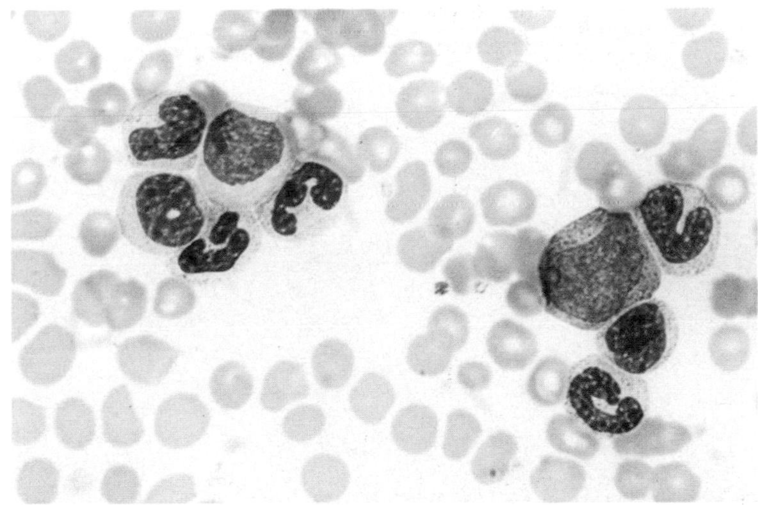

Fig. 3.51 Peripheral blood film of a patient with CGL showing neutrophils and neutrophil precursors. There is one neutrophil with a ring-shaped nucleus.

rather than staining reddish-purple, they stain violet or fail to stain at all. In a neutrophil showing toxic granulation the primary granules remain strongly azurophilic; this may be related to a higher concentration of acid mucosubstances than in normal neutrophils [103]. Degranulation may lead to neutrophils which show toxic granulation also having reduced numbers of granules. Although 'toxic' granulation is characteristic of infection it is non-specific being seen also in the presence of tissue damage of various types. It is also a feature of normal pregnancy and occurs with cytokine therapy (G-CSF and GM-CSF) even in the absence of infection. Other causes of heavy neutrophil granulation are shown in Figs 3.55 and 3.56 and in Table 3.9.

Table 3.8 Some alterations and abnormalities which may be present in neutrophil nuclei

Abnormality	Presence noted
Left shift	Pregnancy Infection, hypoxia, shock
Hypersegmentation	Megaloblastic erythropoiesis Iron deficiency Uraemia Infection Hereditary neutrophil hypersegmentation Myelokathexis [57]
Hyposegmentation	Pelger–Hüet anomaly Bilobed neutrophils with reduced specific granules (lactoferrin deficiency) [64] Non-lobed neutrophils with other congenital anomalies (one case) [65] Acquired or pseudo-Pelger–Hüet anomaly (myelodysplastic syndromes and AML)
Increased nuclear projections	Trisomy D syndrome [66] Associated with large platelets (single family [67]) Associated with a large Y chromosome (drumstick-like) [68] Turner's syndrome [69] As an isolated defect [70] Myelodysplastic syndromes
Ring nuclei	CGL [71] AML [72] Chronic neutrophilic leukaemia [73] Megaloblastic anaemia [74]
Botryoid nucleus	Heat stroke [75] Hyperthermia [76]
Dense chromatin clumping	Myelodysplastic syndromes [77]
Detached nuclear fragments within the cytoplasm	Dysplastic granulopoiesis due to HIV infection or administration of drugs interfering with DNA synthesis*

* B.J. Bain & S.N.W. Wickramasinghe, unpublished observations, 1974.

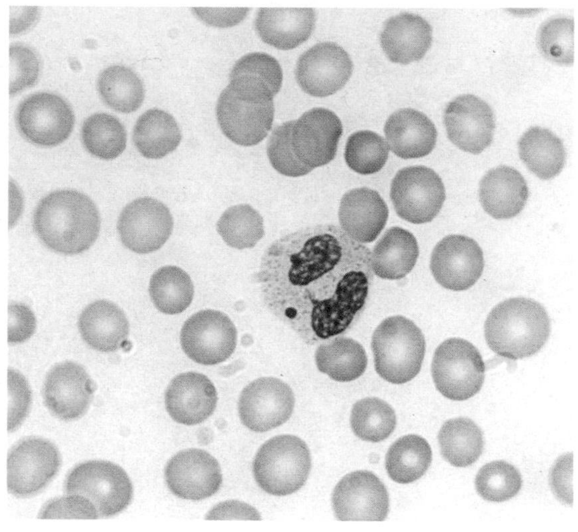

Fig. 3.52 Peripheral blood film of a patient on combination chemotherapy for lymphoma showing a neutrophil with a detached nuclear fragment (Howell–Jolly body-like inclusion).

Abnormal granulation and Auer rods

Abnormal neutrophil granulation (Table 3.10) is seen in a number of inherited conditions including the Chediak–Higashi syndrome and the heterogeneous group of conditions giving rise to the Alder–Reilly anomaly. The Alder–Reilly anomaly occurs as an isolated abnormality, in association with an abnormal peroxidase [104] and as a feature of the mucopolysaccharidoses, Tay–Sachs disease or Batten–Spielmeyer–Vogt disease. The abnormal neutrophils may have heavy granulation resembling toxic granulation or there may be large, clearly abnormal granules (Fig. 3.56). In the Chediack–Higashi syndrome (Fig. 3.57) the abnormal granules are quite variable in their staining characteristics and some may resemble Döhle bodies (see p. 76); at the ultrastructural level, however, they are abnormal granules rather than rough endoplasmic reticulum, being formed by the fusion of primary granules with each other and with secondary granules. There have been reports of abnormal neutrophil granulation resembling that of the Chediak–Higashi syndrome but with atypical features [87]. In an apparently distinct syndrome, abnormal granulation of all

Table 3.9 Some alterations and abnormalities of neutrophil cytoplasm

Abnormality	Presence noted	Abnormality	Presence noted
Reduced granulation	Myelodysplastic syndromes Congenital lactoferrin deficiency [64]	Döhle bodies or similar inclusions	Infection, inflammation, burns Pregnancy G-CSF therapy Myelodysplastic syndromes AML May–Hegglin anomaly Féchtner's syndrome [94] and related anomalies Kwashiorkor [93]
Increased granulation	'Toxic' granulation: pregnancy, infection, inflammation, G-CSF and GM-CSF therapy [85,86] Aplastic anaemia HES Alder–Reilly anomaly Chronic neutrophilic leukaemia [73]	Actin inclusions	Congenital abnormality associated with anaemia and grey skin [95]
Abnormal granulation	Chediak–Higashi syndrome and related anomalies [87,88] Alder–Reilly anomaly AML [89] and myelodysplastic syndromes	Phagocytosed material	
		Bacteria and fungi	Bacterial and fungal infections
		Leishmania	Leishmaniasis
		Cryoglobulin	Multiple myeloma and other cryoglobulinaemias
Vacuolation	Infection, G-CSF therapy, GM-CSF therapy Acute alcohol poisoning [90]; Jordan's anomaly [91] Carnitine deficiency [92] Kwashiorkor [93]	Mucopolysaccharide	Various carcinomas [96]
		Nucleoprotein	Systemic lupus erythematosus [97]
		Melanin	Melanoma [98]
		Bilirubin crystals or amorphous deposits	Severe hyperbilirubinaemia [99,100]
		Cystine crystals	Cystinosis [101]
		Erythrocytes	Autoimmune haemolytic anaemia, paroxysmal cold haemoglobinuria [102], incompatible blood transfusion, potassium chlorate poisoning

mature myeloid cells was associated with bile duct atresia and livedo reticularis [88]. Giant bright blue inclusions composed of actin have been described in the neutrophils and other leucocytes of an infant with anaemia and grey skin discoloration [95] (Fig. 3.58). Occasional patients with myelodysplastic syndromes or with AML have giant granules in neutrophils, which are morphologically similar to those of the Chediack–Higashi syndrome [89].

The Auer rod which is seen in haematological malignancies, specifically AML and refractory anaemia with excess of blasts in transformation (one of the myelodysplastic syndromes), is formed by fusion of primary granules. Auer rods are usually confined to blast cells (Fig. 3.59) but occasionally they are seen in maturing cells, including neutrophils, which are part of the neoplastic clone.

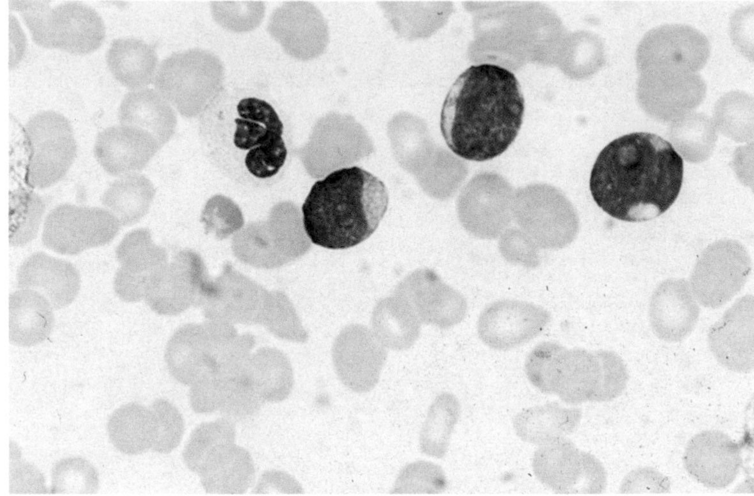

Fig. 3.53 Peripheral blood film of a patient with AML showing three blasts and a hypogranular neutrophil.

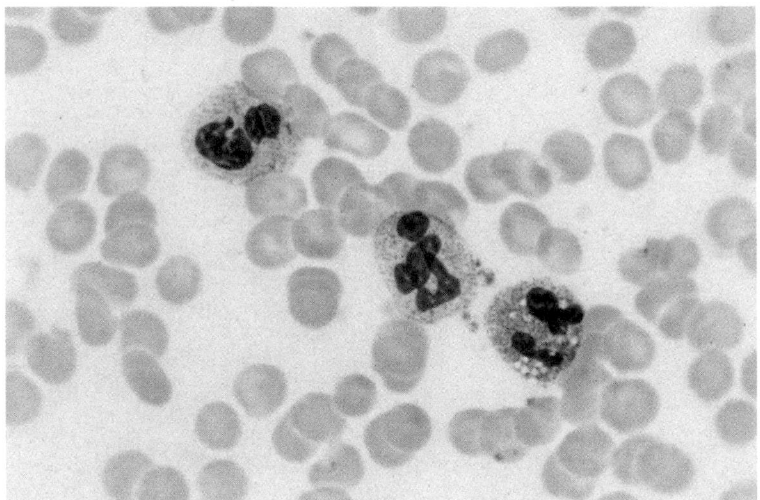

Fig. 3.54 Three neutrophils in the peripheral blood film of a patient with bacterial infection showing toxic granulation and vacuolation.

Vacuolation

Neutrophil vacuolation may occur as the result of fusion of granules with a phagocytic vacuole with subsequent exocytosis of the contents of the secondary lysosome. This is usually a feature of infection (see Fig. 3.54) and partial degranulation of the neutrophil may also be apparent. Vacuolation of neutrophils can also occur as a toxic effect following ethanol ingestion [90] but this is much less often observed than ethanol-induced vacuolation of myeloid precursors. A rare cause of neutrophil vacuolation (together with vacuolation of neutrophil precursors, monocytes and some eosinophils, basophils and lymphocytes) is a familial defect designated as Jordan's anomaly [91,105]; the vacuoles are due to dissolution of lipid [105]. Inheritance appears to be autosomal recessive [92]. Jordan's anomaly may represent carnitine deficiency [92].

Döhle bodies and similar inclusions

Döhle bodies are small, pale-blue or blue–grey cytoplasmic inclusions, single or multiple, often found towards the periphery of the cell (Fig. 3.60).

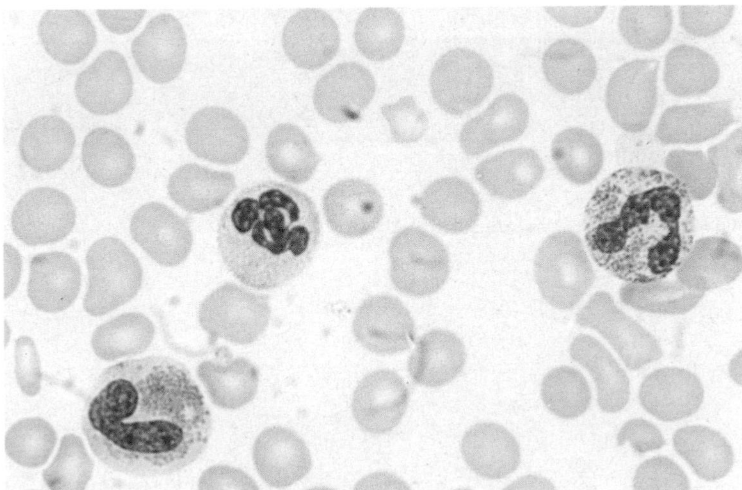

Fig. 3.55 Peripheral blood film of a patient with idiopathic HES showing a normal neutrophil, a neutrophil with abnormally heavy granulation and a hypogranular band eosinophil.

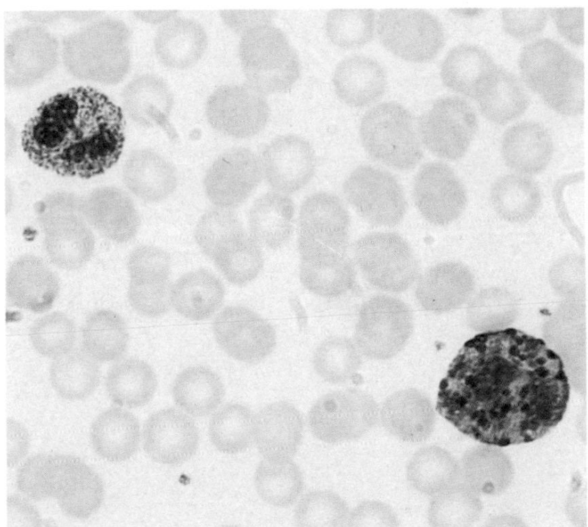

Fig. 3.56 Peripheral blood film of a patient with the Maroteaux–Lamy syndrome showing the Alder–Reilly anomaly of neutrophils. The neutrophil has granules which resemble toxic granulation. The other granulocyte is probably an eosinophil with granules having very abnormal staining characteristics. Courtesy of Mr A. Dean, Nottingham.

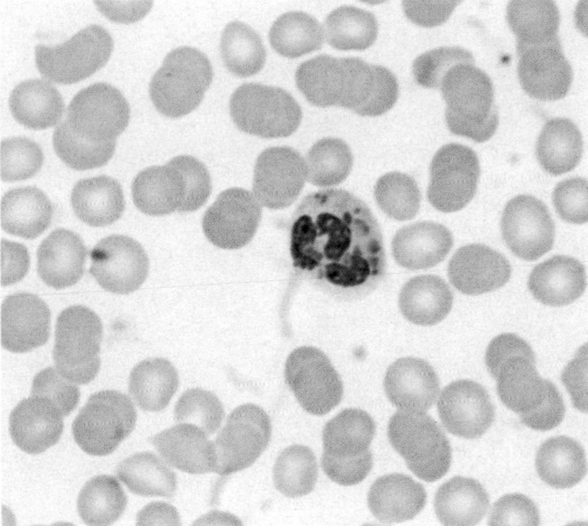

Fig. 3.57 Peripheral blood film of a patient with the Chediak–Higashi syndrome showing a neutrophil with giant and abnormally staining granules. Courtesy of Dr J. McCallum, Kircaldy.

They usually measure only 1–2 μm in diameter but may be up to 5 μm. At the ultrastructural level they are composed of stacks of endoplasmic reticulum together with glycogen granules. Their ribosomal component is indicated by pink staining with a methyl green-pyronin stain and by destruction by ribonuclease; they are seen better in films made from non-anticoagulated blood [106]. Döhle bodies are associated with pregnancy, infective and inflammatory states, burns and administration of cytokines such as G-CSF and GM-CSF. They may be seen in the myelodysplastic syn-

Table 3.10 Inherited conditions in which leucocytes have abnormal granules or cytoplasmic inclusions

Abnormality	Associated features	Morphology of granules or inclusions	Nature of granules or inclusions	Cells affected
Chediak–Higashi anomaly*	Anaemia Neutropenia Thrombocytopenia Jaundice Neurological abnormalities Recurrent infections	Giant granules with colour ranging from grey to red	Abnormal primary granules (specific granules are normal)	Neutrophil Eosinophil Basophil Monocyte Lymphocyte Melanocyte Renal tubule Many other body cells
Alder–Reilly anomaly*	Tay–Sachs disease Mucopoly-saccharidoses such as: Hunter's syndrome† Sanfilippo syndrome Morquio's syndrome Scheie's syndrome Maroteaux–Lamy syndrome	Dark red or purple inclusions which may resemble toxic granules: Inclusions or vacuoles in lymphocytes	Mucopolysaccharide or other abnormal carbohydrate	Neutrophil Eosinophil Basophil Monocyte (rarely) Lymphocyte
May–Hegglin anomaly‡	Thrombocytopenia Giant platelets	Resemble Döhle bodies	Amorphous area of cytoplasm containing structures related to ribosomes	Neutrophil Eosinophil Basophil Monocyte

* autosomal recessive (AR) inheritance.
† Hunter's syndrome is sex-linked recessive.
‡ autosomal dominant (AD) inheritance.

dromes and in AML, and have been described in pernicious anaemia, polycythaemia rubra vera (PRV), CGL, haemolytic anaemia, Wegener's granulomatosis, and following use of anti-cancer chemotherapeutic agents [107].

Large inclusions resembling Döhle bodies, often numerous and sharply defined, are a feature of the May–Hegglin anomaly which is also characterized by thrombocytopenia and giant platelets (Fig. 3.61); they are often spindle- or crescent-shaped, randomly distributed in the cell rather than near the cell margin, and more intensely staining than Döhle bodies. At the ultrastructural level these inclusions differ from the Döhle bodies of reactive states; they appear as an amorphous area largely devoid of organelles, often incompletely surrounded by a single strand of rough endoplasmic reticulum and containing a few dense rods and spherical particles which are probably ribosomes [108].

Inclusions resembling Döhle bodies but differing from them ultrastructurally have also been associated with the features of Alport's or Epstein's syndrome. The name Fechtner's syndrome has been proposed [94].

In normal subjects Döhle bodies are rare. In one study they were seen in three of 20 healthy subjects with an average frequency of 0.1 per 100

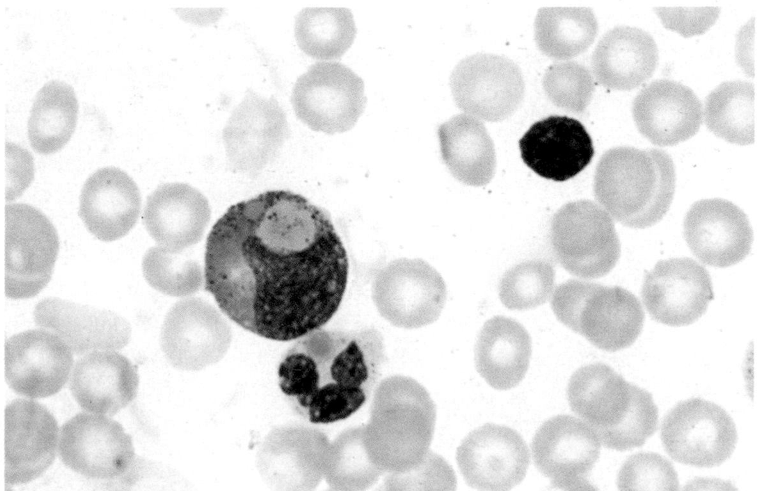

Fig. 3.58 Bone marrow film of a patient with giant actin inclusions (Brandalise's syndrome) showing blue inclusions in a neutrophil and a promyelocyte. Similar inclusions were present in peripheral blood neutrophils and also in eosinophils, basophils, monocytes and lymphocytes. Courtesy of Dr. R.C. Ribeiro, Memphis.

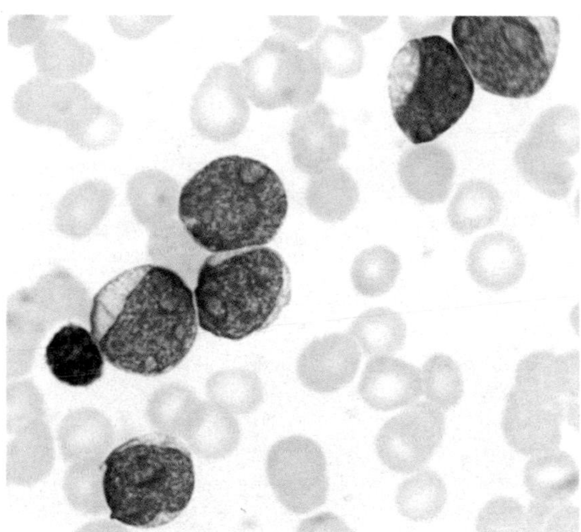

Fig. 3.59 Peripheral blood film of a patient with AML showing blasts, one of which contains an Auer rod.

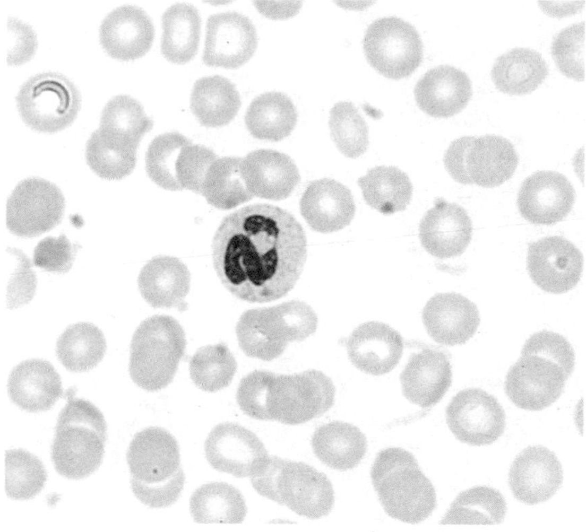

Fig. 3.60 Peripheral blood film of a patient with septicaemia showing a Döhle body in a neutrophil.

cells [107]. In pregnancy, the number of Döhle bodies per 100 cells increases in parallel with the WBC [106]; the increased frequency persists into the post-partum period.

Exogenous neutrophil inclusions

Since neutrophils are phagocytes they may contain inclusions which represent phagocytosed material such as microorganisms (see pp. 107–25) or cryoglobulin. Cryoglobulin (Fig. 3.62) may be seen as single or multiple round, weakly basophilic inclusions or as a single large inclusion which displaces the nucleus. Phagocytosis of cryoglobulin occurs *in vitro*, when the blood is left standing, rather than *in vivo* [109]. Abnormal mucopolysaccharide, which circulates in the blood of patients with malignant diseases, may be

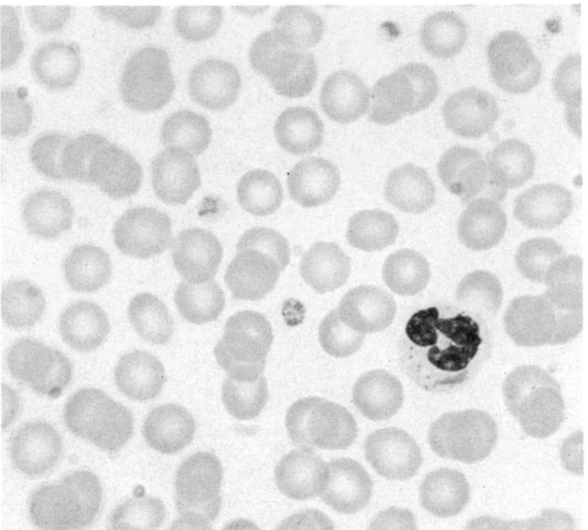

Fig. 3.61 Peripheral blood film of a patient with the May–Hegglin anomaly showing a May–Hegglin inclusion which resembles a Döhle body. Large platelets are also apparent. Courtesy of Dr N. Parker, London.

ingested by neutrophils; the blood film may also show amorphous or fibrillar deposits [96]. Malarial pigment is occasionally observed in neutrophils (Fig. 3.63) but is more commonly present in monocytes. The formation of lupus erythematosus (LE) cells is usually an *in vitro* phenomenon but they may be seen in the peripheral blood of patients with severe lupus erythematosis [97]. Square or rectangular crystals of cystine can be seen in peripheral blood leucocytes in cystinosus but are more readily detected with phase-contrast microscopy [101]. Large cytoplasmic inclusions were observed in a case of colchicine poisoning [110].

Neutrophils may also ingest red cells. This has been observed in autoimmune haemolytic anaemia and in other patients with a positive direct antiglobulin test and also in patients with defective red cells, as in sickle cell anaemia and sickle cell/haemoglobin C disease and in any severe haemolytic anaemias.

Other abnormalities of neutrophil morphology

Macropolycytes

A macropolycyte is about twice the size of a normal neutrophil (Fig. 3.64); its diameter is 15–25 μm rather than 12–15 μm and analysis of its DNA content shows that it is tetraploid rather than diploid, the number of lobes present being increased proportionately. Some macropolycytes are binucleated (Fig. 3.65). Occasional macropolycytes are seen in the blood of healthy subjects.

(a)

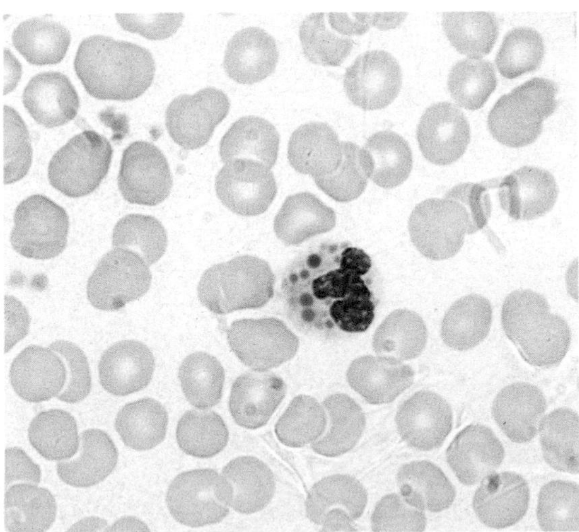

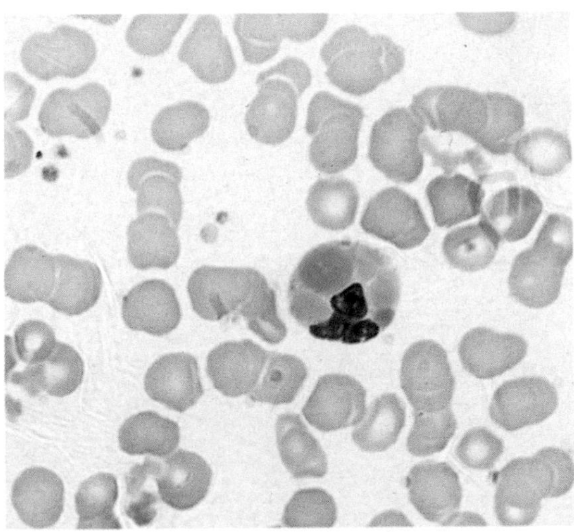

(b)

Fig. 3.62 Peripheral blood film of a patient with cryoglobulinaemia showing cryoglobulin which has been ingested by neutrophils and appears as (a) small round inclusions, and (b) large masses filling the cytoplasm and displacing the nucleus. Some extracellular cryoglobulin is also present. Courtesy of Mr A. Dean.

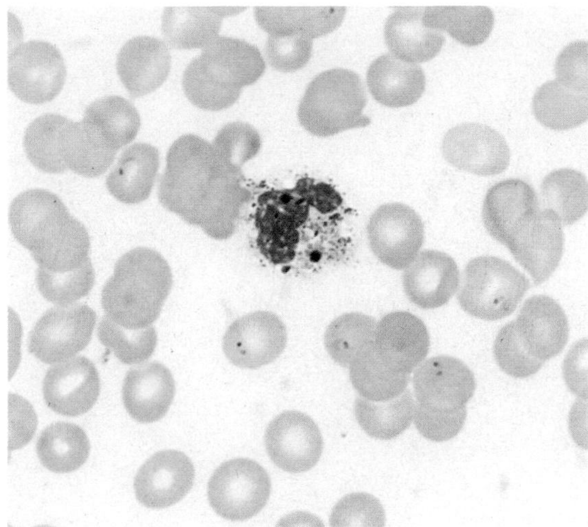

Fig. 3.63 Peripheral blood film of a patient with *Plasmodium falciparum* malaria showing malarial pigment in a neutrophil and ring forms of the parasite within red cells.

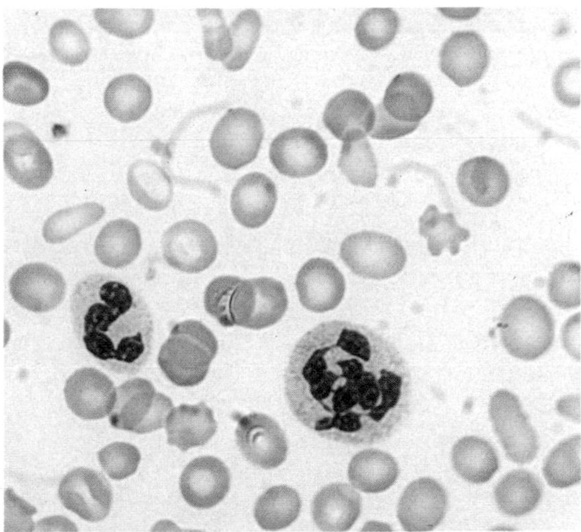

Fig. 3.64 Peripheral blood film of a patient with a myelodysplastic syndrome showing a macropolycyte which is twice the size of the adjacent normal neutrophil. The nucleus is also twice normal size and shows increased nuclear segmentation. In addition the film shows anisochromasia.

Increased numbers are seen in an inherited (autosomal dominant) condition in which 1–2% of neutrophils are giant with six- to 10-lobed nuclei,

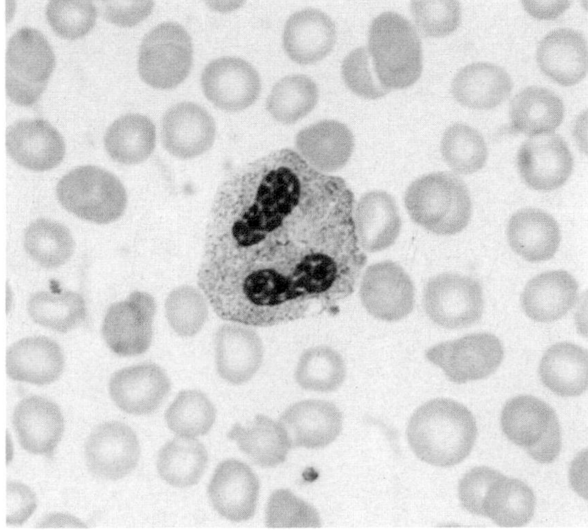

Fig. 3.65 Peripheral blood film of a patient with CLL and reversible chlorambucil-induced myelodysplasia showing a binucleated tetraploid neutrophil. Courtesy of Dr P.C. Srivastava, Burton on Trent.

or with twin mirror-image nuclei [111]. Macropolycytes have been observed following the administration of G-CSF [85] and are present in increased numbers in megaloblastic anaemia. They have also been reported in chronic infection, CGL and other myeloproliferative disorders, and following the administration of cytotoxic drugs and antimetabolites. Most macropolycytes have staining characteristics which are the same as those of other neutrophils but in megaloblastic anaemia macropolycytes may be seen which have a more open chromatin pattern and do not have an increased number of lobes [112]. Patients with HIV infection may have not only binucleate macropolycytes and macropolycytes with an open chromatin pattern but also circulating giant metamyelocytes (Fig. 3.66), cells which are characteristic of megaloblastic anaemia and are usually seen only in the bone marrow.

Necrobiotic neutrophils

Necrobiotic neutrophils are cells which have died in the peripheral blood by a process known as apoptosis or 'programmed cell death'. Occasionally such cells are seen in the blood of healthy subjects and are recognized by their dense, homogeneous

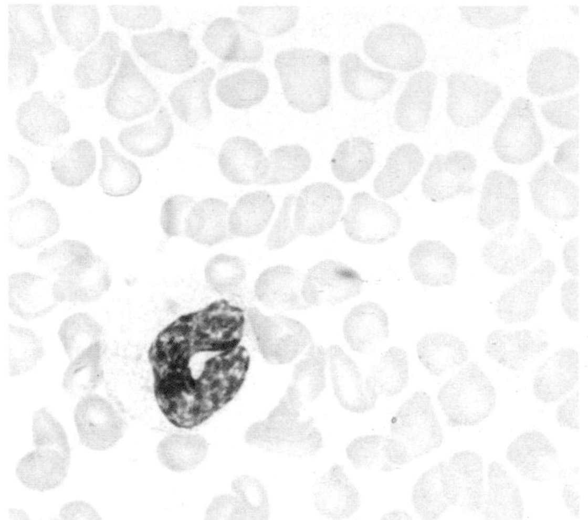

Fig. 3.66 Peripheral blood film of a patient with AIDS showing a hypogranular tetraploid giant metamyelocyte.

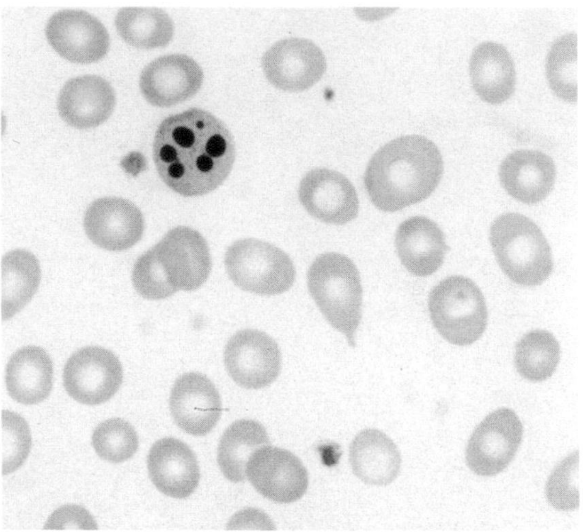

Fig. 3.67 Peripheral blood film of a patient with megaloblastic anaemia showing a necrobiotic (apoptotic) neutrophil. The chromatin has condensed and the nucleus has fragmented into rounded pyknotic masses. The film also shows anisocytosis, macrocytosis and a tear drop poikilocyte.

(pyknotic) nuclei which eventually become completely round, often multiple, dense masses; the cytoplasm shows prominent acidophilia (Fig. 3.67). The frequency of necrobiotic neutrophils is increased in some patients with AML. If blood is left at room temperature for a long time a similar change can occur as an *in vitro* artefact (see p. 43). Leucocytes which have degenerated to the extent that nuclear material is no longer apparent have been designated as necrotic; this is generally an artefact consequent on prolonged storage.

Neutrophil aggregation

Aggregation of neutrophils with or without aggregation of platelets develops *in vitro* in some patients when EDTA-anticoagulated blood is allowed to stand. This is an antibody-mediated time-dependent phenomenon which is not of any clinical significance although it may lead to erroneous automated WBCs. Neutrophil aggregation has also been observed as a transient phenomenon in association with infectious mononucleosis [113] and in acute bacterial infection (Fig. 3.68). Occasionally, it is observed in a patient over many months or years and may then be associated with autoimmune disease (Fig. 3.69). In some patients when the cause is a cold-acting antibody, red cell agglutinates coexist.

Neutrophil fragmentation

Fragmentation of leucocytes, mainly immature cells, is sometimes observed in AML. Fragmentation of neutrophils has also been observed, in association with microangiopathic haemolytic anaemia, in a patient with clot formation at the tip of a dialysis catheter [114]. The mechanism is likely to have been mechanical damage to neutrophils.

The eosinophil

The eosinophil (Fig. 3.70) is slightly larger than the neutrophil with a diameter of 12–17 μm. The nucleus is usually bilobed but occasional nuclei are trilobed, the average lobe count being about 2.3. In females, eosinophils may have drumsticks (Fig. 3.71), but as the frequency of drumsticks is related to the degree of lobulation of the nucleus they are quite infrequent. Eosinophil granules are spherical and considerably larger than those of

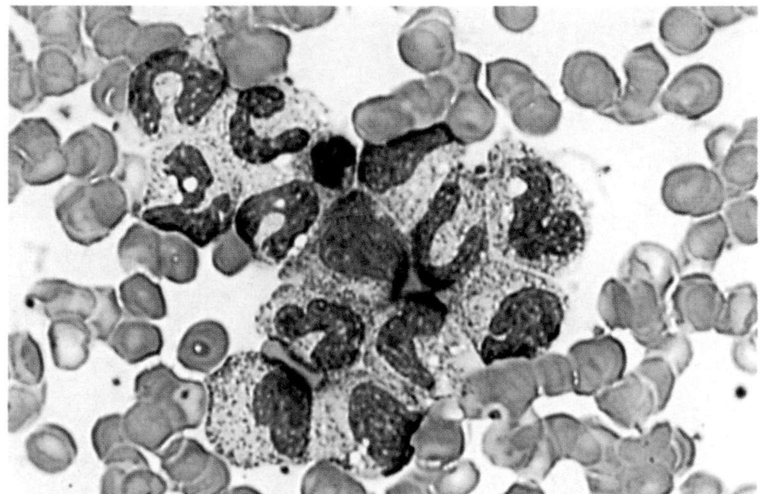

Fig. 3.68 Peripheral blood film of a patient with overwhelming sepsis showing neutrophil aggregation, left shift, toxic granulation and neutrophil vacuolation.

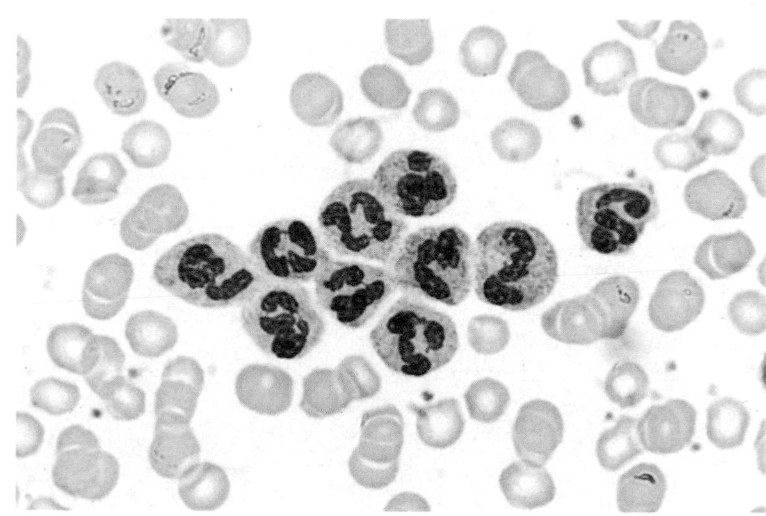

Fig. 3.69 Peripheral blood film of a patient with rheumatoid arthritis showing neutrophil aggregation caused by a cold antibody. In this patient *in vitro* neutrophil aggregation was observed for more than a decade and often led to inaccurate automated WBCs.

neutrophils; they pack the cytoplasm and stain reddish-orange. The cytoplasm of eosinophils is weakly basophilic, ribosomes and rough endoplasmic reticulum being more abundant than in mature neutrophils; when degranulation occurs the pale blue cytoplasm is visible. Very occasional eosinophils in healthy subjects contain some granules with basophilic staining characteristics.

Abnormalities of eosinophil nuclei

Eosinophils may show nuclear hypersegmentation (Fig. 3.72), hyposegmentation (Fig. 3.73) or ring-shaped nuclei (Fig. 3.74). Hypersegmentation can occur as a hereditary phenomenon [115]; in one family hypersegmented eosinophils were also poorly granulated [116] without any apparent clinical defect. Reduced eosinophil lobulation occurs in the Pelger–Hüet (Fig. 3.73) anomaly and has also been observed in lactoferrin deficiency [64].

Hypersegmentation, hyposegmentation and ring-shaped nuclei can all occur as acquired abnormalities. Hyposegmentation of eosinophil nuclei occurs as an acquired phenomenon in myeloproliferative disorders including idiopathic

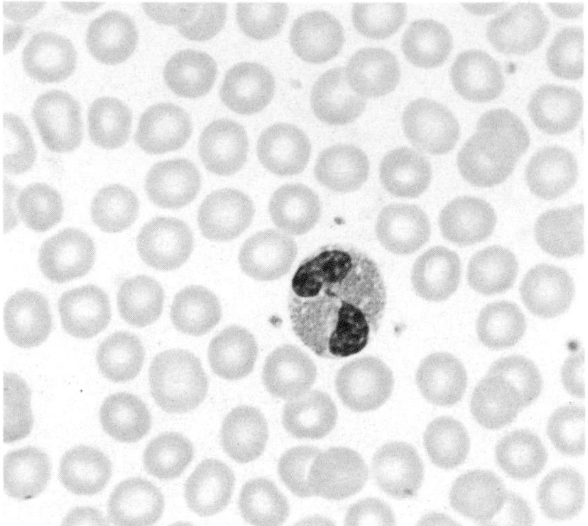

Fig. 3.70 An eosinophil in the peripheral blood film of a healthy subject.

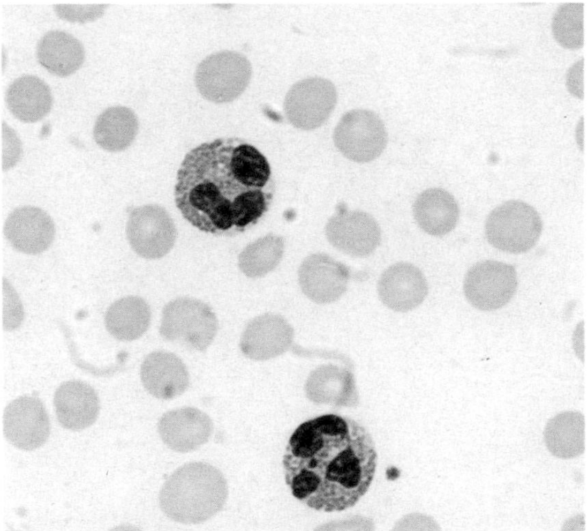

Fig. 3.71 Peripheral blood film of a female with idiopathic HES showing two eosinophils, one of which has a drumstick.

myelofibrosis and in the myelodysplastic syndromes (Fig. 3.75). In the latter group of disorders the chromatin may be clumped and the nuclei entirely or largely non-lobed [117]; this may be regarded as an acquired Pelger–Hüet anomaly confined to eosinophils. Patients with the idiopathic hypereosinophilic syndrome (HES) have

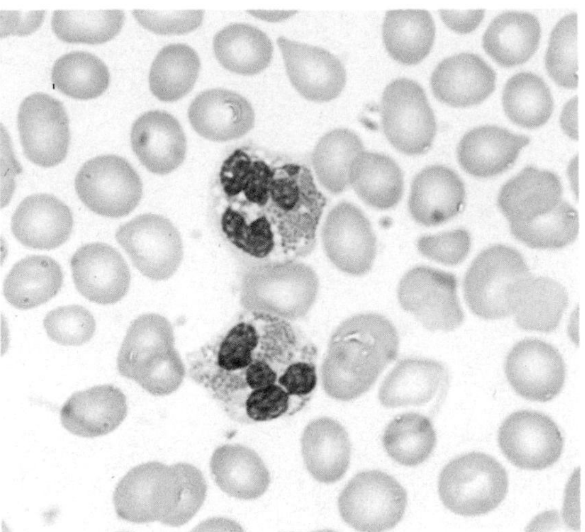

Fig. 3.72 Peripheral blood film of a patient with idiopathic HES showing eosinophil hypersegmentation. Both eosinophils have nuclei with four lobes.

increased numbers of both hypersegmented and hyposegmented eosinophils. Ring eosinophils are seen in the idiopathic HES but also in a variety of other conditions [118]. They appear to have no specific significance.

Abnormalities of eosinophil granules and cytoplasm

Abnormal eosinophil granules may be seen, together with abnormal neutrophil granules in a variety of inherited conditions including the Chediak–Higashi syndrome (Fig. 3.76) and the Alder–Reilly anomaly (see Fig. 3.56 and Table 3.10). In the Alder–Reilly anomaly eosinophil granules may be grey–green or purple on Romanowsky staining [78]. In the Chediak–Higashi syndrome some granules are blue–grey. A further abnormality, confined to eosinophils and basophils, has been noted in one family, the inheritance being autosomal dominant [115]; inclusions were grey or grey–blue. Cytoplasmic inclusions are present in eosinophils in the May–Hegglin anomaly and in the actin inclusion (Baralise's) syndrome [95].

In acquired disorders of granulopoiesis it is not uncommon to see eosinophils in which some granules have eosinophilic staining character-

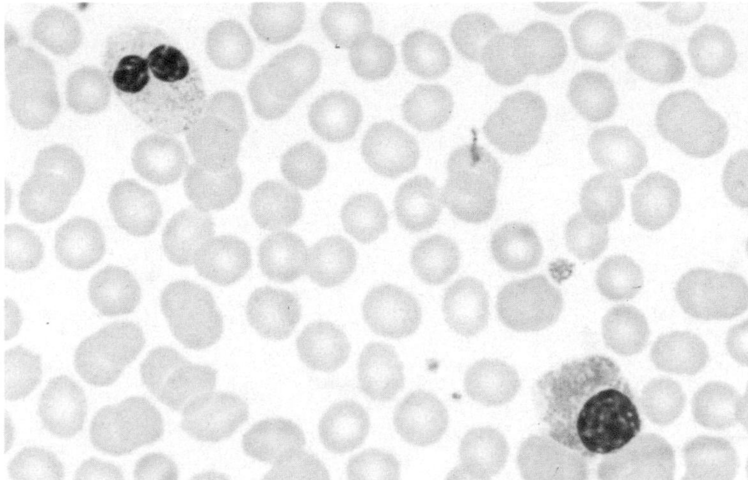

Fig. 3.73 Peripheral blood film of a patient with the inherited Pelger–Hüet anomaly showing a bilobed neutrophil and a non-lobed eosinophil.

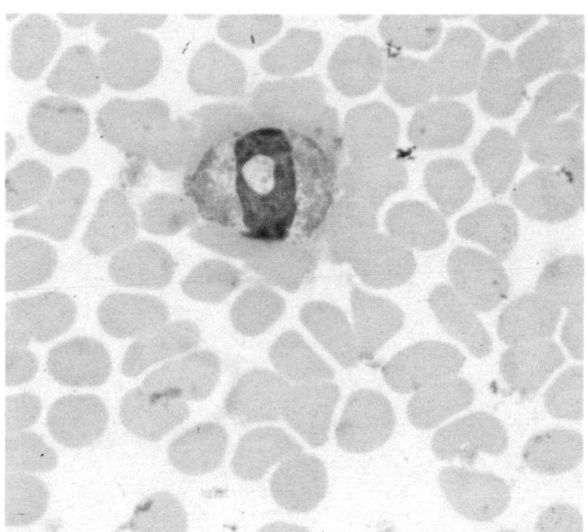

Fig. 3.74 Peripheral blood film of a patient with cyclical oedema with eosinophilia showing an eosinophil with a ring-shaped nucleus.

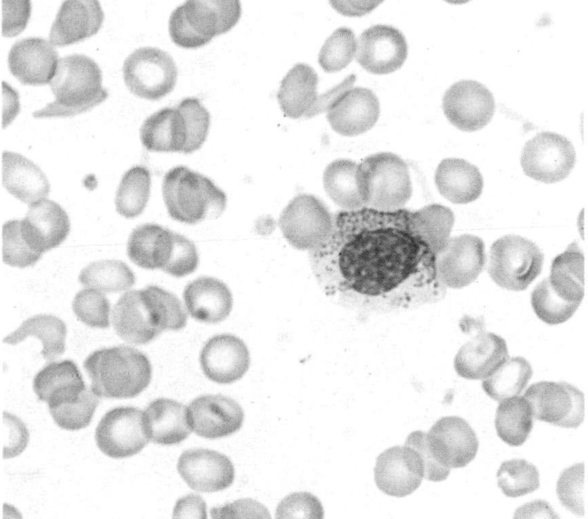

Fig. 3.75 Peripheral blood film of a patient with a myelodysplastic syndrome showing a non-lobulated and hypogranular eosinophil.

istics. This is a sign of cytoplasmic immaturity. Such cells are increased in frequency in CGL (Fig. 3.77), eosinophilic leukaemia and certain categories of AML in which eosinophils are part of the leukaemic clone, particularly cases of acute myelomonocytic leukaemia with eosinophilia associated with inversion of chromosome 16. In all the above cases the abnormal granules are shown on ultrastructural examination to be eosinophil granules with unusual staining characteristics but recent evidence has shown that in some patients with CGL there are also hybrid cells with a mixture of granules of eosinophil type and basophil type [119].

In acquired disorders, eosinophils may be vacuolated or wholly or partly agranular. Hypogranularity could result from defective formation of eosinophil granules in dysmyelopoietic states

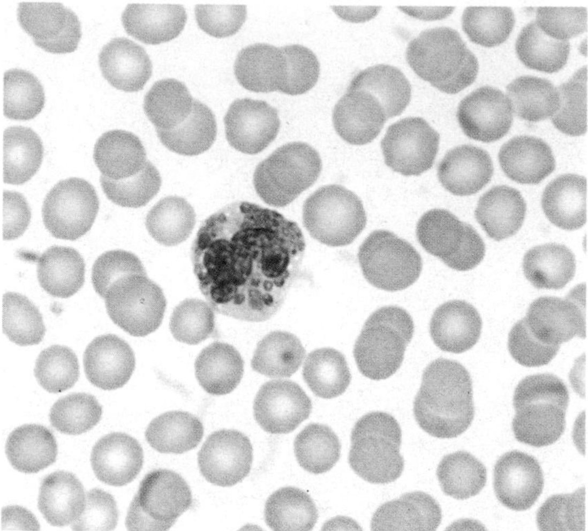

Fig. 3.76 Peripheral blood film of a patient with the Chediak–Higashi syndrome showing an abnormally granulated eosinophil. Courtesy of Dr J. McCallum.

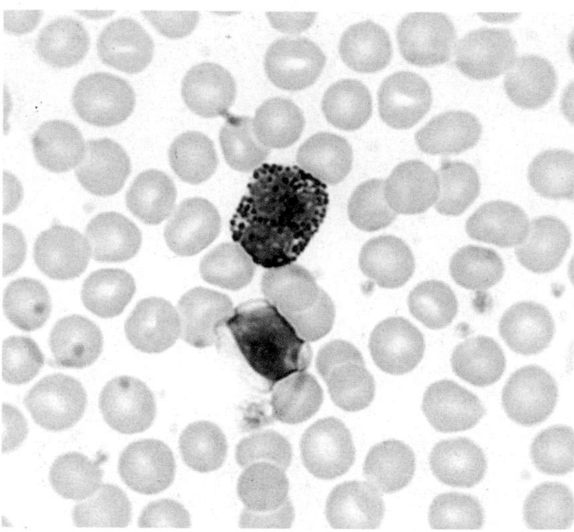

Fig. 3.78 A basophil and a small lymphocyte in the peripheral blood film of a healthy subject.

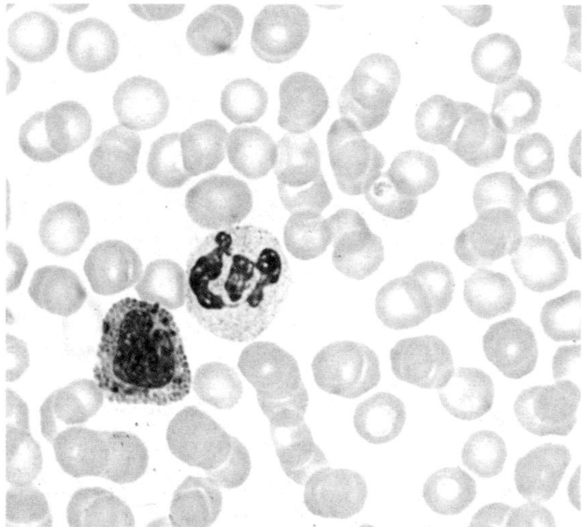

Fig. 3.77 Peripheral blood film of a patient with CGL showing a normal neutrophil and an eosinophil with some basophilic granules.

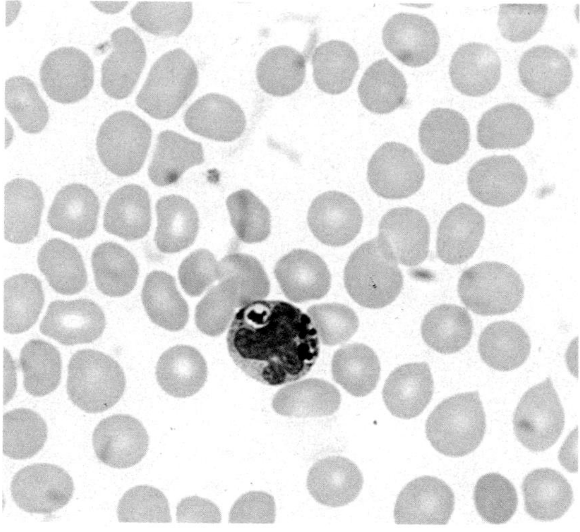

Fig. 3.79 Peripheral blood film of a patient with the Chediak–Higashi syndrome showing an abnormal basophil. Courtesy of Dr J. McCallum.

but since it is usually accompanied by vacuolation it appears likely that in most instances it results from degranulation. Although vacuolation and hypogranularity are characteristic of idiopathic HES the changes are quite non-specific. They can occur also when there is a reactive eosinophilia.

The basophil

The basophil (Fig. 3.78) is of similar size to the neutrophil (10–14 μm in diameter). The nucleus is usually obscured by purple–black granules which are intermediate in size between those of the neutrophil and those of eosinophil. Basophils have abnormal granules in various inherited conditions (Fig. 3.79; also see Table 3.10).

Granules can be reduced in number in myeloproliferative disorders and in the myelodysplastic syndromes (Fig. 3.80), and degranulation can occur in acute allergic conditions (such as urticaria and anaphylactic shock), and during post-prandial hyperlipidaemia. A reduction in the number of granules can also be artefactual since basophil granules are highly water-soluble.

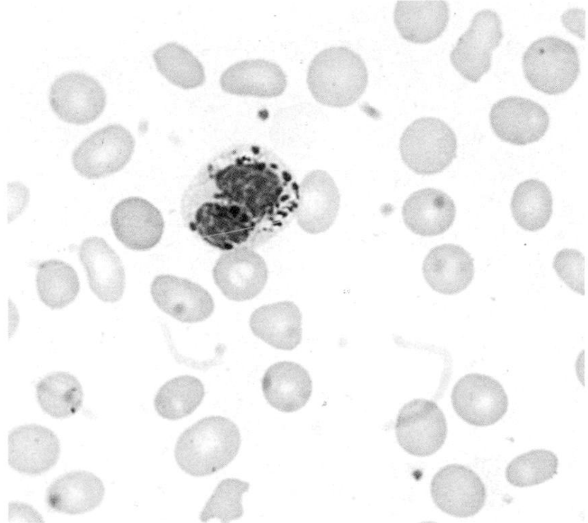

Fig. 3.80 Peripheral blood film of a patient with a myelodysplastic syndrome showing a hypogranular basophil.

The lymphocyte

Peripheral blood lymphocytes vary in diameter from 10 to 16 μm. The smaller lymphocytes (10–12 μm), which predominate, usually have scanty cytoplasm and a round or slightly indented nucleus with condensed chromatin (Fig. 3.81). The larger lymphocytes (12–16 μm) which usually constitute about 10% of circulating lymphocytes, have more abundant cytoplasm and the nuclear chromatin is somewhat less condensed (Fig. 3.82). The smaller lymphocytes are usually circular in outline, whereas larger ones may be somewhat irregular. The cytoplasm, being weakly basophilic, stains pale blue. Lymphocytes may have small numbers of azurophilic granules which contain lysosomal enzymes; occasional larger cells with more abundant cytoplasm have a dozen or so quite prominent granules. Such cells have been designated 'large granular lymphocytes' (Fig. 3.83). In healthy subject they sometimes constitute as many as 10–15% of lymphocytes but usually they are less frequent.

Mature lymphocytes have a nucleolus but, because of the condensation of the chromatin, it is not usually visible in small lymphocytes. In large lymphocytes the nucleolus can sometimes be discerned. Because of the chromatin condensation it is similarly difficult to detect sex chromatin in lymphocytes but sometimes it is visible condensed beneath the nuclear membrane in the larger lymphocytes with more dispersed chromatin [59]. The lymphocytes of infants and children are larger and more pleomorphic than those of adults. In general, the functional subsets of lymphocytes cannot be distinguished morphologically, but lymphokine-activated T cells and natural killer cells are found within the population of large granular lymphocytes.

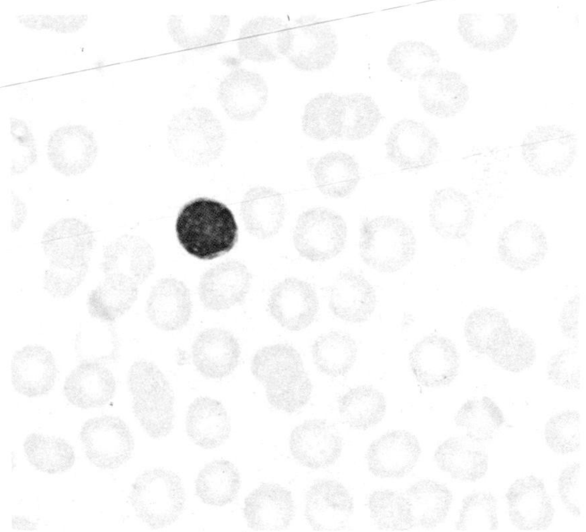

Fig. 3.81 A small lymphocyte in the peripheral blood film of a healthy subject.

Morphological abnormalities of lymphocytes in inherited conditions

Inclusions may be found in lymphocytes in the

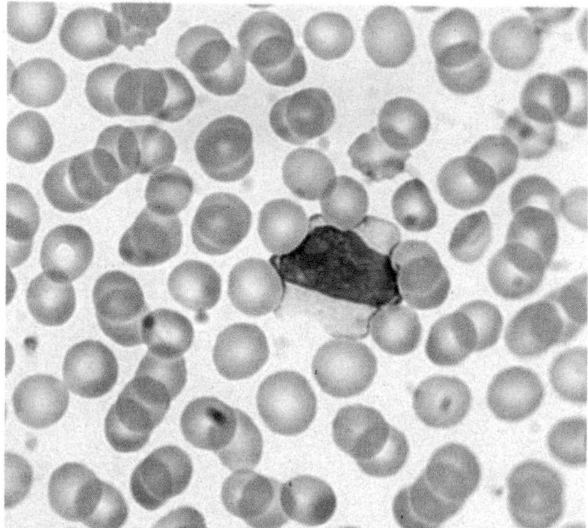

Fig. 3.82 A large lymphocyte in the peripheral blood film of a healthy subject.

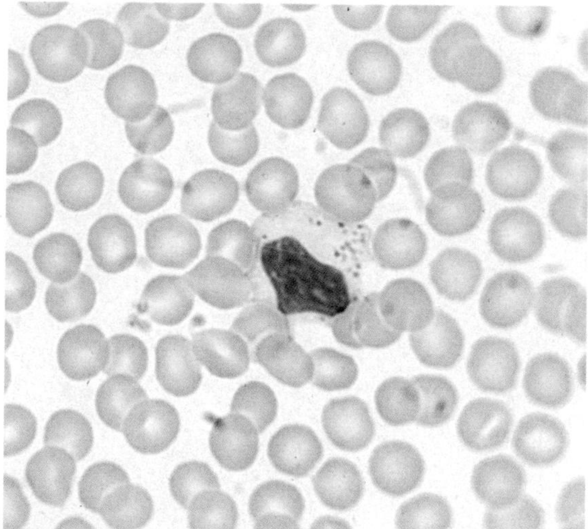

Fig. 3.83 A large granular lymphocyte in the peripheral blood film of a healthy subject.

Chediak–Higashi syndrome and Alder–Reilly anomaly (see Table 3.10). In the Chediak–Higashi syndrome the lymphocyte inclusions can be very large (Fig. 3.84) but in the Alder–Reilly anomaly (Fig. 3.85) they are only a little larger than the granules of normal large granular lymphocytes. Heterozygous carriers of the Chediak–Higashi

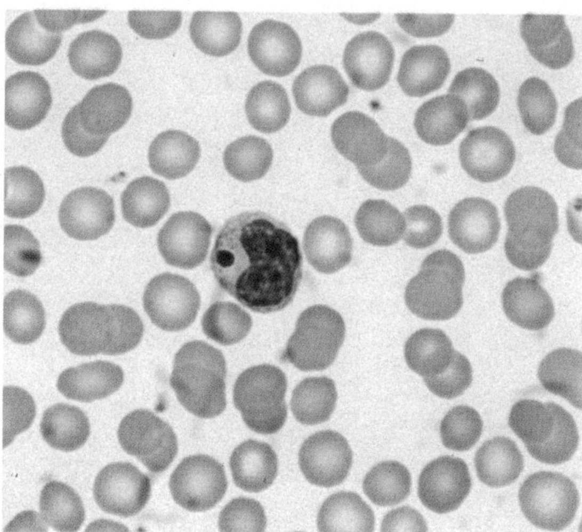

Fig. 3.84 Peripheral blood film of a patient with the Chediak–Higashi syndrome showing a lymphocyte with a large cytoplasmic inclusion. Courtesy of Dr J. McCallum.

syndrome may also have lymphocyte inclusions but only in a small proportion of cells [120]. Occasionally in the Alder–Reilly anomaly, inclusions are found in lymphocytes in the absence of neutrophil abnormalities. Lymphocyte inclusions are usually found when the Alder–Reilly anomaly is consequent on Tay–Sachs disease or on the mucopolysaccharidoses, although they are rare in Morquio's syndrome. Heterozygous carriers for Tay–Sachs disease may have lymphocyte inclusions [78], but in a much lower proportion of lymphocytes than in homozygotes. Alder–Reilly inclusions may be round or comma shaped; they are sometimes surrounded by a halo, and tend to be clustered at one pole of the cell (Fig. 3.85a). When the Alder–Reilly anomaly is due to one of the mucopolysaccharidoses the inclusions stain polychromatically with toluidine blue (Fig. 3.85b) but when the underlying cause is Tay–Sachs disease they do not.

Lymphocyte vacuolation occurs in many inherited metabolic disorders including the following: I-cell disease (Fig. 3.86), the mucopolysaccharidoses, Jordan's anomaly (see p. 80), Niemann–Pick disease, Wolman's disease, Pompe's disease, Tay–Sachs disease, Batten–

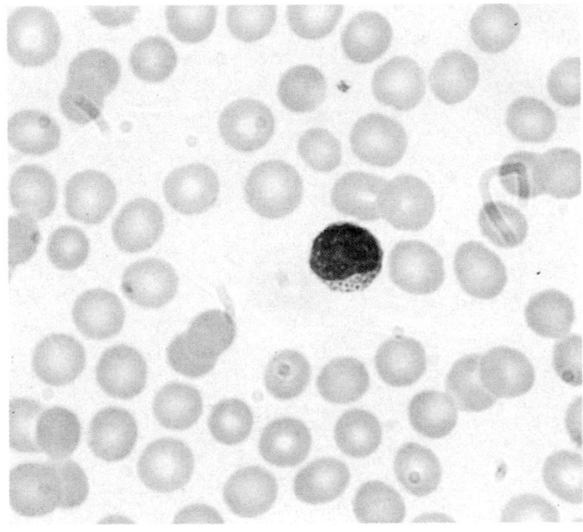
(a)

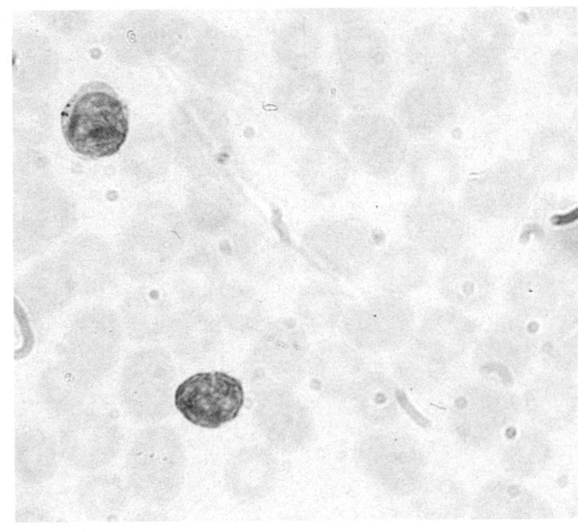
(b)

Fig. 3.85 Peripheral blood film of a patient with the San Filippo's syndrome showing (a) abnormal lymphocyte inclusions which are surrounded by a halo, and (b) blood film of the same patient stained with toluidine blue to show metachromatic staining of the lymphocyte inclusions. Courtesy of Mr A. Dean.

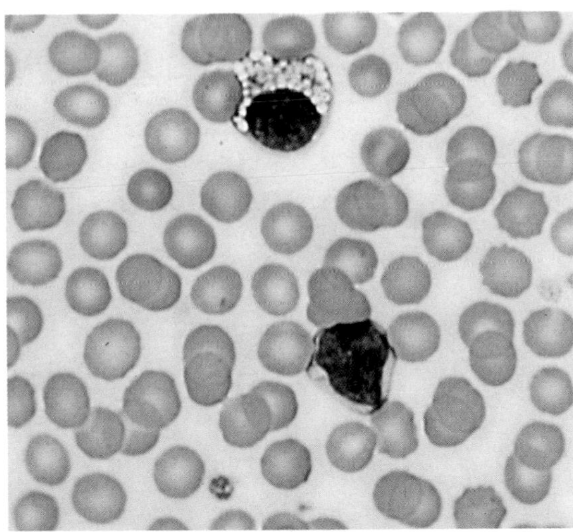

Fig. 3.86 Peripheral blood film of a child with I-cell disease. One of the two lymphocytes shows heavy cytoplasmic vacuolation.

Spielmeyer–Vogt disease and several other rare congenital disorders of metabolism [28,121,122]. In Tay–Sachs disease and Batten–Spielmeyer–Vogt disease heterozygous carriers may also have lymphocyte vacuolation. The metabolic product responsible for vacuolation varies. In some conditions, e.g., Wolman's disease, it is lipid and stains with oil red O, whereas in Pompe's disease it is glycogen and the periodic acid–Schiff (PAS) reaction is positive [92]. In the mucopolysaccharidoses, vacuoles may result from dissolution of abnormal granules. The presence of a pink-staining ring around cytoplasmic vacuoles has been strongly associated with type II mucopolysaccharidosis (Hunter's disease) [123].

Reactive changes in lymphocytes

Lymphocytes can respond to viral infections and other immunological stimuli by an increase in number and cytological alterations. B lymphocytes can transform into plasma cells (Fig. 3.87). Intermediate stages are also seen and are designated plasmacytoid lymphocytes (Fig. 3.88) or Türk cells. Plasmacytoid lymphocytes may contain abundant globular inclusions (Fig. 3.89) composed of immunoglobulin. Such cells have been called 'Mott cells', 'morular cells' or 'grape cells'. Plasmacytoid lymphocytes may also contain crystals of immunoglobulin (Figs 3.90 & 3.91). Both T and B lymphocytes can also transform into immunoblasts, large cells with a central

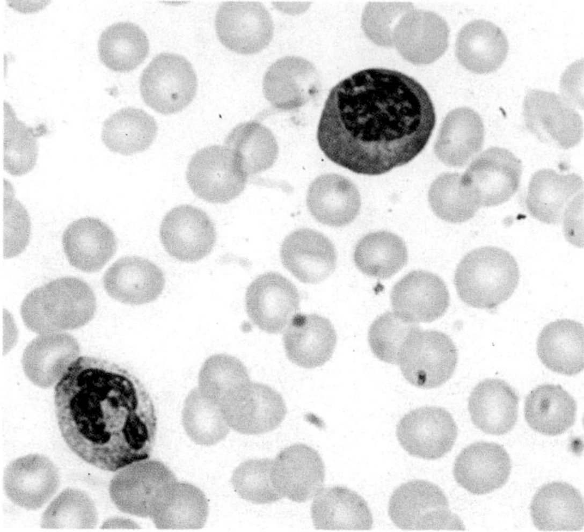

Fig. 3.87 Peripheral blood film of a post-operative patient showing a plasma cell and a neutrophil with toxic granulation and a drumstick.

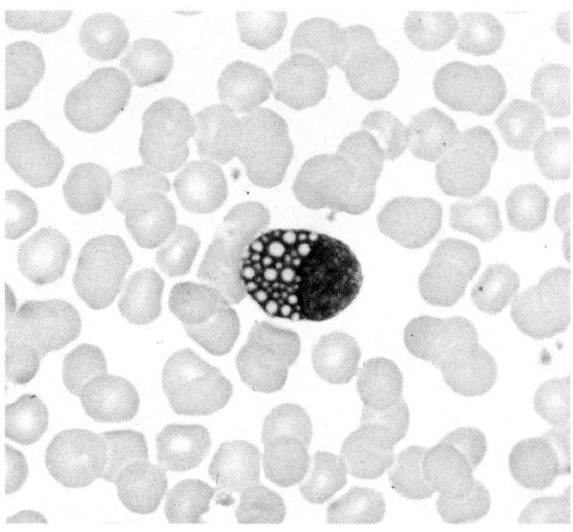

Fig. 3.89 A Mott cell in the peripheral blood.

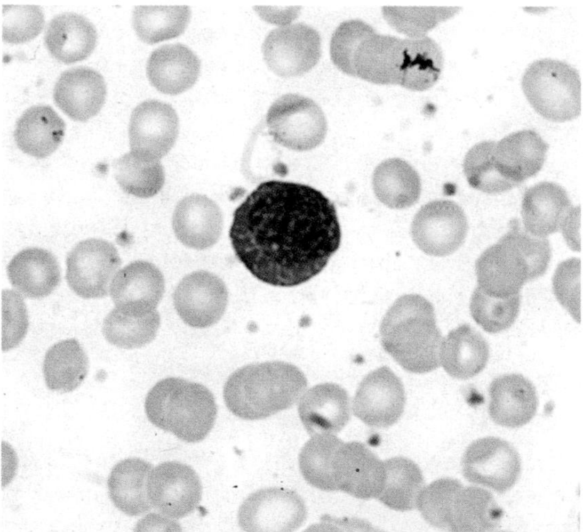

Fig. 3.88 The same peripheral blood film as shown in Fig. 3.87 showing a plasmacytoid lymphocyte.

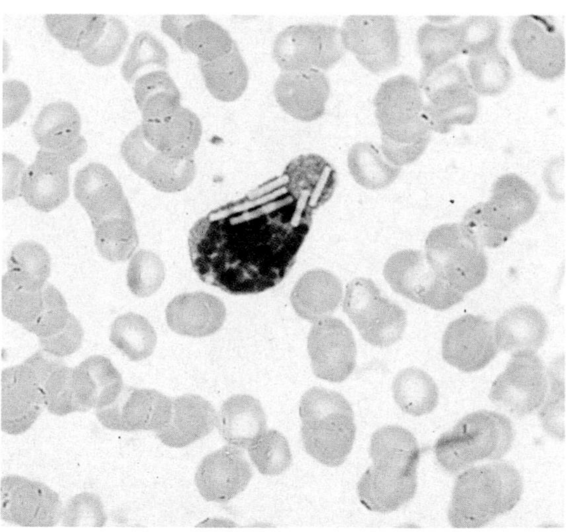

Fig. 3.90 A plasmacytoid lymphocyte containing crystals in the peripheral blood film of a patient with bacterial sepsis.

prominent nucleolus and adundant basophilic cytoplasm (Fig. 3.92). Cells showing other less specific changes in lymphocyte morphology are subsumed under the designation 'atypical lymphocytes' or 'atypical mononuclear cells' (Fig. 3.93). Abnormalities include increased size of the cell, immaturity of the nucleus including lack of chromatin condensation and presence of a nucleolus, irregular nuclear outline or nuclear lobulation, cytoplasmic basophilia, cytoplasmic vacuolation and irregular cellular outline. Multi-lobated lymphocyte nuclei are occasionally seen

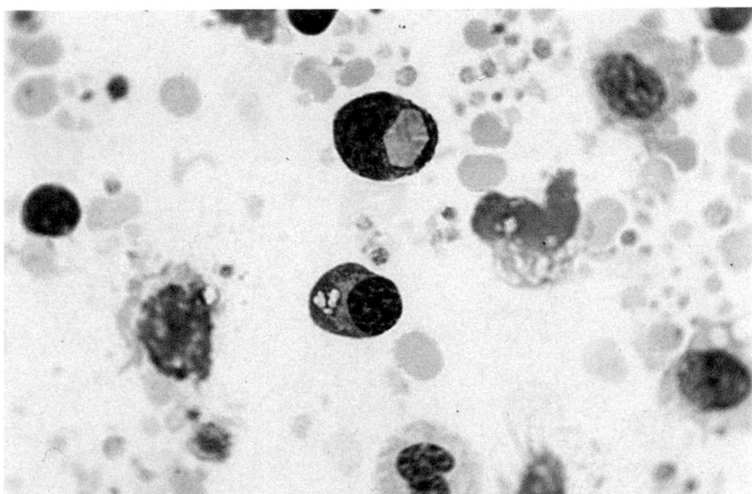

Fig. 3.91 A buffy coat film from the same patient whose peripheral blood film is shown in Fig. 3.90 showing one plasmacytoid lymphocyte containing globular inclusions and another containing a giant crystal.

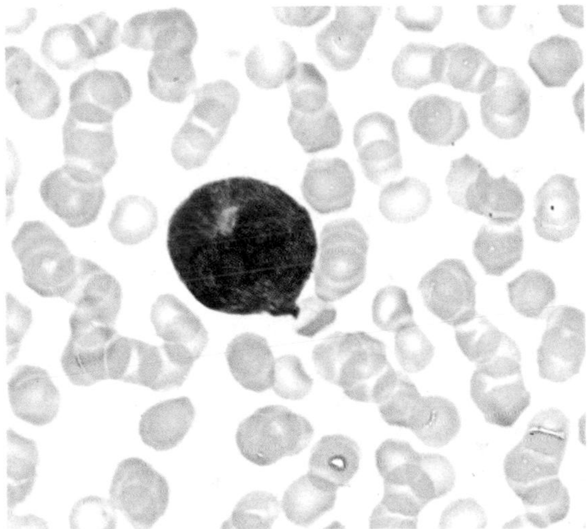

Fig. 3.92 An immunoblast in the peripheral blood film of a patient with infectious mononucleosis.

in reactive conditions [124], although they are more typical of adult T-cell leukaemia/lymphoma (ATLL) (see p. 308). The commonest cause of large numbers of atypical lymphocytes is infectious mononucleosis which is discussed, together with other causes of atypical lymphocytes, on p. 268. Lymphocytes with a clover leaf-shaped nucleus are characteristic of ATLL but can also be seen in carriers of the human T-cell lymphotropic virus type I (HTLV-I) and in infectious mononucleosis, HIV infection and rickettsial infection [124]. Binucleated lymphocytes have been reported after low-dose irradiation and binucleated lymphocytes and lymphocytes with bilobed nuclei in polyclonal B-cell lymphocytosis of cigarette smokers (Fig. 3.94). Infection with the Epstein–Barr virus (EBV) is suspected as a cofactor in the causation of B lymphocytosis of smokers [125]. The number of large granular lymphocytes may also increase as a reactive phenomenon, e.g., in association with chronic viral infection.

Lymphocyte morphology in lymphoproliferative disorders

In most lymphoproliferative disorders the neoplastic cells are cytologically abnormal. Abnormalities show some overlap with those seen in reactive conditions but the majority of lymphoid neoplasms can be recognized as such on cytology alone. Typical features of different conditions are described in Chapter 9.

The plasma cell

Plasma cells are usually tissue cells but, on occasions, they may be present in the peripheral blood (see Figs 3.41 & 3.87). They range in size from somewhat larger than a small lymphocyte

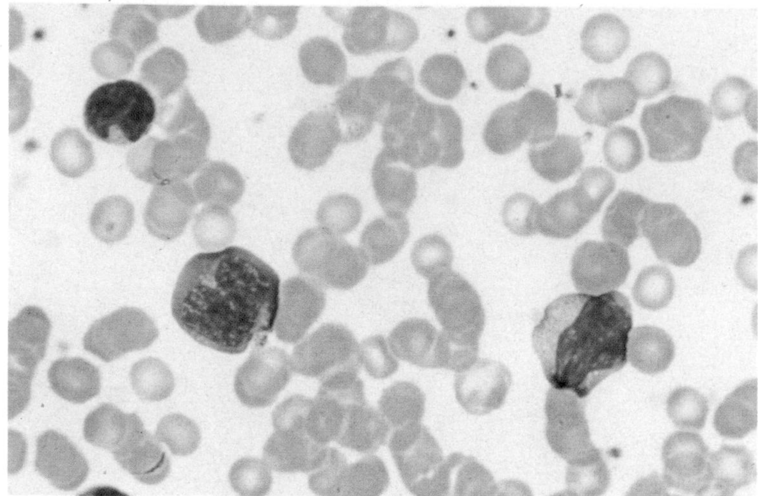

Fig. 3.93 Atypical lymphocytes in the peripheral blood film of a patient with cytomegalovirus infection.

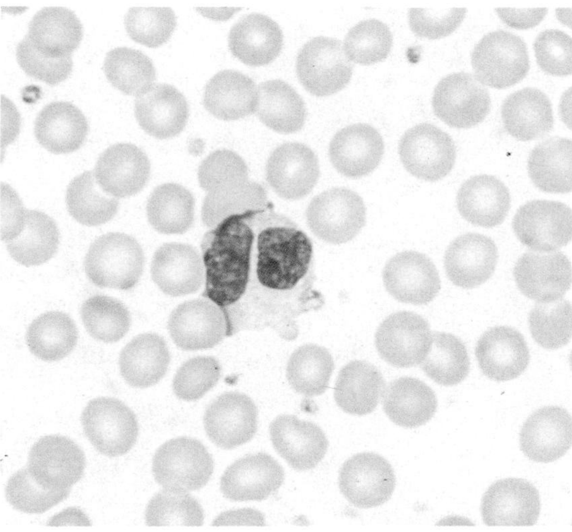

Fig. 3.94 A binucleated lymphocyte in the peripheral blood film of a female cigarette smoker.

(8–10 μm) up to a diameter of about 20 μm and are oval in shape with eccentric nuclei, coarsely clumped chromatin, a moderate amount of strongly basophilic cytoplasm and a less basophilic Golgi zone adjacent to the nucleus. The clock-face chromatin pattern which is seen in tissue sections stained with haematoxylin and eosin is less apparent in circulating plasma cells stained with a Romanowsky stain. Plasma cells may contain secretory products which appear as round or globular inclusions or, less often, crystals.

Circulating plasma cells may be either reactive (to infection or other immunological stimulus) or neoplastic (multiple myeloma, plasma cell leukaemia and related conditions).

The monocyte lineage

The monocyte

The monocyte (Fig. 3.95) is the largest normal peripheral blood cell with a diameter of about 12–20 μm. It has an irregular, often lobulated nucleus and opaque greyish-blue cytoplasm with fine azurophilic granules. The cell outline is often irregular and the cytoplasm may be vacuolated. Sex chromatin may be seen condensed beneath the nuclear membrane [59].

Monocytes may contain abnormal inclusions in various inherited conditions (Fig. 3.96; see also Table 3.10). Since they are phagocytic they are occasionally found to have ingested red cells (Fig. 3.97), cryoglobulin (Fig. 3.98), microorganisms (see pp. 109 and 121) and, rarely, melanin [98] or bilirubin [99]. Following the ingestion and breakdown of malarial parasites there may be residual malarial pigment in the cytoplasm (Fig. 3.99).

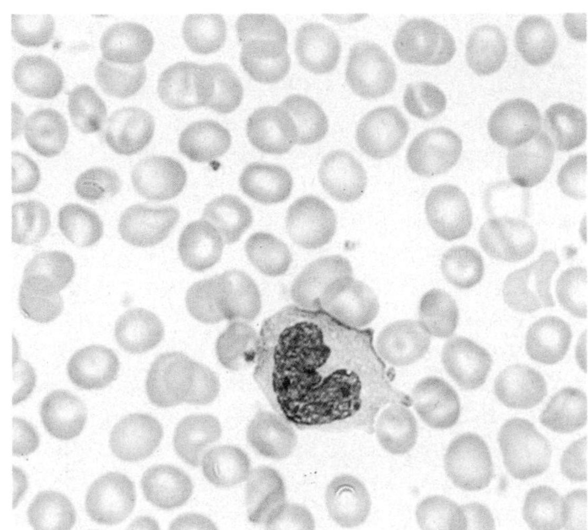

Fig. 3.95 A normal monocyte in the peripheral blood film of a healthy subject.

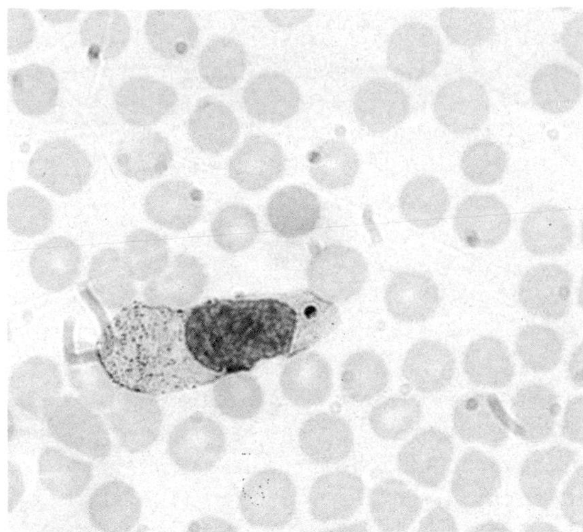

Fig. 3.96 Peripheral blood film of a patient with the Maroteaux–Lamy syndrome showing a monocyte with an abnormal cytoplasmic inclusion. Courtesy of Mr A. Dean.

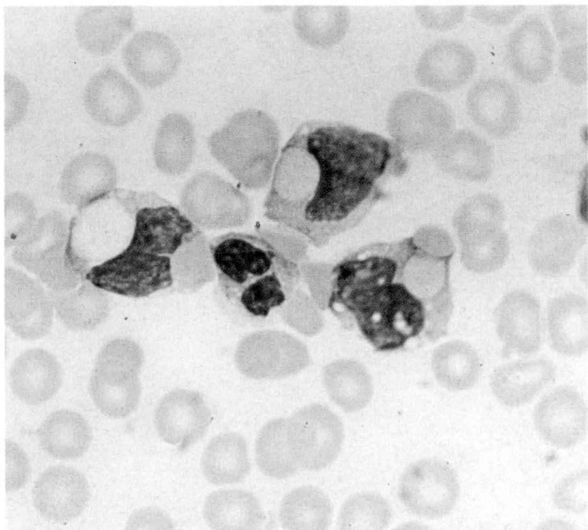

Fig. 3.97 Peripheral blood film of a patient with chronic renal failure taken during haemodialysis showing erythrocytes which have been phagocytosed by monocytes. The patient had a positive direct antiglobulin test but no overt haemolysis.

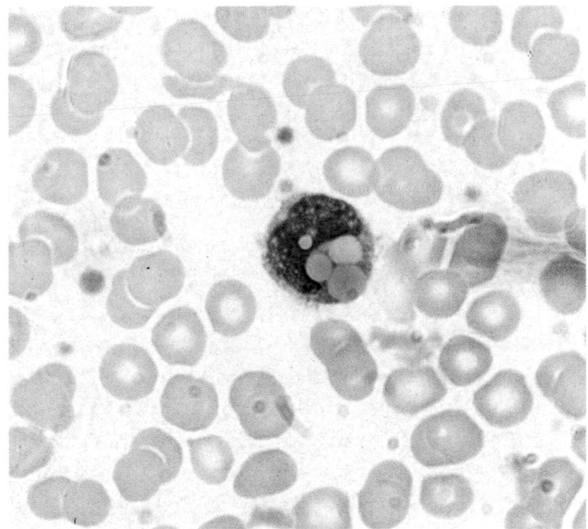

Fig. 3.98 Peripheral blood film of a patient with cryoglobulinaemia showing cryoglobulin within a monocyte. Courtesy of Mr A. Dean.

Monocyte precursors

Monocyte precursors, designated promonocytes and monoblasts, are not normally present in the peripheral blood. Promonocytes have more basophilic cytoplasm and more prominent azurophilic granules than monocytes. They are seen occasionally in reactive conditions as well as in

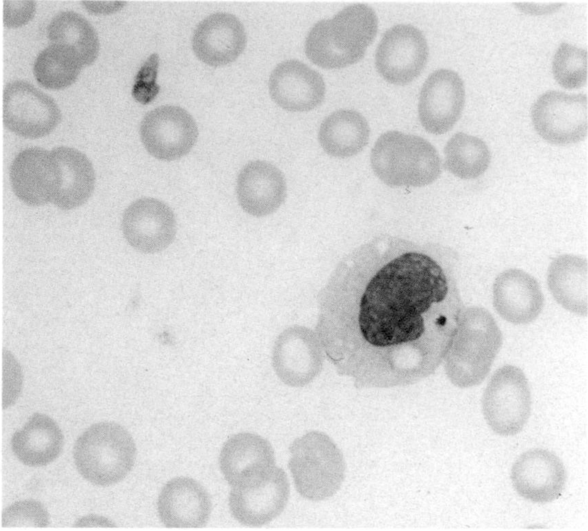

Fig. 3.99 Peripheral blood film of a patient with malaria showing malarial pigment within a monocyte. The film also shows a *Plasmodium falciparum* gametocyte.

leukaemias. Monoblasts are very large cells with voluminous agranular cytoplasm and a large round or lobulated nucleus. They are only seen in the peripheral blood in acute leukaemia with monocytic differentiation (see p. 281).

The macrophage

Monocytes usually develop into macrophages (also called histiocytes) in tissues rather than in the blood. However, occasionally circulating cells with the characteristics of macrophages are seen (Fig. 3.100) [126]. They are associated with a variety of infective and inflammatory states (such as subacute bacterial endocarditis and tuberculosis), malignant disease and parasitic diseases. They may be a little larger than a monocyte or may be very large and multinucleated [101]. The cytoplasm may contain haemopoietic cells, recognizable cellular debris or amorphous debris. In certain inherited metabolic disorders foamy macrophages containing lipid are present in the peripheral blood [122]. Circulating phagocytic cells are also sometimes seen in malignant histiocytosis and acute monocytic leukaemia.

Granulocyte precursors

Granulocytes are generally produced in the bone marrow from myeloblasts, with the intervening stages being promyelocytes, myelocytes and metamyelocytes. On occasion, granulocyte precursors are seen in the blood. The appearance of appreciable numbers of such cells is designated a left shift. If NRBC are also present the blood film is described as leucoerythroblastic. The appearance in the peripheral blood of leucocytes of an earlier stage of development than the metamyelocyte is usually regarded as abnormal unless the blood is from a pregnant woman or a neonate. However, if buffy coat preparations are made metamyelocytes and/or myelocytes are found in about 80% of healthy subjects with a frequency of about one in 1000 granulocytes [127].

The myeloblast

The myeloblast measures 12–20 μm and has a high nucleocytoplasmic ratio and a round or slightly oval nucleus (see Fig. 3.53). The cell is usually somewhat oval and the outline may be slightly irregular. The nucleus has a diffuse chromatin pattern and one to five (most often two or three) not very prominent nucleoli. The cytoplasm is pale blue. A myeloblast is often defined as a cell which has no granules visible by light microscopy, although ultrastructural examination and cytochemistry show that granules are actually present. It is now becoming more common for cells with a relatively small number of granules but without the other characteristics of promyelocytes (see below) to also be included in the myeloblast category, in accordance with the recommendations made by the French–American–British (FAB) group in relation to the diagnosis of AML [128]. Although a myeloblast does have characteristic cytological features it is not always possible to make the distinction between an agranular myeloblast and a lymphoblast on an MGG-stained film.

Circulating myeloblasts in haematological neoplasms may show abnormal cytological features such as the presence of Auer rods (see Fig. 3.59) or cytoplasmic vacuoles. The presence of

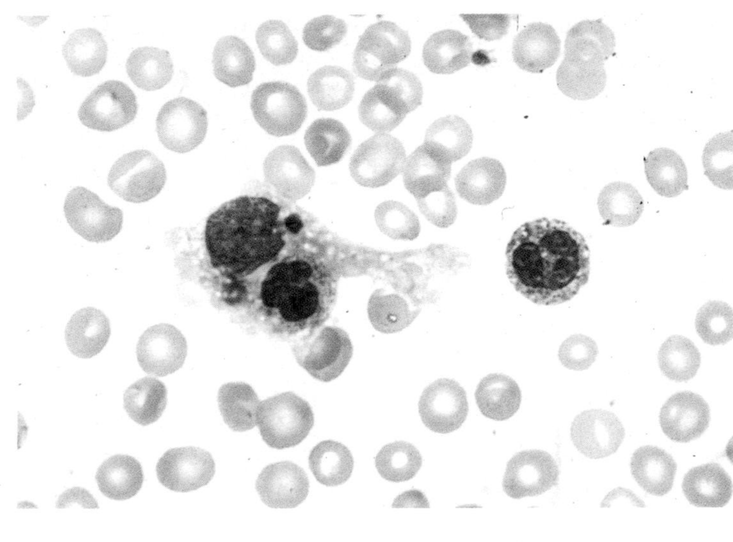

Fig. 3.100 A phagocytic macrophage in a peripheral blood film. Courtesy of Dr Z. Currimbhoy, Bombay.

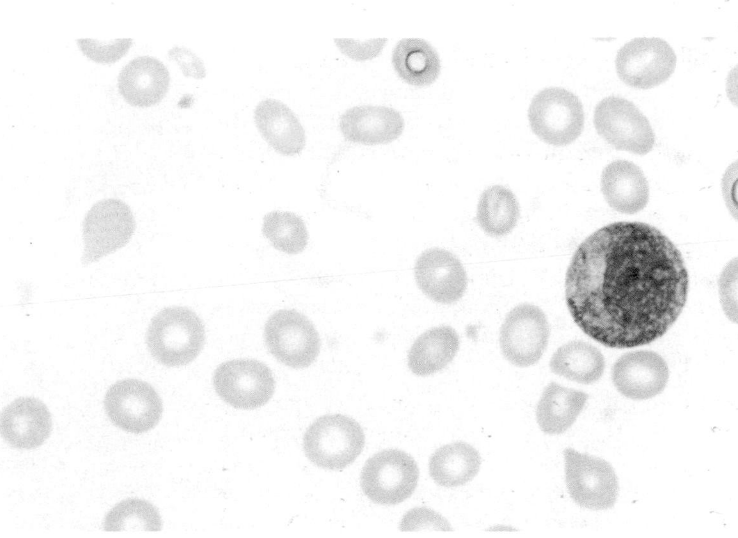

Fig. 3.101 A promyelocyte in the peripheral blood film of a patient with megaloblastic anaemia. The nucleolus and the Golgi zone are readily detectable. The film also shows anisocytosis and tear drop poikilocytes.

even one blast cell with an Auer rod indicates the existence of a myeloid neoplasm.

The promyelocyte

The promyelocyte is larger than the myeloblast with a diameter of 15–25 μm (Fig. 3.101). The cell is round or slightly oval. In comparison with the myeloblast, the nucleocytoplasmic ratio is lower and the cytoplasm is more basophilic. The nuclear chromatin shows only slight condensation and nucleoli are apparent. (Clumped or condensed chromatin, known as heterochromatin is genetically inactive, whereas diffuse euchromatin is genetically active; cellular maturation is associated with progressive condensation of chromatin.) The promyelocyte nucleus is oval with an indentation in one side. The Golgi zone is apparent as a much less basophilic area adjacent to the nuclear indentation. The promyelocyte contains primary or azurophilic granules which surround the Golgi zone and are scattered through the remainder of the cytoplasm.

Morphologically abnormal promyelocytes may be seen in the peripheral blood in several subtypes of AML (see p. 279).

The myelocyte

The myelocyte is smaller than the promyelocyte, measuring 10–20 μm in diameter. It can be identified as belonging to the neutrophil, eosinophil or basophil lineage by the presence of specific or secondary granules with the staining characteristics of these cell lines (Figs 3.102–3.104). Eosinophil myelocytes may have some granules with basophilic staining characteristics. The myelocyte nucleus is oval and sometimes has a slight indentation in one side. Chromatin shows a moderate degree of coarse clumping and nucleoli are not apparent. The cytoplasm is more acidophilic than that of the promyelocyte and the Golgi zone is much less apparent. Neutrophil and eosinophil myelocytes may appear in the blood in reactive conditions and in leukaemias. The presence of basophil myelocytes in the peripheral blood is essentially confined to the leukaemias. In acute leukaemias, circulating myelocytes may show morphological abnormalities such as hypogranularity or abnormally large granules.

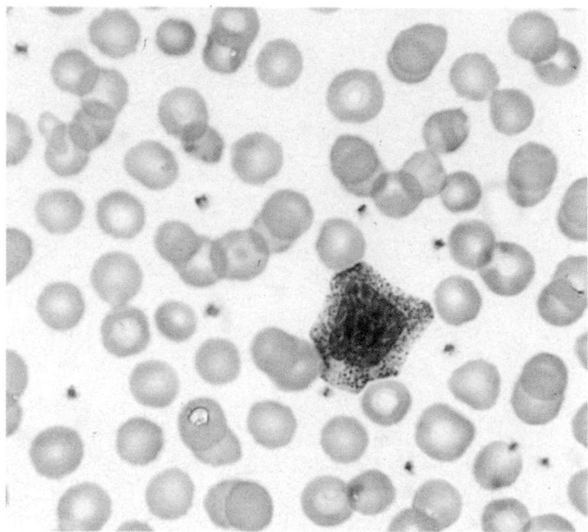

Fig. 3.102 A neutrophil myelocyte in the peripheral blood film of a healthy pregnant woman.

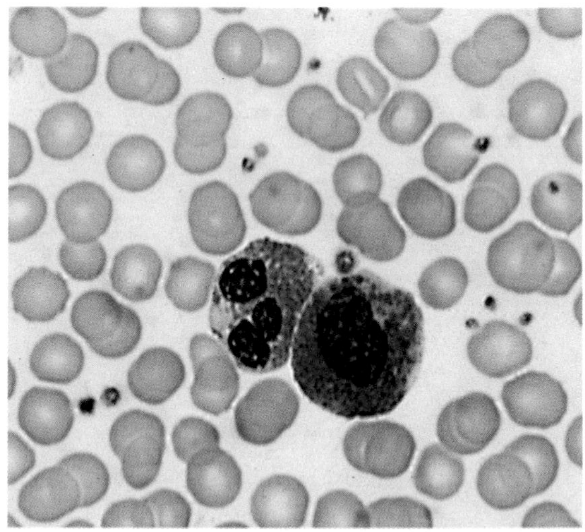

Fig. 3.103 An eosinophil and an eosinophil myelocyte in the peripheral blood film of a patient with CGL.

The metamyelocyte

The metamyelocyte measures 10–12 μm in diameter. Its chromatin is clumped and its nucleus is definitely indented or U-shaped (Fig. 3.105). Protein synthesis has stopped. A neutrophil metamyelocyte has acidophilic cytoplasm while that of an eosinophil myelocyte is weakly basophilic. Small numbers of neutrophil metamyelocytes are occasionally seen in the blood in healthy subjects. They are commonly present in reactive conditions. Some eosinophil metamyelocytes may be seen in patients with eosinophilia.

The mast cell

Mast cells are essentially tissue cells. They are extremely rare in the peripheral blood of normal subjects. They are large cells with a diameter of 20–30 μm. The cellular outline is somewhat irregular. The cytoplasm is packed with basophilic granules which do not obscure the central nucleus (Fig. 3.106). The nucleus is relatively small and round or, more often, oval with a dispersed chromatin pattern. In systemic mastocytosis and

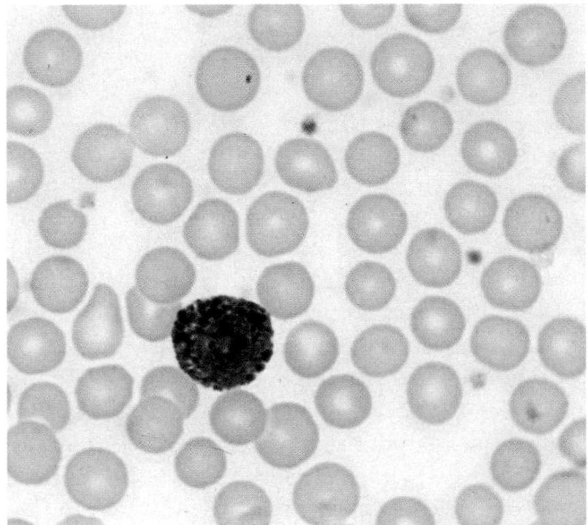

Fig. 3.104 A basophil myelocyte in the peripheral blood film of a patient with CGL.

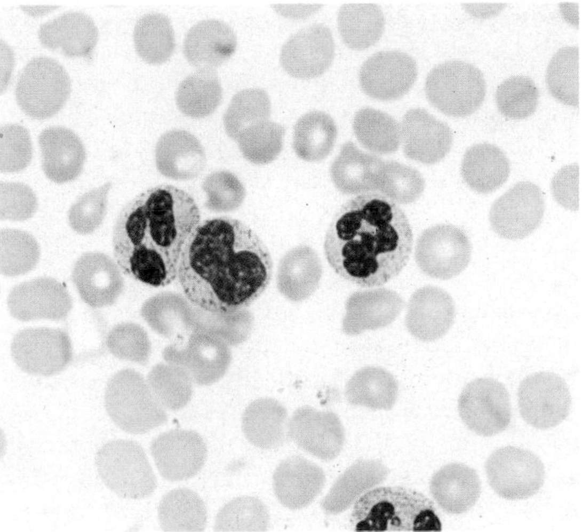

Fig. 3.105 A metamyelocyte and two neutrophils in the peripheral blood film of a patient with CGL.

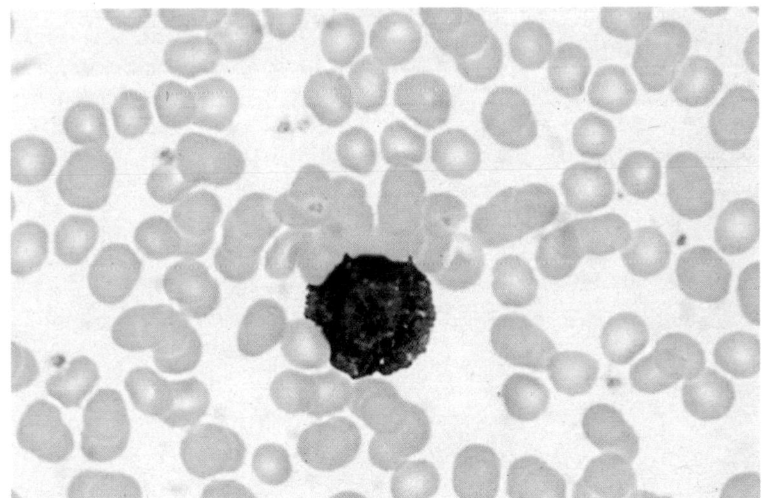

Fig. 3.106 A mast cell in the peripheral blood film of a patient having a health check for non-specific symptoms.

in mast cell leukaemia (see p. 280) circulating mast cells are cytologically quite abnormal and may have lobulated nuclei, scanty granules or a denser chromatin pattern.

Disintegrated cells

The finding of more than a small percentage of disintegrated cells in a blood film is of significance. It may indicate that several days have elapsed since the blood was taken from the patient and the specimen is unfit for testing. When disintegration of cells is due to prolonged storage the granulocytes are smeared preferentially and, if an attempt is made to perform a differential count, there will appear to be neutropenia.

If disintegration of cells occurs in films made from fresh blood it indicates that cells are abnormally fragile. Disintegrated lymphocytes, usually called 'smear cells' or 'smudge cells', are common in CLL (Fig. 3.107). Their presence is of some use in diagnosis since they are not common in non-Hodgkin's lymphoma from which a distinction may have to be made. The fact that these cells are intact *in vivo* and are smeared during preparation of the film is demonstrated by the fact that they are not present if a film of the same blood is made by centrifugation. Although smeared lymphocytes are characteristic of CLL they are not pathognomonic, being seen occasionally in non-Hodgkin's lymphoma and even sometimes in reactive conditions such as whooping cough. Other abnormal cells, e.g., blast cells in AML, may also disintegrate on spreading the blood film. The term 'basket cell' has been applied to a very large, spread out smear cell. Disintegrated cells, if at all frequent, should be included in the differential count (see p. 23).

Platelets and circulating megakaryocytes

When platelets are examined in a blood film an assessment should be made of their number (by relating them to the number of red cells), size and morphology. The film should be examined for platelet aggregates or platelet satellitism. Megakaryocytes are seen, although rarely, in the blood of healthy people. Their number is increased in certain disease states.

Platelets

Normal platelets

The normal platelet measures 1–3 μm in diameter. Platelets contain fine azurophilic granules which may be dispersed throughout the cytoplasm or concentrated in the centre; in the latter case the central granule-containing cytoplasm is known as the granulomere and the peripheral, weakly basophilic agranular cytoplasm as the hyalomere (see Fig. 3.13). Platelets contain several different types of granules of which the α-granules are the equivalent of the azurophilic granules seen on light microscopy.

In EDTA-anticoagulated blood, platelets generally remain separate from one another whereas in native blood they show a tendency to aggregate (see Figs 1.6–1.8). In Glanzmann's thrombasthenia, a severe inherited defect of platelet aggregation, the normal tendency of platelets to aggregate when films are made from native blood is completely absent.

Abnormalities of platelet size

Platelet size can be assessed by comparing the

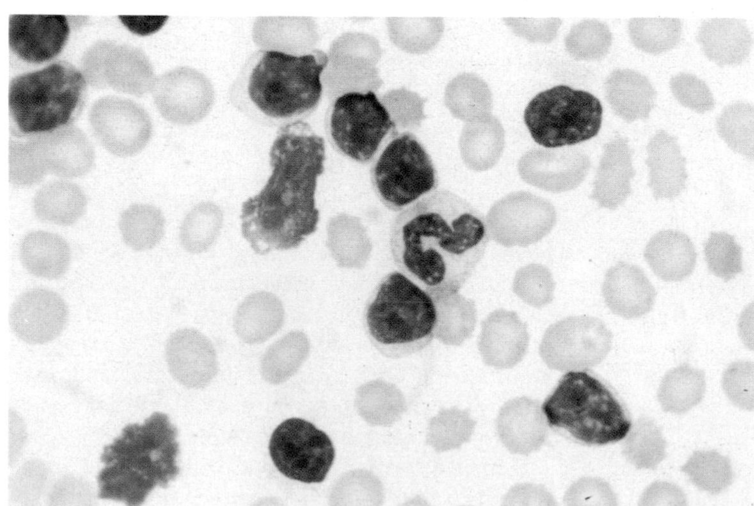

Fig. 3.107 Intact lymphocytes and several disintegrated cells (smear cells or smudge cells) in the peripheral blood film of a patient with CLL.

diameter of the platelets with the diameter of erythrocytes, or platelet diameter can be measured by means of an ocular micrometer.

Platelet size in healthy subjects varies inversely with the platelet count but this variation is not sufficiently great to be detected when a blood film is examined by light microscopy. A sufficient size increase to be detectable microscopically occurs in certain congenital abnormalities of thrombopoiesis and in certain disease states (Table 3.11). Large platelets (i.e., those with a diameter greater than 4 μm) are designated macrothrombocytes. Particularly large platelets with diameters similar to those of red cells or lymphocytes are often referred to as giant platelets (Fig. 3.108). When platelet turnover is increased, platelets are usually large. The absence of large platelets in patients with thrombocytopenia is therefore of diagnostic significance; it suggests that there is a defect of platelet production. Decreased platelet size is less common than increased size but it is a feature of the Wiskott–Aldrich syndrome (Fig. 3.109).

Other abnormalities of platelet morphology and distribution

Platelets which are lacking in α-granules appear grey or pale blue. This occurs as a rare congenital defect known as the grey platelet syndrome [132]. More commonly, apparently agranular platelets result from discharge of platelet granules *in vivo* or *in vitro* or from formation of defective platelets by dysplastic megakaryocytes (Fig. 3.110). If venepuncture is difficult, stimulation of platelets may cause granule release. This is sometimes associated with platelet aggregation so that masses of agranular platelets may be seen. Rarely, a similar phenomenon is caused by a plasma factor causing *in vitro* platelet degranulation and aggregation [133]; in one patient the factor originated from a leiomyosarcoma [134]. Cardiopulmonary bypass can cause release of α-granules with the agranular platelets continuing to circulate. In hairy cell leukaemia, agranular platelets probably result from degranulation within abnormal vascular channels, pseudosinuses lined by hairy cells, which are present in the spleen and other organs. Some agranular platelets are commonly present in the

Table 3.11 Some causes of large platelets

	Inheritance
Congenital	
Bernard–Soulier syndrome*	AR
Heterozygous carriers of Bernard–Soulier syndrome [129]	
Epstein's syndrome (associated with hereditary deafness and nephritis)* [130]	AD
Mediterranean macrothrombocytosis* [47]	Uncertain
Chediak–Higashi anomaly	AR
May–Hegglin anomaly	AD
Associated with increased nuclear projections in neutrophils [67]	AD
In occasional families with Marfan's syndrome and other inherited connective tissue defects [131]	Varied
Grey platelet syndrome* [132]	AR
Hereditary thrombocytopenia with giant platelets but without other morphological abnormality or associated disease*	AR or AD
Acquired	
Immune thrombocytopenic purpura, primary and secondary*	
Thrombotic thrombocytopenic purpura (TTP)*	
Disseminated intravascular coagulation*	
Myeloproliferative disorders — PRV, CGL (chronic phase or in transformation),* idiopathic myelofibrosis,* essential thrombocythaemia	
Myelodysplastic syndromes*	
Megakaryoblastic leukaemia*	
Postsplenectomy and hyposplenic states (including sickle cell anaemia)	

* May also have thrombocytopenia.
AD, autosomal dominant; AR, autosomal recessive.

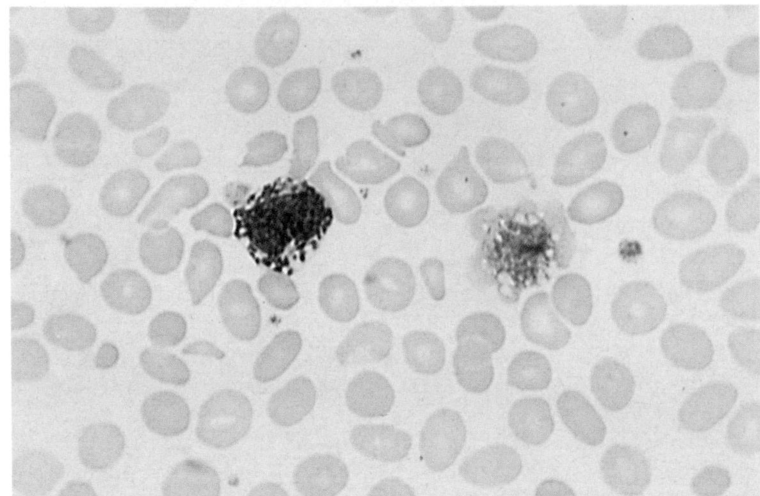

Fig. 3.108 A giant platelet, almost as large as the adjacent basophil, in the peripheral blood of a patient with idiopathic myelofibrosis. The film also shows a platelet of normal size. The red cells show poikilocytosis.

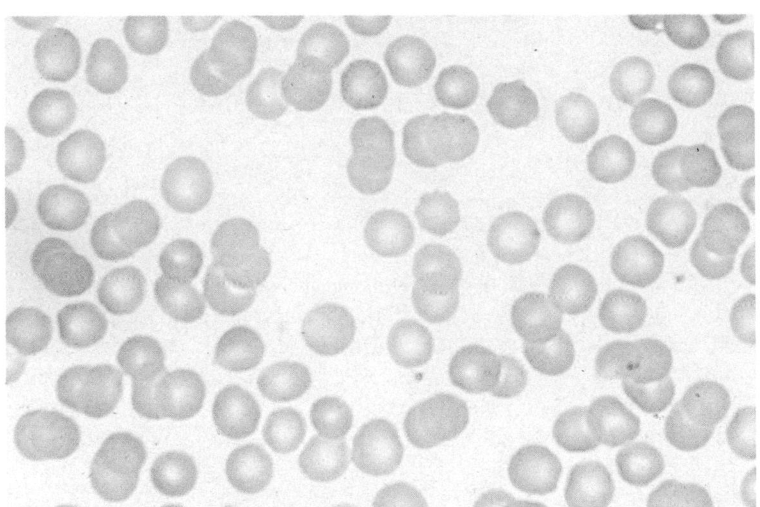

Fig. 3.109 The peripheral blood film of a patient with Wiskott–Aldrich syndrome showing thrombocytopenia and small platelets.

myelodysplastic syndromes and are likely to indicate defective thrombopoiesis. Agranular platelets in the myeloproliferative disorders may result either from defective thrombopoiesis or from discharge of granules from hyperaggregable platelets. In both myelodysplastic and myeloproliferative conditions platelets may be giant and of abnormal shape, features again indicative of abnormal thrombopoiesis. In the May–Hegglin anomaly platelets may not only be larger than normal but also of unusual shape, e.g., cigar-shaped [135].

Various particles, e.g., the parasites of *Plasmodium vivax* [136], may be found within platelets. This is unlikely to represent phagocytosis; it is probably equivalent to emperipolesis, a phenomenon in which white cells and other particles enter the surface connected membrane system of the megakaryocyte.

Platelet aggregation may be consequent on platelet stimulation during skin-prick or venepuncture, or be immunoglobulin mediated. When there is incipient clotting of blood the platelets

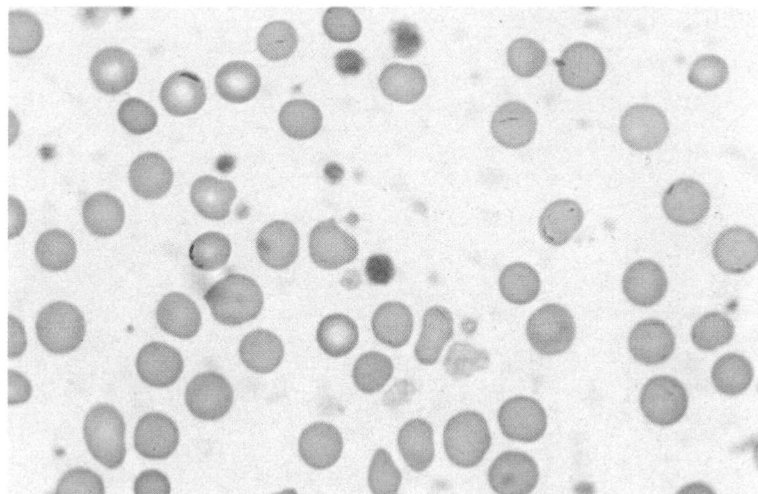

Fig. 3.110 The peripheral blood film of a patient with CGL showing a mixture of normally granulated and agranular platelets. There is also platelet anisocytosis.

may be partly degranulated and the blood film may, in addition, show fibrin strands. Platelet aggregation occurring as an *in vitro* phenomenon, particularly in EDTA-anticoagulated blood, is mediated by a cold antibody with specificity against platelet glycoprotein IIb/IIIa [137]. This antibody is not known to be of any clinical significance. It is important to note the presence of aggregates since they are often associated with a factitiously low platelet count.

Platelet satellitism (Fig. 3.111) is an *in vitro* phenomenon occurring particularly in EDTA-anticoagulated blood. It is induced by a plasma factor, usually either IgG or IgM. Platelets adhere to and encircle neutrophils and some may be phagocytosed [138]. Neutrophils can be joined together by a layer of platelets. Platelet satellitism does not appear to be of any clinical significance, although it may lead to a factitiously low platelet count.

Megakaryocytes

Megakaryocytes are rarely seen in the blood of healthy adults. They are released by the bone marrow but most are trapped in the pulmonary capillaries. However, the fact that they are detectable, albeit in low numbers, in venous blood arising from parts of the body lacking haemopoietic marrow indicates that some can pass through the pulmonary capillaries. Since their concentration is, on average, only between five and seven per millilitre they are more likely to be seen in buffy coat preparations or when special concentration procedures are carried out. In healthy subjects, 99% of the megakaryocytes in peripheral venous blood are almost bereft of cytoplasm (Fig. 3.112) but rare cells with copious cytoplasm are seen. The number of megakaryocytes is increased in the blood of neonates and young infants and also post-partum, post-operatively and in patients with infection, inflammation, malignancy, disseminated intravascular coagulation and myeloproliferative disorders [139–142]. The proportion of intact megakaryocytes with plentiful cytoplasm is increased in infants [140] and in patients with idiopathic myelofibrosis and CGL [142].

Abnormal megakaryocytes and megakaryoblasts may be seen in the blood in pathological conditions. Micromegakaryocytes are seen in some patients with myelodysplastic syndromes, idiopathic myelofibrosis (Fig. 3.113) and CGL, particularly CGL in transformation. They are small diploid mononuclear cells with a diameter of 7–10 μm, which are not always immediately identifiable as megakaryocytes. The nucleus is round or slightly irregular with dense chromatin. Cytoplasm varies from scanty to moderate in amount; when scanty, the nucleus may appear 'bare' but electron microscopy shows that such cells usually have a thin rim of cytoplasm.

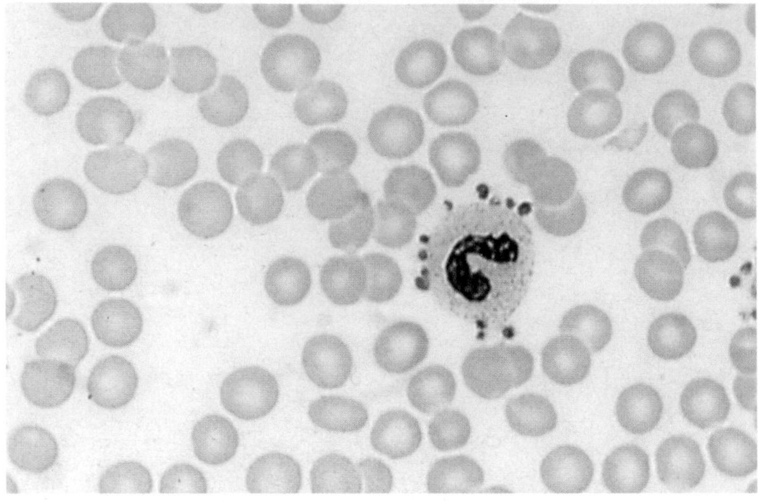

Fig. 3.111 Platelet satellitism.

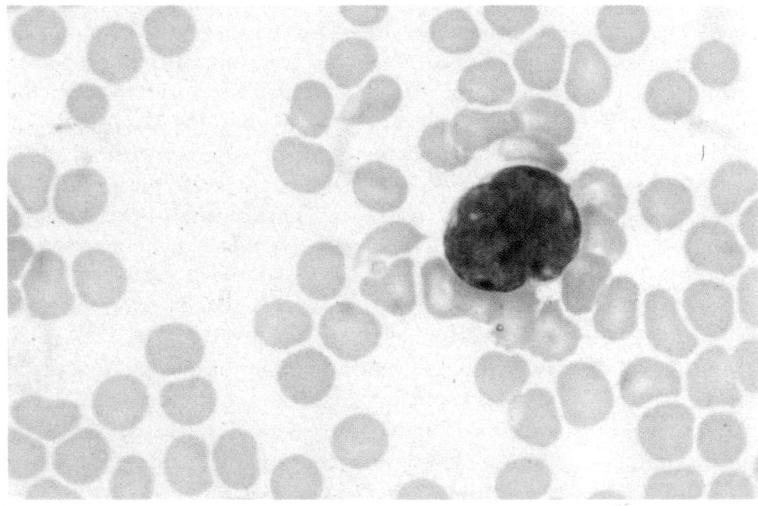

Fig. 3.112 A bare megakaryocyte nucleus in the peripheral blood film of a healthy subject; the size and lobulation of the nucleus indicates its origin from a polyploid megakaryocyte.

Cytoplasm is weakly basophilic. There may be cytoplasmic vacuolation or a few or numerous cytoplasmic granules. Sometimes there are small cytoplasmic protrusions or 'blebs'.

Megakaryoblasts (Fig. 3.114) vary from about 10 μm in diameter up to about 15–20 μm or larger. Smaller ones may resemble lymphoblasts and have no distinguishing features. Larger megakaryoblasts have a diffuse chromatin pattern and cytoplasmic basophilia varying from weak to moderately strong. Cytoplasm varies from scanty to moderate in amount and may form blebs. Megakaryoblasts are often not identifiable as such by cytology alone.

Blood film in healthy subjects

Healthy adult

The blood film in a normal adult shows only slight variation in size and shape of red cells (see Figs 3.13 & 3.42). White cells which are normally present are neutrophils, neutrophil band forms, eosinophils, basophils, lymphocytes and

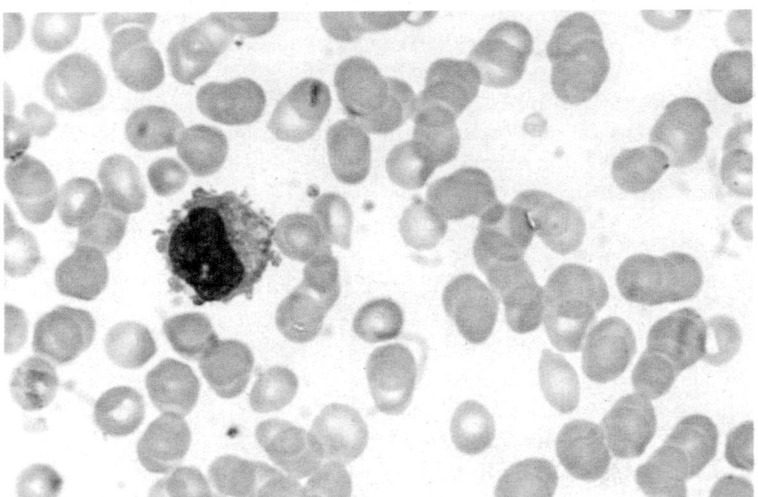

Fig. 3.113 A micromegakaryocyte in the peripheral blood film of a patient with idiopathic myelofibrosis.

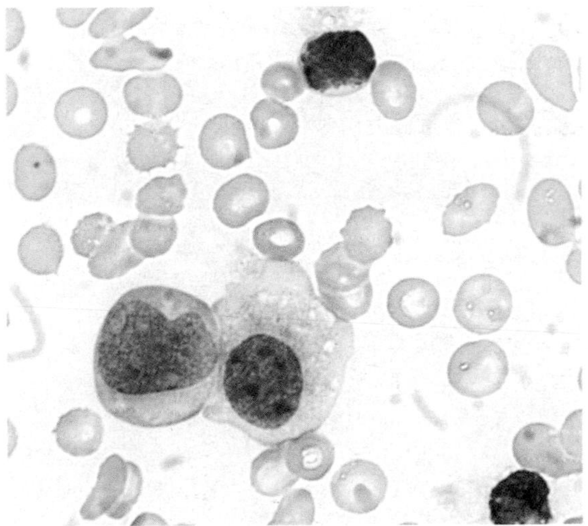

Fig. 3.114 Peripheral blood film of a patient with megakaryoblastic transformation of CGL showing three megakaryoblasts. One of these is large with no distinguishing features, another shows some maturation and has cytoplasm which resembles that of a platelet while the third resembles a lymphoblast. The lineage was confirmed by ultrastructural cytochemistry.

monocytes. Metamyelocytes and myelocytes are rare. Megakaryocytes, usually in the form of almost bare nuclei, are very rare. Platelets are present in such numbers that the ratio of red cells to platelets is of the order of 10–40 : 1.

Pregnancy

During pregnancy the red cells show more variation in size and shape than is seen in non-pregnant women. The MCV also increases, being greatest around 30–35 weeks of gestation. This change occurs independently of any deficiency of vitamin B_{12} or folic acid, although there is an increased need for folic acid during pregnancy. The Hb falls, the lowest concentration being at 30–34 weeks of gestation. Although both iron and folic acid deficiency have an increased prevalence during pregnancy this commonly observed fall in the Hb is not due to a deficiency state, and in fact occurs despite an increase in the total red cell mass. It is consequent on an even greater increase in the total plasma volume. The erythrocyte sedimentation rate (ESR) and rouleaux formation are also increased. Polychromatic cells are more numerous and the reticulocyte count is increased with peak levels of 6% at 25–30 weeks.

The WBC, neutrophil count and monocyte count rise with neutrophils commonly showing toxic granulation and Döhle bodies. A left shift occurs: band forms, metamyelocytes and myelocytes are common, and occasional promyelocytes and even myeloblasts may be seen. The WBC and neutrophil count continue to rise till term. The absolute lymphocyte and eosinophil counts fall.

The platelet count and platelet size do not usually change during normal pregnancy, but the platelet count may fall and the mean platelet volume (MPV) may rise if pregnancy is complicated by toxaemia. Pregnancy-associated thrombocytopenia of unknown mechanism occurs in a small proportion of women with an uncomplicated pregnancy. Normal ranges for haematological parameters during pregnancy are given in Table 5.12.

Infancy and childhood

In normal infants and children red blood cells are hypochromic and microcytic in comparison with those of adults and the MCV and MCH are lower. Iron deficiency is common in infancy and childhood but the difference from adult norms is present even when there is no iron deficiency. The male–female difference in Hb, RBC and PCV/Hct is not present before puberty.

The lymphocyte count of children is higher than that of adults and lymphocyte percentage commonly exceeds the neutrophil percentage ('reversed differential'). A greater proportion of large lymphocytes is commonly observed and some of these may have visible nucleoli. Reactive changes in lymphocytes in response to infection and other immunological stimuli are far commoner than in adults and even apparently completely healthy children may have a few 'atypical' lymphocytes.

Normal ranges for haematological parameters during infancy and childhood are given in Tables 5.9–5.11.

Neonate

The blood film of a healthy neonate shows hyposplenic features (see below), specifically Howell–Jolly bodies, acanthocytes and spherocytes. Spherocytes are, however, more numerous than in a hyposplenic adult. The WBC, neutrophil, monocyte and lymphocyte counts are much higher in the neonate than in the older child or adult. NRBC are much more common and myelocytes are not uncommon. Hb, RBC and PCV are much higher than at any other time after birth and the consequent high viscosity of the blood leads to poor spreading so that the blood film appears 'packed'. This physiological polycythaemia also leads to a very low ESR. Red cell size is increased in comparison with older infants, children and adults. The reticulocyte count is high during the first 3 days after birth [143].

Physiological changes in haematological variables occur in the first days and weeks of life. There is a rise, on average of about 60% of initial counts, in the WBC and the neutrophil count, with peak levels being reached at about 12 hours after birth [144]. By 72 hours the count has fallen back to below that observed at birth. The lymphocyte count falls to its lowest level at about 72 hours and then rises again [144]. By the end of the first week the number of neutrophils has usually fallen below the number of lymphocytes. If there has been late clamping of the umbilical cord there are also rises in Hb, PCV and RBC due to 'autotransfusion' from the placenta followed by reduction of plasma volume. NRBC usually disappear from the blood by about the fourth day in healthy term babies and by the end of the first week most of the myelocytes and metamyelocytes have also disappeared. Band form are also more numerous during the first few days than thereafter, a plateau being reached by the fifth day.

Normal ranges for the neonatal period are given in Tables 5.7 and 5.8.

Premature neonate

Many haematological variables in premature babies differ from those of full-term babies (see above). Their blood films show greater numbers of NRBC, metamyelocytes, myelocytes, promyelocytes and myeloblasts. Hyposplenic features are much more marked than in term babies (Fig. 3.115) and may persist for the first few months of life. Premature babies often develop eosinophilia between the second and third weeks after birth [145].

Hyposplenism

Splenectomy in haematologically normal subjects produces characteristic abnormalities of the blood count and film. The same abnormalities are seen if the spleen is congenitally absent, suffers atrophy or extensive infarction, or becomes non-functional for any reason. Occasionally, if the spleen is

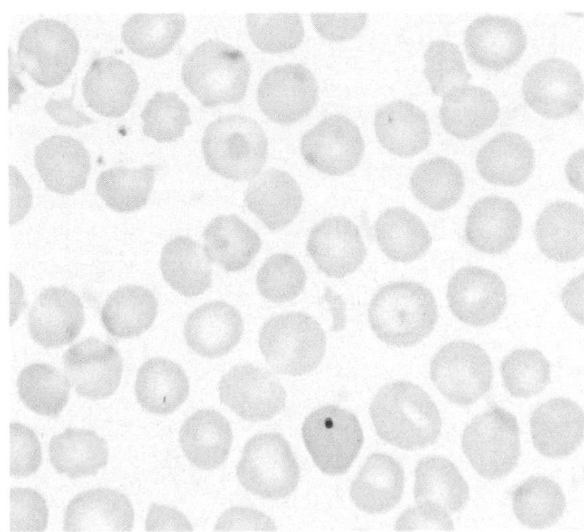

Fig. 3.115 Peripheral blood film from a premature but healthy infant, showing macrocytosis (relative to the film of an adult), a Howell–Jolly body in a polychromatic cell, target cells and schistocyte.

heavily infiltrated by abnormal cells, features of hyposplenism are seen in the presence of splenomegaly.

Immediately after splenectomy there is a thrombocytosis and a marked neutrophil leucocytosis. If infection occurs post-splenectomy the neutrophilia and left shift are very marked. After recovery from surgery the neutrophil count falls to nearly normal levels and the platelet count falls to high normal or somewhat elevated levels – platelet counts of around $500–600 \times 10^9/l$ may persist. A lymphocytosis and a monocytosis persist indefinitely – the lymphocytosis is usually moderate but levels up to $10 \times 10^9/l$ are occasionally seen [146]. Sometimes large granular lymphocytes are increased (see Fig. 9.7). In normal subjects the Hb does not change post-splenectomy but the red cell morphology is altered (see Figs 3.32 & 3.36). Abnormal features include target cells, acanthocytes, Howell–Jolly bodies, small numbers of Pappenheimer bodies (the presence of siderotic granules being confirmed on a stain for iron), occasional NRBC and small numbers of spherocytes. Small vacuoles may be seen in Romanowsky-stained films; on interference phase contract microscopy these appear as 'pits' or 'craters' but in fact they are autophagic vacuoles [147]. The reticulocyte count is increased. Special stains show small numbers of Heinz bodies. Some large platelets may be noted and the mean platelet volume is higher, in relation to the platelet count, than in non-splenectomized subjects.

In patients with underlying haematological disorders a greater degree of abnormality is often seen post-splenectomy. When there is anaemia

Table 3.12 Some causes of hyposplenism

Physiological
Neonatal period (particularly in premature babies) Old age
Pathological
Congenital
Congenital absence or hypoplasia (may be hereditary [148]; may be associated with situs invertus and cardiac anomalies; occurs in reticular agenesis and Fanconi's anaemia [149]; may be caused by maternal coumarin intake)
Congenital polysplenism [150]
Acquired
Splenectomy
Splenic infarction (sickle cell anaemia, sickle cell/haemoglobin C disease and other sickling disorders; essential thrombocythaemia; PRV; following splenic torsion; consequent on acute infection [151])
Splenic atrophy (associated with coeliac disease, dermatitis herpetiformis, ulcerative colitis [152], Crohn's disease [152] and tropical sprue [153]; autoimmune splenic atrophy including that associated with autoimmune thyroid disease, systemic lupus erythematosus [154] and autoimmune polyglandular disease [155]; graft-versus-host disease [156]; following splenic irradiation [157] or Thorotrast administration [158])
Splenic infiltration or replacement (amyloidosis, sarcoidosis, leukaemia and lymphoma (occasionally); carcinoma [159] and sarcoma [160] (rarely))
Functional asplenia, e.g., caused by reticuloendothelial overload (early in the course of sickle cell disease, severe haemolytic anaemia and immune-complex or autoimmune disease) [161]

which persists post-splenectomy a marked degree of thrombocytosis is usual. If Heinz bodies are being formed (e.g., because of an unstable haemoglobin or because an oxidant drug is administered) large numbers are seen when the pitting action of the spleen is lacking. If there is erythroblast iron overload (e.g., in sideroblastic anaemia or in thalassaemia major) Pappenheimer bodies are very numerous. If the bone marrow is megaloblastic or dyserythropoietic Howell–Jolly bodies are particularly large and numerous.

Some of the causes of hyposplenism are given in Table 3.12.

Circulating non-haemopoietic cells

Endothelial cells

Endothelial cells (Figs 3.116 & 3.117) are most likely to be detected if blood films are made from the first drop of blood in a needle; this was particularly noted when needles were re-used and were sometimes barbed [162]. Endothelial cells may appear singly or in clusters. They are large cells, often elongated, with diameters of 20–30 μm and a large amount of pale blue or blue–grey cytoplasm. The nucleus is round to oval with a diameter of 10–15 μm and one to three light blue nucleoli. Nuclei may appear grooved.

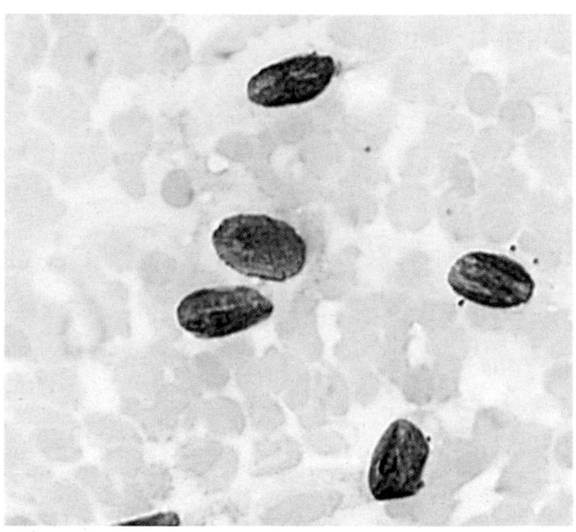

Fig. 3.116 Endothelial cells obtained by scraping the vena cava during post-mortem examination. Courtesy of Dr Marjorie Walker, London.

Increased numbers of endothelial cells are present in conditions with vascular injury (e.g., rickettsial infection, peripheral vascular disease, cytomegalovirus infection, thrombotic thrombocytopenia purpura (TTP), sickle cell disease and following coronary angioplasty) but even in such circumstances they are very infrequent [163].

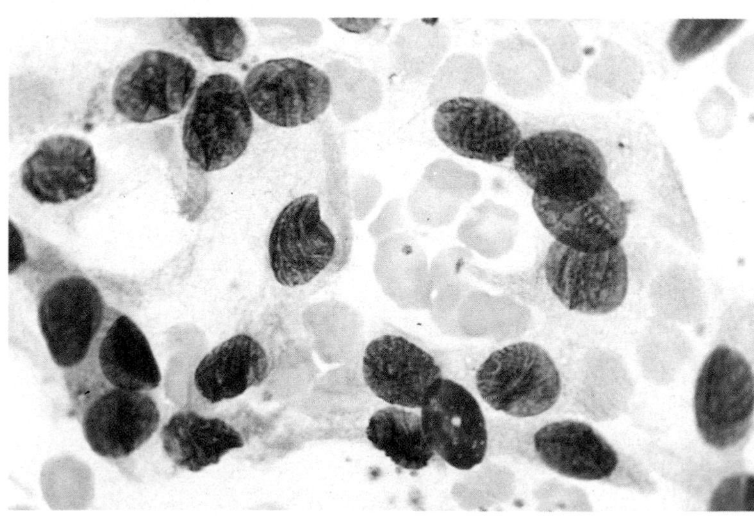

Fig. 3.117 Endothelial cells in a peripheral blood film made from a venous blood sample.

Epithelial cells

When blood is obtained by skin puncture, epithelial cells from the skin may occasionally be present in the blood film. They are large cells with a small nucleus and large amounts of sky-blue featureless cytoplasm (Fig. 3.118a). Some are anucleate (Fig. 3.118b).

Non-haemopoietic malignant cells

In various small cell tumours of childhood, tumour cells can circulate in the blood in appreciable numbers and be mistaken for the lymphoblasts of ALL. Such circulating cells have been described in neuroblastoma, rhabdomyosarcoma and medulloblastoma [164–166]. In rhabdomyosarcoma, syncytial masses of tumour cells have been seen [167]. Carcinoma cells can also circulate in the blood but usually in such small numbers that they are unlikely to be noted unless special concentration procedures are employed [168]. Rarely, they may be seen on routine blood films (Fig. 3.119). Even more rarely a 'leukaemia' of carcinoma cells occurs. 'Carcinocythaemia' has been most often observed in both carcinoma of the lung and breast [169] (Fig. 3.120). Malignant cells in the blood may be in clusters, sometimes large enough clusters to be visible macroscopically (see Fig. 3.4).

In patients with advanced Hodgkin's disease small numbers of Reed–Sternberg cells and mononuclear Hodgkin's cells may rarely be noted in the blood [170]. Even more rarely abnormal cells may be present in such numbers as to constitute a Reed–Sternberg cell leukaemia. In one such patient the total WBC was 140×10^9/l with 92% malignant cells [171]. These included typical Reed–Sternberg cells (giant cells with a diameter of 12–40 μm with mirror-image nuclei and giant nucleoli), and multinucleated and mononuclear Hodgkin's cells, also with giant nucleoli.

Microorganisms in blood films

In patients with bacterial, fungal or parasitic infections microorganisms may be observed free between cells or within red cells, neutrophils or monocytes. They are visible on an MGG-stained films but special stains aid in their identification. The only microorganisms which are observed

(a)

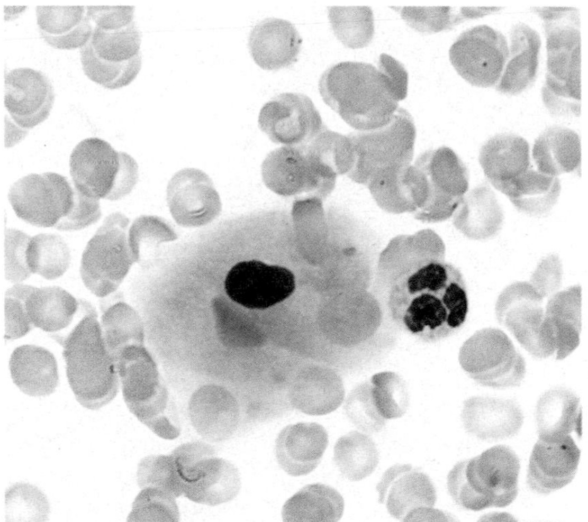

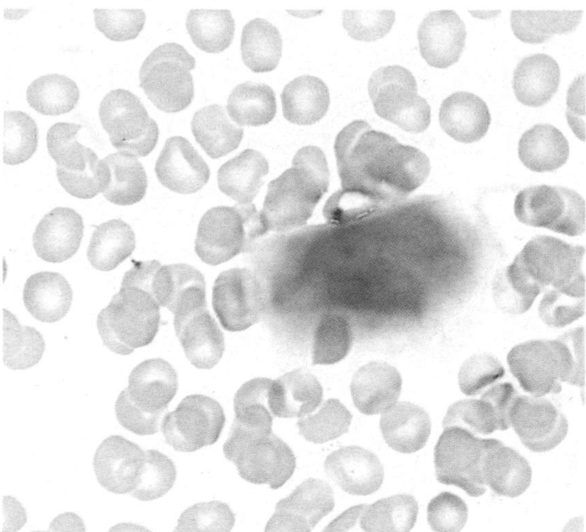

(b)

Fig. 3.118 Epithelial cells in a peripheral blood film prepared from a drop of blood obtained by finger prick: (a) nucleated epithelial cell, and (b) anucleate epithelial cell.

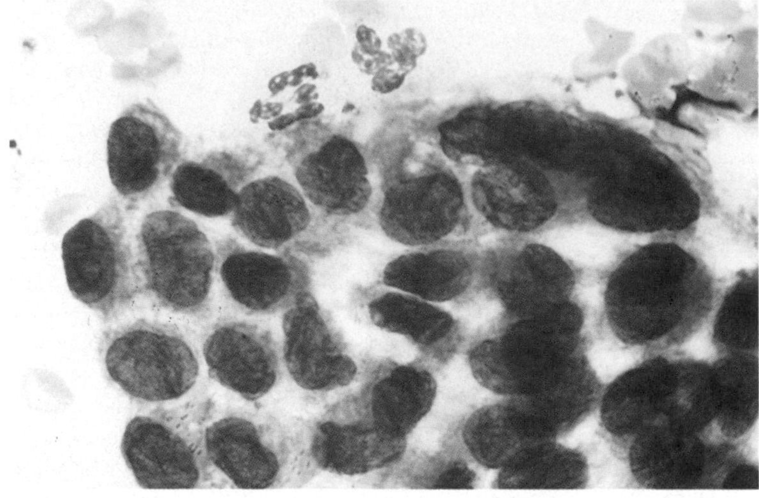

Fig. 3.119 Malignant cells in the routine peripheral blood film of a patient subsequently found to have widespread metastatic adenocarcinoma.

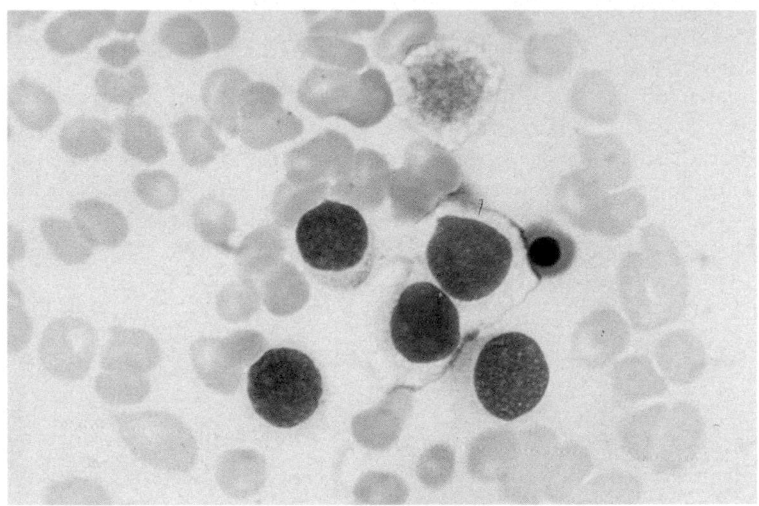

Fig. 3.120 Malignant cells in the peripheral blood of a patient with a past history of carcinoma of the breast, subsequently found to have widespread metastatic disease.

fairly frequently are malarial parasites but the fortuitous observation of other microorganisms in a blood film can also be diagnostically useful, leading to earlier diagnosis and treatment.

Bacteria

In bartonellosis or Oroya fever (Fig. 3.121a), a disease confined to South America, the causative organism, a flagellated bacillus, is present within red cells and infection leads to spherocytosis and haemolytic anaemia. The organisms, *Bartonella bacilliformis*, stain deep red or purple on an MGG stain [172]. Haemotropic bacilli, *Tropheryma whippelii*, have also been reported recently in Whipple's disease in hyposplenic subjects (Fig. 3.121b).

In louse- and tick-borne relapsing fevers the causative spirochaetes, *Borrelia recurrentis*, *Borrelia duttoni*, *Borrelia turicata*, *Borrelia parkerii* or *Borrelia hermsii*, are observed free between cells (Fig. 3.122). Organisms can be detected in the peripheral blood film in 70% of cases of tick-borne relapsing fever [173]. When Borrelia are being sought a thick film is useful.

It is quite uncommon for bacteria other than

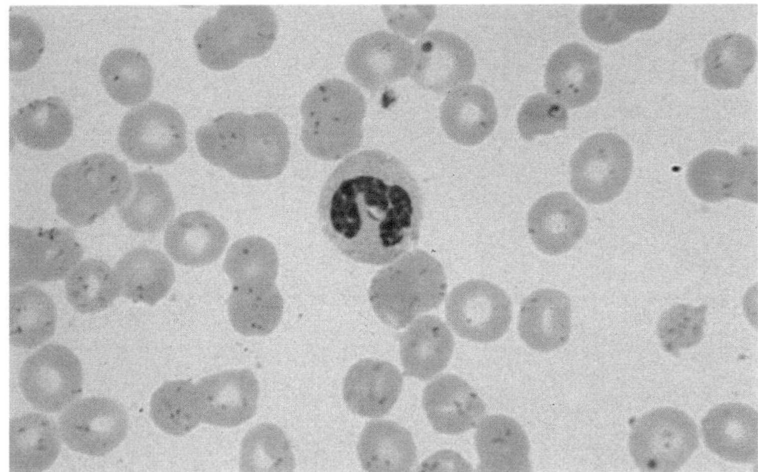

(a)

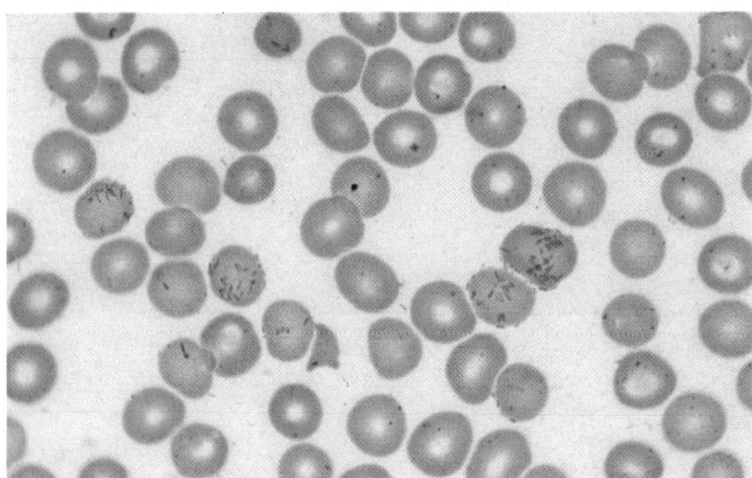

(b)

Fig. 3.121 (a) Peripheral blood film showing multiple small rod-shaped bacilli associated with erythrocytes in a patient with bartonellosis. There is also a red cell containing a Howell–Jolly body. Courtesy of Dr D. Swirsky and Professor Sir John Dacie, London. (b) Peripheral blood film from a hyposplenic patient with Whipple's disease showing a red cell fragment, a red cell containing a Howell–Jolly body and several red cells with which are associated numerous delicate rod-shaped bacilli. Wright's stain. Courtesy of Dr B.J. Patterson, Toronto.

Borrelia to be noted in routine blood films. When present they are most often observed within neutrophils or, occasionally, free between cells. When they are being deliberately sought a buffy coat preparation makes detection more likely. Bacteria are most often seen in hyposplenic or immunosuppressed subjects and in those with indwelling intravenous lines or overwhelming infections. Bacteria which have been observed within neutrophils in routine peripheral blood films include streptococci, staphylococci, *Streptococcus pneumoniae* (pneumococcus), *Neisseria meningitidis* (meningococcus; Fig. 3.123), *Clostridium perfringens*, *Yersinia pestis*, *Bacteroides distasonis* [174], Corynebacterium [174], *Capnocytophaga canimorsus* (previously known as the DF-2 organism), *Klebsiella oxytoca* [175], *Ehrlichia chaffeensis* [176] and *Ehrlichia phagocytophila* [177]. Ehrlichia have also been observed within monocytes and atypical lymphocytes [178]. The plague bacillus, *Yersinia pestis*, is found extracellularly [179]. Bacteria in peripheral blood films may have characteristic features which give a clue to their identity. They can be identified as cocci or bacilli and, following a Gram stain, as Gram negative or Gram positive. Spore forming

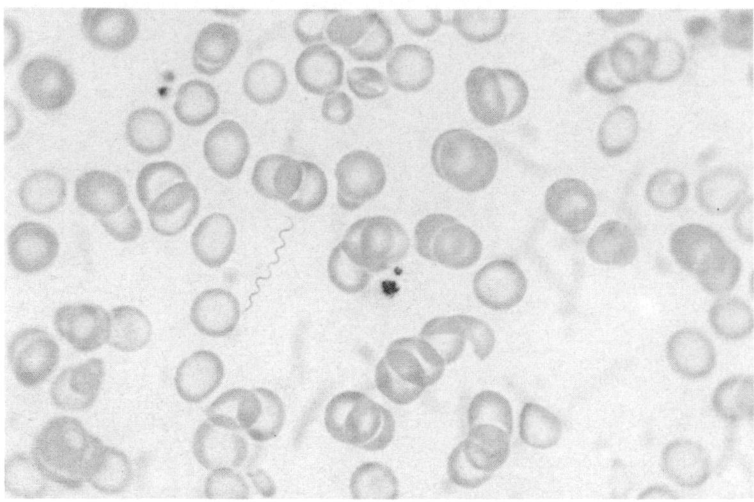

Fig. 3.122 *Borrelia recurrentis* in the peripheral blood of a child with relapsing fever.

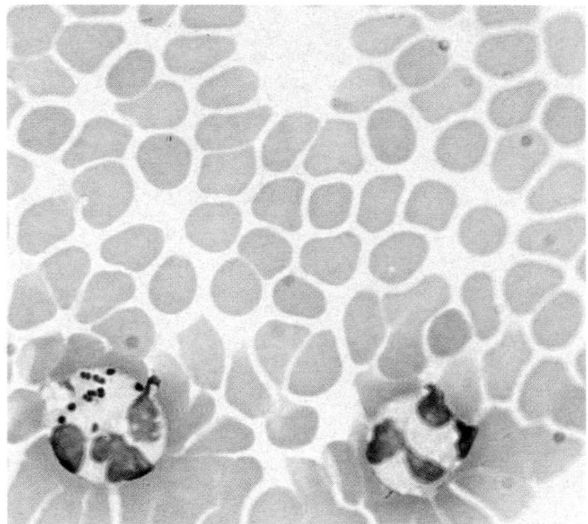

Fig. 3.123 A neutrophil containing diplococci from a patient with fatal *Neisseria meningitidis* septicaemia.

by Clostridia has been observed [180]. Yersinia may be bipolar in a Romanowsky stain [179]. Erhlichia may appear as small single organisms or as morulae containing a number of elemental bodies. Bacteria which have colonized indwelling venous lines despite antibiotic therapy may be morphologically abnormal, appearing filamentous as a consequence of failure of septation (Fig. 3.124) [175]. The finding of bacteria in a blood film is usually highly significant. The exception is with cord blood samples which are often collected in circumstances in which bacterial contamination is likely; if they are left at room temperature and delay occurs in delivery to the laboratory it is not uncommon to see bacteria in stained films.

Fungi

Fungi have also been observed in peripheral blood films, particularly in patients with indwelling central venous lines who are also neutropenic or have defective immunity. They may be observed free or within neutrophils or monocytes. Fungi which have been observed in neutrophils include *Candida albicans, Candida parapsilosis* [181] (Fig. 3.125), *Hansenula anomala* [182], *Histoplasma capsulatum, Cryptococcus neoformans* [183] and *Penicillium marneffei* (Fig. 3.126) [184] and in monocytes *Histoplasm capsulatum* and *Penicillium marneffei* [184]. In febrile neutropenic patients a search of the peripheral blood film can confirm a diagnosis of systemic fungal infection some days in advance of positive cultures in a significant proportion of patients [182].

Parasites

Some parasites, such as malaria parasites and babesiae, are predominantly blood parasites, while

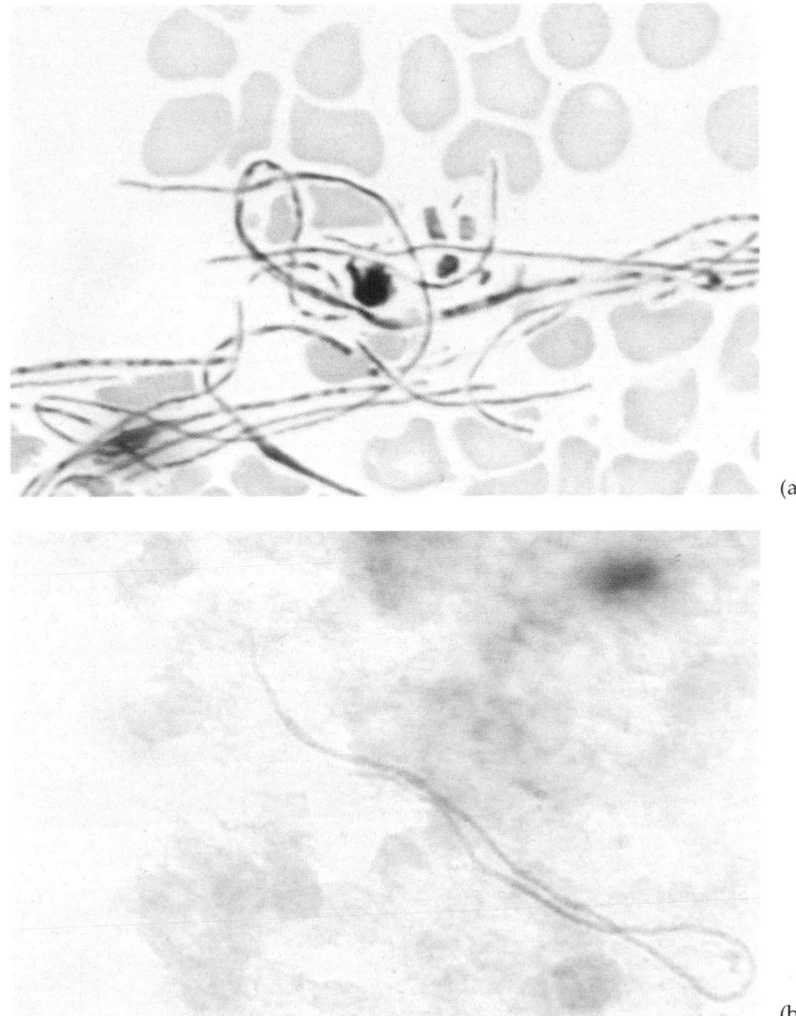

Fig. 3.124 *Klebsiella oxytoca* in a film of blood obtained from an indwelling venous line, showing failure of septation (a) MGG stain, and (b) Gram stain. Courtesy of Dr Carol Barton and Mr J. Kitaruth, Reading.

other, such as filariae, have part of their life cycle in the blood. Parasites which may be detected in the blood film are listed with their geographical distribution in Tables 3.13 and 3.14.

Malaria and babesiosis

Although malaria parasites may be detected in MGG-stained blood films, their detection and identification is facilitated by Leishmann or Giemsa staining at a higher pH. A thick film is preferable for detection of parasites and a thin film for identification of the species. A thick film should be examined for at least 5 minutes before being considered negative. If only a thin film is available it should be examined for at least 15 minutes, or until 100–200 high power fields have been examined, before being considered negative. Partially immune subjects are particularly likely to have a low parasite count so that a prolonged search may be required for parasite detection. In patients with a strong suspicion of malaria whose initial films are negative, repeated blood examinations may be needed. *Plasmodium falciparum* is associated with the highest parasite counts with sometimes 10–40% of red cells being parasitized;

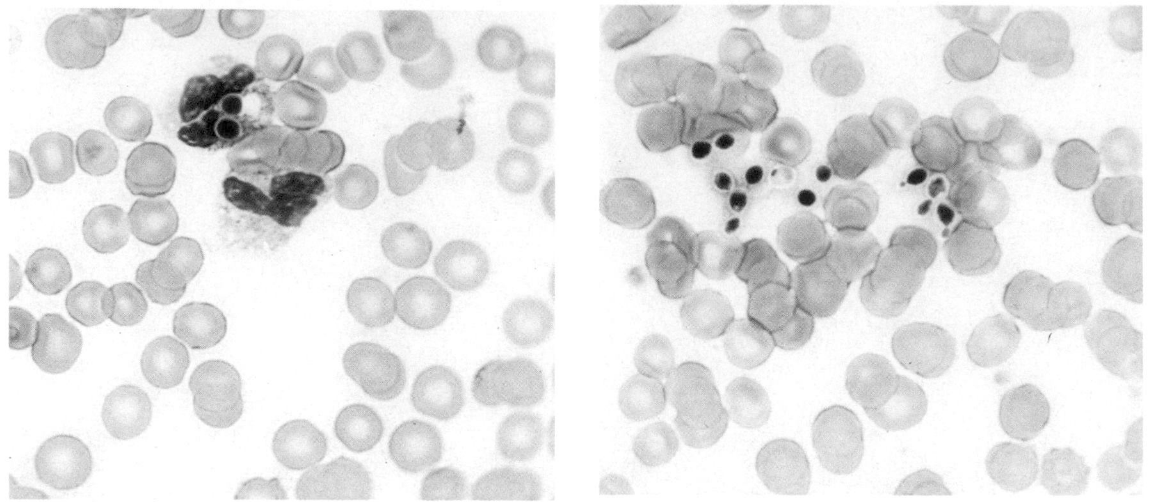

(a) (b)

Fig. 3.125 *Candida parapsilosis* in a peripheral blood film (a) within neutrophils, and (b) free between red cells. Several organisms are budding. Courtesy of Dr B. Vadher and Dr Marilyn Treacy, London.

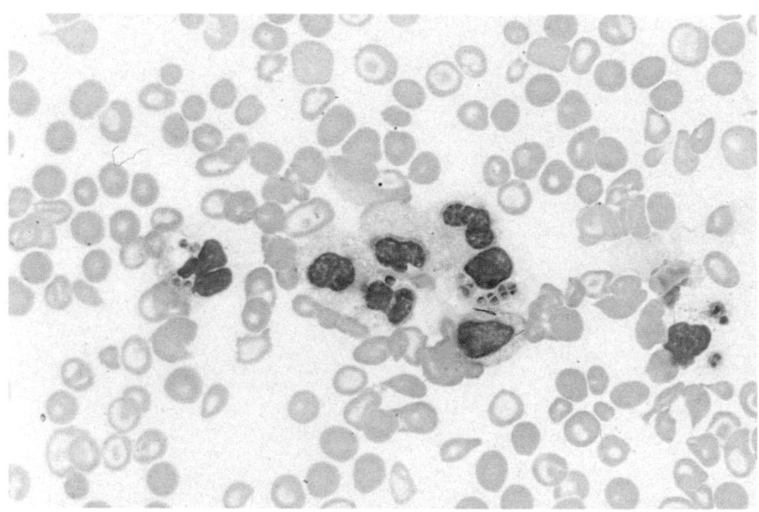

Fig. 3.126 *Penicillium marneffei* in the peripheral blood of a patient with AIDS. Courtesy of Dr K.F. Wong, Hong Kong.

paradoxically, patients may be seriously ill with no parasites being detectable on initial blood examination. This is consequent on parasitized red cells being sequestered in tissues. When *Plasmodium falciparum* is detected, a count of the proportion of cells which are parasitized should be made to allow monitoring during therapy. A failure of the parasite count to fall indicates a drug-resistant parasite. Useful features in distinguishing between the four species are summarized in Fig. 3.127 and illustrated in Figs. 3.128–3.131. Associated abnormalities which may be noted in the films of patients with malaria are anaemia, thrombocytopenia, atypical lymphocytes, phagocytosis of parasitized and non-parasitized red cells by monocytes, and malaria pigment in monocytes and occasionally in neutrophils. Malaria pigment in leucocytes is mainly associated with *Plasmodium falciparum* malaria. The histograms or scatter plots of automated full

Table 3.13 Protozoan parasites which may be detected in blood films

Parasite	Disease or common name	Usual distribution
Sporozoans		
Plasmodium falciparum	Malignant tertian malaria	Widespread in tropics and subtropics, particularly in Africa
Plasmodium vivax	Benign tertian malaria	Widespread in tropics and occurs also in some temperate zones; not West Africa
Plasmodium malariae	Quartan malaria	Scattered in the tropics
Plasmodium ovale	Benign tertian malaria	Tropical West Africa; scattered foci elsewhere including tropical Asia, New Guinea and the Western Pacific
Babesia microti	Babesiosis	North-Eastern coastal USA, West Coast and Mid-West
Babesia divergens	Babesiosis	Europe [187]
Haemoflagellates		
Trypanosoma brucei rhodesiense	Sleeping sickness	East Africa
Trypanosoma brucei gambiense	Sleeping sickness	Tropical West and Central Africa
Trypanosoma cruzi	South American trypanosomiasis or Chagas' disease	Wide area of Central and South America
Trypanosoma rangeli	Non-pathogenic	Central and South America
Leishmania donovani	Visceral leishmaniasis or kala azar	India, China, Central Asia, Central and Northern Africa, Portugal, the Mediterranean littoral, Central and South America

blood counters may be abnormal in the presence of malarial parasites.

Babesia is a rare parasite of man and can easily be confused with malaria parasites. The trophozoites are small rings, similar to those of *Plasmodium falciparum*, 1–5 μm in diameter with one or two chromatin dots and scanty cytoplasm. Sometimes they are pyriform (pear-shaped) and either paired (Fig. 3.132a) or with the pointed ends of four parasites being in contact to give a Maltese cross formation (Fig. 3.132b). Babesiosis occurs particularly but not exclusively in hyposplenic subjects in whom 25% or more of cells may be parasitized. In those with a functioning spleen the level of parasitaemia is usually low. The method of detection is by thick and thin films, as for malaria. There is often associated thrombocytopenia.

Haemoflagellates

The morphological features of haemoflagellates which may be found in the peripheral blood are summarized in Fig. 3.133. Trypanosomes may be

	General features and changes in red cells	Early trophozoite (ring form)	Mature trophozoite
Plasmodium vivax	Red cells much enlarged, irregular and pale with fine red stippling (Schuffner's dots); usually low or moderate parasitaemia; all stages of life cycle often present; sometimes multiple parasites per cell	Thick rings, 1/3–1/2 the diameter of the red cell 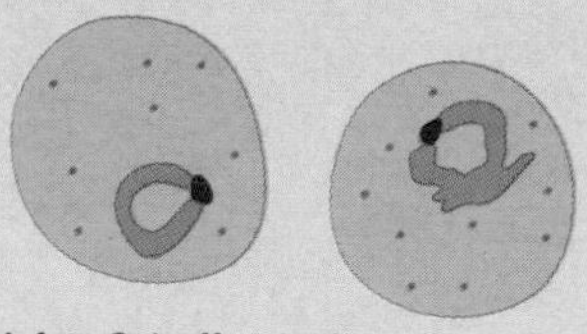 A few Schuffner's dots Accolé (shoulder) forms and double dots less common than with *P. falciparum*	Ameboid rings, 1/2–2/3 the diameter of the red cell Pale blue or lilac parasite with prominent central valuole 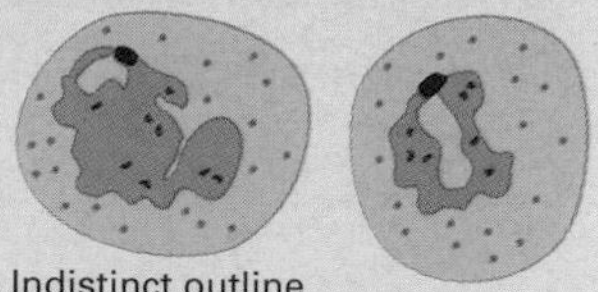 Indistinct outline Scattered fine yellowish-brown pigment granules or rods
Plasmodium ovale	Red cells enlarged but not as much as with *P. vivax*; cells pale and some are oval or pear-shaped; some are ragged (fimbriated) at one or both ends; fine to coarse red stippling (Schuffner's dots); low parasitaemia; often fewer stages present than with *P. vivax*	Thick, compact rings, 1/3–1/2 the diameter of the red cell 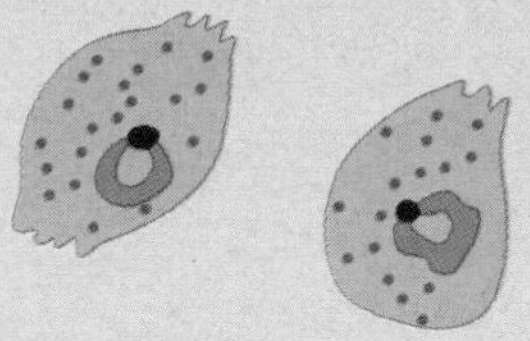 Numerous Schuffner's dots but paler than with *P. vivax*	Thick rings, less irregular than those of *P. vivax*, 1/3–1/2 the diameter of the red cell 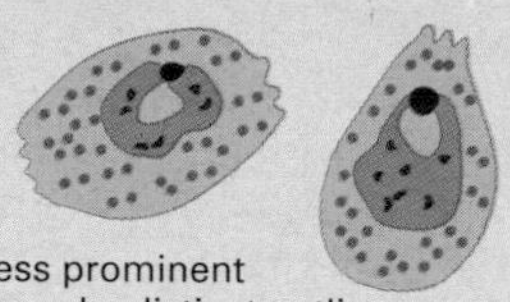 Less prominent vacuole, distinct outline Yellowish-brown pigment which is coarser and darker than that of *P. vivax* Schuffner's dots prominent
Plasmodium falciparum	Cells not enlarged; staining characteristics usually unaltered but sometimes there are some pale cells; sometimes multiple parasites per cell and heavy parasitaemia (10–40% of cells); often only ring forms are present	Delicate rings, 1/6–1/4 the diameter of the red cell 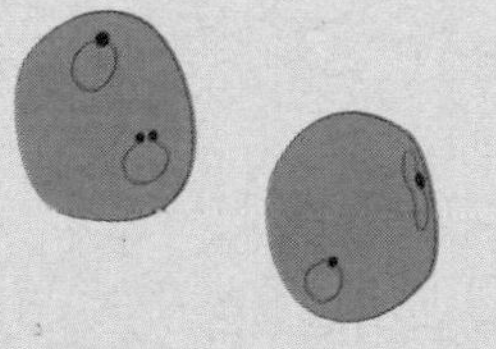 Double dots and accolé forms common	Fairly delicate rings, 1/3–1/2 the diameter of the red cell 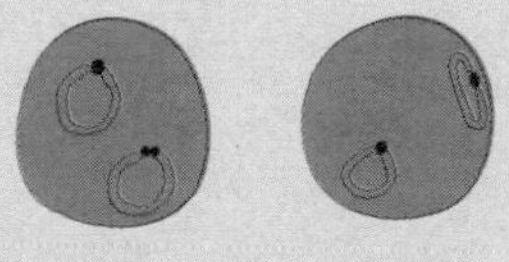 Red-mauve stippling (Maurer's dots or clefts) may be present Mature trophozoites are less often present in peripheral blood than ring forms
Plasmodium malariae	Cells not enlarged, sometimes contracted; staining characteristics not altered; lowest degree of parasitaemia; multiple parasites per cell rare; no stippling unless overstained; all stages usually present	Small, thick, compact rings Small chromatin dot which may be inside the ring 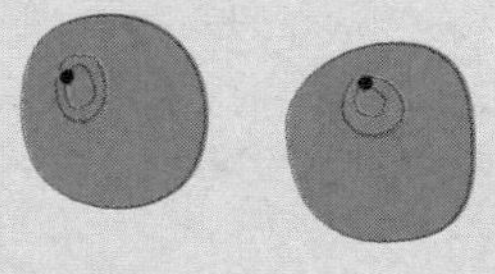 Double dots and accolé forms rare	Ameboid form more compact than *P. vivax* Sometimes angular or band forms 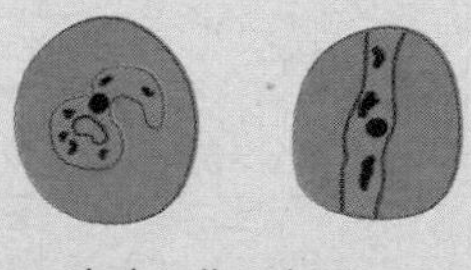 Heavy, dark yellow-brown pigment No stippling unless overstained

Fig. 3.127 Features which are useful in distinguishing between the different species of malaria parasites.

Early schizont	Late schizont	Gametocyte: Macrogametocyte	Gametocyte: Microgametocyte
Rounded or irregular Ameboid Loose central mass of fine yellowish-brown pigment 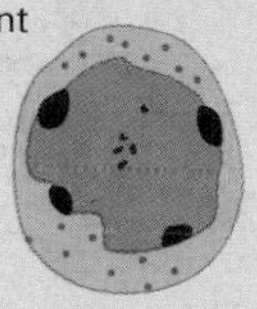 Schizont almost fills cell Schuffner's dots	12–24 (usually 16–24) medium-sized merozoites 1–2 clumps of peripheral pigment 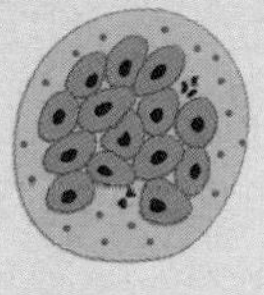 Schizont almost fills cell Schuffner's dots	Round or ovoid, almost fills enlarged cell Blue cytoplasm 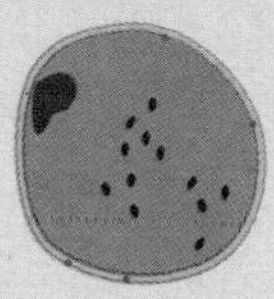 Eccentric compact red nucleus Scattered pigment	Round or ovoid, as large as a normal red cell but does not fill the enlarged red cell 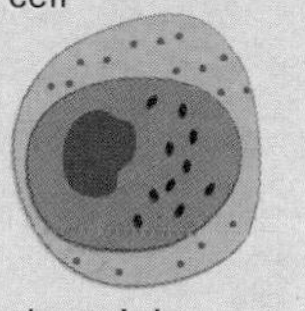 Faintly staining Larger, lighter red central or eccentric nucleus Fine, scattered pigment
Round, compact Darkish brown pigment, heavier and coarser than that of *P. vivax* 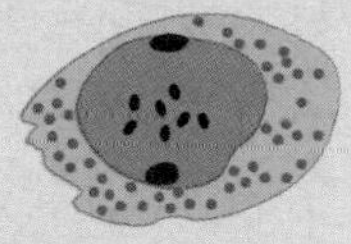 Schuffner's dots	6–12 (usually 8) large merozoites arranged irregularly like a bunch of grapes 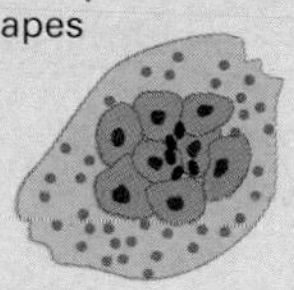 Central pigment Schuffner's dots	Similar to *P. vivax* but somewhat smaller 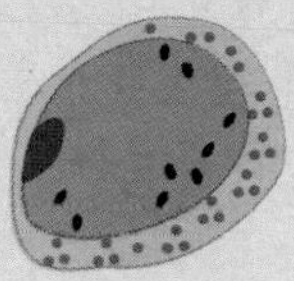 Pigment coarser and blacker, scattered but mainly near the periphery	Similar to *P. vivax* but smaller 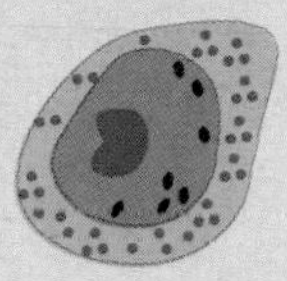
Not usually seen in blood Very small, ameboid Scattered light brown to black pigment	Not usually seen in blood 8–32 (usually few) very small merozoites; grouped irregularly Peripheral clump of coarse dark brown pigment	Sickle or crescent shaped Deforms cell which often appears empty of haemoglobin 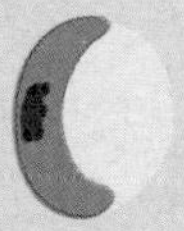 Blue cytoplasm Compact central nucleus with pigment aggregated around it	Oval or crescentic with blunted ends Pale blue or pink 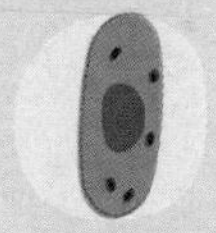 Large pale nucleus with pigment more scattered than in macrogametocyte
Compact, round, fills red cell 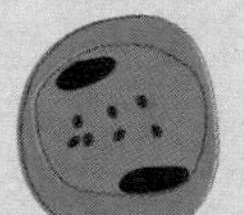 Coarse dark yellow-brown pigment	6–12 (usually 8–10) large merozoites, arranged symmetrically, often in a rosette or daisy head formation 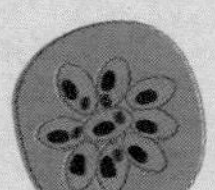 Central coarse dark yellowish-brown pigment	Similar to *P. vivax* but smaller, round or oval, almost fills cell, blue with a dark nucleus 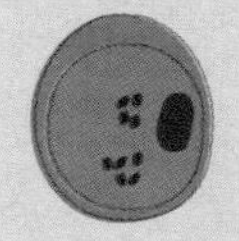 Prominent pigment concentrated at centre and periphery	Similar to *P. vivax* but smaller, pink or paler blue than macrogametocyte with a larger, paler nucleus 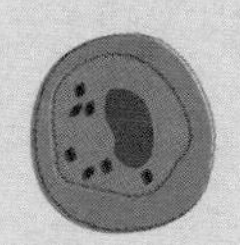 Prominent pigment

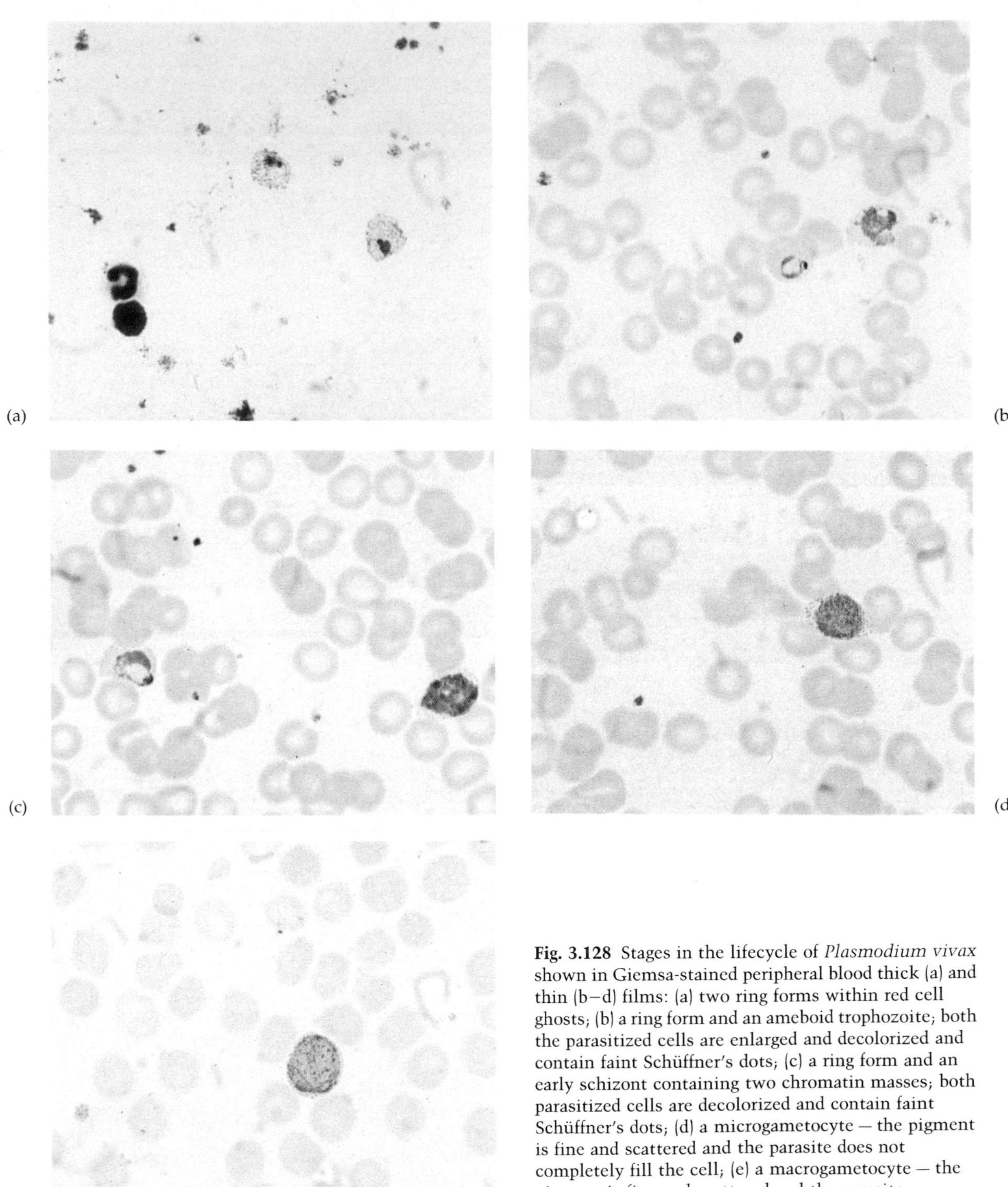

Fig. 3.128 Stages in the lifecycle of *Plasmodium vivax* shown in Giemsa-stained peripheral blood thick (a) and thin (b–d) films: (a) two ring forms within red cell ghosts; (b) a ring form and an ameboid trophozoite; both the parasitized cells are enlarged and decolorized and contain faint Schüffner's dots; (c) a ring form and an early schizont containing two chromatin masses; both parasitized cells are decolorized and contain faint Schüffner's dots; (d) a microgametocyte – the pigment is fine and scattered and the parasite does not completely fill the cell; (e) a macrogametocyte – the pigment is fine and scattered and the parasite completely fills the cell and is larger than the non-parasitized red cells.

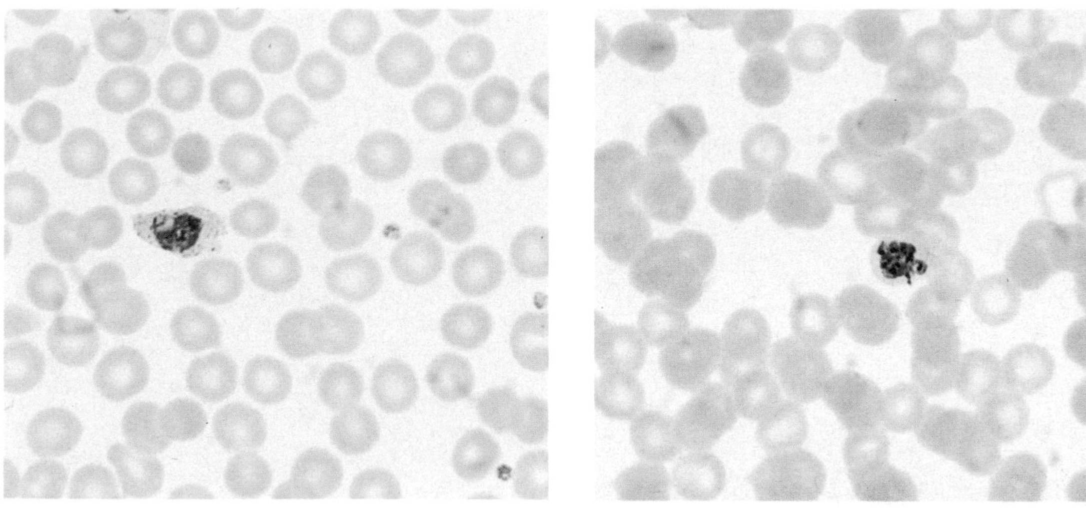

Fig. 3.129 Stages in the lifecycle of *Plasmodium ovale* in Giemsa-stained thin films: (a) a late trophozoite in an enlarged, decolorized and oval red cell which has a fimbriated end; pigment is coarser and darker than in *Plasmodium vivax*, the parasite is more compact and Schüffner's dots are more prominent; (b) a schizont containing eight merozoites; coarse pigment is clustered centrally.

Table 3.14 Nematode (family Filarioidea) parasites which may be detected in blood films

Parasite	Disease or common name	Usual distribution
Wucheria bancrofti	Filariasis — end stage may be elephantiasis	Widespread in tropics and subtropics, particularly Asia, Polynesia, New Guinea, Africa and Central and South America
Brugia malayi	Filariasis — end stage may be elephantiasis	India, South-East Asia, China, Japan
Loa loa	Eye worm or calabar swellings	African equatorial rainforest and its fringes
Mansonella perstans	Persistent filariasis, usually non-pathogenic	Tropical Africa, Central and South America
Mansonella ozzardi	Ozzard's filariasis, usually non-pathogenic	Central and South America, West Indies
Onchocerca volvulus	Onchocerciasis (river blindness)	Central and West Africa and Sudan, Central America

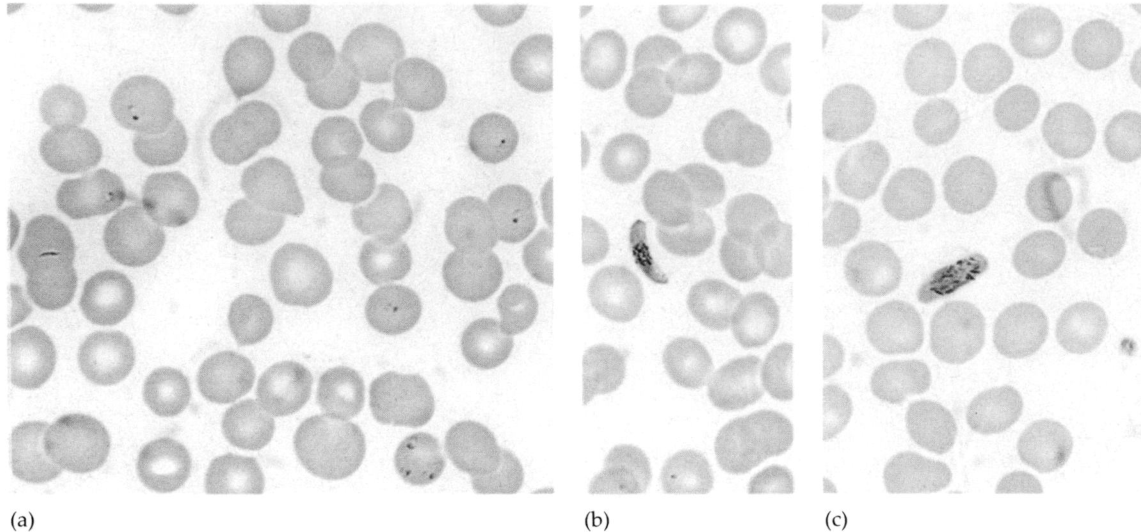

(a) (b) (c)

Fig. 3.130 Stages in the lifecycle of *Plasmodium falciparum* in Giemsa-stained thin films; the cells are not enlarged or decolorized: (a) delicate early ring form with two or more parasites per cell being common; (b) macrogametocyte — the parasite is sickle-shaped with a compact nucleus and pigment clustered centrally; (c) a microgametocyte which is broader and less curved than the macrogametocyte with a more diffuse nucleus and less concentrated pigment.

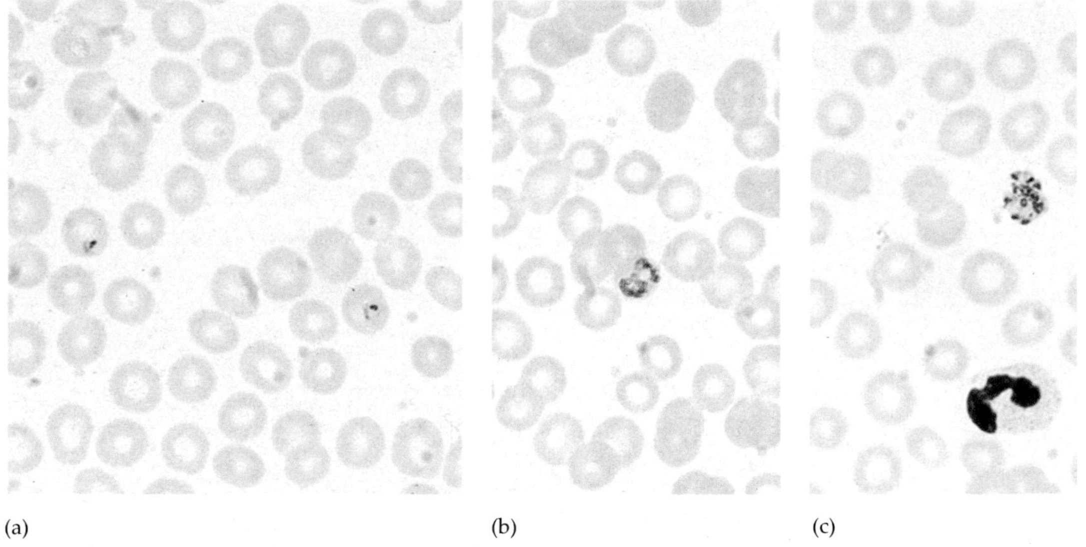

(a) (b) (c)

Fig. 3.131 Stages in the lifecycle of *Plasmodium malariae* in Giemsa-stained thin films; red cells are not enlarged or decolorized (a) early ring forms which are small but less delicate than those of *Plasmodium falciparum*; one parasite has a chromatin dot within the ring; (b) ameboid trophozoite with coarse dark-brown pigment; (c) schizont with about seven merozoites in a daisy-head arrangement with central coarse brown pigment.

(a) 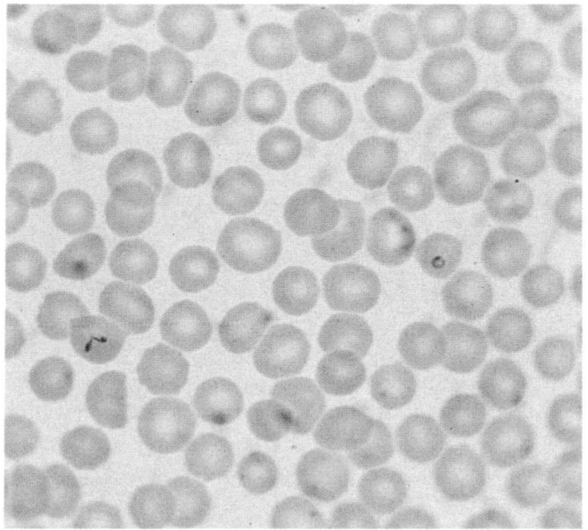 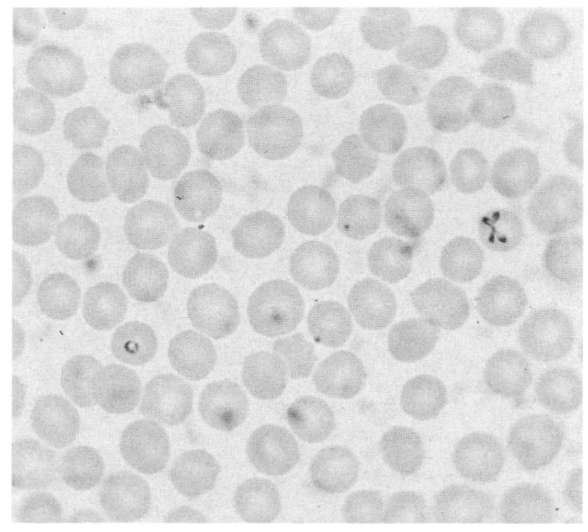 (b)

Fig. 3.132 Blood film from a splenectomized monkey parasitized by *Babesia microti*: (a) a single ring form and a pair of pyriform parasites; (b) a single ring form and four pyriform parasites in a tetrad or Maltese cross formation. Courtesy of Mr J. Williams, London.

detected in the peripheral blood as motile, extracellular parasites. They have a slender body and move by means of a flagellum extending from the kinetoplast at the rear end of the parasite to the front end where the flagellum is free (Figs 3.134 & 3.135); the flagellum is joined to the body by an undulating membrane. The parasite may be seen moving in a wet preparation when a drop of anticoagulated blood is placed on a slide, beneath a coverslip, for microscopic examination. They may also be detected in fixed preparations such as thick or thin films or buffy coat films. Scanty parasites are more readily detected by examining the sediment of 10–20 ml of haemolysed blood. *Trypanosoma brucei rhodesiense* and *Trypanosoma brucei gambiense* (Fig. 3.134) are morphologically identical but their geographical distributions differ (see Table 3.13). Examination of the peripheral blood is more likely to be useful in the case of *Trypanosoma brucei rhodesiense*. Concentration techniques may be needed with *Trypanosoma brucei gambiense*, or parasites may be undetectable in the blood, lymph node puncture being required for diagnosis.

Trypanosoma cruzi (Fig. 3.135) differs morphologically from the African parasites. It is rarely detected by direct examination of the blood, concentration procedures usually being required. It can be distinguished on morphological grounds from the non-pathogenic *Trypanosoma rangeli* which has a similar geographical distribution (see Fig. 3.133).

Leishmania donovani, the causative organism of kala azar, may be detected in monocytes or neutrophils in the peripheral blood, in thick or thin films or in buffy coat preparations (Fig. 3.136). Examination of a peripheral blood film may avoid the need for a bone marrow or splenic aspiration but these procedures are much more sensitive than peripheral blood examination. Associated features which may be noted in patients with kala azar are anaemia, leucopenia, neutropenia, thrombocytopenia and increased rouleaux formation.

Filaria

In filariasis, adult worms residue in tissues and

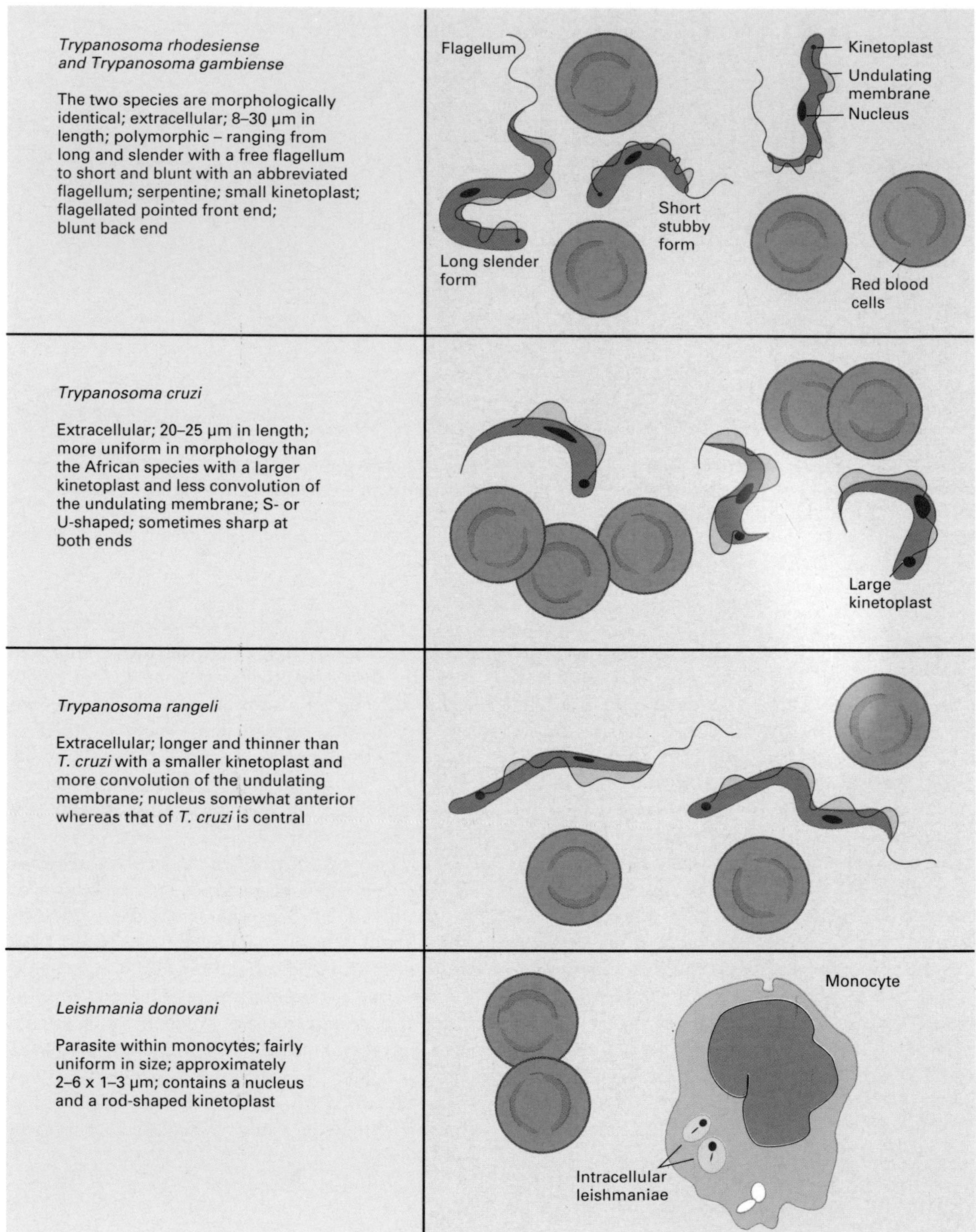

Fig. 3.133 Summary of the morphological features of haemoflagellates.

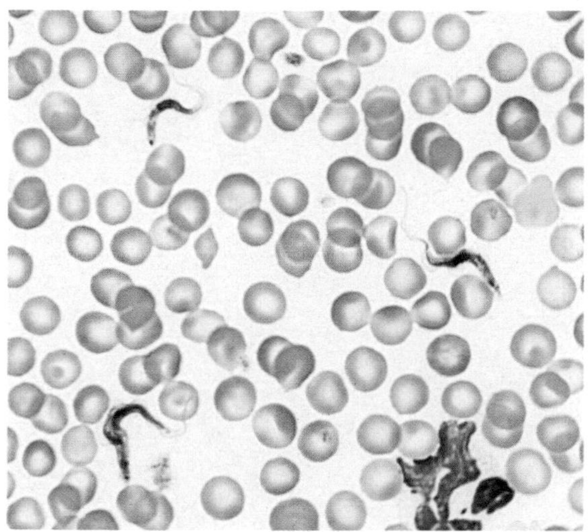

Fig. 3.134 *Trypanosoma brucei gambiense*; the parasites are serpentine with a small kinetoplast (×384).

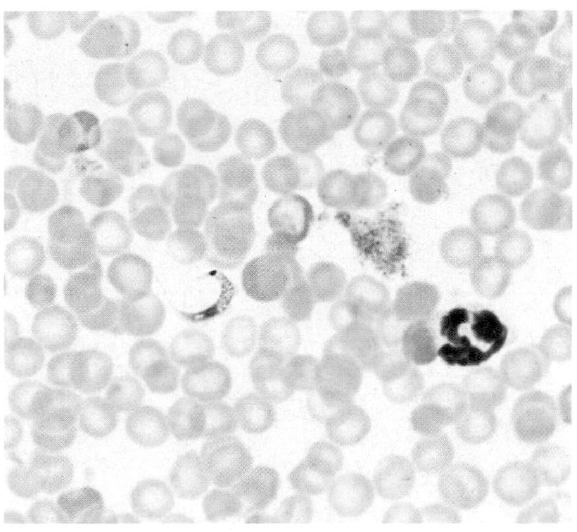

Fig. 3.135 *Trypanosoma cruzi*; the parasite is curved but not usually serpentine and has a large kinetoplast (×384).

(a)

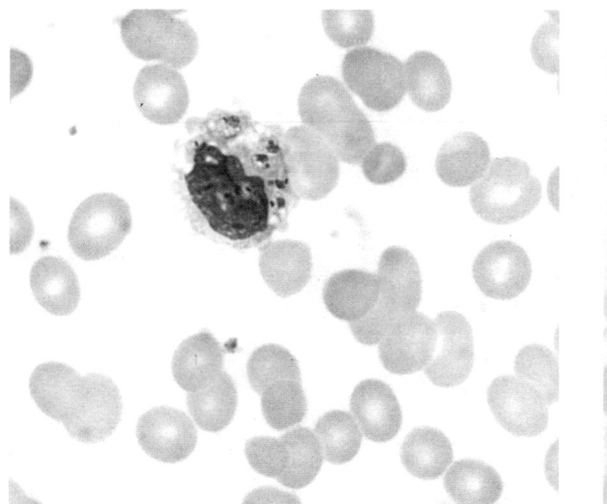

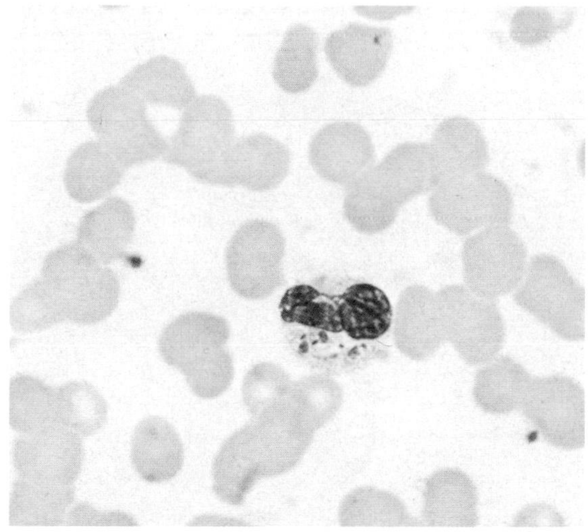

(b)

Fig. 3.136 *Leishmanii donovani* in (a) a monocyte, and (b) a neutrophil in the peripheral blood of a patient with AIDS.

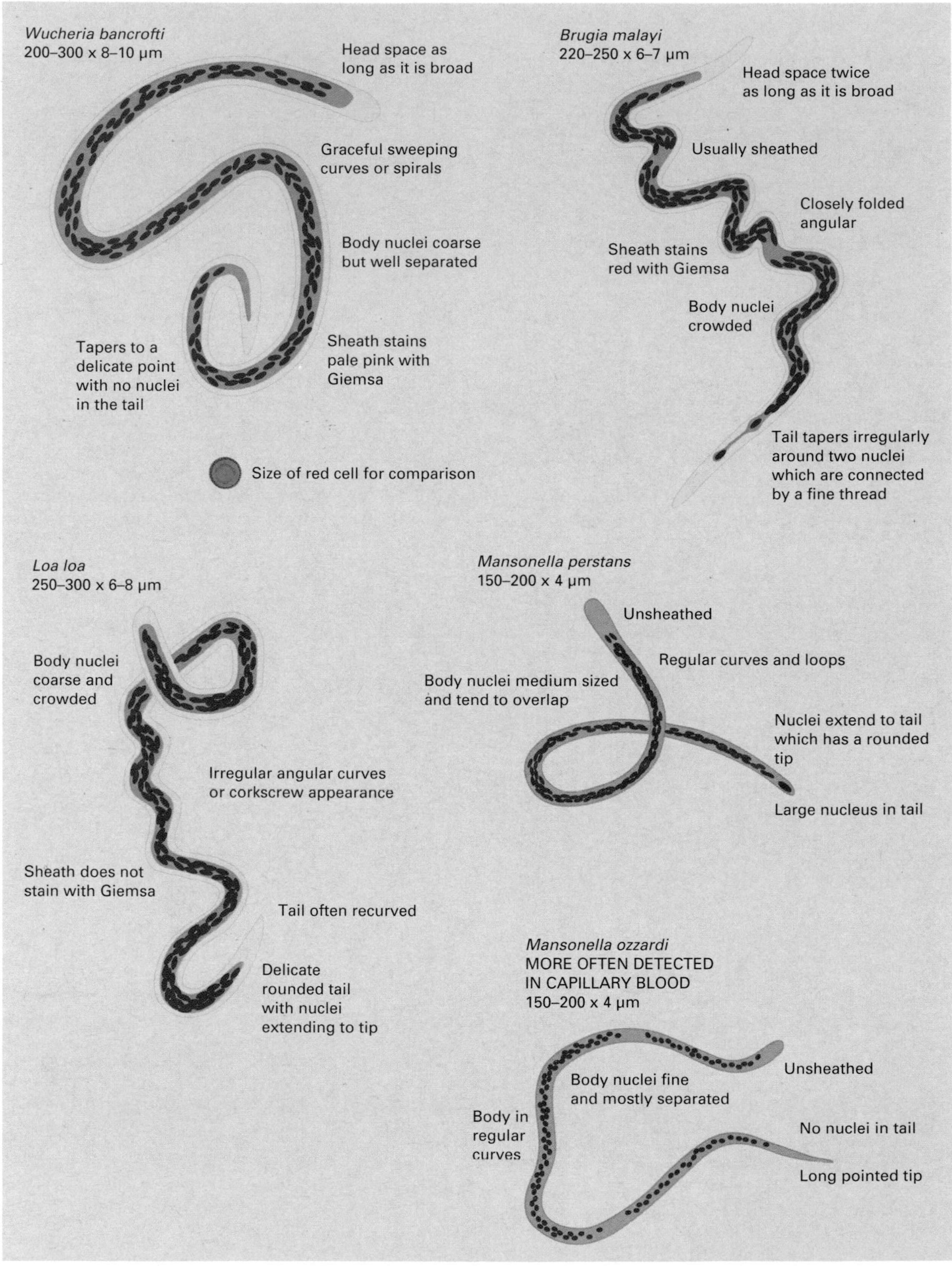

Fig. 3.137 Morphological features which are useful in distinguishing between the microfilariae of different species of filariae.

release microfilariae into the blood stream. Microfilariae are detectable during the acute phase of the disease, but are not detectable in patients with chronic tissue damage but without active disease. As the microfilariae are motile, examination of a wet preparation is often useful; they can also be detected in thick and thin films. Repeated blood examinations may be needed and blood specimens must be obtained at an appropriate time for the species being sought: *Wucheria bancrofti* and *Brugia malayi* release their microfilariae at night, whereas those of *Loa loa* are released during the day. *Mansonella ozzardi* is non-periodic. It lives in skin capillaries so may be more readily identified in capillary blood [186]. *Mansonella perstans* is usually non-periodic but release may be noctural or, less often, diurnal.

Morphological features which are useful in distinguishing the various microfilariae are summarized in Fig. 3.137 and illustrated in Figs 3.138–3.141. In general, pathogenic filariae are sheathed and non-pathogenic are non-sheathed. However, *Brugia malayi* is sometimes seen unsheathed [186]. *Brugia timori*, which is confined to Lesser Sunda Island of Indonesia, is similar to *Brugia malayi* but it is longer with fewer body kinks, a longer space at the head end, less dense nuclei and less intense staining [186]. *Onchocerca volvulus* is occasionally seen in the blood, especially in heavy infections and after therapy [186].

Microfilariae moving through tissues are responsible for the syndrome known as tropical eosinophilia in which respiratory symptoms are

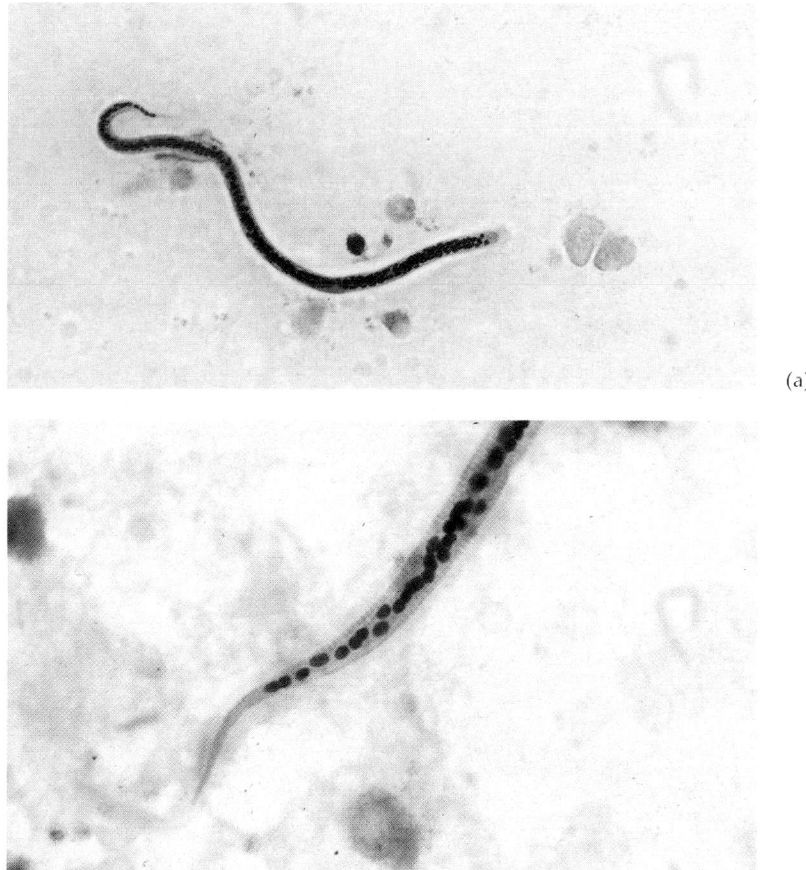

Fig. 3.138 Microfilariae of *Wucheria bancrofti* in thick films: (a) microfilaria showing the negative impression of the sheath (×365); (b) tail of a microfilaria showing that the nuclei do not extend into the tail (×912).

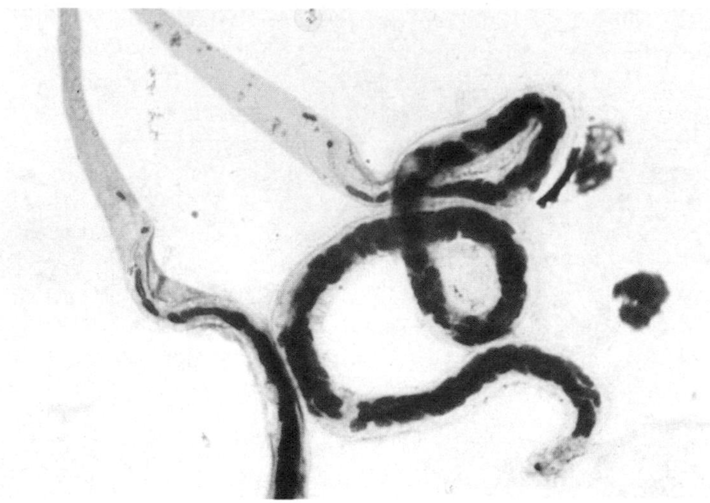

Fig. 3.139 Microfilariae of *Brugia malayi* in thick film showing the widely separated tail nuclei (×912). Courtesy of Dr S. Abdalla, London.

(a)

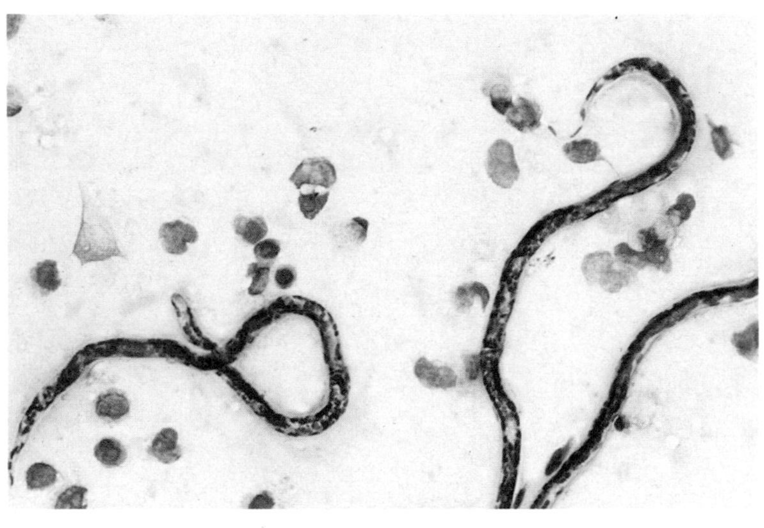

(b)

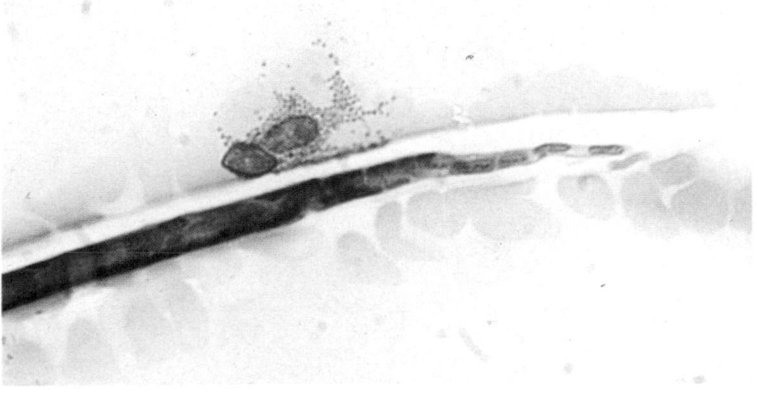

Fig. 3.140 Microfilariae of *Loa loa*: (a) a thick film showing the head and tail of microfilariae; nuclei extend to the tail (×365); (b) the tail of a microfilaria in a thin film showing the negative impression of the sheath; the nuclei extend to the tail (×912).

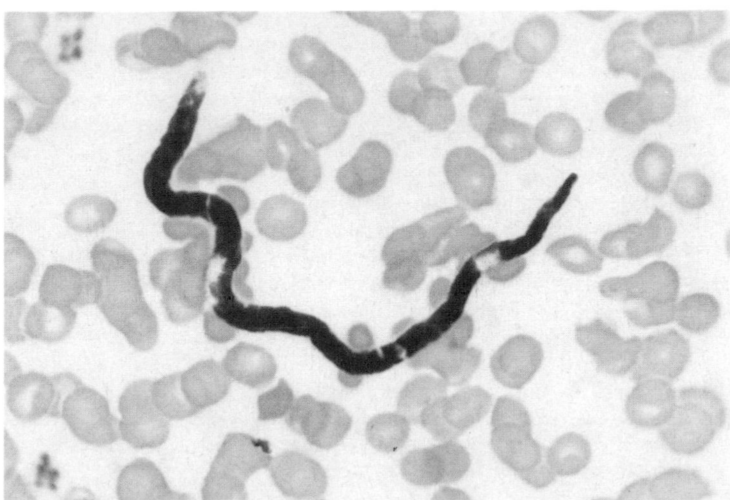

Fig. 3.141 Microfilaria of *Mansonella perstans* in a thin film (×912). Courtesy of Dr S. Abdalla.

associated with eosinophilia, increased rouleaux formation and an elevated ESR. However, microfilariae are not usually detectable in the blood of patients with tropical eosinophilia.

References

1 Bain BJ, Selection, care and maintenance of a microscope. In: Machin SJ, Mackie I, Patterson K, Cavill I, Contreras M, Knight R, eds. *Laboratory Haematology*. Edinburgh: Churchill Livingstone, 1995.

2 Bain BJ, Liesner R. Pseudo-pyropoikilocytosis: a striking artefact. *J Clin Pathol* 1995 (in press).

3 Sheehan RG, Frenkel EP. Influence of hemoglobin phenotype on the mean erythrocyte volume. *Acta Haematol* 1983; 69: 260–5.

4 Maggio A, Gagliano F, Siciliano S. Hemoglobin phenotype and mean erythrocyte volume in Sicilian people. *Acta Haematol* 1984; 71: 214.

5 Kaplan E, Zuelzer WW, Neel JV. Further studies on haemoglobin C alone and in combination with sickle cell anemia. *Blood* 1953; 8: 735–46.

6 Fairbanks VF, Gilchrist GS, Brimhall B, Jereb JA, Goldston EC. Hemoglobin E trait reexamined: a cause of microcytosis and erythrocytosis. Blood 1979; 53: 109–15.

7 Bird AR, Wood K, Leisegang F, Mathew CG, Ellis P, Hartley PS, Karabus CD. Hemoglobin E variants: a clinical, haematological and biosynthetic study of four South African families. *Acta Haematol* 1984; 72: 135–7.

8 Stavem P, Romslo I, Hovig T, Rootwelt K, Emblem R. Ferrochelatase deficiency of the bone marrow in a syndrome of congenital microcytic anaemia with iron overload of the liver and hyperferraemia. *Scand J Haematol* 1985; 34: 204–6.

9 Tulliez M, Testa U, Rochant H, Henri A, Vainchenker W, Toubol J, Breton-Gorius J, Dreyfus B. Reticulocytosis, hypochromia, and microcytosis: an unusual presentation of the preleukaemic syndrome. *Blood* 1982; 59: 293–9.

10 Ruocco L, Baldi A, Cecconi N, Marini A, Azzarà A, Ambrogi F, Grassi B. Severe pancytopenia due to copper deficiency. *Acta Haematol* 1986; 76: 224–6.

11 Simon SR, Branda RF, Tindle BF, Burns SL. Copper deficiency and sideroblastic anemia associated with zinc ingestion. *Am J Hematol* 1988; 28: 181–3.

12 Ramadurai J, Shapiro C, Kozloff M, Telfer M. Zinc abuse and sideroblastic anemia. *Am J Hematol* 1993; 42: 227–8.

13 How J, Davidson RJL, Bewsher PD. Red cell changes in hyperthyroidism. *Scand J Haematol* 1979; 23: 323–8.

14 Hillman RS, Finch CA. *Red Cell Manual*, 5th edn. Philadelphia: FA Davis, 1985.

15 Larrick JW, Hyman ES. Acquired iron deficiency anemia caused by an antibody against the transferrin receptor. *N Engl J Med* 1984; 311: 214–18.

16 Porter KG, McMaster D, Elmes ME, Love AHG. Anaemia and low serum copper during zinc therapy. *Lancet* 1977; ii: 774.

17 Helman N, Rubenstein LS. The effects of age, sex, and smoking on erythrocytes and leukocytes. *Am J Clin Pathol* 1975; 63: 35–44.

18 Eastham RD, Jancar J. Macrocytosis in Down's syndrome and during long term anticonvulsant therapy. *J Clin Pathol* 1970; 23: 296–8.

19 Cauchi MN, Smith MB. Quantitative aspects of red cell size variation during pregnancy. *Clin Lab Haematol* 1981; 4: 149–54.

20 Rees MI, Worwood M, Thompson PW, Gilbertson C, May A. Red cell dimorphism in a young man with a constitutional chromosomal translocation t(11;22) (p15.5;q11.21). *Br J Haematol* 1994; 87: 386–95.
21 Perrotta AL, Finch CA. The polychromatophilic erythrocyte. *Am J Clin Pathol* 1972; 57: 471–7.
22 Rowles PM, Williams ES. Abnormal red cell morphology in venous blood of men climbing at high altitude. *Br Med J* 1983; 286: 1396.
23 Bessis M. *Living Blood Cells and their Ultrastructure*, trans. Weed RI. Berlin: Springer-Verlag, 1973.
24 Wolf PL, Koett J. Hemolytic anemia in hepatic disease with decreased erythrocyte adenosine triphosphate. *Am J Clin Pathol* 1980; 73: 785–8.
25 Shilo S, Werner D, Hershko C. Acute hemolytic anemia caused by severe hypophosphatemia in diabetic ketoacidosis. *Acta Haematol* 1985; 73: 55–7.
26 McGrath KM, Zalcberg JR, Slonin J, Wiley JS. Intralipid induced haemolysis. *Br J Haematol* 1982; 50: 376–8.
27 Austin RF, Desforges JF. Hereditary elliptocytosis: an unusual presentation of hemolysis in the newborn associated with transient morphologic abnormalities. *Pediatrics* 1969; 44: 196–200.
28 Nurse GT, Coetzer TL, Palek J. The elliptocytoses, ovalocytoses and related disorders. *Baillière's Clin Haematol* 1992; 5: 187–207.
29 Farolino DL, Rustagi PK, Currie MS, Doeblin TD, Logue GL. Teardrop-shaped cells in autoimmune hemolytic anemia. *Am J Hematol* 1986; 21: 415–18.
30 Miwa S, Fujii H, Tani K, Takahashi K, Takegawa S, Fujinami N, Sakurai M, Kubo M *et al.* Two cases of red cell aldolase deficiency associated with hereditary hemolytic anemia in a Japanese family. *Am J Hematol* 1981; 11: 425–37.
31 Carlyle RF, Nichols G, Rowles PM. Abnormal red cells in blood of men subjected to simulated dives. *Lancet* 1979; i: 1114–16.
32 Feo CT, Tchernia G, Subtil E, Leblond PF. Observations of echinocytosis in eight patients: a phase contrast and SEM study. *Br J Haematol* 1978; 40: 519–26.
33 Kay MM, Bosman GJ, Lawrence C. Functional topography of band 3: specific structural alteration linked to functional aberrations in human erythrocytes. *Proc Natl Acad Sci USA* 1988; 85: 492–6.
34 Doll DC, Lest AF, Dayhoff DA, Loy TS, Ringenberg QS, Yarbro JW. Acanthocytosis associated with myelodysplasia. *J Clin Oncol* 1989; 7: 1569–72.
35 Palek J, Jarolim P. Clinical expression and laboratory detection of red blood cell membrane protein mutations. *Semin Hematol* 1993; 30: 249–83.
36 Bassen FA, Kornzweig AL. Malformation of the erythrocytes in a case of atypical retinitis pigmentosa. *Blood* 1950; 5: 381–7.
37 Estes JW, Morley TJ, Levine IM, Emerson CP. A new hereditary acanthocytosis syndrome. *Am J Med* 1967; 42: 868–81.
38 Sakai T, Mawatari S, Iwashita H, Goto I, Kuroiwa Y. Choreoacanthocytosis. *Arch Neurol* 1981; 38: 335.
39 Udden MM, Umeda M, Hirano Y, Marcus DM. New abnormalities in the morphology, cell surface receptors and electrolyte balance in In(1u) erythrocytes. *Blood* 1987; 69: 52–7.
40 McGrath KM, Collecutt MF, Gordon A, Sawers RJ, Faragher BS. Dehydrated hereditary stomatocytosis — a report of two families and a review of the literature. *Pathology* 1984; 16: 146–50.
41 Reinhardt WH, Gössi U, Bütikofer P, Ott P, Sigrist H, Schatzmann H-J, Lutz HU, Straub PW. Haemolytic anaemia in analpha-lipoproteinaemia (Tangier disease): morphological, biochemical, and biophysical properties of the red blood cell. *Br J Haematol* 1989; 72: 272–7.
42 Godin DV, Garnett ME, Hoag G, Wadsworth LD, Frohlich J. Erythrocyte abnormalities in hypoalphalipoproteinemia syndrome resembling fish eye disease. *Eur J Haematol* 1988; 41: 176–81.
43 Miller DR, Rickles FR, Lichtman MA, La Celle PL, Bates J, Weed R. A new variant of hereditary hemolytic anemia with stomatocytosis and erythrocyte cation abnormality. *Blood* 1971; 38: 184–204.
44 Davidson RJ, How J, Lessels S. Acquired stomatocytosis: its prevalence and significance in routine haematology. *Scand J Haematol* 1977; 19: 47–53.
45 Wislöff F, Boman D. Acquired stomatocytosis in alcoholic liver disease. *Scand J Haematol* 1979; 23: 43–50.
46 Mallory DM, Rosenfield RE, Wong KY, Heller C, Rubinstein P, Allen FH, Walker ME, Lewis M. Rh_{mod}, a second kindred (Craig). *Vox Sang* 1976; 30: 430–40.
47 von Behrens WE. Splenomegaly, macrothrombocytopenia and stomatocytosis in healthy Mediterranean subjects. *Scand J Haematol* 1975; 14: 258–67.
48 Valentine WN. Hemolytic anemia and inborn errors of metabolism. *Blood* 1979; 54: 549–59.
49 Eichner ER. Erythroid karyorrhexis in the peripheral blood smear in severe arsenic poisoning: a comparison with lead poisoning. *Am J Clin Pathol* 1984; 81: 533–7.
50 Mathy KA, Koepke JA. The clinical usefulness of segmented vs. stab neutrophil criteria for differential leukocyte counts. *Am J Clin Pathol* 1974; 61: 947–58.
51 Akenzua GI, Hui YT, Milner R, Zipursky A. Neutrophil and band counts in the diagnosis of

neonatal infections. *Pediatrics* 1974; 54: 38–42.
52 Christensen RD, Rothstein G. Pitfalls in the interpretation of leukocyte counts of newborn infants. *Am J Clin Pathol* 1978; 72: 608–11.
53 Christensen RD, Rothstein G, Anstall HB, Bybee B. Granulocyte transfusions in neonates with bacterial infection, neutropenia, and depletion of mature bone marrow neutrophils. *Pediatrics* 1981; 70: 1–6.
54 Chanarin I. *Megaloblastic Anaemias*, 2nd edn. St Louis: CV Mosby, 1979.
55 Edwin E. The segmentation of polymorphonuclear neutrophils. *Acta Med Scand* 1967; 182: 401–10.
56 Davidson WM. Inherited variations in leukocytes. *Semin Haematol* 1968; 5: 255–74.
57 Hess U, Ganser A, Schnürch H-G, Seipelt G, Ottman OG, Falk S, Schulz G, Hoelzer D. Myelokathexis treated with recombinant human granulocyte-macrophage colony-stimulating factor (rhGM-CSF). *Br J Haematol* 1992; 80: 254–6.
58 Davidson WM, Smith DR. A morphological sex difference in the polymorphonuclear neutrophil leucocytes. *Br Med J* 1954; ii: 6–7.
59 Murthy MSN, Emmerich von H. The occurrence of the sex chromatin in white blood cells of young adults. *Am J Clin Pathol* 1958; 30: 216–27.
60 Davidson WM, Fowler JF, Smith DR. Sexing the neutrophil leucocytes in natural and artificial chimaeras. *Br J Haematol* 1958; 4: 231–8.
61 Mittwoch U. The incidence of drumsticks in patients with three X chromosomes. *Cytogenetics* 1963; 2: 24–33.
62 Tomonaga M, Matsuura G, Watanabe B, Kamochi Y, Ozono N. Leukocyte drumsticks in chronic granulocytic leukaemia and related disorders. *Blood* 1961; 18: 581–90.
63 Archer RK, Engisch HJC, Gaha T, Ruxton J. The eosinophil leucocyte in the blood and bone marrow of patients with Down's anomaly. *Br J Haematol* 1971; 21: 271–6.
64 Strauss RG, Bove KE, Jones JF, Mauer AM, Fulginiti VA. An anomaly of neutrophil morphology with impaired function. *N Engl J Med* 1974; 290: 478–84.
65 Plum CM, Warburg M, Danielsen J. Defective maturation of granulocytes, retinal cysts and multiple skeletal malformations in a mentally retarded girl. *Acta Haematol* 1978; 59: 53–63.
66 Huehns ER, Lutzner M, Hecht F. Nuclear abnormalities of the neutrophils in D_1(13–15)-trisomy syndrome. *Lancet* 1964; i: 589–90.
67 Girolami A, Fabris F, Caronato A, Randi ML. Increased numbers of pseudodrumsticks in neutrophils and large platelets. A 'new' congenital leukocyte and platelet morphological abnormality. *Acta Haematol* 1980; 64: 324–30.
68 Moore CM, Weinger RS. Pseudo-drumsticks in granulocytes of a male with a Yqh+ polymorphism. *Am J Hematol* 1980; 8: 411–14.
69 Gibson BES. Inherited disorders. In: Hann IM, Gibson BES, Letsky EA, eds. *Fetal and Neonatal Haematology*. London: Baillière Tindall, 1991.
70 Seman G. Sur une anomalie constitutionnelle héréditaire du noyau des polynucléaires neutrophiles. *Rev d'Hématol* 1959; 14: 409–12.
71 Langenhuijsen MMAC. Neutrophils with ring shaped nuclei in myeloproliferative disorders. *Br J Haematol* 1984; 58: 227–30.
72 Stavem P, Hjort PF, Vogt E, Van der Hagen CB. Ring-shaped nuclei of granulocytes in a patient with acute erythroleukaemia. *Scand J Haematol* 1969; 6: 31–2.
73 Kahoh T, Saigo K, Yamagishi M. Neutrophils with ring-shaped nuclei in chronic neutrophilic leukaemia. *Am J Clin Pathol* 1986; 86: 748–51.
74 Craig A. Ring neutrophils in megaloblastic anaemia. *Br J Hematol* 1988; 67: 247–8.
75 Hernandez JA, Aldred SW, Bruce JR, Vanatta PR, Mattingly TL, Sheehan WW. 'Botryoid' nuclei in neutrophils of patients with heat stroke. *Lancet* 1980; ii: 642–3.
76 Neftel KA, Müller OM. Heat-induced radial segmentation of leucocyte nuclei: a non-specific phenomenon accompanying inflammatory and necrotizing diseases. *Br J Haematol* 1981; 48: 377–82.
77 Gustke SS, Becker GA, Garancis JC, Geimer NF, Pisciotta AV. Chromatin clumping in mature leukocytes: a hitherto unrecognized abnormality. *Blood* 1970; 35: 637–58.
78 Brunning RD. Morphologic alterations in nucleated blood and marrow cells in genetic disorders. *Hum Pathol* 1970; 1: 99–124.
79 Skendzel LP, Hoffman GC. The Pelger anomaly of leukocytes: forty cases in seven families. *Am J Clin Pathol* 1962; 37: 294–301.
80 Ardeman S, Chanarin I, Frankland AW. The Pelger–Hüet anomaly and megaloblastic anemia. *Blood* 1963; 22: 472–6.
81 Klein A, Hussar AE, Bornstein S. Pelger–Hüet anomaly of leukocytes. *N Engl J Med* 1955; 253: 1057–62.
82 Parmley RT, Tzeng DY, Baehner RL, Boxer LA. Abnormal distribution of complex carbohydrates in neutrophils of a patient with lactoferrin deficiency. *Blood* 1983; 62: 538–48.
83 Deutsch PH, Mandell GL. Reversible Pelger–Hüet anomaly associated with ibuprofen therapy. *Arch Intern Med* 1985; 145: 166.
84 Schmitz LL, McClure JS, Letz CE, Dayton V, Weisdorf DJ, Parkin JL, Brunning RD. Morphologic and quantitative changes in blood and marrow

cells following growth factor therapy. *Am J Clin Pathol* 1994; 101: 67–75.

85 Campbell LJ, Maher DW, Tay DLM, Boyd AW, Rockman S, McGrath K, Fox RM, Morstyn G. Marrow proliferation and the appearance of giant neutrophils in response to recombinant human granulocyte colony stimulating factor (rhG-CSF). *Br J Haematol* 1992; 80: 298–304.

86 Ryder JW, Lazarus HM, Farhi DC. Bone marrow and blood findings after marrow transplantation and rhGM-CSF therapy. *Am J Clin Pathol* 1992; 97: 631–7.

87 Gale PF, Parkin JL, Quie PG, Pettitt RE, Nelson RP, Brunning RD. Leukocyte granulation abnormality associated with normal neutrophil function and neurological abnormality. *Am J Clin Pathol* 1986; 86: 33–49.

88 Newburger PE, Robinson JM, Pryzansky KB, Rosoff PM, Greenberger JS, Tauber AI. Human neutrophil dysfunction with giant granules and defective activation of the respiratory burst. *Blood* 1983; 61: 1247–57.

89 Van Slyck EJ, Rebuck JW. Pseudo-Chediak–Higashi anomaly in acute leukemia. *Am J Clin Pathol* 1974; 62: 673–8.

90 Davidson RJ, McPhie JL. Cytoplasmic vacuolation of peripheral blood cells in acute alcoholism. *J Clin Pathol* 1980; 33: 1193–6.

91 Jordans GHW. The familial occurrence of fat containing vacuoles in the leucocytes diagnosed in two brothers suffering from dystrophia musculorum progressiva. *Acta Med Scand* 1953; 145: 419–23.

92 Hann IM, Rankin A, Lake BD, Pritchard J. *Colour Atlas of Paediatric Haematology*. Oxford: Oxford University Press, 1983.

93 Schopfer K, Douglas SD. Fine structural studies of peripheral blood leucocytes from children with kwashiorkor: morphological and functional studies. *Br J Haematol* 1976; 32: 573–7.

94 Peterson LC, Rao KV, Crosson JT, White JG. Fechtner syndrome — a variant of Alport's syndrome with leukocyte inclusions and macrothrombocytopenia. *Blood* 1985; 65: 397–406.

95 Ribeiro RC, Howard TH, Brandalise S, Behm FG, Parham DM, Wang WC, Crist WM, Parmley RT. Giant actin inclusions in hematopoietic cells associated with transfusion-dependent anemia and grey skin colouration. *Blood* 1994; 83: 3717–26.

96 Nosanchuk J, Terzian J, Posso M. Circulating mucopolysaccharide (mucin) in two adults with metastatic adenocarcinoma. *Arch Pathol Lab Med* 1987; 111: 545–8.

97 Chomet B, Kirshen MM, Schaefer G, Mudrik P. The finding of the LE (lupus erythematosus) cells in smears of untreated, freshly drawn peripheral blood. *Blood* 1953; 8: 1107–9.

98 Weil SC, Holt S, Hrisinko MA, Little L, De Backer N. Melanin inclusions in peripheral blood leukocytes of a patient with malignant melanoma. *Am J Clin Pathol* 1985; 84: 679–81.

99 Sen Gupta PC, Ghosal SP, Mukherjee AK, Maity TR. Bilirubin crystals in neutrophils of jaundiced neonates and infants. *Acta Haematol* 1983; 70: 69–70.

100 Smith H. Unidentified inclusions in haemopoietic cells, congenital atresia of the bile ducts and livedo reticularis in an infant. A new syndrome? *Br J Haematol* 1967; 13: 695–705.

101 Miale JB. *Laboratory Medicine: Hematology*, 6th edn. St Louis: CV Mosby, 1982.

102 Hernandez JA, Steane SM. Erythrophagocytosis by segmented neutrophils in paroxysmal cold hemoglobinuria. *Am J Clin Pathol* 1984; 81: 787–9.

103 Schofield KP, Stone PCW, Beddall AC, Stuart J. Quantitative cytochemistry of the toxic granulation blood neutrophil. *Br J Haematol* 1983; 53: 15–22.

104 Presentey B. Alder anomaly accompanied by a mutation of the myeloperoxidase structural gene. *Acta Haematol* 1986; 75: 157–9.

105 Rosenszajn L, Klajman A, Yaffe D, Efrati P. Jordan's anomaly in white blood cells. *Blood* 1966; 28: 258–65.

106 Abernathy MR. Döhle bodies associated with uncomplicated pregnancy. *Blood* 1966; 27: 380–5.

107 Itoga T, Laszlo J. Döhle bodies and other granulocytic alterations during chemotherapy with cyclophosphamide. *Blood* 1962; 20: 668–74.

108 Jenis EH, Takeuchi A, Dillon DE, Ruymann FB, Rivkin S. The May–Hegglin anomaly: ultrastructure of the granulocyte inclusion. *Am J Clin Pathol* 1971; 55: 187–96.

109 Volpé R, Ogryzlo MA. The cryoglobulin inclusion cell. *Blood* 1955; 10: 493–6.

110 Powell HC, Wolf PL. Neutrophilic leukocyte inclusions in colchicine intoxication. *Arch Pathol Lab Med* 1976; 100: 136–8.

111 Kapff CT, Jandl JH. *Blood: atlas and sourcebook of hematology*, Boston: Little, Brown, 1981.

112 Cooke WE. The macropolycyte. *Br Med J* 1927; i: 12–13.

113 Guibaud S, Plumet-Leger A, Frobert Y. Transient neutrophil aggregation in a patient with infectious mononucleosis. *Am J Clin Pathol* 1971; 80: 883–4.

114 Nand S, Bansal VK, Kozeny G, Vertuno L, Remlinger KA, Jordan JV. Red cell fragmentation syndrome with the use of subclavian hemodialysis catheters. *Arch Intern Med* 1985; 145: 1421–3.

115 Tracey R, Smith H. An inherited anomaly of human eosinophils and basophils. *Blood Cells* 1978; 4: 291–300.

116 Presentey BZ. A new anomaly of eosinophilic

granulocytes. *Am J Clin Pathol* 1968; 49: 887–90.

117 Kay NE, Nelson DA, Gottleib AJ. Eosinophilic Pelger–Hüet anomaly with myeloproliferative disorder. *Am J Clin Pathol* 1973; 60: 663–8.

118 Bain BJ. The significance of ring eosinophils in humans. *Br J Haematol* 1989; 73: 580–1.

119 Weil SC, Hrisinko MA. A hybrid eosinophilic–basophilic granulocyte in chronic granulocytic leukaemia. *Am J Clin Pathol* 1987; 87: 66–70.

120 Douglas SD, Blume RS, Wolff SM. Fine structural studies of leukocytes from patients and heterozygotes with the Chediak–Higashi syndrome. *Blood* 1969; 33: 527–40.

121 Groover RV, Burke EC, Gordon H, Berdon WE. The genetic mucopolysaccharidoses. *Semin Haematol* 1972; 9: 371–402.

122 Kolodny EH. Clinical and biochemical genetics of the lipidoses. *Semin Haematol* 1972; 9: 251–71.

123 Maier-Redelsperger M, Stern M-H, Maroteaux P. Pink rings lymphocyte: a new cytologic abnormality characteristic of mucopolysaccharidosis type II (Hunter disease). *Pediatrics* 1988; 82: 286–7.

124 Iwasaki H, Ueda T, Uchida M, Nakamura T, Takada N, Mahara F. Atypical lymphocytes with a multilobated nucleus from a patient with tsutsugamushi disease (scrub typhus) in Japan. *Am J Hematol* 1991; 36: 150–1.

125 Chow K C, Nacilla JQ, Witzig TE, Li C-Y. Is persistent polyclonal B lymphocytosis caused by Epstein Barr virus? A study with polymerase chain reaction and *in situ* hybridization. *Am J Hematol* 1992; 41: 270–5.

126 Currimbhoy Z. An outbreak of an infection associated with circulating activated monocytes and haemophagocytes in children in Bombay, India. *Am J Pediatr Hematol Oncol* 1991; 13: 274–9.

127 Efrati P, Rozenszajn L. The morphology of buffy coats in normal human adults. *Blood* 1960; 15: 1012–19.

128 Bennett JM, Catovsky D, Daniel MT, Flandrin G, Galton DAG, Gralnick HR, Sultan C. Proposals for the classification of the myelodysplastic syndromes. *Br J Haematol* 1982; 51: 189–99.

129 Hicsönmez G, Ozkaynak F. Diagnosis of heterozygous state for Bernard–Soulier disease. *Acta Haematol* 1984; 71: 285–6.

130 Epstein CJ, Sahud MA, Piel CF, Goodman JR, Bernfield MR, Kushner JH, Ablin AR. Hereditary macrothrombocytopathia, nephritis and deafness. *Am J Med* 1972; 52: 299–310.

131 Estes JW. Platelet size and function in the heritable disorders of connective tissues. *Ann Intern Med* 1968; 68: 1237–49.

132 Raccuglia G. Gray platelet syndrome. A variety of qualitative platelet disorder. *Am J Med* 1971; 51: 818–27.

133 Mant MJ, Doery JCG, Gauldie J, Sims H. Pseudothrombocytopenia due to platelet aggregation and degranulation in blood collected in EDTA. *Scand J Haematol* 1975; 15: 161–70.

134 Stavem P, Kjaerheim A. *In vitro* platelet stain preventing (degranulating) effect of various substances. *Scand J Haematol* 1977; 18: 170–6.

135 Hamilton RW, Shaikh BS, Ottie JN, Storch AE, Saleem A, White JG. Platelet function, ultrastructure and survival in the May–Hegglin anomaly. *Am J Clin Pathol* 1980; 74: 663–8.

136 Fajardo LF, Tallent C. Malaria parasites within human platelets. *JAMA* 1974; 229: 1205–7.

137 Casonato A, Bertomoro A, Pontara E, Dannhauser D, Lazzaro AR, Girolami A. EDTA dependent pseudothrombocytopenia caused by antibodies against the cytoadhesive receptor of platelet gpIIB/IIIA. *J Clin Pathol* 1994; 47; 625–30.

138 Yoo D, Weems H, Lessin LS. Platelet to leukocyte adherence phenomenon. *Acta Haematol* 1982; 68: 142–8.

139 Hansen M, Pedersen NT. Circulating megakaryocytes in patients with pulmonary inflammation and in patients subjected to cholecystectomy. *Scand J Haematol* 1979; 23: 211–16.

140 Pederson NT, Petersen S. Megakaryocytes in the foetal circulation and in cubital venous blood in the mother before and after delivery. *Scand J Haematol* 1980; 25: 5–11.

141 Pederson NT, Cohn J. Intact megakaryocytes in the venous blood as a marker for thrombopoiesis. *Scand J Haematol* 1981; 27: 57–63.

142 Pederson NT, Laursen B. Megakaryocytes in cubital venous blood in patients with chronic myeloproliferative disorders. *Scand J Haematol* 1983; 30: 50–8.

143 Lowenstein ML. The mammalian reticulocyte. *Int Rev Cytol* 1959; 9: 135–74.

144 Xanthou M. Leucocyte blood picture in full-term and premature babies during neonatal period. *Arch Dis Child* 1970; 45: 242–9.

145 Gibson EL, Vaucher Y, Corrigan JJ. Eosinophilia in premature infants: relationship to weight gain. *J Pediatr* 1984; 95: 99–101.

146 Wilkinson LS, Tang A, Gjedsted A. Marked lymphocytosis suggesting chronic lymphocytic leukemia in three patients with hyposplenism. *Am J Med* 1983; 75: 1053–6.

147 Holyroyde CP, Gardner FH. Acquisition of autophagic vacuoles by human erythrocytes: physiological role of the spleen. *Blood* 1970; 36: 566–75.

148 Kevy SV, Tefft M, Vawter GF, Rosen FS. Hereditary splenic hypoplasia. *Pediatrics* 1968; 42: 752–7.

149 Garriga S, Crosby WH. The incidence of leukemia in families of patients with hypoplasia of the marrow. *Blood* 1959; 14: 1008–14.

150 Rodin AE, Sloan JA, Nghiem QX. Polysplenia with severe congenital heart disease and Howell–Jolly bodies. *Am J Clin Pathol* 1972; 58: 127–34.
151 Eshel Y, Sarova-Pinhas I, Lampl Y, Jedwab M. Autosplenectomy complicating pneumococcal meningitis in an adult. *Arch Intern Med* 1991; 151: 998–9.
152 Ryan FP, Smart RC, Holdsworth CD, Preston FE. Hyposplenism in inflammatory bowel disease. *Gut* 1978; 19: 50–5.
153 Corazza GR, Gasbarrini G. Defective spleen function and its relation to bowel disease. *Clin Gastroenterol* 1983; 12: 651–69.
154 Dillon AM, Stein HB, English RA. Splenic atrophy in systemic lupus erythematosus. *Ann Intern Med* 1982; 96: 40–3.
155 Friedman TC, Thomas PM, Fleisher TA, Feuillan P, Parker RI, Cassorla F, Chrousos GP. Frequent occurrence of asplenia and cholelithiasis in patients with autoimmune polyglandular disease type 1. *Am J Med* 1991; 91: 625–30.
156 Kahls P, Panzer S, Kletter K, Minar E, Stain-Kos M, Walter R, Lechner K, Hinterberger W. Functional asplenia after bone marrow transplantation: a late complication related to extensive chronic graft-versus-host disease. *Ann Intern Med* 1988; 109: 461–4.
157 Dailey MO, Coleman CN, Fajardo LF. Splenic injury caused by therapeutic irradiation. *Am J Surg Pathol* 1981; 5: 325–31.
158 Bensinger TA, Keller AR, Merrell LF, O'Leary DS. Thorotrast-induced reticuloendothelial blockade in man. *Am J Med* 1971; 51: 663–8.
159 Kurth D, Deiss A, Cartwright GE. Circulating siderocytes in human subjects. *Blood* 1969; 34: 754–64.
160 Steinberg MH, Gatling RR, Tavassoli M. Evidence of hyposplenism, in the presence of splenomegaly. *Scand J Haematol* 1983; 31: 437–9.
161 Sunder-Plassmann G, Geissler K, Penner E. Functional asplenia and vasculitis associated with anti-neutrophil cytoplasmic antibodies. *N Engl J Med* 1992; 327: 437–8.
162 Shanberge JN. Accidental occurrence of endothelial cells in peripheral blood smears. *Am J Clin Pathol* 1954; 25: 460–4.
163 George F, Brouqui P, Bofta M-C, Mutin M, Drancourt M, Brisson C, Raoult D, Sampol J. Demonstration of *Rickettsia conorii*-induced endothelial injury *in vivo* by measuring circulating endothelial cells, thrombomodulin, and von Willebrand factor in patients with Mediterranean spotted fever. *Blood* 1993; 82: 2109–16.
164 Christensen WN, Ultmann JE, Mohos SC. Disseminated neuroblastoma in an adult presenting with the picture of thrombocytopenic purpura. *Blood* 1956; 11: 273–8.
165 Nunez C, Abboud SL, Leman NC, Kemp JA. Ovarian rhabdomyosarcoma presenting as leukemia. *Cancer* 1983; 52: 297–300.
166 Pollak ER, Miller HJ, Vye MV. Medulloblastoma presenting as leukemia. *Am J Clin Pathol* 1981; 76: 98–103.
167 Krause JR. Carcinocythemia. *Arch Pathol Lab Med* 1979; 103: 98.
168 Melamed MR, Cliffton EE, Seal SH. Cancer cells in the peripheral venous blood. A quantitative study of cells of problematic origin. *Am J Clin Pathol* 1962; 37: 381–8.
169 Brace W, Bain B, Walker M, Catovsky D. Teaching cases from the Royal Marsden Hospital: an elderly patient with unusual circulating cells. *Leuk Lymphoma* 1995; 18: 529–30.
170 Bouroncle BA. Sternberg–Reed cells in the peripheral blood of patients with Hodgkin's disease. *Blood* 1966; 27: 544–56.
171 Sinks LF, Clein GP. The cytogenetics and cell metabolism of circulating Reed–Sternberg cells. *Br J Haematol* 1966; 12: 447–53.
172 Dooley JR. Haemotropic bacteria in man. *Lancet* 1980; ii: 1237–9.
173 Le CT. Tick-borne relapsing fever in children. *Pediatrics* 1980; 66: 963–6.
174 Lawrence C, Brown ST, Freundlich LF. Peripheral blood smear bacillemia. *Am J Med* 1988; 85: 111–13.
175 Fife A, Hill D, Barton C, Burden P. Gram negative septicaemia diagnosed on peripheral blood smear appearances. *J Clin Pathol* 1993; 47: 82–4.
176 Rynkiewicz DL, Liu LX. Human ehrlichiosis in New England. *N Engl J Med* 1994; 330: 292–3.
177 Chen S-M, Dumler JS, Bakken JS, Walker DH. Identification of a granulocytotropic *Ehrlichia* species as the etiologic agent of human disease. *J Clin Microbiol* 1994; 32: 589–95.
178 McDade JE. Ehrlichiosis — a disease of animals and humans. *J Infect Dis* 1990; 161: 609–17.
179 Mann JM, Hull HF, Schmid GP, Droke WE. Plague and the peripheral smear. *JAMA* 1984; 251: 953.
180 Kuberski TT. Intraleukocytic spore formation and leukocytic vacuolization during *Clostridium perfringens* septicemia. *Am J Clin Pathol* 1977; 68: 794–6.
181 Monihan JM, Jewell TW, Weir GT. *Candida parapsilosis* diagnosed by peripheral blood smear. *Arch Pathol Lab Med* 1986; 110: 1180–1.
182 Girmenia C, Jaalouk G. Detection of *Candida* in blood smears of patients with hematologic malignancies. *Eur J Haematol* 1994; 52: 124–5.
183 Yao YDC, Arkin CF, Doweiko JP, Hammer SM. Disseminated cryptococcosis diagnosed on peripheral blood smear in a patient with acquired

immunodeficiency syndrome. *Am J Med* 1990; 89: 100–2.

184 Wong KF, Tsang DNC, Chan JKC. Bone marrow diagnosis of penicilliosis. *N Engl J Med* 1994; 330: 717–18.

185 Spach DH, Liles WC, Campbell GL, Quick RE, Anderson DE, Fritsche TR. Tick-borne diseases in the United States. *N Engl J Med* 1993; 329: 936–47.

186 Learning Bench Aid No 3. *Microscopical Diagnosis of Lymphatic Filariasis, Loiasis, Onchocerciasis.* Tropical Health Technology, Doddington, Cambridgeshire.

187 Hoffbrand AV, Pettit JE. *Sandoz Atlas, Clinical Haematology.* London: Gower, 1988.

CHAPTER 4

Detecting Erroneous Blood Counts

Automated blood counts may be inaccurate and it is the responsibility of the laboratory staff performing a count or authorizing a report to detect inaccuracies whenever possible.

The validation of an automated count requires: (i) knowledge that an instrument is capable of measuring all variables accurately, that it has been correctly calibrated and that quality control procedures indicate normal functioning; and (ii) assessment of each individual count as to whether it is likely to be correct or that, alternatively, it requires further review. If the first set of conditions has been met then it may be possible to validate counts by means of a computer program, either built into the automated counter or developed to fit the specifications of an individual laboratory. Counts can be computer-validated if: (i) all measurements fall within predetermined limits (which may be somewhat wider than the reference limits for that measurement) and there are no 'flags'; or (ii) measurements fall outside predetermined limits but nevertheless have not changed significantly in comparison with previous measurements on that individual. When results do not meet either set of criteria they should be individually assessed in relation to the clinical details and, if necessary, further steps should be taken to validate the results. These further steps may include: (i) examination of the histograms produced by an automated instrument to establish the likely reason for anomalous results or 'flags'; (ii) examination of the blood specimen, e.g., to check the date and time when venesection was performed, to confirm that the specimen was of adequate volume and to detect clots, fibrin strands, hyperlipidaemia or haemolysis; (iii) examination of a blood film; or (iv) various combinations of these procedures. Which procedures are necessary depends on the nature of the abnormality shown on the automated count and the safeguards that are already built into the instrumentation, e.g., to confirm the identity of the patient and detect specimens of inadequate volume or containing clots. Opinions differ as to whether blood films should always be examined in conjunction with the initial blood count from a patient or whether an automated count with no 'flags' can be accepted as valid evidence that there is no significant haematological abnormality. The latter policy will miss some abnormalities of clinical significance but not many. Regrettably, the time when it was possible to examine a blood film in conjunction with all blood counts appears to have passed, under the pressure of economic factors. Validation of a count before it is released also includes ensuring that results have been produced for all tests required, i.e., that no result has been 'voted out' because of poor replicate counts or because it is beyond the linearity limits of the instrument.

Blood count results should be assessed as to probability in the light of the clinical details. For example, cytopenia could be accepted without further review in a patient known to have had recent chemotherapy. Similarly, an increased WBC with a 'left shift' flag could be accepted in a post-partum or post-operative patient. Counts which have 'flags' indicating the presence of blast cells, atypical lymphocytes or NRBC require microscopic review. Whether flags for 'left shift' or 'immature granulocytes' always require review is a matter of individual laboratory policy. Blood count results which are unexpected or which fall a long way outside reference limits generally require further attention. An abnormal MCHC is a useful indicator of factitious results since it is derived from all measured red cell variables, i.e., Hb, RBC and MCV or Hct. It is thus sensitive to erroneous measurements in any of these three variables caused, for example, by hyperlipidaemia, intravascular haemolysis, non-lysis of red cells in the Hb channel and red cell agglutination. A markedly elevated MCV is also often factitious. Recognized causes of factitious results are summarized in Table 4.1. Some occur with all instruments while others are specific to a methodology. Laboratory workers should be familiar with the factitious results which are likely with the particular instrument they are operating. The rest of this chapter will deal with factitious results other than those consequent on technical errors or instrument and reagent malfunction.

It should be noted that factitious results are more likely to have been reported for instruments which have been in use for a long time or have been studied in detail. The lack of reported factitious results for other instruments does not indicate that they do not occur.

Table 4.1 Some causes of inaccurate automated blood counts

Fault in specimen collection or storage	Blood from wrong patient – blood specimen and request form relate to different patients
	Specimen diluted (e.g., taken from above intravenous infusion or excess liquid EDTA relative to volume of blood)
	Specimen taken into too high a concentration of EDTA
	Specimen haemoconcentrated due to prolonged application of tourniquet
	Specimen partly clotted
	Specimen lysed
	Specimen inadvertently heated or frozen
	Aged blood
Faulty sampling	Failure to prime instrument
	Inadequate mixing
	Specimen of inadequate volume
	Aspiration probe blocked, e.g., by clot from previous sample
	Carry-over from preceding very abnormal specimen (minor with modern instruments)
Faulty calibration	
Faulty maintenance, other instrument malfunction, reagent failure	
Inaccuracy inherent in specific methodologies	Underestimation of MCV by impedance counters in the presence of hypochromia
Inaccuracy due to unusual specimen characteristics	For example, erroneous Hb or red cell indices caused by cold agglutinins or hyperlipidaemia or factitious 'neutropenia' caused by peroxidase deficiency

Errors in automated WBC

Errors which may occur in automated WBCs are summarized in Tables 4.2 and 4.3. The only common causes of erroneous counts are factitiously high counts caused by NRBC, platelet aggregates or non-lysis of red cells. Factitiously low counts are uncommon, unless the blood has taken many days to reach the laboratory.

Erroneous WBCs are usually detected because of instrument 'flags' and improbable results for the WBC or other measurements, or by abnor-

Table 4.2 Some causes of a falsely high WBC

Cause	Instruments on which fault can occur
NRBC	All
Numerous giant platelets	All
Non-lysis of red cells	
Uraemia	Technicon H.6000 and H.1* series
Fetal and neonatal specimens	Technicon H.6000 and H.1* series, Cell-Dyn (optical channels), some Toa-Sysmex
Abnormal haemoglobins (e.g., AS, SS, AC, AE, AD, AO^{Arab})	Technicon H.1* series, some Toa-Sysmex
Liver disease	Toa-Sysmex (some)
Cold agglutinins	Coulter
Platelet aggregates	Coulter and Technicon
Cryoglobulinaemia and cryofibrinogenaemia	Coulter and Toa-Sysmex
Paraproteinaemia	Coulter and Toa-Sysmex
Fibrin strands	Coulter
Hyperlipidaemia	Coulter
Malaria parasites	Coulter and Toa-Sysmex
Unstable haemoglobin	Coulter

* Basophil channel gives accurate WBC but differential counts are erroneous.

Table 4.3 Some causes of a falsely low WBC

Cause	Instruments on which abnormality can occur
Cell lysis caused when blood is more than 3 days old	Coulter, Cobas Argos 5 Diff and probably other
Leucocyte or leucocyte and platelet aggregation due to an antibody or to alteration of the cell membrane	Coulter, Toa-Sysmex, Technicon H-6000 and H.1 series
Potent cold agglutinin	Coulter

malities detectable on instrument scatter plots or histograms. For example, an erroneous WBC consequent on a cold agglutinin would usually be accompanied by an improbably high MCV and MCHC. Neutrophil aggregation may be indicated by an elevated peroxidase score (HPX) on a Technicon H-6000 counter [1] or by an abnormal cloud at the top of the neutrophil area of the Coulter STKS or Technicon H.1 series of instruments.

With the latest automated impedance counters it may be impossible to determine an accurate WBC when there are numerous NRBC since some but not all of the RBC are included in the 'WBC'. If an accurate count is needed it is necessary to perform a total nucleated cell count, either in a haemocytometer or on a back-up instrument with adjustable thresholds, and then correct the count for the number of NRBC by counting their percentage on a blood film. Non-lysis of red cells is mainly a problem when the WBC is measured by light-scattering technology. Impedance counters usually produce an accurate result. The observation of factitious elevation of the WBC caused by non-lysis of red cells can be clinically useful since it may be indicative of a previously undiagnosed haemoglobinopathy. This has been noted with Technicon H.6000 and, to a lesser extent, H.1 series instruments and on the differential count channel of Toa-Sysmex instruments.

Factitious counts caused by platelet aggregates can usually be prevented by taking the blood specimen into citrate rather than EDTA. Erroneous counts caused by cryoproteins and cold agglutinins can be rectified by keeping the specimen warm. Aggregation of leucocytes is often time-dependent and is sometimes caused by a cold antibody, so that keeping the specimen warm and performing the blood count rapidly after phlebotomy can produce an accurate count. When erroneous counts are due to causes other than white cell clumping, haemocytometer counts will be accurate.

Table 4.4 Some causes of a falsely high Hb estimate

Cause	Instruments on which fault can occur	Detection
High WBC	All, but to a variable extent	Check whenever WBC is very high
Hyperlipidaemia, endogenous or due to parenteral nutrition	Coulter, Technicon	Improbable results for MCH and MCHC or flagging of MCHC/CHCM discrepancy; fuzzy red cell outlines on blood films
Paraprotein or hypergammaglobulinaemia	Coulter	MCH and MCHC slightly elevated
Cryoglobulinaemia	Coulter	MCH and MCHC slightly elevated

Errors in haemoglobin concentration and red cell indices

Haemoglobin concentration

Errors which may occur in automated measurements of the Hb and red cell indices are shown in Tables 4.4–4.6. Such erroneous results are usually suspected from a markedly elevated MCV, a markedly abnormal MCHC or a discrepancy between MCHC and CHCM.

Erroneous estimations of Hb (see Table 4.4) are most often consequent on turbidity caused by a high WBC or lipid in the plasma, either endogenous lipid [2] or that consequent on parenteral nutrition [3]. The degree of elevation of the WBC which causes an erroneous Hb varies greatly between instruments since it is dependent on the strength of the lytic agent which is employed in the WBC/Hb channel. The problem can be circumvented if separate channels are used for the WBC and the Hb, as in the latest Toa-Sysmex instruments, since a more powerful lytic agent can then be used. The instrument operator should be aware of the degree of leucocytosis which is likely to make Hb erroneous on a specific instrument and results should then be checked by manual techniques. The haemolysate is centrifuged before absorbance is read so that turbidity caused by the presence of cellular debris does not affect the reading. Erroneous results from hyperlipidaemia may be suspected when red cell indices are improbable or red cells on stained blood films have fuzzy outlines. This error can be confirmed by examining the plasma, after either centrifugation or red cell sedimentation, and noting the milky appearance. The problem can be dealt with by performing a microhaematocrit and a 'blank' measurement using the patient's plasma. A correction is then as follows:

$$\text{true Hb} = \text{measured Hb} - [\text{'Hb' of lipaemic plasma} \times (1 - \text{Hct})]$$

Alternatively, the plasma can be carefully removed and replaced by an equal volume of isotonic fluid before repeating the automated count. Similarly, the use of a plasma blank permits the correction of minor errors caused by the presence of a paraprotein or polyclonal hypergammaglobulinaemia. With the Technicon H.1 series of instruments a correct Hb can be calculated from CHCM and a microhaematocrit when there is lipid or other interfering substances in the plasma. The errors introduced into the Hb estimation by marked hyperbilirubinaemia and the presence of high levels of carboxyhaemoglobin are not of such magnitude as to be of practical importance and can therefore be ignored.

Table 4.5 Some causes of inaccurate estimates of RBC, MCV and Hct

Fault	Cause	Instruments on which fault can occur	Fault	Cause	Instruments on which fault can occur
Falsely high RBC	WBC very high	Coulter Technicon		WBC very high	Coulter
	Numerous large platelets	Coulter		Hyperosmolar states	Coulter
	Hyperlipidaemia (not consistently)	Coulter		Excess K_2EDTA	Technicon H.1 series
	Cryoglobulinaemia, cryofibrinogenaemia	Coulter	Falsely low MCV	Hypochromic red cells	All impedance instruments, Technicon H.6000
Falsely low RBC	Cold agglutinins	Coulter and Technicon		Increase in ambient temperature	Coulter
	EDTA-dependent panagglutination	Coulter		Hypo-osmolar states	Coulter
	In vitro red cell lysis due to mishandling of specimen or very abnormal red cells	All	Falsely high Hct	Factitious elevation of MCV (except when due to a cold agglutinin)	See above
	Extreme microcytosis or fragmentation causing red cells to fall below the lower threshold	Coulter		Factitious reduction of RBC	See above
Falsely high MCV	Storage of blood at room temperature	Most instruments, to a varying extent (see text)	Falsely low Hct	Factitious reduction of MCV	See above
	Cold agglutinins and EDTA-dependent agglutination	Coulter and Technicon		Factitious reduction of RBC by extreme microcytosis or *in vitro* red cell lysis	See above
				Cold agglutinin	Coulter

RBC, MCV and Hct

Errors in the RBC, MCV and Hct are summarized in Table 4.5. Impedance and earlier light-scattering instruments have an intrinsic error which leads to the MCV of hypochromic cells being underestimated and their MCHC being overestimated. This can also lead to two apparent populations on a red cell size histogram with blood samples which, on a Technicon H.1 series counter, show a single population of cells on a histogram of red cell size but two populations on a histogram of red cell haemoglobinization.

Storage of blood at room temperature may cause errors in the MCV and Hct. Coulter instruments usually give stable measurements unless blood has been stored for several days but a 6 fl rise by 24 hours has been observed with another impedance counter, the Toa-Sysmex NE-8000 [4]. With the Technicon H.1 series of instruments a rise in the MCV starts after about 8 hours; by 24 hours the average rise varies between 4–5 and 7–8 fl, depending on the ambient temperature. The MCV on the Cobas Argos Diff 5 rises by about 2 fl by 24 hours [5]. A low MCHC, without any corresponding hypochromia being detectable on a blood film, can indicate that an elevation in the MCV is caused by red cell swelling as a consequence of storage.

When blood samples are processed without delay, errors in the RBC, MCV and Hct (excluding those which are intrinsic to the methodology) are most often caused by cold agglutinins. Impedance counters are prone to more major errors for this reason than are current light-scattering Technicon instruments. The factitious elevation of MCV is consequent on the doublets and triplets which pass through the aperture being counted and sized as if they were single cells. The RBC is factitiously low both for this reason and because, with some counters, larger agglutinates are above the upper threshold for red cells and are excluded from the count. The size of doublets and triplets is also underestimated. For these reasons although MCV (Hct × 1000/RBC) is overestimated, Hct is underestimated. The underestimation of Hct means that there is a factitious elevation of MCH and MCHC. Erroneous counts can generally be eliminated by warming the sample before processing. When the cold agglutinin is very potent it may be necessary to both warm the blood specimen and predilute the sample for analysis in warmed diluent.

Other causes of factitious errors in the RBC, MCV and Hct are uncommon. Various changes in plasma osmolality lead to artefacts in MCV measurement by impedance counters. If a cell is in a hyperosmolar environment *in vivo* due, e.g., to severe hypernatraemia or severe hyperglycaemia, then the cytoplasm of the cell will also be hyperosmolar. When the blood is diluted within the automated counter in a medium of much lower osmolality then the more rapid movement of water than of electrolytes, glucose or urea across the cell membrane will lead to acute swelling of the cell which is reflected in the measured MCV. Since the Hct is calculated from the MCV it will also be increased whereas the MCHC is correspondingly reduced. This phenomenon may occur in hypernatraemic dehydration [6], severe uraemia [6] and in hyperglycaemia, e.g., due to uncontrolled diabetes mellitus [7]. Not only may factitious macrocytosis be produced but true microcytosis may be masked. The converse error of a falsely low MCV and Hct with elevation of the MCHC may be seen in patients with hyponatraemia [6] such as may be seen in chronic alcoholics and patients with inappropriate secretion of antidiuretic hormone. The factitious reduction of MCV in hypo-osmolar states can lead to masking of a true macrocytosis as well as factitious microcytosis. This error can be eliminated in instruments with a predilute mode by diluting the sample and allowing time for equilibration of solutes across the red cell membrane. A control sample should be prediluted and tested in parallel since, although the osmolality of the recommended diluent differs between instruments, it is often somewhat hypertonic so that the MCV of cells from normal subjects may also alter on predilution.

With the Technicon H.1 series of instruments, factitious macrocytosis can result from cell swelling which is induced by taking a small volume of blood into excess K_2EDTA. A hypochromia 'flag' also occurs [8].

If microcytosis is severe, some red cells may fall below the lower threshold of the instrument and, as these cells are excluded from the measurements, the MCV is overestimated. In the case of impedance counters this is usually more than counteracted by the fact that the cells are likely to be hypochromic and the inherent error of the methodology leads to the size of those cells which fall above the threshold being underestimated (see p. 136). If there are normochromic red cell fragments falling below the lower threshold the MCV will be overestimated without any counterbalancing effect being expected. Neither of these artefacts is of practical importance.

Inaccuracies in the Hct are those expected from inaccuracies in the RBC and MCV.

MCH and MCHC

Errors which may occur in the MCH and MCHC are summarized in Table 4.6. Errors in these variables are consequent on errors in the primary measurements from which they are derived. Mechanisms have been explained above. The inherent error of impedance counting leads to the MCHC being a very stable variable which fails to reflect true changes occurring in red cells. This is paradoxically useful since abnormalities of the MCHC are commonly factitious and therefore serve to alert the laboratory worker to the possibility of an erroneous result. In the case of current Technicon instruments, true abnormality of the MCHC is commoner but so is a factitious reduction consequent on swelling of cells as blood ages. A discrepancy between MCHC and CHCM serves as a flag since the latter variable is measured directly and thus is not affected by errors in Hb estimation.

Table 4.6 Some causes of inaccurate MCH and MCHC estimations

Fault	Cause	Instruments on which fault can occur
MCH falsely high	Factitious elevation of Hb	See Table 4.4
	Factitious reduction of RBC	See Table 4.5
	Intravascular haemolysis with free haemoglobin in plasma	All instruments
MCHC falsely high or true fall of MCHC masked	Factitious elevation of Hb	See Table 4.4
	Intravascular haemolysis with free haemoglobin in plasma or *in vitro* lysis of red cells	All instruments
	Factitious reduction in Hct or the product of MCV and RBC	See Table 4.5
	Hypo-osmolar states	Coulter
MCHC falsely low	Factitious elevation of MCV (except when caused by cold agglutinins)	See Table 4.5
	Factitious elevation of RBC by numerous giant platelets	All instruments
	Hyperosmolar states	Coulter instruments

Errors in platelet counts

The causes of erroneous platelet counts are summarized in Table 4.7. Factitiously low platelet counts are quite common as a consequence either of partial clotting of the specimen or of platelet aggregation or satellitism (see p. 102). Platelet aggregation may be due to activation of platelets during a difficult venepuncture or may be mediated by an antibody, which is either an IgG or IgM EDTA-dependent antibody or an EDTA-independent antibody. Platelet satellitism is also an antibody-mediated EDTA-dependent phenomenon. Neither *in vitro* aggregation nor platelet satellitism is of any significance *in vivo* but the detection of all factitiously low platelet counts is very important in order to avoid unnecessary investigation and treatment of the patient. There have been instances in which a factitiously low platelet count has led to a mistaken diagnosis of idiopathic thrombocytopenic purpura (ITP) and consequent corticosteroid treatment and even splenectomy.

The accuracy of any unexpectedly low platelet counts must always be confirmed. The specimen should be examined with an orange stick to detect any small clots or fibrin strands and the instrument histograms and scatter plots should be assessed. Some instruments are able to detect fibrin strands or small clots and flag their presence. The presence of platelet aggregates may also be flagged and an abnormal cluster or band of particles may be apparent in scattergrams. The

Table 4.7 Some causes of inaccurate automated platelet counts

Cause	Instrument on which observed
Falsely low platelet counts	
Partial clotting of specimen	All
Activation of platelets during venepuncture with consequent aggregation	All
EDTA-induced platelet aggregation	All
Platelet satellitism	All
Giant platelets falling above upper threshold for platelet count	All
Falsely high platelet counts	
Microcytic red cells or red cell fragments falling below upper threshold for the platelet count	All
White cell fragments counted as platelets	All
Haemoglobin H disease	Coulter
Cryoglobulin	Coulter, Technicon H.1 series

presence of an abnormal cluster along the top of the neutrophil box with the H.1 series may indicate the occurrence of platelet satellitism. However, not all falsely low platelet counts are flagged or associated with abnormal scattergrams. For example, platelet aggregates may be so large that they are the same size as white cells and are thus not identified. It is therefore important to examine a blood film for the presence of fibrin strands, platelet aggregates, platelet satellitism and giant platelets whenever a platelet count is unexpectedly low. Falsely low counts should be deleted from reports since clinical staff often do not realize that a comment such as 'platelet aggregates' is likely to mean that the platelet count is wrong. When platelet aggregation is antibody-mediated, accurate counts can usually be obtained on specimens taken into citrate or heparin rather than EDTA (but the effect of dilution must be allowed for). Some such antibodies are cold antibodies, so performing a count rapidly on a specimen which has been kept warm can also produce a valid count. Alternatively, if the platelet count is clearly normal, the comment 'platelet count normal on film' may be acceptable and obviate the need to obtain a further blood specimen.

It may be impossible to obtain an accurate automated platelet count in the presence of numerous giant platelets, in which case a haemocytometer count is required.

If a low platelet count is supported by the blood film, but is nevertheless unexpected, a repeat specimen should be obtained with careful attention to venepuncture technique before the count is regarded as a valid result on which management decisions should be based.

Falsely elevated platelet counts are much less common than falsely reduced counts. They are usually due to the presence of marked microcytosis (e.g., in haemoglobin H disease) or to the presence of red cell fragments (e.g., in microangiopathic haemolytic anaemia or severe burns) so that a significant numbers of red cells fall below the upper threshold for platelets. Even with variable thresholds and fitted curves it may not be possible to separate very small red cells or fragments from platelets. An accurate platelet count despite the presence of red cell fragments or microcytes can be produced by a Sysmex R-1000 Reticulocyte Analyzer. The RNA of both platelets and reticulocytes is stained with the fluorescent dye, auramine, and the two populations are then separated by gating [9]. Microcytic red cells do not take up the dye since they do not contain RNA.

Occasionally, falsely elevated platelet counts are caused by other particles of a similar size to platelets. The counting of fragments of white cell cytoplasm as platelets has been described in AML [10], hairy cell leukaemia [11] and lymphoma [12]. The counting of red and white cell fragments as platelets may have serious implications in acute leukaemia as a severe thrombocytopenia may be masked and left untreated [13].

When platelets are distributed evenly in a blood film, the platelet count can be validated by counting the ratio of platelets to red cells and calculating the platelet count indirectly from the RBC.

Errors in automated differential counts

Automated differential counts should be regarded as a means of screening blood samples for an abnormality and producing a differential count when there are only numerical abnormalities. Instruments may show systematic inaccuracies or may be inaccurate only with abnormal specimens of various types.

When mean automated counts for different leucocyte categories are compared with mean manual counts it is not uncommon for automated instruments to show inaccuracies which are statistically significant but too small to be of practical importance. Even when a discrepancy is larger it is not necessarily a practical problem as long as differential counts on patient samples are compared with a carefully derived reference range for the same instrument.

It is often not possible to obtain an accurate automated count on blood specimens with abnormal characteristics, e.g., if there are cells present for which the instrument does not have recognition criteria. The philosophy differs between instrument manufacturers as to whether counts on such samples are usually rejected (STKS and Toa-Sysmex NE-8000) or whether a count is usually produced but is 'flagged' (Technicon H.2 series and Cell-Dyn 3000) [14]. A possible disadvantage of the latter policy is that there are some laboratory workers with an inclination to believe any figure produced by a laboratory instrument, even if it is flagged. However, of more concern is the occurrence of inaccurate counts which are not flagged. All instruments fail to flag some samples containing NRBC, immature granulocytes, atypical lymphocytes and even, occasionally, blast cells.

Storage of blood at room temperature, e.g., during transport from outlying clinics or satellite hospitals, leads to inaccurate measurements but the time taken for such inaccuracy to occur differs according to the instruments and the cell type. Storage effects are generally greater with impedance counters than with cytochemical light-scattering instruments. The effect of storage is a great deal less if the specimen can be stored at 4° C when any delay in analysis is anticipated.

Two- and three-part differential counts on impedance-based automated full blood counters

Inevitably two- and three-part differential counts do not identify an increase of eosinophils or basophils and two-part differential counts do not identify monocytosis. The loss of clinically useful information is not great since most differential counts are performed to detect abnormalities of neutrophil or lymphocyte counts. The 'monocyte' or 'mononuclear cell' count is also not very accurate since some eosinophils, basophils and neutrophils are counted in this category [15]. Automated three-part differential counts on Coulter counters and other impedance instru-

Table 4.8 Some causes of inaccurate differential WBC on Technicon H.1, H.2 and H.3 instruments

Mechanism	Nature of factitious result
Non-lysis of red cells (see p. 134)	Elevation of 'lymphocyte' count and reduction of neutrophil count (see Fig. 4.1)
Neutrophil peroxidase deficiency	Reduction of neutrophil count; increase of monocyte and LUC counts (see Fig. 4.2)
Eosinophil peroxidase deficiency	Reduction of eosinophil count; increase of neutrophil, monocyte or LUC count (see Fig. 4.3)
Monocyte peroxidase deficiency	Reduction of monocyte count and increase of LUC count (see Fig. 4.4)
Neutrophil cluster misidentified as eosinophils	Reduction of neutrophil count and elevation of eosinophil count (see Fig. 4.5)
Large cell residues in basophil channel due to presence of NRBC, blast cells, lymphoma cells or other abnormal cells	Elevation of 'basophil' count (see Fig. 4.6)
Ageing of sample (more than 24 hours)	'Left shift' flag

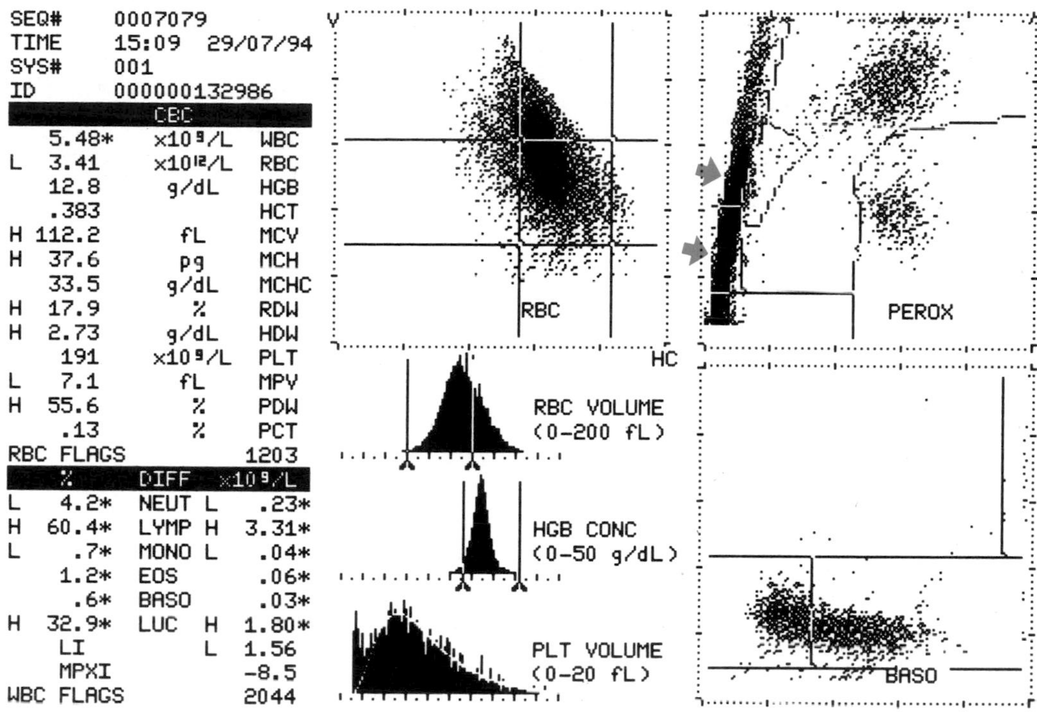

Fig. 4.1 Technicon H.2 histograms and scatter plots showing an erroneous differential count caused by failure of lysis of neonatal red cells. The peroxidase channel WBC of $75.8 \times 10^9/l$ has been rejected in favour of the basophil channel WBC of $5.48 \times 10^9/l$ but the differential count has been derived from the peroxidase channel where many of the non-lysed red cells have been counted as lymphocytes or LUC. This has led to a factitious neutropenia. The erroneous differential count was flagged. The plots also illustrate the increased size of fetal red cells.

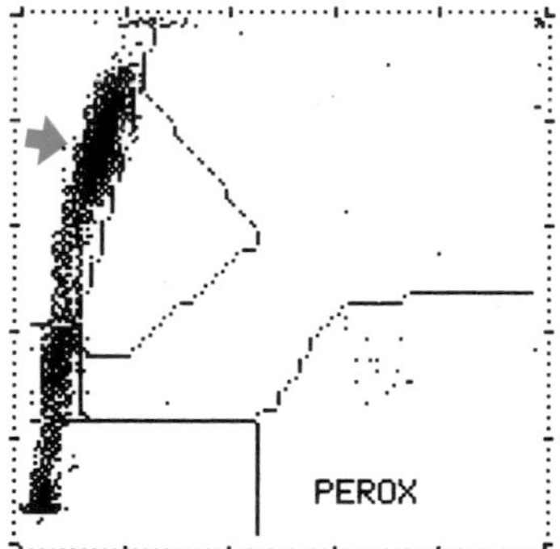

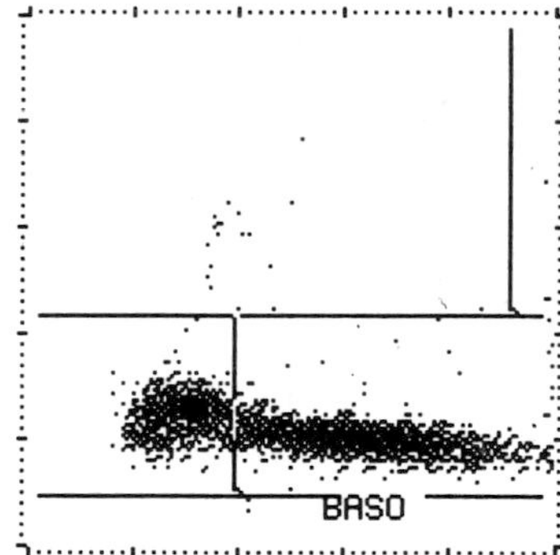

Fig. 4.2 Technicon H.2 white cell scatter plots from a patient with severe neutrophil peroxidase deficiency leading to an erroneous neutrophil count. Virtually all the neutrophils have been classified as large unstained (i.e., peroxidase-negative) cells and the neutrophil count was zero. The basophil lobularity channel, however, shows a normal number of granulocytes.

ments may be inaccurate within 30 minutes of venesection and become inaccurate again when the blood has been stored at room temperature for more than 6 hours. There is then a fall in the neutrophil count and a rise in the 'mononuclear cell' count which is progressive with time.

The majority (but not all) of specimens containing NRBC, blast cells, immature granulocytes and atypical lymphocytes are flagged by impedance-based three-part automated differential counters.

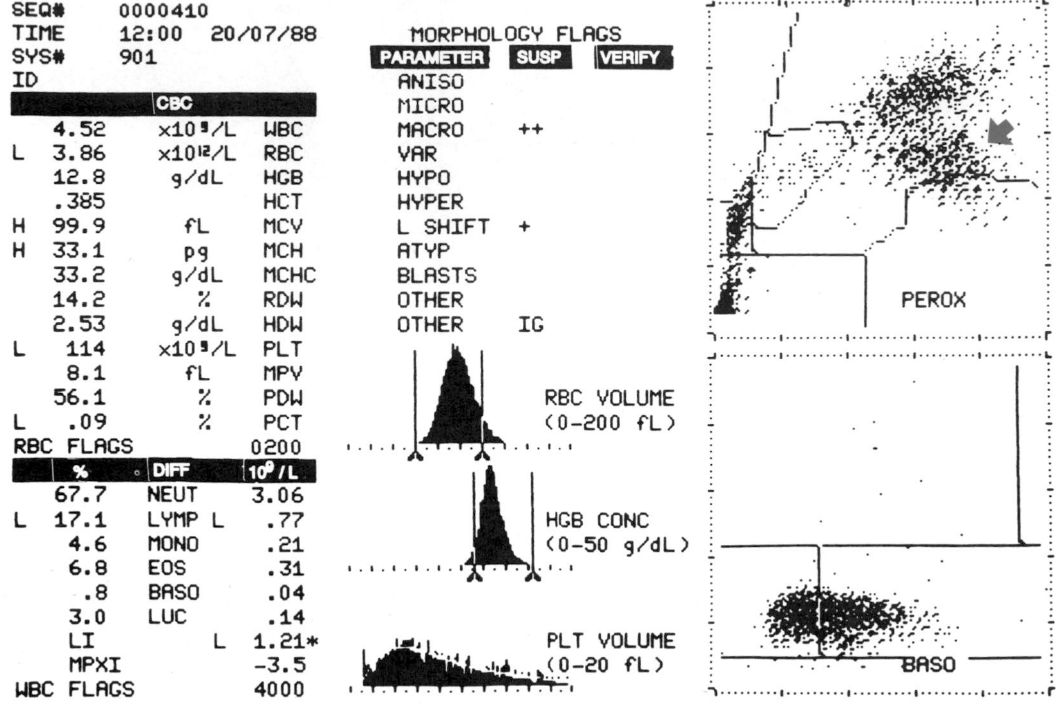

Fig. 4.3 Technicon H.2 white cell scatter plots from a patient with partial eosinophil peroxidase deficiency showing an eosinophil cluster which has not been recognized. About two-thirds of the eosinophils have been classified as neutrophils.

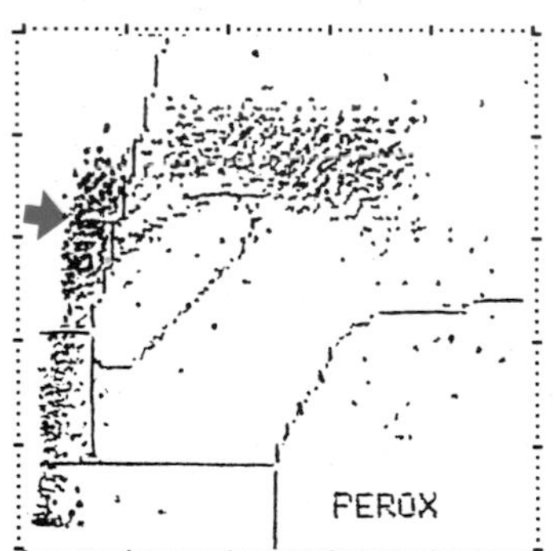

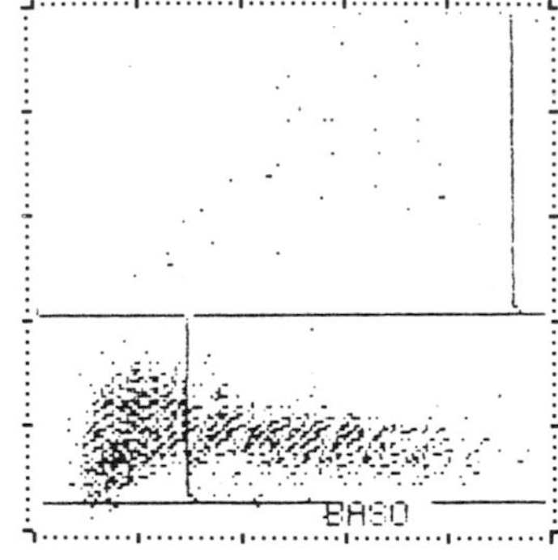

Fig. 4.4 Technicon H.2 white cell scatter plots from a patient with monocyte peroxidase deficiency causing an erroneous monocyte count. Almost all the monocytes have been counted as LUC. The automated monocyte count was $0.09 \times 10^9/l$ while the manual count was $0.5 \times 10^9/l$.

Five-part differential counts

Differential count of Technicon H.1 series

Since the Technicon H.1 series of instruments base the differential WBC on peroxidase cytochemistry in addition to light scattering they can produce erroneous counts as a result of inherited or acquired deficiency of peroxidase in neutrophils, eosinophils or monocytes. Some of the factitious results which have been observed with these instruments are shown in Table 4.8 and illustrated in Figs 4.1–4.6.

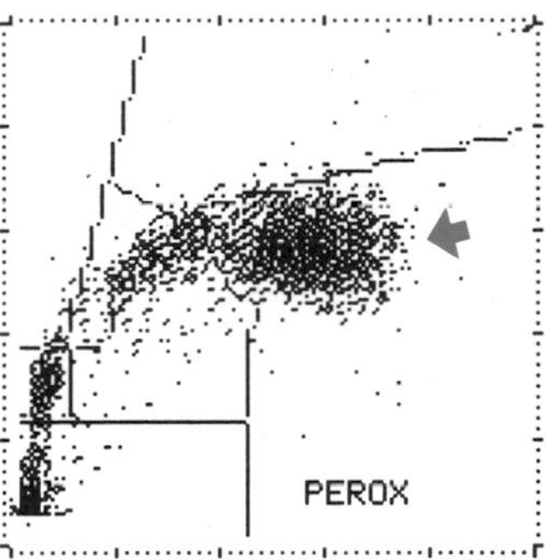

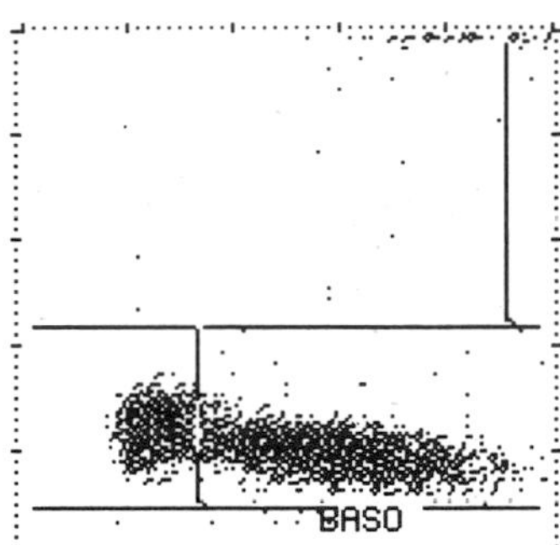

Fig. 4.5 Technicon H.1 white cell scatter plots showing neutrophils which have caused less forward light scatter than normal and have been misclassified as eosinophils.

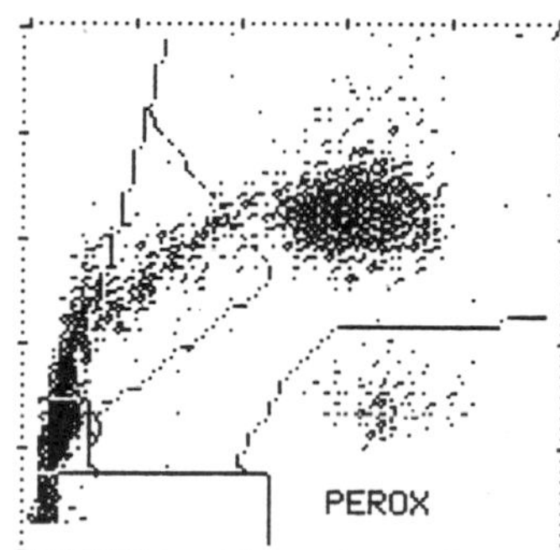

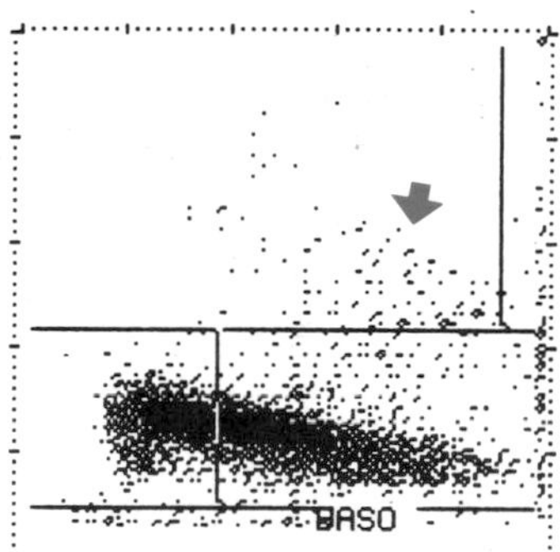

Fig. 4.6 Technicon H.2 white cell scatter plots from a patient with follicular lymphoma showing pseudobasophilia as a consequence of lymphoma cells being misclassified as basophils.

Five-part differential counts on Coulter, Toa-Sysmex and other instruments

Some systematic inaccuracies in counts have been reported. One study of the Coulter STKS five-part differential [14] found an overestimation of lymphocyte numbers and an underestimation of monocyte numbers. In another study, the STKS gave less accurate granulocyte and lymphocyte counts in HIV-infected patients than in other subjects [16]; some granulocyte counts were falsely low and lymphocyte counts were more scattered than with a Coulter S Plus IV three-part differential. Cobas instruments have been observed to overestimate monocyte counts [17].

Storage effects differ between instruments. The accuracy of the Coulter STKS differential count shows some deterioration after 6–8 hours of room temperature storage with a significant fall in the monocyte and eosinophil counts and a rise in the lymphocyte count [18]. Some Toa-Sysmex instruments, e.g., the NE-8000, have shown a marked rise in the monocyte count after 8 hours room temperature storage and a rise in the neutrophil count after 24 hours [19]. The Cobas Argos 5 Diff shows a significant rise in the lymphocyte count and a fall in the counts of other types of leucocyte between 6 and 24 hours [20]. Technicon H.1 series instruments have a relatively stable differential count with on average no more than 1–2% change in any category of leucocyte by 72 hours. The effects of storage may differ for certain types of specimen. A study with the Sysmex NE-8000 counter found that in HIV-positive patients the lymphocyte count fell after 24 hours of room temperature storage [21].

Blood specimens with abnormal characteristics can give rise to inaccurate counts, as shown in Table 4.9.

Errors in automated reticulocyte counts

Automated reticulocyte counts may be falsely elevated when there is autofluorescence or

Table 4.9 Some causes of inaccurate automated differential white cell counts on impedance and impedance/light-scattering instruments

Fault	Effect	Instrument on which observed
Neutrophil aggregation	Falsely low WBC and neutrophil percentage, falsely high lymphocyte percentage	All
Non-lysis of red cells	Falsely high WBC and lymphocyte count	
Neonatal red cells		Coulter STKS [22]
Hyperlipidaemia		Coulter STKS
Abnormal haemoglobins (e.g., C, S, D, G)		Toa-Sysmex NE-8000
Obstructive jaundice		Toa-Sysmex NE-8000
Malaria parasites	Falsely high lymphocyte and monocyte counts	Toa-Sysmex NE-8000
Other cells counted as basophils	Falsely high basophil count	
Abnormal lymphocytes in HIV-infected subjects		Coulter STKS [23]
Type of specimen not specified		Coulter STKS [18]
Myeloblasts		Toa-Sysmex NE-8000 [24]
Various abnormal cells		Cell-Dyn 3000 [25]
Basophils counted as lymphocytes in some cases of CGL	Falsely low basophil count	Coulter STKS [18]
Abnormal lymphocytes (CLL) counted as monocytes	Falsely high monocyte count	Cobas Argos 5 Diff
Plasma interference	Falsely high eosinophil count	Coulter STKS [18]
Poor separation of leucocyte clusters	Some eosinophils sometimes counted as neutrophils, some neutrophils sometimes counted as monocytes, pseudobasophilia	Coulter STKS [20,26]
Giant platelets counted as lymphocytes	Falsely high lymphocyte count	Coulter STKS [26]
Some neutrophils counted as monocytes in patients with left shift	Falsely high monocyte count; falsely low neutrophil count	Cobas Helios and Argos [17]

Table 4.10 Some causes of falsely elevated automated reticulocyte counts

Increased autofluorescence
Neonatal samples and post-splenectomy [27]
Heinz bodies [28]
Binding of fluorescent dye to particles other than RNA
High WBC or NRBC count and/or abnormal leucocytes, e.g., in CLL [29]
Howell–Jolly bodies [30]
Irreversibly sickled cells [29]
Cold agglutinins [27]
Large platelets [27]
Malaria parasites

when fluorescence is produced by binding of the fluorochrome to something other than the RNA of reticulocytes, usually DNA or RNA in other cells. Less information is available on erroneous counts with non-fluorescent nucleic acid stains. Some known causes of falsely elevated reticulocyte counts are shown in Table 4.10.

Erroneously low reticulocyte counts have been observed if blood is obtained from a patient after fluorescent retinal angiography has been performed [31].

References

1 Bizzaro N. Granulocyte aggregation is edetic acid and temperature dependent. *Arch Pathol Lab Med* 1993; 117: 528–30.

2 Nosanchuk JS, Roark MF, Wanser C. Anemia masked by triglyceridemia. *Am J Clin Pathol* 1974; 62: 838–9.

3 Nicholls PD. The erroneous haemoglobin–hyperlipidaemia relationship. *J Clin Pathol* 1977; 30: 638–40.

4 Brigden ML, Page NE, Graydon C. Evaluation of the Sysmex NE–8000 automated hematology analyzer in a high-volume outpatient laboratory. *Am J Clin Pathol* 1993; 100: 618–25.

5 Lewis SM, Bainbridge I, McTaggart P, Garvey BJ, England JM, Perry TE. *MDD Evaluation Report: Cobas Argos 5 Diff Automated Hematology Analyser.* London: Medical Devices Directorate, 1992.

6 Beautyman W, Bills T. Osmotic error in measurements of red cell volume. *Lancet* 1974; ii: 905–6.

7 Strauchen JA, Alston W, Anderson J, Gustafson Z, Fajardo LF. Inaccuracy in automated measurement of hematocrit and corpuscular indices in the presence of severe hyperglycemia. *Blood* 1981; 57: 1065–7.

8 Hinchliffe RF, Bellamy GJ, Lilleyman JS. Use of the Technicon H1 hypochromia flag in detecting spurious macrocytosis induced by excessive K_2EDTA concentration. *Clin Lab Haematol* 1992; 14: 268–9.

9 Paterakis G, Konstantopoulos K, Loukopoulos D. Spuriously increased platelet count due to microcyte interference: value of the R–1000 (Sysmex) Reticulocyte Analyzer. *Am J Hematol* 1994; 45: 57–8.

10 Shulman G, Yapit MK. Whole blood platelet counts with an impedance type particle counter. *Am J Clin Pathol* 1980; 73: 104–6.

11 Stass SA, Holloway ML, Slease RB, Schumacher HR. Spurious platelet counts in hairy cell leukemia. *Am J Clin Pathol* 1977; 68: 530–1.

12 Stass SA, Holloway ML, Peterson V, Creegan WJ, Gallivan M, Schumacher HR. Cytoplasmic fragments causing spurious platelet counts in the leukemic phase of poorly differentiated lymphocytic lymphoma. *Am J Clin Pathol* 1979; 71: 125–8.

13 Hammerstrom J. Spurious platelet counts in acute leukaemia with DIC due to cell fragmentation. *Clin Lab Haematol* 1992, 14: 239–43.

14 Bentley SA, Johnson A, Bishop CA. A parallel evaluation of four automated hematology analyzers. *Am J Clin Pathol* 1993; 100: 626–32.

15 Bain BJ. An assessment of the three-population differential count on the Coulter Counter Model S Plus IV. *Clin Lab Haematol* 1986; 8: 347–59.

16 Cohen AJ, Peerschke EIB, Steigbigel RT. A comparison of the Coulter STKS, Coulter S+IV, and manual analysis of white cell differential counts in a human immunodeficiency virus-infected population. *Am J Clin Pathol* 1993; 100: 611–17.

17 Bentley SA, Johnson TS, Sohier CH, Bishop CA. Flow cytometric differential leucocyte analysis with quantification of neutrophil left shift: an evaluation of the Cobas–Helios Analyzer. *Am J Clin Pathol* 1994; 102: 223–30.

18 Robertson EP, Lai HW, Wei DCC. An evaluation of leucocyte analysis on the Coulter STKS. *Clin Lab Haematol* 1992; 14: 53–68.

19 Hu C-Y, Wang C-H, Chuang H-M, Shen M-C. Evaluation of performance for automated differential leucocyte counting on Sysmex NE-8000 by NCCLS recommended protocol H20-T. *Clin Lab Haematol* 1993; 15: 287–99.

20 Sheridan BL, Lollo M, Howe S, Bergeron N. Evaluation of the Roche Cobas Argos 5 Diff automated haematology analyser with comparison with

Coulter STKS. *Clin Lab Haematol* 1994; 16: 117–30.
21 Koepke JA, Smith-Jones M. Lymphocyte counting in HIV-positive individuals. *Sysmex J Int* 1992; 2: 71–4.
22 Fournier M, Adenis C, Fontaine H, Carnaille B, Goudemand J. Evaluation and use of the white blood cell differential provided by the Coulter STKS in a children's hospital. *Clin Lab Haematol* 1994; 16: 33–42.
23 Germain PR, Lammers DB. False basophil counts on the Coulter STKS. *Lab Med* 1994; 25: 376–9.
24 Sivakumaran M, Allen B, Wood JK. Automated differential leucocyte counting on the Sysmex NE-8000 analyser. *Clin Lab Haematol* 1994; 16: 206–7.
25 Cornbleet PJ, Myrick D, Judkins S, Levy R. Evaluation of the CELL-DYN 3000 differential. *Am J Clin Pathol* 1992; 98: 603–14.
26 Cornbleet PJ, Myrick D, Levy R. Evaluation of the Coulter STKS five-part differential. *Am J Clin Pathol* 1993; 99: 72–81.
27 Chin-Yee I, Keeney M, Lohmann RC. Flow cytometric reticulocyte analysis using thiazole orange; clinical experience and technical limitations. *Clin Lab Haematol* 1991; 13: 177–88.
28 Hinchliffe RF. Error in automated reticulocyte counts due to Heinz bodies. *J Clin Pathol* 1993; 46: 878–9.
29 Ferguson DJ, Lee S-F, Gordon PA. Evaluation of reticulocyte counts by flow cytometry in a routine laboratory. *Am J Hematol* 1990; 33: 13–17.
30 Lofsness KG, Kohnke ML, Geier NA. Evaluation of automated reticulocyte counts and their reliability in the presence of Howell–Jolly bodies. *Am J Clin Pathol* 1994; 101: 85–90.
31 Hirata R, Morita Y, Hirai N, Seki M, Imanishi A, Toriumi J, Kawakubo T, Horiuchi T. The effects of fluorescent substances on the measurement of reticulocytes — using automated reticulocyte analyzers R-1000 and R-3000. *Sysmex J Int* 1992; 2: 10–15.

CHAPTER 5

Normal Ranges

The interpretation of any laboratory test result requires assessment as to whether or not the result is normal. 'Normal' means that the results are those expected in that individual when in a state of optimal health (assuming that the person does not have any inherited disorder affecting the blood). Since one rarely has the information to make this assessment, it is necessary instead to consider whether the result is what would be expected in a healthy subject as biologically similar to the particular individual as possible. Test results are conventionally compared with normal ranges, such ranges often being derived from textbooks and sometimes being of obscure origin. More recently test results have been compared with reference ranges. The concepts underlying the derivation of a reference range are as follows.

A reference individual is one selected using defined criteria and coming from a population which includes all individuals who meet those criteria. A reference sample is a number of reference individuals chosen to represent the reference population. Reference values are test results derived from the reference individuals and can be analysed and statistically described: they will fall within certain limits; and they will have a certain distribution with a mean, a median and a mode. The usual method of describing a collection of reference values is in terms of the reference limits which exclude 2.5% of the values at either end of the observed range, i.e., the reference interval represents the central 95% of the observed values. Such a reference interval derived from the sample individuals will be representative of the reference interval of the population from which it is derived; the closeness of fit of the two intervals can be represented by the confidence limits of the mean and each of the reference limits. Closeness of fit is determined by the size of the sample and by whether the reference individuals have been chosen from the reference population in a way which is free of bias. Reference individuals can be derived from the reference population by random sampling or carefully selected to reflect the mix of age, sex, social class and other variables in the reference population. Reference intervals are commonly referred to as 'reference ranges', a readily understandable term although it is not officially recommended.

A reference individual is not necessarily healthy, but if a good state of health is included as a criterion for selection then it is clear that the reference interval may be very similar to a traditional 'normal range', although more carefully defined.

If reference ranges are to be useful in assessing haematology results they should take account of whether test results are influenced by age, sex or ethnic origin and separate ranges should be derived when necessary. Pregnant women would normally be excluded unless deriving a range for application during pregnancy. Reference ranges are often derived from test results obtained in carefully controlled conditions with fasting and rested subjects who have abstained from alcohol, cigarettes and drugs and whose blood specimens are taken at a defined time of day. Such conditions are not often met by patient populations and it may be more useful to use ambulant, non-fasting individuals whose habits reflect those of the population from which they and the patients are drawn. The site of blood sampling and other variations in the technique of obtaining a blood sample affect results of haematological tests (Table 5.1). For this reason blood specimens should be taken in the same manner and using the same anticoagulant (dry or liquid) as in the patient population.

Establishing reference ranges on a population sample is a difficult and expensive procedure which is often beyond the resources of an individual laboratory. Nevertheless, laboratories should, whenever possible, establish their own ranges using their own techniques and instrumentation. Normal ranges can be derived from healthy volunteers, from subjects attending health screening clinics or having annual medical examinations or from staff having pre-employment testing. Hospital staff may not be ideal because their average age is likely to be considerably lower than that of the patient population. First-time blood donors are satisfactory but those who have donated regularly in the past may have depleted iron stores which will affect haematological test results. It is also possible to derive normal ranges from data on patients, based on the assumption that the test results for any measurement will represent a normal and an abnormal population with some overlap. Large numbers are necessary and the statistics are fairly complex [3]. Particular problems exist in deriving ranges for elderly people because of the high prevalence of known and occult disease. It is desirable, if possible, to separate the effects of the increasing incidence of disease from the effects of the ageing process itself. Similarly, it may be difficult in a developing country to select an adequate population sample which is not adversely affected by malnutrition and subclinical disease. In such circumstances it may be necessary to derive normal ranges from 'élite' individuals (such as the army, police force, medical students, doctors, nurses and laboratory workers); such individuals will not be typical of the communities from which they are drawn, but their test results will more closely approximate to those which would be expected in an optimal state of health. Problems also occur in populations with a high prevalence of genetic disease. In deriving ranges for red cell variables it is necessary to exclude subjects with haemoglobinopathies and α- and β-thalassaemia trait. Exclusion of β-thalassaemia

Table 5.1 Some effects of the method of obtaining a blood specimen on haematological variables*

Site for obtaining blood specimen
During the first week of life the Hb, PCV and RBC are approximately 15% higher in heel-prick than in venous specimens;† in older infants, children and adults no consistent differences have been observed between finger-prick and venous specimens but ear-lobe capillary specimens have Hb, PCV and RBC values 6–17% higher than finger-prick or venous specimens. In neonates heel-prick specimens have WBC, neutrophil and lymphocyte counts about 20% higher than arterial or venous samples; counts are most likely to approximate to those of venous blood if there is a free flow of blood and if early drops, excluding the first, are used for the count

Position of the arm
PCV, Hb and RBC are 2–3% higher if the arm is hanging down than if it is at the level of the atrium of the heart

Use of tourniquet
Hb, PCV and RBC are increased by 2–3% by prolonged application of a tourniquet

Nature of anticoagulant
The dilution caused by using a liquid anticoagulant causes a slight reduction of cell counts, Hb and PCV

Prior rest
The Hb, PCV and RBC fall by 5–8% after as little as half an hours bed rest

* For relevant references see Bain [1].
† It has been reported that at birth capillary Hb is higher than cord blood Hb [2] but it appears likely that this observation was consequent on the 20–60 minutes delay which occurred before the capillary sample was obtained.

trait and haemoglobinopathies is not difficult since diagnosis is easy but exclusion of α-thalassaemia trait requires DNA analysis. However, unless this is done it is not possible to distinguish genuine ethnic differences from differences caused by a high prevalence of a genetic abnormality. Thus, subtle differences in Hb and red cell indices between American black and white people are probably attributable to the 25–30% prevalence of α-thalassaemia trait among black people. In deriving reference ranges for children it is desirable to exclude subclinical iron deficiency.

Once a set of test results are available they must be dealt with by statistical techniques which are appropriate for the distribution of the data. If data have a normal (Gaussian) distribution then a mean and SD can be estimated and the mean ±1.96 SD will represent the central 95% of the data. The commonly used mean ±2 SD represents 95.4% of the data. The Hb and the other red cell variables can be treated as if they have a Gaussian distribution, although they are not strictly Gaussian [4]. Other haematological variables have a skewed distribution with a tail of higher values; this is true for the WBC and the absolute counts of various types of leucocytes. If data with this type of distribution are treated inappropriately, as if they were Gaussian, the estimates for both the upper and lower limits will be too low and the lower limit will often be negative. A logarithmic transformation may be appropriate or a more complex transformation may be necessary [5]. If a Gaussian distribution cannot be produced by transformation of the data, a non-parametric analysis must be carried out, i.e., one which makes no assumptions about the distribution. The advantages of using transformation to a Gaussian distribution is that a smaller sample size is adequate, of the order of 36 samples in contrast with the 120 samples which is the smallest adequate sample for non-parametric analysis [6].

Use of the central 95% range is arbitrary but gives a reasonable balance between missing a clinically significant abnormality and misclassifying a normal subject as abnormal. However, comparison of an observed value in a patient with a laboratory's normal range should be done with the constant awareness that for each test 5% of values of healthy subjects will fall outside the normal range. Conversely, an individual may, as a result of a pathological process, have an alteration in a test result away from his or her own normal value while still remaining within the 'normal' range. When previous results are available on patients some attention should be paid to them as well as to whether a result falls outside the laboratory's normal range.

If a laboratory does not derive its own normal ranges but adopts those of others it is incumbent on it to be certain not only that the type of population is similar and the appropriate statistical techniques have been applied but also that the blood sampling techniques and laboratory methods, including the methods of calibrating instruments, are identical.

Haematological variables are affected not only by age, sex, ethnic origin and altitude but also by a number of other biological factors and extraneous influences (Tables 5.2 & 5.3).

Normal ranges for adults

Some reference ranges for red cell and white cell variables for white adults are shown in Tables 5.4 and 5.5. These ranges can also be applied to Indians, Chinese and South-East Asian populations. For red cell variables it also appears appropriate to apply reference ranges for whites to black people since it is likely that the differences observed in population surveys are consequent on undiagnosed α-thalassaemia trait. For leucocyte counts, particularly neutrophil counts, it is necessary to have specific reference ranges applicable to Africans and Afro-Caribbeans (Table 5.6). The lower WBC and neutrophil counts observed in these ethnic groups may be partly explicable on the basis of diet and other extraneous influences but a true biological difference appears to exist. However, the higher eosinophil counts previously reported in Africans and Indians do not represent a biological difference from white people; eosinophilia observed was explicable on the basis of subclinical disease, particularly parasitic infection. Because of superior precision, reference ranges for automated differential leucocyte counts are narrower

Table 5.2 Some demographical factors affecting haematological variables*

Sex

RBC, Hb and PCV are higher in men than in women

Women in the reproductive age range have a higher WBC and neutrophil count than men, whereas in post-menopausal women the WBC is lower than in men

The platelet count is higher in women than in men

Age

Normal values of neonates, infants and children differ widely from those of adults (see Tables 5.7–5.11)

Hb rises in women and falls in men between the fifth and seventh decades

Lymphocyte counts fall in old age

Ethnic origin

WBC and neutrophil counts are lower in black than in white people, are lower in Africans than in West Indians or black Americans (see Table 5.6) and are also lower in Yemenite Jews than in other white people. The lower WBC in black people is not apparent at birth but has appeared by the age of 1 year. WBC and differential counts of Indians, Chinese and South-East Asian populations are the same as those of northern European white people. Eosinophil counts do not differ between healthy subjects of different ethnic groups.

In some studies but not others black people have had lower platelet counts than white people

Geographical location

RBC, Hb and PCV are increased at higher altitude; in one study the response to moderate altitude was a rise in RBC alone with MCV being lower whereas at a greater altitude Hb and PCV also rose [7]

* For further relevant references see Bain [1].

than those for manual differential counts (see Table 5.5). They are also dependent on methodology and thus need to be derived specifically for individual models of instrument. Not even all instruments operating on the same principles give identical results. Locally derived reference

Table 5.3 Some biological factors and common extraneous influences affecting haematological variables*

Diurnal variation

WBC and neutrophil counts are higher in the afternoon than in the morning. The eosinophil count is lowest at 10 a.m. to midday, and up to twice as high between midnight and 4 a.m.

The platelet count is higher in the afternoon and evening

Hb and PCV are higher in the morning than the evening

Pregnancy (see Table 5.12)

WBC, neutrophil and monocyte counts rise during pregnancy; a left shift occurs; lymphocyte, eosinophil and basophil counts fall

RBC, Hb and PCV fall; MCV rises, on average about 6 fl

ESR rises

The neutrophil alkaline phosphatase score rises

The platelet count has been observed to fall during pregnancy but if subjects with pregnancy-related hypertension are excluded there is usually no fall

Labour

During labour there is a further marked rise in WBC and neutrophil count together with a steep fall in the eosinophil count and a slight further fall of the lymphocyte count

Post-partum

WBC and neutrophil count remain markedly elevated for some days post-partum then fall gradually over 4–6 weeks

RBC, Hb and PCV fall to the lowest level at 3–4 days post-partum

Menstruation

WBC, neutrophil and monocyte counts fall steeply during menstruation; a reciprocal change is seen in the eosinophil count; the basophil count falls mid-cycle

Menopause

WBC and neutrophil count fall post-menopausally

Hb rises

Continued

Table 5.3 (*Continued*)

Exercise
WBC and absolute counts of all leucocyte types rise
RBC, Hb and PCV rise
Season
Hb and PCV are somewhat lower in summer [8]
Cigarette smoking [9]
WBC, neutrophil and monocyte counts are higher in smokers
RBC, Hb, PCV, MCV and MCH are higher
The platelet count is higher
ESR is higher
Alcohol intake
MCV and MCH are higher
Heavy alcohol intake can cause anaemia, leucopenia and thrombocytopenia

* For relevant references see Bain [1].

Table 5.4 The 95% ranges for red cell variables in white adults based on 700 healthy subjects, aged between 18 and 60 years, studied by the author. Of the subjects, 350 were male and 350 female; half were studied on Coulter instruments (S and S Plus IV) and half on Technicon instruments (Hemalog 8 and H.2). Except where indicated, the ranges are derived from all 700 subjects

	Male		Female
RBC × 10^{-12}/l	4.32–5.66		3.88–4.99
Hb (g/dl)	13.3–16.7		11.8–14.8
PCV (Hct) (l/l)	0.39–0.5		0.36–0.44
MCV (fl)		82–98*	
MCH (pg)		27.3–32.6	
MCHC (g/dl)		31.6–34.9	
RDW		9.9–15.5†	
		11.6–13.9‡	
HDW		1.82–2.64‡	

* MCV is very dependent on the technology used and the method of instrument calibration so that derivation of normal ranges for individual laboratories is important.
† Coulter S Plus IV, $n = 200$
‡ Technicon H.2, $n = 200$.

ranges are needed for red cell variables for populations living at high altitude. Above 2000 m the Hb is elevated by 1–1.5 g/dl and the RBC and PCV are also elevated [7].

Normal ranges for neonates

Some normal ranges for haematological variables in neonates are shown in Tables 5.7 and 5.8. Ranges applicable to the fetus from 8 weeks of gestation onwards have also been published [23–25]. Published ranges for red cell variables in Indian babies [26] and in Jamaican babies in whom haemoglobinopathies and β-thalassaemia trait had been excluded [14] are similar to those for European neonates whereas Nigerian babies have been observed to have lower RBCs, Hbs and PCVs [15]. Since haemoglobinopathies and thalassaemia trait were not excluded in the latter group, it may be more appropriate to apply ranges for red cell variables derived for white babies to all ethnic groups, including Africans. The lower neutrophil count which is noted in African and West Indians later in life is not apparent in the neonatal period so that the same reference ranges for leucocyte counts can be applied to neonates of all ethnic groups [17,18,27].

The Hb, PCV and RBC in the neonate are considerably influenced by the time of umbilical cord clamping (see Table 5.7), since inflow from the placenta increases the blood volume of the neonate by up to 50–60% during the first few minutes after birth. The rate of transfer of placental blood to the neonate is increased if oxytocin is administered to the mother to stimulate uterine contraction and is decreased if the baby is held above the level of the mother immediately after delivery. During the first few hours of life, plasma volume decreases so that the Hb, PCV and RBC rise appreciably, particularly when late clamping has been practiced. NRBC may be present in appreciable numbers at birth but the count falls rapidly in the first 24 hours. By 4 days they are infrequent. NRBC are more numerous in cord blood of premature infants and infants of diabetic mothers [28], and also when there has been fetal blood loss, haemolysis or intra-uterine hypoxia. The reticulocyte count at birth is higher than at

Table 5.5 95% ranges for automated and manual leucocyte counts in white adults, derived by the author, using data from 700 healthy subjects aged between 18 and 60 years.

	Male	Female	Method and number of subjects
WBC $\times 10^{-9}$/l	3.7–9.5	3.9–11.1	Various methods, $n = 700$
Neutrophils $\times 10^{-9}$/l	1.7–6.1	1.7–7.5	Automated counts, Technicon H.2 $n = 200$
Lymphocytes $\times 10^{-9}$/l	1–3.2		
Monocytes $\times 10^{-9}$/l	0.2–0.6		
Eosinophils $\times 10^{-9}$/l	0.03–0.46		
Basophils $\times 10^{-9}$/l	0.02–0.09		
LUC $\times 10^{-9}$/l	0.09–0.29		
Granulocytes $\times 10^{-9}$/l	1.8–7.5	2.1–8.9	Automated counts, Coulter S Plus IV, $n = 200$
Lymphocytes $\times 10^{-9}$/l	1.15–3.25		
Mononuclear cells $\times 10^{-9}$/l	0.18–0.86		
Neutrophils $\times 10^{-9}$/l	1.5–6.5	1.8–7.4	WBC on Coulter S or S Plus IV; 500-cell manual differential count, $n = 400$
Lymphocytes $\times 10^{-9}$/l	1.1–3.5		
Monocytes $\times 10^{-9}$/l	0.21–0.92		
Eosinophils $\times 10^{-9}$/l	0.02–0.67		
Basophils $\times 10^{-9}$/l	0–0.13		

LUC, large unstained (i.e. peroxidase-negative) cells.

Table 5.6 95% ranges for WBC and automated neutrophil counts (Technicon H.2 counter) for adult African and Afro-Caribbean subjects

	Male			Female		
	WBC ($\times 10^{-9}$/l)	Neutrophil count ($\times 10^{-9}$/l)	*n*	WBC ($\times 10^{-9}$/l)	Neutrophil count ($\times 10^{-9}$/l)	*n*
African	2.8–7.2	0.9–4.2	57	3.0–7.4	1.3–3.7	29
Afro-Caribbean	3.1–9.4	1.2–5.6	38	3.2–10.6	1.3–7.1	39

any other time of life but it drops markedly after birth. There is a steady decline in the RBC, Hb and PCV but, as shown in Table 5.7, an Hb of less than 14 g/dl in the first week of life is indicative of anaemia. The WBC at birth is influenced by the mode of delivery, being lower after an elective caesarean section than after vaginal delivery or when a caesarean section has been peformed after labour has commenced [29]. The WBC and neutrophil counts rise after birth to a peak level at about 12 hours and thereafter fall sharply [18]. The lymphocyte count falls in the first few days of life [19]. The neutrophil count is initially higher than the lymphocyte count. This is reversed between the fourth and seventh days of life.

Maternal smoking causes a small increase in the neonatal Hb, PCV and MCV and a more substantial decrease in the neutrophil count which persists for at least the first few days after birth [30]. Babies which are small for their gestational age also have lower neutrophil counts [31]. Other maternal and fetal factors influencing the neutrophil count in the neonate are shown in Tables 6.4 and 6.20 and causes of polycythaemia

Table 5.7 95% ranges for red cell variables in healthy full-term neonates during the first month of life

	RBC × 10^{-12}/l	Hb (g/dl)	PCV (l/l)	MCV (fl)
White				
Cord blood (early cord clamping) [10]	3.5–6.7	13.7–20.1	0.47–0.59	90–118
Birth to 96 hours				
early cord clamping [11,12]	3.8–6.5	14.2–24	0.46–0.75	101–137
late cord clamping [12]		16.1–24		
1–2 weeks (early cord clamping) [11]	3.2–6.4	12.8–21.8	0.38–0.70	75–149
3–4 weeks (early cord clamping) [11,13]	2.8–5.3	10.1–18.3	0.32–0.55	90–120
Jamaican				
1 day [14]	4.6–7.6	15.7–27.5		90–118
1 week [14]	4–6.9	13.4–22.4		88–116
4 weeks [14]	3.1–5.9	9.5–18.1		83–107
Nigerian				
1 day [15]	2.7–5.3	11.6–19.6	0.32–0.58	113 (mean)
2 weeks [15]	2.35–4.55	9.4–16.8	0.31–0.47	113 (mean)
4 weeks [15]	2.1–3.95	7.5–13.6	0.24–0.41	108 (mean)

Table 5.8 90 or 95% ranges for white cell and NRBC counts for full-term white babies during the first month of life*

	WBC (×10^{-9}/l)	Neutrophil count (×10^{-9}/l)	Lymphocyte count (×10^{-9}/l)	Monocyte count (×10^{-9}/l)	Eosinophil count (×10^{-9}/l)	NRBC count (×10^{-9}/l)
Cord blood [10,16,17]	5–23	1.7–19	1–11	0.1–3.7	0.05–2	0.03–5.4
30 minutes [18,19]		1.9–5.8				
12 hours [16,18]		6.6–23.5				
24 hours [16,18]		4.8–17.1				
48 hours [16,18]		3.8–13.4				
0–60 hours [20]			2–7.3	0–1.9	0–0.8	
72 hours [16,18]		2–9.4				
4 days [16,18,19]		1.3–8	2.2–7.1	0.2–1.8	0.2–1.9	
60 hours to 5 days [18,20]		2–6	1.9–6.6	0–1.7	0–0.8	
7–8 days [16,18,21]	9–18.4	1.8–8	3–9	0.03–0.98	0.16–0.94	0.03–0.11
2 weeks [16,18]		1.7–6				
5 days to 4 weeks [18,20]		1.8–5.4	2.8–9.1	0.09–1.7	0–0.8	
3–4 weeks [16,18]		1.6–5.8				
4 weeks [22]	5–19.5	1–9	4–13.5			

* Data from different series have been amalgamated to include the lowest and highest limits found in different studies. The ranges of Gregory and Hay [16] and Weinberg *et al.* [20] are 90% rather than 95% ranges while the scatter plots of Manroe *et al.* [18] show the full range of counts.

and anaemia in the neonatal period in Tables 6.2 and 6.18.

Premature babies have a lower WBC and lower neutrophil and lymphocyte counts than term babies; NRBC and immature myeloid cells are more numerous and the reticulocyte count is

Table 5.9 95% ranges for red cell variables for white infants and children*

Age	RBC × 10^{-12}/l	Hb (g/dl)	PCV (l/l)	MCV (fl)
2 months [13,18]	2.6–4.3	8.9–13.2	0.26–0.40	75–125§ [18] 84–106‡ [13]
3 months [18,34]	3.1–4.3	9.3–13.8	0.27–0.39	73–103
4 months [13]	3.5–5.1	10.3–14.1	0.32–0.44	76–97
6 months [13,34]	3.9–5.5	9.9†–14.1	0.31–0.41	68–85
1 year [13,34]	4.1–5.3	9.8†–14.1	0.33–0.41	71–84
18 months [34]		9.7†–15.1		
2–5/6 years [13,22,35]	4.23–5.03	9.6†–14.8	0.34–0.40	73–86
5/6–9 years [22,36]	4.31–5.11	10.7–14.6	0.34–0.42	75–88
9–12 years [22,36]	4.31–5.11	11.5–15.4	0.34–0.42	76–91
12–14/15 years [22,35,36]				
male	4.51–5.31	11.5–15.8	0.36–0.46	76–92
female	4.24–5.04	11.7–15.3	0.36–0.44	77–92.5
14–18 years [22,36]				
male		13–17		77–92.5
female		12–15.4		77–92.5

* Data have been amalgamated to include the highest and lowest limits in different series.
† Iron deficiency was largely excluded in most series [13,22,35,36]. However, others have reported that Hb is rarely less than 11 g/dl in children who are not iron deficient [37] and the data of Castriota *et al.* [35] and Dallman *et al.* [22] support this.
‡ MCV calculated from microhaematocrit and RBC [18].
§ MCV measured by impedance counter [13].

higher [19,32]. At birth the Hb and PCV are similar to those of term babies but the RBC is lower and the MCV higher [33]. Neutrophil and lymphocyte counts reach the levels of term babies by about 1 week [19,32]. In premature babies the eosinophil count often becomes elevated 2–3 weeks after birth.

Normal ranges in infants and children

Normal ranges applicable to infants and children are shown in Tables 5.9 and 5.10. The steady decline in RBC, Hb and PCV which follows the early peak continues to a nadir around 2 months of age. There is a simultaneous rapid fall in MCV and MCH. In premature babies the post-natal decline in Hb is more rapid and the nadir is lower (Table 5.11).

The exclusion of children with iron deficiency is important in deriving paediatric normal ranges since one of the purposes of such ranges is to facilitate the diagnosis of iron deficiency. The iron stores of the neonate are adequate to sustain erythropoiesis for 3–5 months, depending on whether the infant was full term or premature and on whether the cord was clamped early or late. Thereafter, iron deficiency is common. Iron deficiency can be excluded by requiring a normal serum ferritin or transferrin saturation, or a normal red cell protoporphyrin concentration, or by administering iron supplements before testing.

The lower WBC and neutrophil counts noted in black adults are apparent in infants by 9–12 months of age [42].

Normal ranges in pregnancy

The changes in haematological variables which occur during pregnancy are discussed on p. 103. Normal ranges are given in Table 5.12. The Hb usually remains above 10 g/dl unless there is iron deficiency or some other complication.

Normal ranges for platelet counts

The manual platelet count is imprecise and both

Table 5.10 95% ranges for total and differential white cell counts for white infants and children

Age	WBC ($\times 10^{-9}$/l)	Neutrophil count ($\times 10^{-9}$/l)	Lymphocyte count ($\times 10^{-9}$/l)	Monocyte count ($\times 10^{-9}$/l)	Eosinophil count ($\times 10^{-9}$/l)	Basophil count ($\times 10^{-9}$/l)	LUC count ($\times 10^{-9}$/l)
9 days–1 year*	7.3–16.6	1.5–6.9	3.4–9.4	0.21–1.64	0.06–0.62	0.02–0.17	0.09–0.61
1 year*	5.6–17	1.5–6.9	2.5–8.6	0.15–1.28	0.06–0.62	0.02–0.12	0.13–0.72
1 year†	6–17.5	1.5–8.5	4–10.5				
2 years*	5.6–17	1.5–6.9	2.2–7.7	0.15–1.28	0.04–1.19	0.02–0.12	0.11–0.68
2 years†	6–17	1.5–8.5	3–9.5				
3 years*	4.9–12.9	1.5–6.9	1.7–5.5	0.15–1.28	0.04–1.19	0.02–0.12	0.09–0.48
4 years*	4.9–12.9	1.8–7.7	1.7–5.5	0.15–1.28	0.09–1.4	0.03–0.12	0.09–0.38
4 years†	5.5–15.5	1.5–8.5	2–8				
5 years*	4.9–12.9	1.8–7.7	1.6–4.3	0.15–1.28	0.09–1.04	0.03–0.12	0.08–0.32
6 years*	4.4–10.6	1.5–5.9	1.6–4.3	0.15–1.28	0.08–1.01	0.02–0.12	0.07–0.26
6 years†	5–14.5	1.5–8	1.5–7				
7 years*	4.4–10.6	1.5–5.9	1.6–4.3	0.15–1.28	0.08–1.01	0.02–0.12	0.07–0.26
4–7 years‡	6.3–16.2	1.6–9	2.2–9.8	0.06–1	0–1.4	0–0.26	
8 years*	3.9–9.9	1.5–5.9	1.4–3.8	0.15–1.28	0.08–1.01	0.02–0.12	0.07–0.26
8 years†	4.5–13.5	1.5–8	1.5–6.8				
9–10 years*	3.9–9.9	1.5–5.9	1.4–3.8	0.15–1.28	0.08 1.01	0.02–0.12	0.07–0.26
10 years†	4.5–13.5	1.8–8	1.5–6.5				
11 years*	3.9–9.9	1.5–5.9	1.4–3.8	0.15–1.28	0.04–0.76	0.02–0.12	0.07–0.26
12–13 years*	3.9–9.9	1.5–5.9	1.4–3.8	0.15–1.28	0.04–0.76	0.02–0.1	0.07–0.26
14 years*	3.9–9.9	1.4–5.6	1.4 3.8	0.15 1.28	0.04–0.76	0.02–0.1	0.07–0.26
8–14 years‡	4.9–13.7	1.4–7.5	1.9–7.6	0.06–0.8	0–0.75	0–0.2	
15–16 years*	3.9–9.9	1.7–5.7	1.4–3.8	0.15 1.28	0.04–0.76	0.02–0.1	0.07–0.26

* Differential count performed on a Hemalog D automated differential counter [21].
† 100-cell manual differential count [38].
‡ 200-cell manual differential count, recalculated to make allowance for skewed distribution [39,40].

Table 5.11 95% ranges for Hb (g/dl) in pre-term but iron-replete babies in the first 6 months of life [41]

	Birthweight 1000–1500 g	Birthweight 1501–2000 g
2 weeks	11.7–18.4	11.8–19.6
4 weeks	8.7–15.2	8.2–15
2 months	7.1–11.5	8–11.4
3 months	8.9–11.2	9.3–11.8
4 months	9.1–13.1	9.1–13.1
6 months	9.4–13.8	10.7–12.6

manual and automated platelet counts are prone to inaccuracy. As a consequence there are considerable discrepancies in published ranges (Table 5.13). It is therefore important for laboratories to establish their own reference ranges for their own methodologies. Platelet counts in Africans have been observed to be lower than those of white people [54,55] but this is less true of West Indians and of Africans living in Britain [50]. This suggests that the low platelet counts observed in Africa are at least in part caused by dietary factors or subclinical disease.

Infants and children have similar platelet counts to adults [24,56]. Neonates, both premature and full term, have similar platelet counts to older children and adults [24,31,56] but babies which are small for gestational age [31] and many sick babies have lower counts.

Normal ranges for reticulocyte counts

When reticulocyte counts are expressed as a per-

Table 5.12 95% ranges for haematological variables during pregnancy

Period of gestation	7–14 weeks	15–22 weeks	23–30 weeks	31–38 weeks
Hb (g/dl)	12.8–13.6*	11.4–13.8*	10.9–13.8*	11.1–13.6*

	First trimester	Second trimester	Third trimester
RBC × 10^{-12}/l	3.52–4.52	3.2–4.41	3.1–4.44
Hb (g/dl)	11–14.3	10–13.7	9.8–13.7
PCV (l/l)	0.31–0.41	0.30–0.38	0.28–0.39
MCV (fl)	81–96	82–97	91–99
WBC × 10^{-9}/l	5.7–13.6	6.2–14.8	5.9–16.9, 5.9–13.7†
Neutrophil count × 10^{-9}/l	3.6–10.1	3.8–12.3	3.9–13.1, 3.7–10.8†
Lymphocyte count × 10^{-9}/l	1.1–3.5	0.9–3.9	1–3.6, 1–3.1†
Monocyte count × 10^{-9}/l	0–1	0.1–1.1	0.1–1.1, 0.3–1.1†
Eosinophil count × 10^{-9}/l	0–0.6	0–0.6	0–0.6, 0.02–0.33†
Basophil count × 10^{-9}/l	0–0.1	0–0.1	0–0.1, 0–0.09†
Platelet count × 10^{-9}/l	174–391	171–409	155–429

All data derived from Balloch *et al.* [3] except for data derived from Cruikshank [43]* and from England and Bain [44]†.

centage, reported normal ranges have been between 0.4 and 2% in one study [57] and 0.8–2.5% and 0.8–4.1% for males and females respectively in another [58]. Later studies with automated reticulocyte counts have not generally found any sex difference in the percentage of reticulocytes. Reticulocyte counts are more meaningfully expressed as absolute numbers. In one study, a mean of 88 × 10^9/l and a range of 18–158 × 10^9/l were found [59]. Reference ranges reported for automated reticulocyte counts have varied considerably, from 19–59 × 10^9/l [60] to 40–140 × 10^9/l [61]. The higher values reported by Chin-Yee *et al.* [61] appear more acceptable since, in this study, automated and manual counts were similar.

References

1 Bain BJ. *Blood Cells: a Practical Guide*. London; Gower, 1989.

2 Moe PJ. Umbilical cord blood and capillary blood in the evaluation of anaemia in erythroblastosis foetalis. *Acta Pediatr Scand* 1967; 56: 391–4.

3 Balloch AJ, Cauchi MN. Reference ranges for haematology parameters in pregnancy derived from patient populations. *Clin Lab Haematol* 1993; 15: 7–14.

4 Giorno R, Clifford JH, Beverly S, Rossing RG. Hematology reference ranges. Analysis by different statistical technics and variations with age and sex. *Am J Clin Pathol* 1980; 74: 765–70.

5 Solberg EK. Statistical treatment of collected reference values and determination of reference limits. In: Gräsbeck R, Alström W, eds. *Reference Values in Laboratory Medicine*. Chichester: John Wiley, 1981.

6 Amador E. Health and normality. *JAMA* 1975; 232: 953–5

7 Ruíz-Argüelles GJ, Sanchez-Medal L, Loria A, Piedras J, Córdova MS. Red cell indices in normal adults residing at altitude from sea level to 2670 meters. *Am J Hematol* 1980; 8: 265–71.

8 Kristal-Boneh E, Froom P, Harari G, Shapiro Y, Green MS. Seasonal changes in red blood cell parameters. *Br J Haematol* 1993; 85: 603–7.

9 Bain BJ. Haematological effects of smoking. *J Smoking Rel Dis* 1992; 3: 99–108.

10 Marks J, Gairdner D, Roscoe JD. Blood formation in infancy. Part III. Cord blood. *Arch Dis Child* 1955; 30: 117–20.

11 Matoth Y, Zaizov R, Varsano I. Postnatal changes in some red cell parameters. *Acta Paediatr Scand* 1971;

Table 5.13 The 95% ranges for platelet counts ($\times 10^{-9}$/l) in healthy adults

Method	Male		Female	Reference
White				
Microscopy	140–440			[45]
	127–351		165–359	[46]
		140–340		
		145–375		[47]
Impedance counting in platelet-rich plasma	143–179		156–417	[48]
Impedance counting		170–430		[49]
in whole blood	168–411		188–445	[50]
	184–370		196–451	[51]
	157–365		164–384	[52]
Light scattering in whole blood		162–346 (Hemalog 8)		(B.J. Bain, unpublished data, 1980)
	143–332		169–358 (H.1)	(B.J. Bain, unpublished data, 1994)
Japanese				
Light scattering in whole blood		130–350		[53]
Africans and West Indians				
Microscopy				
Nigerians	95–278			[54]
	114–322			[54]
Impedance counting				
Zambians	36–258			[55]
Impedance counting				
Africans in London	128–365		166–377	[50]
West Indians in London	210–351		160–411	[50]
Light scattering				
Africans in London	118–297		149–332 (H.1)	(B.J. Bain, unpublished data, 1994)
West-Indians in London	134–332		165–368 (H.2)	(B.J. Bain, unpublished data, 1994)

60: 317–23.

12 Lanzkowsky P. Effects of early and late clamping of umbilical cord on infant's haemoglobin level. *Br Med J* 1960; ii: 1777–82.

13 Saarinem UM, Siimes MD. Developmental changes in red blood cell counts and indices of infants after exclusion of iron deficiency by laboratory criteria and continuous iron supplementation. *J Pediatr* 1978; 92: 412–16.

14 Serjeant GR, Grandison Y, Mason K, Serjeant B, Sewell A, Vaidya V. Hematological indices in normal Negro children: a Jamaican cohort from birth to five years. *Clin Lab Haematol* 1980; 2: 169–78.

15 Scott-Emuakpor AB, Okolo AA, Omene JA, Ukpe SI. The limits of physiological anaemia in the African neonate. *Acta Haematol* 1985; 74: 99–103.

16 Gregory J, Hey E. Blood neutrophil response to bacterial infection in the first month of life. *Arch Dis Child* 1972; 47: 747–53.

17 Chan PCY, Hayes L, Bain BJ. A comparison of the white cell counts of cord bloods from babies of different ethnic origins. *Ann Trop Paediatr* 1985; 5: 153–5.

18 Manroe BL, Weinberg AG, Rosenfeld CR, Brown R. The neonatal blood count in health and disease. I. Reference values for neutrophilic cells. *J Pediatr* 1979; 95: 89–98.

19 Xanthou M. Leucocyte blood picture in full-term and premature babies during neonatal period. *Arch Dis Child* 1970; 45: 242–9.

20 Weinberg AG, Rosenfeld CR, Manroe BL, Browne R. Neonatal blood cell count in health and disease II

values for lymphocytes, monocytes, and eosinophils. *J Pediatr* 1985; 106: 462–6.
21 Cranendonk E, van Gennip AH, Abeling NGGM, Behrendt H, Hart AA. Reference values for automated cytochemical differential count of leukocytes in children 0–16 years old: a comparison with manually obtained counts from Wright-stained smears. *J Clin Chem Clin Biochem* 1985; 23: 663–7.
22 Dallman PR, Siimes MA. Percentile curves for hemoglobin and red cell volume in infancy and childhood. *J Pediatr* 1979; 94: 26–31.
23 Playfair JHL, Wolfendale MR, Kay HEM. The leucocytes of peripheral blood in the human foetus. *Br J Haematol* 1963; 9: 336–44.
24 Millar DS, Davis LR, Rodeck CH, Nicolaides KH, Mibashan RS. Normal blood cell values in the early mid-trimester fetus. *Prenat Diagn* 1985; 5: 367–73.
25 Forestier F, Daffos F, Galactéros F, Bardakjian J, Rainaut M, Beuzard Y. Haematological values of 163 normal fetuses between 18 and 30 weeks of gestation. *Paediatr Res* 1986; 20: 342–6.
26 Aneja S, Manchanda R, Patwari A, Sagreiya K, Bhargava SK. Normal hematological values in newborns. *Indian Pediatr* 1979; 16: 781–6.
27 Ezeilo GC. A comparison of the haematological values of cord bloods of African, European and Asian neonates. *Afr J Med Sci* 1978; 7: 163–9.
28 Green DW, Mimouni F. Nucleated erythrocytes in healthy infants and in infants of diabetic mothers. *J Pediatr* 1990; 116: 129–31.
29 Frazier JP, Cleary TG, Pickering LK, Kohl S, Ross PJ. Leukocyte function in healthy neonates following vaginal and cesarean section deliveries. *J Pediatr* 1982; 101: 269–72.
30 Harrison KL. The effect of maternal smoking on neonatal leucocytes. *Aust NZ J Obstet Gynaecol* 1979; 19: 166–8.
31 McIntosh N, Kempson C, Tyler RM. Blood counts in extremely low birth weight infants. *Arch Dis Child* 1988; 63: 74–6.
32 Coulombel L, Dehan M, Tchernia G, Hill C, Vial M. The number of polymorphonuclear leucocytes in relation to gestational age in the newborn. *Acta Paediatr Scand* 1979; 68: 709–11.
33 Zaizov R, Matoth Y. Red cell values on the first postnatal day during the last sixteen weeks of gestation. *Am J Hematol* 1976; 1: 275–8.
34 Burman D. Haemoglobin levels in normal infants aged 3 to 24 months, and the effect of iron. *Arch Dis Child* 1972; 47: 261–71.
35 Castriota-Scanderberg A, Pedrazzi G, Mercadanti M, Stapane I, Butturini A, Izzi G. Normal values of total reticulocytes and reticulocyte subsets in children and young adults. *Haematologica* 1992; 77: 363–4.
36 Natvig H, Vellar OD, Andersen J. Studies on hemoglobin value in Norway. VII. Hemoglobin, hematocrit and MCHC values among boys and girls aged 7–20 years in elementary and grammar school. *Acta Med Scand* 1967; 182: 183–91.
37 Hunter RE, Smith NJ. Hemoglobin and hematocrit values in iron deficiency in infancy. *J Pediatr* 1972; 81: 710–13.
38 Dallman PR. Blood and blood forming tissues. In Rudolph AM, Hoffman JIE, eds. *Rudolph's Pediatrics*, 19th edn. New York: Appleton & Lange, 1991.
39 Osgood EE, Brownlee IE, Osgood MW, Ellis DM, Cohen W. Total, differential and absolute leukocyte counts and sedimentation rates of healthy children four to seven years of age. *Am J Dis Child* 1939; 58: 61–70.
40 Osgood EE, Brownlee IE, Osgood MW, Ellis DM, Cohen W. Total, differential and absolute leukocyte counts and sedimentation rates of healthy children. Standards for children eight to fourteen years of age. *Am J Dis Child* 1939; 58: 282–94.
41 Lundström U, Siimes MA, Dallman PR. At what age does iron supplementation become necessary in low-birth-weight infants. *J Pediatr* 1977; 91: 878–83.
42 Sadowitz PD, Oski FA. Differences in polymorphonuclear cell counts between healthy white and black infants: response to meningitis. *Pediatrics* 1983; 72: 405–7.
43 Cruikshank JM. Some variations in the normal haemoglobin concentration. *Br J Haematol* 1970; 18: 523–9.
44 England JM, Bain BJ. Annotation: total and differential leucocyte count. *Br J Haematol* 1976; 33: 1–7.
45 Brecher G, Cronkite EP. Morphology and enumeration of human blood platelets. *J Appl Physiol* 1950; 3: 365–77.
46 Sloan AW. The normal platelet count in man. *J Clin Pathol* 1951; 4: 37–46.
47 Miale JB. *Laboratory Medicine Hematology*, 6th edn. St Louis: CV Mosby, 1982.
48 Bain BJ, Forster T. A sex difference in the bleeding time. *Thromb Haemostas* 1980; 43: 131–2.
49 Giles C. The platelet count and mean platelet volume. *Br J Haematol* 1981; 48: 31–7.
50 Bain BJ, Seed M. Platelet count and platelet size in Africans and West Indians. *Clin Lab Haematol* 1986; 8: 43–8.
51 Payne BA, Pierre RV. Using the three-part differential. Part 1. Investigating the possibilities. *Lab Med* 1986; 17: 459–62.
52 Gladwin AM, Trowbridge EA, Slater DN, Reardon D, Martin JF. The size and number of bone marrow megakaryocytes in malignant lymphoma and their

relationship to the platelet count. *Am J Hematol* 1990; 35: 225–31.

53 Takamatsu N, Yamamoto H, Onomura Y, Ichikawa N. A study of the hematological reference ranges and changes with age using the automated hematology analyzer K-1000™. *Sysmex J Int* 1992; 2: 136–45.

54 Essien EM, Usanga EA, Ayeni O. The normal platelet count and platelet factor 3 availability in some Nigerian population groups. *Scand J Haematol* 1973; 10: 378–83.

55 Gill GV, England A, Marshal C. Low platelet counts in Zambians. *Trans R Soc Trop Med Hyg* 1979; 73: 111–12.

56 Sell EJ, Corrigan JJ. Platelet counts, fibrinogen concentrations, and factor V and factor VII levels in healthy infants according to gestational age. *J Pediatr* 1973; 82: 1028–32.

57 Crouch JY, Kaplow LS. Relationship of reticulocyte age to polychromasia, shift cells and shift reticulocytes. *Arch Pathol Lab Med* 1985; 109: 325–9.

58 Deiss A, Kurth D. Circulating reticulocytes in normal adults as determined by the new methylene blue method. *Am J Clin Pathol* 1970; 53: 481–4.

59 Lee GR. Normal blood and bone marrow values in men. In: Wintrobe MM, Lee GR, Boggs DR, Bithell TC, Foerster J, Athens JW, Lukens JN, eds. *Clinical Hematology*, 8th edn. Lea & Febiger, 1981: 1855.

60 Nobes PR, Carter AB. Reticulocyte counting using flow cytometry. *J Clin Pathol* 1990; 43: 675–8.

61 Chin-Yee I, Keeney M, Lohmann C. Flow cytometric reticulocyte analysis using thiazole orange: clinical experience and technical limitations. *Clin Lab Haematol* 1991; 13: 177–88.

CHAPTER 6

Quantitative Changes in Blood Cells

This chapter deals with quantitative changes in blood cells, first the causes of increased cell counts for each lineage then the causes of decreased counts. An increase of a cell type usually results either from redistribution of cells or from increased bone marrow output; occasionally an increased count, most noticeably of red cells, can result from a decrease of plasma volume. A decreased count of any cell type can result from diminished bone marrow output, redistribution, or shortened survival in the circulation.

Polycythaemia

The term polycythaemia, strictly speaking, should indicate an increase in the number of red cells in the circulation but, in practice, the term is used for an increase of the Hb and PCV/Hct above that which is normal for the age and sex of the subject. Usually, the RBC, Hb and PCV/Hct rise in parallel. Conventionally, the term polycythaemia does not refer to an increased RBC if the Hb is normal as may be seen, for example, in thalassaemia trait. A raised Hb can be due to a decreased plasma volume occurring either acutely or chronically. An acute decrease in plasma volume can be caused by shock, when there is a loss of fluid from the intravascular compartment, or by dehydration. A chronic decrease in plasma volume is sometimes due to cigarette smoking but in many cases the cause is unknown. The phenomenon has been referred to as 'stress polycythaemia' but 'pseudopolycythaemia' is a better term since there is no clear relationship to 'stress'.

Alternatively, a raised Hb can be due to true polycythaemia, i.e., to an increase in the total volume of circulating red cells (often referred to, inaccurately, as the 'red cell mass'). True polycythaemia can be primary or secondary. In primary polycythaemia there is an intrinsic bone marrow disorder, either inherited or acquired. Erythropoietin concentration is decreased. In contrast, secondary polycythaemia is generally mediated by increased erythropoietin production, usually occurring either as a physiological response to hypoxia or as a result of inappropriate secretion by a diseased kidney or by a tumour. Causes of polycythaemia are summarized in Table 6.1. The differential diagnosis of PRV is discussed on p. 257. Neonates have higher Hbs than adults but the Hb may rise even higher in pathological conditions. Some causes of polycythaemia which are peculiar to the neonatal period are summarized in Table 6.2.

Neutrophil leucocytosis — neutrophilia

Neutrophil leucocytosis or neutrophilia is the elevation of the absolute neutrophil count above that which would be expected in a healthy subject of the same age, sex, race and physiological status. Healthy neonates have both a higher neutrophil

Table 6.1 Some causes of polycythaemia

Primary

Inherited

Erythroid progenitor cells with enhanced sensitivity to erythropoietin [1]

Acquired

Polycythaemia rubra vera (PRV) (primary proliferative polycythaemia)
Essential or idiopathic erythrocytosis

Secondary

Caused by tissue hypoxia

Inherited

Inadequate oxygen-carrying capacity
- Caused by congenital deficiency of NAD-linked or NADH-linked methaemoglobin reductase with consequent methaemoglobinaemia
- Haemoglobin M (structurally abnormal haemoglobins with tendency to form methaemoglobin)

Impaired release of oxygen from haemoglobin
- High affinity haemoglobins including some methaemoglobins and some cases of hereditary persistence of fetal haemoglobin
- Oxygen affinity of haemoglobin increased by very low levels of 2,3-DPG consequent on deficiency of diphosphoglycerate mutase or, occasionally, deficiency of phosphofructokinase [2]

Acquired

Hypoxia
- Residence at high altitude
- Cyanotic heart disease
- Chronic hypoxic lung disease
- Sleep apnoea and other hypoventilation syndromes including morbid obesity (Pickwickian syndrome)
- Hepatic cirrhosis (consequent on pulmonary arteriovenous shunting) [3]

Inadequate oxygen-carrying capacity
- Chronic carbon monoxide poisoning [4] or heavy cigarette smoking
- Chronic methaemoglobinaemia or sulphaemoglobinaemia caused by drugs or chemicals

Consequent on inappropriate synthesis of erythropoietin (proven or presumptive) [5,6]

Inherited

Familial inappropriate increase of erythropoietin synthesis [7]

Acquired

Renal lesions including carcinoma (hypernephroma), Wilms' tumour, renal adenoma, renal haemangioma, renal sarcoma, renal cysts including polycystic disease of the kidney, renal artery stenosis, renal vein thrombosis, post-transplant polycythaemia, hydronephrosis, horseshoe kidney, nephrocalcinosis (including that caused by hyperparathyroidism), Bartter's syndrome
Cerebellar haemangioblastoma
Hepatic lesions including hepatoma, hepatic hamartoma, hepatic angiosarcoma, hepatic haemangioma
Uterine fibroids
Tumours of the adrenal gland, ovary, lung, thymus
Androgen administration or androgen-secreting tumours in women
Cushing's syndrome and primary aldosteronism

Unknown mechanisms

Inherited

Some familial cases [8]

Acquired

Excessive erythrocytosis at altitude (Monge's disease)
Associated with POEMS syndrome [9]

2,3-DPG, 2,3-diphosphoglycerate; POEMS, Polyendocrinopathy, Organomegaly, Endocrinopathy, M-protein, Skin changes syndrome.

count than is normal at other stages of life and a left shift. Similarly, women in the reproductive age range have somewhat higher neutrophil counts than men; the count varying with the menstrual cycle. During pregnancy, a marked rise in the neutrophil count occurs and this is further accentuated during labour and the post-partum period. In addition, pregnancy is associated with a left

Table 6.2 Some causes of polycythaemia of particular importance in or peculiar to the neonatal period

Intra-uterine twin to twin transfusion
Intra-uterine maternal to fetal transfusion
Placental insufficiency and intrauterine hypoxia
Small-for-dates babies
Post-mature babies
Maternal pregnancy-associated hypertension
Maternal smoking
Maternal diabetes mellitus
Chromosomal abnormalities
Down's syndrome
Trisomy 13 syndrome
Trisomy 18 syndrome
Neonatal thyrotoxicosis
Congenital adrenal hyperplasia

shift (with myelocytes and even a few promyelocytes appearing in the blood), with 'toxic' granulation and with Döhle bodies.

Neutrophil leucocytosis is usually due to redistribution of white cells or increased bone marrow output. Rarely, there is a prolongation of the period a neutrophil spends in the circulation. Exercise can alter the distribution of white cells within the circulation with cells which were previously marginated against the endothelium being mobilized into the circulating blood. Vigorous exercise can double the neutrophil count. The absolute number of lymphocytes, monocytes, eosinophils and basophils also increases but because of the more striking increase in neutrophil numbers the increase of other cell types may go unnoticed. If exercise is both severe and prolonged a left shift can occur, indicating that there is then increased bone marrow output in addition to redistribution. Patients do not usually undergo severe exercise before having a blood sample taken but adrenaline administration and epileptiform convulsions can mobilize neutrophils similarly and even severe pain can have an effect on the neutrophil count. Corticosteroids also alter neutrophil kinetics. The output from the bone marrow is increased and there is a concomitant decrease in egress to the tissues. A rise in the WBC starts within a few hours of intravenous administration or within 1 day of oral administration. WBCs as high as $20 \times 10^9/l$ occur, the elevation being predominantly due to neutrophilia but with some increase also in the absolute monocyte count, and with a fall in the absolute eosinophil and lymphocyte counts. Adrenaline and corticosteroids do not cause toxic granulation, Döhle bodies, left shift or neutrophil vacuolation.

Neutrophilia in pathological conditions is usually consequent on increased output from the bone marrow which more than compensates for any increased egress to the tissues. The major causes of neutrophilia are shown in Table 6.3 and some causes of particular importance in the neonatal period in Table 6.4.

Eosinophil leucocytosis — eosinophilia

Eosinophil leucocytosis or eosinophilia is the elevation of the eosinophil count above levels observed in healthy subjects of the same age with no history of allergy. Eosinophil counts are higher in neonates than in adults. A slow decline in the eosinophil count occurs in elderly people. Eosinophil counts are the same in men and women. Contrary to earlier reports, they do not differ between different ethnic groups. High eosinophil counts previously reported in Indians and Africans are attributable to environmental influences.

The absolute eosinophil count is increased with vigorous exercise but not out of proportion to the increase in other leucocytes.

Some of the causes of eosinophilia are shown in Tables 6.5 and 6.6, the commonest being allergic diseases (particularly asthma, hayfever and eczema) and, in some parts of the world, parasitic infection. Allergic conditions causing eosinophilia are usually readily apparent from the patient's medical history, but in the case of parasitic infections the laboratory detection of eosinophilia may be the finding which leads to the correct diagnosis. In hospital patients eosinophilia can be a useful sign of drug allergy. When the eosinophil count is greatly elevated (greater than $10 \times 10^9/l$) the likely causes are far fewer (Table 6.7).

The laboratory detection of eosinophilia in patients with lung disease (Table 6.8) is important in indicating relevant diagnostic possibilities and in excluding conditions such as Wegener's granulomatosis, which are not associated with eosinophilia. In patients with symptoms suggestive of obstructive airways disease the presence of eosino-

Table 6.3 Some causes of neutrophil leucocytosis

Inherited

Hereditary neutrophilia [10]

Inherited deficiency of CR3 complement receptors [11]

Deficient surface expression of leucocyte adhesion molecules [12,13]

Acquired

Infections
- Many acute and chronic bacterial infections, including miliary tuberculosis and some rickettsial infections, e.g., Rocky Mountain spotted fever and some cases of typhus
- Some viral infections, e.g., chickenpox, herpes simplex infection, rabies, poliomyelitis, St Louis encephalitis virus infection, Eastern equine encephalitis virus infection, hantavirus infection [14]
- Some fungal infections, e.g., actinomycosis, coccidioidomycosis, North American blastomycosis
- Some parasitic infections, e.g., liver fluke, hepatic amoebiasis, filariasis, some *Pneumocystis carinii* infections

Tissue damage, e.g., trauma, surgery (particularly splenectomy), burns, acute hepatic necrosis, acute pancreatitis

Tissue infarction, e.g., myocardial infarction, pulmonary embolism causing pulmonary infarction, sickle cell crisis, atheroembolic disease

Acute inflammation and severe chronic inflammation, e.g., gout, pseudogout (calcium pyrophosphate crystal deposition disease), rheumatic fever, rheumatoid arthritis, Still's disease, ulcerative colitis, polyarteritis nodosa, familial Mediterranean fever, scleroderma, familial cold urticaria

Acute haemorrhage

Acute hypoxia

Heat stress [15]

Metabolic and endocrine disorders, e.g., diabetic ketoacidosis, acute renal failure, Cushing's syndrome, thyrotoxic crisis

Malignant disease (particularly but not only when there is extensive disease or tumour necrosis), e.g., carcinoma, sarcoma, melanoma, Hodgkin's disease

Myeloproliferative and leukaemic disorders, e.g., chronic granulocytic leukaemia (CGL), chronic myelomonocytic leukaemia (CMML), neutrophilic leukaemia, acute myeloid leukaemia (AML) (not commonly), other rare leukaemias, polycythaemia rubra vera (PRV) (primary proliferative polycythaemia), essential thrombocythaemia, idiopathic myelofibrosis (early in the disease process), systemic mastocytosis

Post-neutropenia rebound, e.g., following dialysis-induced neutropenia, recovery from agranulocytosis and cytotoxic chemotherapy, treatment of megaloblastic anaemia

Administration of cytokines such as G-CSF, GM-CSF, IL-1, IL-3 [16], IL-6 [17]

Administration of drugs, e.g., adrenaline, corticosteroids, lithium, clozapine [18]

Poisoning by various chemicals and drugs

Envenomation, e.g., scorpion bite [19] or 'killer bee' attack [20]

Hypersensitivity reactions including those due to drugs

Cigarette smoking

Vigorous exercise

Acute pain, epileptic convulsions, electric shock, paroxysmal tachycardia

Eclampsia and pre-eclampsia (pregnancy-associated hypertension)

Kawasaki's disease

Sweet's syndrome [21]

Neuroleptic malignant syndrome [22]

philia usually indicates a reversible or asthmatic component, although it does not necessarily indicate allergic rather than other triggering factors [45]. In uncomplicated asthma the eosinophil count is rarely in excess of 2×10^9/l. Higher levels, often in association with deteriorating pulmonary function, may indicate either allergic aspergillosis or the Churg–Strauss syndrome. The Churg–Strauss syndrome is a variant of polyarteritis nodosa which is characterized by pulmonary infil-

Table 6.4 Significant causes of neutrophilia in the neonate

Maternal factors
Smoking
Fever
Prolonged intrapartum oxytocin administration
Administration of dexamethasone

Fetal factors
Stressful delivery
Birth asphyxia or other hypoxia
Crying
Physiotherapy
Pain, e.g., lumbar puncture
Hypoglycaemia
Seizures
Infection
Haemolysis
Intraventricular haemorrhage
Meconium aspiration syndrome
Hyaline membrane disease with pneumothorax

Table 6.5 Some of the commoner causes of eosinophilia

Allergic diseases, e.g., atopic eczema, asthma, allergic rhinitis (hayfever), acute urticaria, allergic bronchopulmonary aspergillosis and other bronchoallergic fungal infections

Drug hypersensitivity (particularly to gold, sulphonamides, penicillin, nitrofurantoin)

Parasitic infection (particularly when tissue invasion has occurred), e.g., schistosomiasis, trichinosis, strongyloidiasis, filariasis, cysticercosis, echinococcosis (hydatid cyst), toxocariasis (infection by *Toxocara canis* or *Toxocara catis*, visceral larva migrans), dirofilariasis (infection by dog heartworm, *Difilaria immitis*), epidemic eosinophilic enteritis (infection by *Ancylostoma caninum*) [23], lung fluke (*Paragonimus westermani*) infection [24], *Blastocystis hominus* infection [25], enteric infection by *Isospora belli* or *Dientamoeba fragilis* [26]

Skin diseases, e.g., pemphigus, bullous pemphigoid, herpes gestationalis, eosinophilic pustular folliculitis [27]

trates and eosinophilia, neither of which is typical of classical polyarteris nodosa [46]. Patients are also seen with some features of classical polyarteritis nodosa and some of the Churg–Strauss syndrome: this has been referred to as 'chronic necrotizing vasculitis' or 'the overlap syndrome'. Eosinophilia of $1.5 \times 10^9/l$ or more is an important criterion in making the diagnosis of the Churg–Strauss syndrome or the overlap syndrome.

In some patients with eosinophilia and pulmonary infiltration no underlying condition can be found. Many such patients have a condition known as eosinophilic pneumonia; its cause is unknown, but chest radiology shows distinctive peripheral infiltration and there is a predictable response to corticosteroid therapy. The combination of the characteristic X-ray appearance with eosinophilia has been considered sufficient to make the diagnosis [47] whereas in the minority of patients lacking eosinophilia a lung biopsy is needed to establish the diagnosis.

Eosinophilia is a rare manifestation of non-haemopoietic malignancy. It is usually associated with widespread malignant disease but rarely may provide a clue to a localized tumour. Eosinophilia may also occur as a reaction to lymphoid malignancy, particularly Hodgkin's disease, T-lineage non-Hodgkin's lymphoma and T-acute lymphoblastic leukaemia (T-ALL). Eosinophilia associated with lymphoid malignancy has been observed up to 1 year in advance of other evidence of the disease, and may recur some weeks before relapse can be detected.

In a minority of cases, eosinophilia is neoplastic rather than reactive. Eosinophilia is present in 80% of cases of CGL and in a lower percentage of other myeloid leukaemias and myeloproliferative disorders. It occurs occasionally in AML and rarely in the myelodysplastic syndromes. In some patients with leukaemia, differentiation is predominantly to eosinophils and the term 'eosinophilic leukaemia' is then applicable (see p. 277).

There remains a group of patients with persistent, moderate or marked eosinophilia for which no cause can be found despite detailed investigation. This condition is designated the 'idiopathic hypereosinophilic syndrome (HES)' (see p. 272).

Table 6.6 Some of the less common and rare causes of eosinophilia

Hereditary eosinophilia	Angioimmunoblastic lymphadenopathy [34]
Myeloid leukaemias, e.g., CGL and some other chronic myeloid leukaemias (CMLs), systemic mastocytosis and less often other chronic myeloproliferative disorders, AML (particularly FAB categories M2Eo and M4Eo), eosinophilic leukaemia	Administration of cytokines, e.g., GM-CSF or IL-2, IL-3 or IL-5
Lymphoproliferative disorders, e.g., acute lymphoblastic leukaemia (B and T lineage), non-Hodgkin's lymphoma (particularly T-cell), Hodgkin's disease, mycosis fungoides and Sézary's syndrome, angioimmunoblastic lymphadenopathy, angiolymphoid hyperplasia with eosinophilia	Immune deficiency states and other conditions with recurring infections, e.g., Wiskott–Aldrich syndrome, Job's syndrome, infantile genetic agranulocytosis, HIV infection, particularly if complicated by HTLV-II infection [26]
Non-haematological malignant disease, e.g., carcinoma, sarcoma, glioma, mesothelioma, malignant melanoma, hepatoma, metastatic pituitary tumour [28]	Cyclical neutropenia
Bowel disease, e.g., eosinophilic enteritis, Crohn's disease, ulcerative colitis	Cyclical eosinophilia with angioedema
Autoimmune and connective tissue disorders, e.g., Churg–Strauss variant of polyarteritis nodosa, systemic necrotizing vasculitis (variant of polyarteritis nodosa), rheumatoid arthritis, eosinophilic fasciitis (some cases caused by L-tryptophan) [29], eosinophilic cellulitis [30], progressive systemic sclerosis [31], systemic lupus erythematosus, chronic active hepatitis [32] sclerosing cholangitis (uncommonly) [33]	Miscellaneous, e.g., recovery from some bacterial and viral infections, premature neonates during the first few weeks of life, scarlet fever, tuberculosis, coccidioidomycosis, *Pneumocystis carinii* infection, disseminated histoplasmosis [35], propanolol administration, drug abuse including cocaine inhalation [36,37], toxic oil syndrome [38], L-tryptophan toxicity [39], haemodialysis, atheroembolic disease [40], chronic graft-versus-host disease, thrombocytopenia with absent radii syndrome, chronic pancreatitis, Omenn's syndrome (familial histiocytic reticulosis) [41], HIV infection [42]
	Unknown, i.e. idiopathic hypereosinophilic syndrome (HES) [26]

Table 6.7 Some causes of marked eosinophilia

Parasitic infections, e.g., toxocariasis, trichinosis, tissue migration by larvae of ascaris, ankylostoma or strongyloides
Drug hypersensitivity
Churg–Strauss variant of polyarteritis nodosa
Hodgkin's disease
Idiopathic HES
Eosinophilic leukaemia

Basophil leucocytosis — basophilia

Some of the causes of basophilia are shown in Table 6.9. The detection of basophil leucocytosis is useful in making the distinction between a myeloproliferative disorder and a reactive condition since only in myeloproliferative disorders and certain leukaemias is a marked increase in the basophil count at all common. A rising basophil count in CGL is of prognostic significance since it often indicates an accelerated phase of the disease and impending blast transformation. The occurrence of basophilia in association with ALL may indicate that the patient is Philadelphia-positive and in AML may indicate Philadelphia-positivity or the presence of the t(6;9)(p23;q34.3) translocation, both karyotypic abnormalities being of adverse prognostic significance. Basophilic leukaemia is often Philadelphia-positive and in this case should be regarded as a variant of CGL.

Lymphocytosis

Lymphocytosis is an increase in the absolute lymphocyte count above what would be expected

Table 6.8 Some causes of eosinophilia with pulmonary infiltration

Parasitic infections, e.g., toxocariasis, filariasis, schistosomiasis, larval migration stage of strongyloidiasis, ascariasis, ankylostomiasis
Asthma
Allergic bronchopulmonary aspergillosis
Hypersensitivity reactions to drugs and chemicals, including those due to zinc, chromium or beryllium
Churg–Strauss variant of polyarteritis nodosa and systemic necrotizing vasculitis
Infections
Tuberculosis (rarely), brucellosis [43] cooccidioidomycosis (rarely), histoplasmosis [43], *Pneumocystis carinii* pneumonia (rarely)
Sarcoidosis [43]
Hodgkin's disease [43]
Cocaine pneumonitis
Cytokine (GM-CSF) administration [44]
Chronic idiopathic eosinophilic pneumonia
Idiopathic HES

Table 6.9 Some causes of basophil leucocytosis

Myeloproliferative and leukaemic disorders
Chronic granulocytic leukaemia (almost invariably)
Other chronic myeloid leukaemias
Acute myeloid leukaemia (very rarely)
Polycythaemia rubra vera
Essential thrombocythaemia
Idiopathic myelofibrosis
Systemic mastocytosis
Some cases of Philadelphia-positive ALL
Basophilic leukaemia
Reactive basophilia
Myxoedema (hypothyroidism)
Ulcerative colitis
Hypersensitivity states
Oestrogen administration
Hyperlipidaemia
Idiopathic hypereosinophilic syndrome
Administration of IL-3 [16]

in a healthy subject of the same age. Since the lymphocyte counts of infants and children are considerably higher than those of adults it is particularly important to use age-adjusted reference ranges. There are no gender or ethnic differences in the lymphocyte count. In an adult, a count greater than $3.5 \times 10^9/l$ may be considered abnormal. Some of the causes of lymphocytosis are shown in Table 6.10.

In assessing a lymphocytosis it is important to consider cytology as well as the lymphocyte count and both should be assessed in relation to the age and clinical features of the patient. Children are more prone than adults to both lymphocytosis and reactive changes in lymphocytes and even apparently healthy children may have some lymphocytes showing atypical features.

Lymphocytosis can occur without there being any cytological abnormality. This is usual when lymphocytosis is due to redistribution of lymphocytes (e.g., following exercise or adrenaline injection or as an acute response to severe stress), in endocrine abnormalities and in 'acute infectious lymphocytosis' (see Table 6.10). Cytological abnormalities are also uncommon in whooping cough but sometimes there are cleft cells resembling those of follicular lymphoma [67]. In other viral and bacterial infections there are often minor changes in lymphocytes, such as a visible nucleolus or increased cytoplasmic basophilia, which are often referred to as 'reactive changes'. Infectious mononucleosis and to a lesser extent other conditions are associated with much more striking reactive changes, the abnormal cells being referred to as 'atypical lymphocytes' or 'atypical mononuclear cells' (see p. 268). Post-splenectomy lymphocytosis is usually mild with only minor atypical features. Sometimes post-splenectomy lymphocytosis is consequent on an increase in large granular lymphocytes. It is important to realize that post-splenectomy counts can be in excess of $10 \times 10^9/l$ and misdiagnosis as a lymphoproliferative disorder has occurred. Many heavy cigarette smokers have a mild lymphocytosis without cytological abnormalities. A minority of smokers, mainly women, have a persistent polyclonal B-cell lymphocytosis associated with characteristic atypical features, specifically bilobed nuclei and binuclearity, in a proportion of cells. EBV infection may be a cofactor in the latter syndrome [60]. An increase of large granular lymphocytes can occur as a reactive change, e.g., in chronic hepatitis B or chronic EBV infection, sometimes without an increase in the total lymphocyte count.

Table 6.10 Some causes of lymphocytosis

Viral infections including measles (rubeola), German measles (rubella), mumps, chickenpox (varicella), influenza, infectious hepatitis (hepatitis A), infectious mononucleosis (EBV infection), infectious lymphocytosis (infection by certain Coxsackie viruses, adenoviruses types 1, 2 and 5, and echovirus 7 [48–52]), cytomegalovirus infection, HIV infection, infection by HTLV-I and HTLV-II [53]
Certain bacterial infections including whooping cough (pertussis, infection by *Bordatella pertussis*), brucellosis, tuberculosis, syphilis, plague (*Yersinia pestis* infection) [54], rickettsial infections including scrub typhus (*Rickettsia tsutsugamushi*) and murine typhus (*Rickettsia typhi*) [55,56] and bacterial infections in infants and young children
Hyperreactive malarial splenomegaly [57]
Transient stress-related lymphocytosis, e.g., associated with myocardial infarction, cardiac arrest, trauma, obstetric complications, sickle cell crisis [58,59]
Adrenaline injection
Vigorous muscular contraction, e.g., vigorous exercise, status epilepticus
Cigarette smoking causing either T-lymphocytosis (common) or persistent polyclonal B-lymphocytosis (uncommon) [60]
Administration of cytokines, e.g., IL-3 [16] or G-CSF [61]
Allergic reactions to drugs
Serum sickness
Splenectomy
Endocrine disorders, e.g., Addison's disease, hypopituitarism, hyperthyroidism [62]
β-Thalassaemia intermedia [63]
Gaucher's disease [64]
Thymoma [65]
Hodgkin's disease [66]
Lymphoid leukaemias and other lymphoproliferative disorders, e.g., CLL, non-Hodgkin's lymphoma, Hodgkin's disease (rarely), ATLL, hairy cell leukaemia and hairy cell variant leukaemia, Waldenström's macroglobulinaemia, heavy chain disease, mycosis fungoides and Sézary's syndrome, large granular lymphocyte leukaemia

In lymphoproliferative disorders, lymphocytosis is usually caused by the presence of considerable numbers of lymphoma cells in the peripheral blood. However, occasionally, e.g., in Hodgkin's disease, there is a lymphoma-associated polyclonal reactive lymphocytosis [66]. Neoplastic lymphocytes almost always show cytological abnormalities. The exception is large granular lymphocyte leukaemia in which the neoplastic cells are usually cytologically indistinguishable from normal cells. It is often said that in CLL there is an increase in apparently normal, mature lymphocytes but in fact subtle abnormalities are present. The specific cytological features of this and other lymphoproliferative disorders are described in Chapter 9. In general, lymphoproliferative disorders have distinctive cytological features and can thus be readily distinguished from reactive changes in lymphocytes. An exception may occur in some low-grade non-Hodgkin's lymphomas, particularly mantle cell lymphoma, some cases of which have neoplastic cells which can be confused with reactive lymphocytes. For this reason the term 'reactive changes' should be used with circumspection.

Monocytosis

Monocytosis is an increase of the monocyte count above what would be expected in a healthy subject of the same age. The absolute monocyte count is higher in neonates than at other stages of life. A rise occurs in pregnancy in parallel with the rise in the neutrophil count. Some of the common causes of monocytosis are shown in Table 6.11.

In examining a film of a patient with an unexplained monocytosis other evidence of chronic infection or myelodysplasia should be sought. The presence of promonocytes and blasts suggest either AML with monocytic differentiation or malignant histiocytosis.

Plasmacytosis

Plasmacytosis is the appearance in the blood of appreciable numbers of plasma cells. These may be reactive or neoplastic. Some of the causes of plasmacytosis are shown in Table 6.12.

In reactive plasmacytosis the number of circu-

Table 6.11 Some causes of monocytosis [68]

Chronic infection including miliary tuberculosis [69] and congenital syphilis [70]
Chronic inflammatory conditions including Crohn's disease, ulcerative colitis, rheumatoid arthritis and systemic lupus erythematosus
Carcinoma [71]
Administration of cytokines including G-CSF, GM-CSF, M-CSF and IL-3 [16,72]
Myeloproliferative and leukaemic conditions including CMML and other myelodysplastic conditions, CGL*, atypical CML, juvenile myeloid leukaemia, systemic mastocytosis, AML, malignant histiocytosis
Cyclical neutropenia, chronic idiopathic neutropenia
Long-term haemodialysis [73]
Lymphomatoid granulomatosis [74]

* Absolute but not relative monocytosis.

Table 6.12 Some causes of peripheral blood plasmacytosis

Reactive
Bacterial and viral infections and immunizations
Hypersensitivity reaction to drugs
Streptokinase administration
Serum sickness
Systemic lupus erythematosus
Angioimmunoblastic lymphadenopathy
Neoplastic
Multiple myeloma and plasma cell leukaemia
γ-heavy chain disease
Waldenström's macroglobulinaemia (rarely)

lating plasma cells is usually low but occasionally quite considerable numbers are present. A case of serum sickness due to tetanus antitoxin, for example, was found to have $3.2 \times 10^9/l$ plasma cells [75]. In reactive plasmacytosis the plasma cells are usually mature but occasionally plasmablasts are present. Plasma cells may contain vacuoles or, occasionally, crystals. Atypical lymphocytes and plasmacytoid lymphocytes may also be present and cells of other lineages may show reactive changes.

Table 6.13 Some causes of thrombocytosis

Primary
Essential thrombocythaemia (all cases)
Chronic granulocytic leukaemia (most cases)
Idiopathic myelofibrosis (early in the disease course)
Polycythaemia rubra vera (many cases)
Myelodysplastic syndromes (a minority of cases, e.g., in the 5q-syndrome and in some cases of sideroblastic anaemia)
AML (a minority of cases, particularly acute megakaryoblastic leukaemia)
Transient abnormal myelopoiesis in neonates with Down's syndrome (some cases)
Secondary
Infection
Inflammation
Haemorrhage
Surgery and trauma
Malignant disease
Kawasaki's disease [76]
Iron deficiency
Rebound after cytotoxic chemotherapy
Rebound after alcohol withdrawal
Following treatment of severe megaloblastic anaemia
Severe haemolytic anaemia, particularly after unsuccessful splenectomy
Associated with multicentric angiofollicular hyperplasia [77], Castleman's disease [78] and POEMS [78]
Adrenaline administration
Vinca alkaloid administration
Following administration of IL-3 [16], IL-6 [79], or erythropoietin to premature infants [80]
Associated with vitamin E administration in premature infants [81]
Associated with infantile cortical hyperostosis [82]
In infants of drug-abusing mothers [83]
Redistributional
Splenectomy and hyposplenism
Unknown mechanism
Tidal platelet dysgenesis

POEMS, polyendocrinopathy, organomegaly, endocrinopathy, M-protein, skin changes syndrome.

Neoplastic plasma cells usually show more cytological abnormality than those produced in reactive states. The haematological features of multiple myeloma and its differential diagnosis are discussed on p. 304.

Thrombocytosis

Thrombocytosis is an increase of the platelet count above what would be expected in a healthy subject of the same age and sex. Use of the term 'thrombocythaemia' is usually restricted to a thrombocytosis occurring as the consequence of a myeloproliferative disorder; the term 'essential thrombocytosis' is synonymous. Thrombocytosis is usually consequent on increased marrow production of platelets, either autonomous or reactive. Following splenectomy, and in hyposplenism, thrombocytosis is due to redistribution of platelets. Some of the causes of thrombocytosis are shown in Table 6.13 and the causes of a marked increase in the platelet count in Table 6.14. It should be noted that as more and more routine platelet counts are performed on very sick patients the percentage of even very high platelet counts which are reactive is increasing and myeloproliferative disorders are now responsible for only 10–15% of counts greater than $1000 \times 10^9/l$.

Blood film and count

Increased platelet size, platelet anisocytosis, the presence of poorly granulated platelets, circulating megakaryocyte nuclei or micromegakaryocytes and an increased basophil count are all suggestive of a primary bone marrow disease rather than a reactive thrombocytosis. Large platelets are also seen in hyposplenism whereas in reactive thrombocytosis platelets are generally small and normally granulated. The blood film may also show abnormalities of other lineages which indicate the correct diagnosis. The features of hyposplenism should be specifically sought.

The degree of elevation of the platelet count is of some use in the differential diagnosis. Counts of greater than $1500 \times 10^9/l$ are usually indicative of a myeloproliferative disorder but reactive thrombocytosis with counts as high as $2000 \times 10^9/l$ [86] and even $6000 \times 10^9/l$ [87] have been reported. In primary thrombocytosis the automated blood count may show an increased MPV and PDW, indicative of increased platelet size and platelet anisocytosis, respectively. In secondary or reactive thrombocytosis the MPV and PDW are more often normal.

Further tests

The cause of reactive thrombocytosis is usually readily apparent from the clinical history. When the cause is not apparent a bone marrow aspirate, trephine biopsy and cytogenetic analysis are indicated. Indirect evidence favouring a reactive thrombocytosis includes increased ESR, fibrinogen concentration and concentration of factor VIII and von Willebrand's factor. It can sometimes be difficult to distinguish iron deficiency with a marked reactive thrombocytosis from PRV with complicating iron deficiency and in these circumstances a judicious trial of iron therapy may be needed.

Table 6.14 Some causes of markedly elevated platelet counts

	Platelet count		
	$>1000 \times 10^9/l$ [84] n = 102 (%)	$>900 \times 10^9/l$ [85] n = 526 (%)	$>1000 \times 10^9/l$ [86] n = 280 (%)
Malignant disease	45	27	11.5
Splenectomy or hyposplenism	40	20	16
Myeloproliferative disorder	28	26	14
Infection or inflammation	30	19	26
Connective tissue disorder	2	9	
Iron deficiency	4		
Trauma			11.5
Blood loss			5
Rebound			2.5

Anaemia

Anaemia can be due to: (i) defective production of red cells; (ii) reduced red cell survival in the circulation due to haemolysis or blood loss; (iii) increased pooling of essentially normal red cells in a large spleen; or (iv) sequestration of abnormal red cells such as those in sickle cell anaemia or sickle cell/haemoglobin C disease, in the spleen or, less often, in the liver. Anaemia may be an isolated abnormality or there may be pancytopenia (see p. 175).

Blood film and count

The blood film and count commonly give a clue to the cause of the anaemia by showing microcytosis, macrocytosis or a specific type of poikilocyte. Red cell disorders associated with these features are discussed in Chapter 8. The presence

Table 6.15 Some causes of normocytic normochromic anaemia (other than conditions which usually cause pancytopenia which are listed in Table 6.25)

Causative conditions	Peripheral blood features which may be useful in diagnosis
Early iron deficiency*	A few hypochromic cells may be present, RDW increased
Anaemia of chronic disease*	Increased rouleaux and ESR, occasionally increased platelet count or WBC, RDW often normal
Lead poisoning*	Basophilic stippling, some cases have polychromasia
Double deficiency of iron and vitamin B_{12} or folic acid*†	Hypersegmented neutrophils, increased RDW
Blood loss	If blood loss is severe and acute, anaemia is leucoerythroblastic; polychromasia, reticulocytosis and increased RDW develop within a few days
Non-spherocytic haemolytic anaemia*	Occasional poikilocytes, polychromasia, increased reticulocyte count, RDW increased (see p. 238)
Some congenital dyserythropoietic anaemias†	Striking anisocytosis and poikilocytosis (see p. 254)
Paroxysmal nocturnal haemoglobinuria	Sometimes other cytopenias – particularly a low WBC, low NAP score, polychromasia in some cases
Myelodysplastic syndromes†	Other features of myelodysplastic syndromes (see p. 285)
Renal failure	Sometimes keratocytes or schistocytes
Liver failure†	Target cells, stomatocytes, acanthocytes, other cytopenias
Hypothyroidism†	Sometimes acanthocytes
Addison's disease and hypopituitarism	Lymphocytosis, eosinophilia, neutropenia, monocytopenia
Hyperparathyroidism	Nil
Anorexia nervosa	Acanthocytes, other cytopenia, poikilocytosis, basophilic stippling
Pure red cell aplasia†	Normal RDW, reticulocytes very low or absent
Pearson's syndrome (mitochondrial cytopathy)† [88]	Nil

* Can also be microcytic.
† Can also be macrocytic.

of polychromasia suggests an adequate bone marrow response to anaemia and indicates that anaemia may have been caused by haemolysis or haemorrhage. The differential diagnosis of a normocytic, normochromic anaemia and the peripheral blood features which may be helpful in suggesting the diagnosis are summarized in Table 6.15. Causes of pure red cell aplasia are detailed in Table 6.16. In some anaemic patients the blood film is leucoerythroblastic, i.e., granulocyte precursors and NRBC are present. In these cases the differential diagnosis is more limited, as summarized in Table 6.17. A leucoerythroblastic blood film is normal in the neonatal period and pregnant women occasionally have NRBC in addition to the more usual granulocyte precursors. Otherwise a leucoerythroblastic blood film, other than during an acute illness, is likely to indicate serious underlying disease.

In the perinatal period, the conditions responsible for anaemia differ somewhat from those operating later in life (Table 6.18). In the fetus and neonate, haemolytic anaemia may be consequent on transplacental passage of antibodies (alloantibodies or, less often, autoantibodies) or on intrauterine infections by microorganisms which in later life do not usually cause anaemia (e.g., cytomegalovirus infection, toxoplasmosis, syphilis and rubella) [96]. The consequences of anaemia also differ from those at other periods of life. Severe anaemia in the fetus can lead to hydrops fetalis, a condition characterized by gross oedema of the fetus and placenta, often leading to intra-uterine death. In the neonate, because of the immaturity of the liver, severe haemolysis can lead to marked hyperbilirubinaemia with consequent brain damage. The identification of anaemia, particularly haemolytic anaemia, in the fetus and neonate is therefore of considerable importance.

Table 6.16 Some causes of pure red cell aplasia

Constitutional (Diamond–Blackfan syndrome)
Transient erythroblastopenia of childhood
Hereditary transcobalamin II deficiency [89]
Associated with CLL or large granular lymphocyte leukaemia, thymoma, or autoimmune disease such as systemic lupus erythematosus or autoimmune polyglandular syndrome
Pregnancy-associated [90]
Chronic parvovirus infection
Myelodysplastic syndromes (e.g., refractory anaemia)
ABO-incompatible bone marrow transplantation [91]

Table 6.17 Some causes of leucoerythroblastic anaemia

Bone marrow infiltration in carcinoma, lymphoma (Hodgkin's disease, non-Hodgkin's lymphoma), CLL, multiple myeloma, ALL or other malignant disease
Myeloproliferative disorders, particularly idiopathic myelofibrosis and CGL
AML and the myelodysplastic syndromes
Bone marrow granulomas, e.g., in miliary tuberculosis
Storage diseases
Acute haemolysis (including erythroblastosis fetalis)
Shock, e.g., due to severe haemorrhage
Severe infection
Rebound following bone marrow failure or suppression
Crises of sickle cell anaemia
Bone marrow infarction
Thalassaemia major
Severe megaloblastic anaemia
Systemic lupus erythematosus [92]
Severe nutritional rickets [93]
Marble bone disease (osteopetrosis)

Further tests

When the cause of anaemia is not apparent from the clinical history or the blood film and count other tests are needed. Those most likely to be useful are: (i) a reticulocyte count; (ii) serum iron and either transferrin concentration or serum ferritin assay; (iii) serum B_{12} and red cell folate assays; and (iv) tests of renal; thyroid and hepatic function. If these investigations do not reveal the cause of the anaemia a bone marrow aspirate is indicated. When there is an unexplained leucoerythroblastic anaemia, other than during an acute illness, a bone marrow aspirate and trephine biopsy is indicated without delay.

In the neonate, serological tests on mother and baby, haematological assessment of both parents and G6PD assay may be useful.

Table 6.18 Some causes of anaemia of importance in the fetus and neonate

Fetus and neonate
Haemolysis due to transplacental passage of alloantibodies, e.g., rhesus or Kell antibodies
Haemoglobin Bart's hydrops fetalis
Parvovirus infection
Severe inherited haemolytic anaemias: G6PD deficiency (sometimes following maternal ingestion of oxidants), triose phosphate isomerase deficiency, glucose phosphate isomerase deficiency, pyruvate kinase deficiency) [94]
Congenital leukaemia [95]
Fetomaternal haemorrhage
Twin-to-twin haemorrhage

Neonate
Haemorrhage from the cord or the placenta or internal haemorrhage during or as a consequence of birth
Haemolytic disease of the newborn
Transient severe haemolysis in hereditary elliptocytosis
Haemolysis associated with disseminated intravascular coagulation caused by sepsis
Removal of inappropriately large amounts of blood for laboratory testing
Congenital infections including, rarely, congenital malaria
Prematurity

Neutropenia

Neutropenia is a reduction of the absolute neutrophil count below that which would be expected in a subject of the same age, sex, physiological status and ethnic origin. It is particularly important to use an appropriate reference range in black people, to avoid a misdiagnosis of neutropenia, since Africans and, to a lesser extent black American and Afro-Caribbeans, have neutrophil counts much lower than those of white people. Neutropenia may be an isolated phenomenon or part of a pancytopenia. Mechanisms of neutropenia include: (i) inadequate production by the bone marrow because of bone marrow replacement or ineffective granulopoiesis; (ii) destruction by bone marrow macrophages and other reticuloendothelial cells in haemophagocytic syndromes; (iii) defective release from the bone marrow as in myelokathexis; (iv) redistribution within the vasculature as occurs early during haemodialysis; (v) pooling in the spleen; (vi) shortened intravascular lifespan as in immune neutropenias; and (vii) rapid egress to the tissues when the bone marrow output cannot increase adequately, as in neonates with sepsis.

An unexpected apparent neutropenia on an automated counter should always be confirmed on a blood film since it may be factitious (see Chapter 4). The detection of unexpected neutropenia by the laboratory can be of vital importance, since drug-induced agranulocytosis can be rapidly fatal. In many clinical circumstances the likely cause of neutropenia will be readily apparent from the patient's medical history, including the history of drug intake. When the history and examination of the blood film do not reveal the cause, bone marrow investigation is usually necessary. The causes of neutropenia are summarized in Tables 6.19 and 6.20.

Table 6.19 Some inherited disorders causing neutropenia

Congenital aleukocytosis (reticular agenesis)
Infantile genetic agranulocytosis (Kostmann's syndrome)
Neutropenia with pancreatic exocrine deficiency and dyschondroplasia (Shwachman's syndrome)
Neutropenia with pancreatic exocrine deficiency and sideroblastic erythropoiesis (Pearson's syndrome) [88]
Familial benign neutropenia
Familial severe neutropenia
Congenital dysgranulopoietic neutropenia [97]
Myelokathexis [98]
Lazy leucocyte syndrome
Chediak–Higashi syndrome
Dyskeratosis congenita with neutropenia
Associated with X-linked agammaglobulinaemia (one-third of cases)
Associated with cartilage–hair hypoplasia
Blackfan–Diamond syndrome, during the course of the disease [99]
Associated with certain inborn errors of metabolism (idiopathic hyperglycinaemia, isovaleric acidaemia, methylmalonic acidaemia, type Ib glycogen storage disease [100], carnitine deficiency [101]

Table 6.20 Some acquired disorders causing neutropenia

Infections
- Viral infections, e.g., measles, mumps, rubella, influenza, infectious hepatitis, infectious mononucleosis, cytomegalovirus infection, yellow fever, dengue fever, Colorado tick fever, parvovirus infection (occasionally), advanced HIV infection (AIDS)
- Bacterial infections, e.g., typhoid, paratyphoid, brucellosis, tularaemia [102], some cases of miliary tuberculosis [69], some Gram-negative infections (early in the disease process), overwhelming bacterial infection, bacterial infection in neonates, rickettsial infections including scrub typhus [103], rickettsial pox [104] and some cases of typhus
- Protozoal infection, e.g., malaria, kala-azar, trypanosomiasis
- Fungal infections, e.g., histoplasmosis [105]

Drugs, e.g., alkylating agents and other anti-cancer and related drugs (including azathioprine and zidovudine), idiosyncratic reaction to drugs (most common with antithyroid drugs, sulphonamides, chlorpromazine, gold), interferon

Irradiation

Bone marrow replacement, e.g., in ALL, multiple myeloma, or carcinoma

Idiopathic and secondary myelofibrosis

Ineffective granulopoiesis, e.g., in most cases of AML and MDS

Megaloblastic anaemia

Aplastic anaemia

Paroxysmal nocturnal haemoglobinuria

Acute anaphylaxis

Hypersplenism

Haemophagocytic syndromes

Immune neutropenia
- Alloimmune neutropenia in neonates, as a consequence of maternal antibody

Autoimmune neutropenia [106]
- Isolated autoimmune neutropenia
- Immune neutropenia associated with autoimmune haemolytic anaemia, autoimmune thrombocytopenia, systemic lupus erythematosus, rheumatoid arthritis (Felty's syndrome), scleroderma, hyperthyroidism, chronic active hepatitis, polyarteritis nodosa, primary biliary cirrhosis, thymoma, Hodgkin's disease, non-Hodgkin's lymphoma, angioimmunoblastic lymphadenopathy, large granular lymphocyte leukaemia, viral infection (chronic parvovirus infection [107], HIV infection, infectious mononucleosis), Castleman's disease, Sjögren's syndrome, mannosidosis, hypogammaglobulinaemia
- Autoimmune panleucopenia [108]
- Autoimmune pure white cell aplasia [109]

Cyclical neutropenia, including adult onset cyclical neutropenia associated with large granular lymphocyte leukaemia

Haemodialysis and filtration leukopheresis (early during the procedures)

Endocrine disorders, e.g., hypopituitarism, Addison's disease, hyperthyroidism [62]

Alcoholism [110]

Copper deficiency [111]

Hypercarotenaemia [112]

Associated with transient erythroblastopenia of childhood [113]

Intravenous immunoglobulin infusion in infants [114]

Rhesus disease of the newborn [114]

Babies born to hypertensive mothers [114,115]

Babies with asphyxia neonatorum [115]

Extracorporeal membrane oxygenation in neonates [116]

Administration of erythropoietin to premature babies [80]

Eosinopenia

Eosinopenia is a reduction of the eosinophil count below what would be expected in a healthy subject of the same age. Eosinopenia is rarely noted on a routine blood film and cannot be detected on a routine 100-cell differential cell count since the eosinophil is a relatively infrequent cell and the reference limits include zero. Since the introduction of automated differential counts eosinopenia is far more often noted. However, it is a common non-specific abnormality so its detection is not of much clinical significance.

A physiological fall in the eosinophil count occurs during pregnancy and there is a further fall during labour. Common causes of a low eosinophil count are shown in Table 6.21. Rare causes which have been reported include thymoma, pure eosinophil aplasia [117], and apparent autoimmune destruction of eosinophils and basophils [118].

Basopenia

Basopenia is a reduction in the basophil count below that which would be expected in a healthy subject. Some of the causes are shown in Table 6.22. Basophils are so infrequent in normal blood that their reduction is not likely to be noticed on inspection of the film or on a routine 100-cell or even 500-cell differential count. Basopenia can be detected on automated differential counters since they have reference ranges for basophils which do not include zero. However, the observation of basopenia has not yet been found to be of any great importance in diagnosis.

Lymphocytopenia (lymphopenia)

Lymphopenia or, more correctly, lymphocytopenia, is a reduction of the lymphocyte count below what would be expected in a healthy subject of the same age. Lymphocytopenia is extremely common as part of the acute response to stress although it is often overshadowed by the coexisting changes in neutrophils. It is more likely to be noticed when an automated differential count is performed and counts are expressed in absolute numbers. With the increasing importance of the diagnosis of AIDS, characterized by increasingly severe lymphopenia with disease progression, it is important to realize how common this abnormality is in acutely ill patients regardless of the nature of the underlying illness. Causes of lymphocytopenia are summarized in Table 6.23.

Table 6.21 Some causes of eosinopenia

Acute stress including trauma, surgery, burns, epileptiform convulsions, acute infections, acute inflammation, myocardial infarction, anoxia and exposure to cold
Cushing's syndrome
Drugs including corticosteroids and ACTH, adrenaline and other β-agonists, histamine, aminophylline
Haemodialysis (during procedure)

Table 6.22 Some causes of basopenia

Acute stress including infection and haemorrhage
Cushing's syndrome and administration of ACTH
Anaphylaxis, acute urticaria and other acute allergic reactions
Hyperthyroidism
Progesterone administration

Thrombocytopenia

Thrombocytopenia is a reduction of the platelet count below the level expected in a healthy subject of the same age and sex. Ethnic origin may aso be relevant since lower platelet counts have been observed in Africans and Afro-Caribbeans. Thrombocytopenia may be congenital or acquired and due to reduced production or to increased destruction, consumption or extravascular loss. The causes are summarized in Table 6.24.

Blood film and count

In unexplained congenital thrombocytopenia both platelet size and granularity and white cell morphology should be assessed. A number of inherited conditions have thrombocytopenia associated with morphological abnormalities of platelets or neutrophils (see p. 78). In acquired thrombocytopenia platelet size is also relevant since increased platelet consumption or destruction with increased bone marrow output is associated with increased platelet size whereas bone marrow failure is associated with small or normal sized platelets. Red cells should be assessed for any evidence of a microangiopathic haemolytic anaemia which may be associated with thrombocytopenia caused by a thrombotic microangiopathy. The blood film should be examined for blast cells, immature

Table 6.23 Some causes of lymphocytopenia

Acute stress including trauma, surgery, burns, acute infection, fulminant hepatic failure
Acute and chronic renal failure (including patients on dialysis)
Cushing's syndrome and the administration of corticosteroids or ACTH
Carcinoma (particularly with advanced disease)
Hodgkin's disease (particularly with advanced disease)
Some non-Hodgkin's lymphomas
Angioimmunoblastic lymphadenopathy
AIDS – the end stage of HIV infection
Cytotoxic and immunosuppressive therapy including use of antilymphocyte and antithymocyte globulin
Clozapine therapy [18]
Irradiation
Alcoholism [110]
Rheumatoid arthritis [119] and systemic lupus erythematosus [120]
Sarcoidosis [121]
Aplastic anaemia and agranulocytosis
The myelodysplastic syndromes [122]
Anorexia nervosa [123]
Intestinal lymphangiectasia and Whipple's disease
Iron-deficiency anaemia [124]
Chronic platelet apheresis [125]
Graft-versus-host disease
Administration of 'Lorenzo's oil' [126]
Certain rare congenital syndromes including reticular dysgenesis, severe combined immunodeficiency, Swiss type agammaglobulinaemia, some case of thymic hypoplasia (di George's syndrome) and ataxia telangiectasia

granulocytes or NRBC which may be indicative of leukaemia or bone marrow infiltration.

The automated blood count shows an increased MPV and PDW when there is increased platelet consumption or destruction and a low MPV when there is failure of bone marrow output.

Other tests

In congenital thrombocytopenia the patient should be assessed for evidence of associated congenital defects and other family members should be assessed for platelet number and morphology and other evidence of inherited abnormalities.

In acquired thrombocytopenia not readily explained by the clinical circumstances a bone marrow aspiration, tests for autoantibodies (antinuclear factor, anti-DNA antibodies and the lupus anticoagulant) and coagulation tests to exclude disseminated intravascular coagulation can be useful. Testing for HIV antibodies should be considered.

Pancytopenia

Pancytopenia is a combination of anaemia (with reduction of RBC), leucopenia and thrombocytopenia. Leucopenia is usually mainly due to a reduction in the neutrophil count although the numbers of other granulocytes, monocytes and lymphocytes are often also reduced.

Pancytopenia is usually caused by bone marrow replacement or failure but is sometimes consequent on splenic pooling or peripheral destruction of mature cells. Some of the causes of pancytopenia are shown in Table 6.25. In hospital practice, pancytopenia is most often consequent on cytotoxic or immunosuppressive drug therapy.

Blood film and count

When the aetiology is not readily apparent from the clinical history the blood film should be carefully examined for blast cells, dysplastic features in any cell lineage, lymphoma cells, hairy cells, myeloma cells, rouleaux, macrocytes or hypersegmented neutrophils, NRBC and immature granulocytes. Blast cells should be specifically sought along the edges of the film. Blast cells and hairy cells may be very infrequent but the presence of even small numbers is significant.

Differential diagnosis

The presence of dysplastic features in the absence of administration of cytotoxic drugs suggests either MDS or HIV infection. Macrocytosis may be present in liver disease and alcohol abuse, megaloblastic anaemia, hypoplastic and aplastic anaemias, MDS and following cytotoxic chemotherapy. Poikilocytic red cells and a leucoerythroblastic blood film (see Table 6.17) suggest bone marrow infiltration or idiopathic myelofibrosis. A low

Table 6.24 Some causes of thrombocytopenia (excluding conditions which usually cause pancytopenia)

Failure of platelet production

Congenital
May–Hegglin anomaly
Bernard–Soulier syndrome
Epstein's syndrome (thrombocytopenia with deafness and renal disease)
Other inherited thrombocytopenias, some with large platelets and some with platelets of normal size
Megakaryocytic hypoplasia, inherited or due to intra-uterine events (including some cases of trisomy 13 and trisomy 18 syndromes)
Fanconi's anaemia

Acquired
Following bone marrow damage by some of the drugs which can cause aplastic anaemia or as the first manifestation of aplastic anaemia
Thiazide administration
Myelodysplastic syndromes
Severe iron deficiency (rarely)
Parvovirus infection (rarely)
Interferon therapy
Paroxysmal nocturnal haemoglobinuria
Alcohol abuse [127]
Autoimmune [127]
Idiopathic acquired amegakaryocytic thrombocytopenia

Increased platelet consumption or destruction

Immune mechanisms

Congenital
Alloimmune thrombocytopenia
Transplacental transfer of maternal autoantibody
Maternal drug hypersensitivity

Acquired
Autoimmune thrombocytopenic purpura as an isolated abnormality or associated with other autoimmune disease (systemic lupus erythematosus, rheumatoid arthritis, autoimmune haemolytic anaemia (Evans' syndrome), with a lymphoproliferative disease (CLL, non-Hodgkin's lymphoma, Hodgkin's disease, large granular lymphocyte leukaemia), with sarcoidosis [128] or with angioimmunoblastic lymphadenopathy
Drug-induced immune thrombocytopenia including heparin-induced thrombocytopenia
Post-infection thrombocytopenia, particularly after rubella but also after chickenpox, infectious mononucleosis, other viral infections and vaccinations
Immune thrombocytopenia associated with HIV infection
Immune thrombocytopenia associated with cytomegalovirus infection [129], Mycoplasma infection [130], scarlet fever (β-haemolytic streptococcal infection) [131]
Post-transfusion purpura
Cocaine abuse [132]
Anaphylaxis
Onyalai [133]

Non-immune mechanisms

Congenital
Schulman–Upshaw syndrome [134,135]

Acquired
Disseminated intravascular coagulation
Thrombotic microangiopathy (TTP and related conditions, see Table 8.3)
Associated with certain viral infections (e.g., viral haemorrhagic fevers, hantavirus infection, dengue fever and Colorada tick fever (coltivirus infection), acute infection by HIV), riskettsial infections (e.g., Rocky Mountain spotted fever, malignant Mediterranean spotted fever), bacterial infections (e.g., Brazilian haemorrhagic fever (*Haemophilus aegyptis* infection) and relapsing fever (*Borrelia recurrentis* infection)) and protozoal infections (malaria and babesiosis)
Extracorporeal circulation
Massive transfusion
Kaposi's sarcoma [136]
DDAVP therapy in type IIB von Willebrand's disease

Redistribution of platelets

Congenital
Hypersplenism

Acquired
Administration of Lorenzo's oil [126,137]
Hypersplenism (including acute sequestration in sickle cell disease)
Hypothermia [138]

Uncertain or complex mechanisms

Congenital
Wiskott–Aldrich syndrome
The grey platelet syndrome
Chediak–Higashi anomaly
Cyclical thrombocytopenia and tidal platelet dysgenesis

Continued on p. 177

Table 6.24 (*Continued*)

Mediterranean macrothrombocytosis
Some cases of type IIB von Willebrand's disease
Congenital infections (toxoplasmosis, cytomegalovirus infection, rubella, syphilis, listeriosis, Coxsackie B infection, herpes simplex virus infection)
Associated with severe rhesus haemolytic disease of the newborn
Babies of hypertensive mothers [114]
Associated with certain inborn errors of metabolism (idiopathic hyperglycinaemia, methylmalonic acidaemia, isovaleric acidaemia [139]
Acquired
Phototherapy in the neonate [140]
Mechanical ventilation in the neonate [141]
Neonatal herpes simplex infection
Associated with cyanotic congenital heart disease
Graves' disease [142]
Pregnancy-associated thrombocytopenia
IL-2 therapy [143]
Monge's disease (inappropriate altitude-related polycythaemia) [144]
Paracetamol (acetaminophen) overdose [145]

reticulocyte count indicates failure of bone marrow output whereas an elevated reticulocyte count suggests peripheral destruction, e.g., paroxysmal nocturnal haemoglobinuria or immune destruction of cells.

The FBC may show an elevated MCV and elevated RDW. An appropriately increased MPV suggests peripheral platelet destruction whereas a reduced MPV despite thrombocytopenia suggests failure of bone marrow output.

Further tests

A reticulocyte count is indicated and a bone marrow aspirate is usually necessary. Unless a cellular aspirate is obtained, a trephine biopsy is also required. Bone marrow aspiration is needed urgently if the clinical history suggests the possibility of a haemophagocytic syndrome, acute infection or the rapid onset of megaloblastic anaemia. In the latter condition macrocytes and hypersegmented neutrophils may be infrequent or absent and only the bone marrow aspirate reveals the diagnosis. The other tests which are needed will be determined by the results of these

Table 6.25 Some causes of pancytopenia

Inherited disorders
Inherited conditions causing aplastic anaemia: Fanconi's anaemia, dyskeratosis congenita, xeroderma pigmentosa, some cases of Shwachman's syndrome
Marble bone disease (osteopetrosis)
Inherited metabolic disorders: mannosidosis, Gaucher's disease, adult Nieman–Pick disease, methylmalonic aciduria, oxalosis, isovaleric acidaemia, α-methyl β-hydroxybutyric aciduria, propionic acidaemic [146–148]
Other rare inherited conditions: some cases of Pearson's syndrome [88] and pancytopenia associated with necrotizing encephalopathy [149]
Acquired disorders
Aplastic and hypoplastic anaemias including: idiopathic, virus-induced, drug-induced and chemical-induced aplastic anaemia; bone marrow aplasia preceding ALL; bone marrow aplasia associated with thymoma and large granular lymphocyte leukaemia; graft-versus-host disease; irradiation; use of alkylating agents and other anti-cancer and related drugs
Bone marrow infiltration including in ALL, AML (ineffective haemopoiesis also contributes), multiple myeloma, carcinoma, non-Hodgkin's lymphoma and hairy cell leukaemia, hairy cell variant leukaemia
Clonal disorders of haemopoiesis: the myelodysplastic syndromes, paroxysmal nocturnal haemoglobinuria, acute myelofibrosis, advanced idiopathic myelofibrosis
Secondary myelofibrosis, e.g., caused by carcinomatous infiltration
Ineffective haemopoiesis: acute or severe megaloblastic anaemia; arsenic poisoning [150]
Haemophagocytic syndromes
AIDS
Systemic lupus erythematosus
Combined immunocytopenia [151]
Severe or chronic graft-versus host disease [152]
Drug-induced immune pancytopenia (e.g., caused by phenacetin, para-amino salicylic acid, sulphonamides, rifampicin and quinine)
Hypersplenism
Acute infections: some cases of acute HIV infection [153], parvovirus [154], ehrlichiosis [155], brucellosis [156] and miliary tuberculosis, cytomegalovirus infection in bone marrow transplant recipients [157]
Fusariosis [62]
Wilson's disease [158]
Hyperthyroidism (rarely) [159]
Alcohol toxicity [110]
Copper deficiency [160]

initial investigations and by the specific diagnosis which is suspected.

References

1 Juvonen E, Ikkala E, Fyhrquist F, Ruutu T. Autosomal dominant erythrocytosis caused by increased sensitivity to erythropoietin. *Blood* 1991; 78: 3066–9.

2 Tanaka KR, Zerez CR. Red cell enzymopathies of the glycolytic pathway. *Semin Hematol* 1990; 27: 165–85.

3 Hutchinson DCS, Sapru RP, Sumerling MD, Donaldson GWK, Richmond J. Cirrhosis, cyanosis and polycythemia: multiple pulmonary arteriovenous anastomoses. *Am J Med* 1968; 45: 139–51.

4 di Marco AT. Carbon monoxide poisoning presenting as polycythemia. *N Engl J Med* 1989; 319: 874.

5 Hammond D, Winnick S. Paraneoplastic erythrocytosis and ectopic erythropoietins. *Ann N Y Acad Sci* 1974; 230; 219–27.

6 Souid AK, Dubanshy AS, Richman P, Sadowitz PD. Polycythemia: a review article and a case report of erythrocytosis secondary to Wilms' tumor. *Pediatr Hematol Oncol* 1993; 10: 215–21.

7 Distelhorst CW, Wagner DS, Goldwasser E, Adamson JW. Autosomal dominant familial erythrocytosis due to anomalous erythropoietin production. *Blood* 1981; 58: 1155–8.

8 Emanuel PD, Eaves CJ, Broudy C, Papayannopoulo T, Moore MR, D'Andrea AD, Prchal JF, Eaves AC *et al.* Familial and congenital polycythemia in three unrelated families. *Blood* 1992; 79: 3019–30.

9 Nakanishi T, Sobue I, Tokokura Y, Nishitani H, Kuroiwa Y, Satayoshi E, Tsubaki T, Igata A *et al.* The Crow–Fukase syndrome: a study of 102 cases in Japan. *Neurology* 1984; 34: 712–20.

10 Herring WB, Smith LG, Walker RI, Herion JC. Hereditary neutrophilia. *Am J Med* 1974; 56: 729–34.

11 Malech HL, Gallin JI. Current concepts: immunology, neutrophils in human disease. *N Engl J Med* 1987; 317: 687–94.

12 Arnaout MA. Structure and function of the leukocyte adhesion molecules CD11/CD18. *Blood* 1990; 75: 1037–50.

13 Etzione A, Frydman M, Pollack S, Avidor I, Phillips ML, Paulson JC, Gershoni-Baruch R. Recurrent severe infections caused by a novel leukocyte adhesion deficiency. *N Engl J Med* 1992; 327: 1789–92.

14 Duchin JC, Koster FT, Peters CJ, Simpson GL, Tempest B, Zaki SR, Kziazek TG, Rollin PE *et al.* Hantavirus pulmonary syndrome. *N Engl J Med* 1994; 330: 949–55.

15 Keatinge WR, Coleshaw SRK, Easton JC, Coller F, Mattock MB, Chelliah R. Increased platelet and red cell counts, blood viscosity, and plasma cholesterol levels during heat stress, and mortality from coronary and cerebral thrombosis. *Am J Med* 1986; 81: 795–800.

16 Ganser A, Lindemann A, Siepelt G, Ottman OG, Herrmann F, Eder M, Frisch J, Schulz G *et al.* Effects of recombinant human interleukin-3 in patients with normal haematopoiesis and in patients with bone marrow failure. *Blood* 1990; 76: 666–76.

17 Asano S, Okano A, Ozawa K, Nakahata T, Ishibashi T, Koike K, Kimura H *et al. In vivo* effects of recombinant human interleukin-6 in primates: stimulated production of platelets. *Blood* 1990; 75: 1602–5.

18 Gershon SL. Clozapine – deciphering the risks. *N Engl J Med* 1993; 329: 204–5.

19 Berg RA, Tarantino MD. Envenomation by scorpion *Centruroides exilicauda* (*C. sculpturatus*): severe and unusual manifestations. *Pediatrics* 1991; 87: 930–3.

20 Franca FOS, Benvenuti LA, Fan HW, Dos Santos DR, Hain SH, Picchi-Martins FR, Cardoso JLC, Kamiguti AS *et al.* Severe and fatal mass attack by 'killer' bees (Africanized honey bee – *Apis mellifera scutellata*) in Brazil: clinicopathological studies with measurement of serum venom concentrations. *Q J Med* 1994; 87: 269–82.

21 Cooper PH, Innes DJ, Greer KE. Acute febrile neutrophilic dermatosis (Sweet's syndrome) and myeloproliferative disorders. *Cancer* 1983; 51: 1518–26.

22 Rosenberg MR, Green M. Neuroleptic malignant syndrome: review of response to therapy. *Arch Intern Med* 1989; 149: 1927–31.

23 Prociv P, Croese J. Epidemic eosinophilic enteritis in north Queensland caused by common dog hookworm, *Ancylostoma caninum. Aust NZ J Med* 1990; 20: 439.

24 Burton K, Yogev R, London N, Boyer K, Shulman ST. Pulmonary paragonimiasis in Laotian refugee children. *Pediatrics* 1982; 70: 246–8.

25 Sheehan DJ, Raucher BG, McKitrick JC. Association of *Blastocystis hominis* with signs and symptoms of human disease. *J Clin Microbiol* 1986; 24: 548–50.

26 Weller PF, Bubley GJ. The idiopathic hypereosinophilic syndrome. *Blood* 1994; 83: 2759–79.

27 Darmstadt GL, Tunnessen WW, Sweren RJ. Eosinophilic pustular folliculitis. *Pediatrics* 1992; 89: 1095–8.

28 Lowe D, Jorizzo J, Hutt MSR. Tumour-associated eosinophilia: a review. *J Clin Pathol* 1981; 34: 1343–8.

29 Case records of the Massachusetts General Hos-

pital. Case 18–1992. *N Engl J Med* 1992; 326: 1204–12.

30 Wells GC, Smith NP. Eosinophilic cellulitis. *Br J Dermatol* 1979; 100: 101–9.

31 Don IJ, Khettry U, Canoso JJ. Progressive systemic sclerosis with eosinophilia and a fulminant course. *Am J Med* 1978; 65: 346–8.

32 Panush RS, Wilkinson LS, Fagin RR. Chronic active hepatitis associated with Coombs-positive hemolytic anemia. *Gastroenterology* 1973; 64; 1015–19.

33 Neeman A, Kadish U. Marked eosinophilia in a patient with primary sclerosing cholangitis. *Am J Med* 1987; 83: 378–9.

34 Cullen MH, Stansfield AG, Oliver RTD, Lister TA, Malpas JS. Angio-immunoblastic lymphadenopathy: report of ten cases and review of the literature. *Q J Med* 1979; 48: 151–77.

35 Bullock WE, Artz RP, Bhathena D, Tung KSK. Histoplasmosis: association with circulating immune complexes, eosinophilia, and mesangiocapillary glomerulonephritis. *Arch Intern Med* 1979; 139: 700–2.

36 Mayron LW, Alling S, Kaplan E. Eosinophilia and drug abuse. *Ann Allergy* 1972; 30: 632–7.

37 Rubin RB, Neugarten J. Cocaine-associated asthma. *Am J Med* 1990; 88: 438–9.

38 Gabriel LC, Escribano LM, Villa E, Leiva C, Valdes MD. Ultrastructural studies of blood cells in toxic oil syndrome. *Acta Haematol* 1968; 75: 165 70.

39 Kilbourne EM, Swygert LA, Philen RM, Sun RK, Auerbach SB, Miller L, Nelson DE *et al.* Interim guidance on the eosinophilia–myalgia syndrome. *Ann Intern Med* 1990; 112: 85–7.

40 Carvajal JA, Anderson R, Weiss L, Grismer J, Berman R. Atheroembolism. An etiologic factor in renal insufficiency, gastrointestinal haemorrhages, and peripheral vascular diseases. *Arch Intern Med* 1967; 119: 593–9.

41 Omenn GS. Familial reticuloendotheliosis with eosinophilia. *N Engl J Med* 1965; 273: 427–32.

42 van der Graaf W, Borleffs JCC. Eosinophilia in patients with HIV infection. *Eur J Haematol* 1994; 52: 246–7.

43 Crofton JW, Livingstone JL, Oswald NC, Roberts ATM. Pulmonary eosinophilia. *Thorax* 1952; 7: 1–35.

44 Donhuijsen K, Haedicke C, Hattenberger C, Freund M. Granulocyte-macrophage colony-stimulating factor-related eosinophilia and Loeffler's endocarditis. *Blood* 1992; 79: 2798.

45 Schatz M, Wasserman S, Patterson R. The eosinophil and the lung. *Arch Intern Med* 1982; 142: 1515–19.

46 Fauci AS, Harley JB, Roberts WC, Ferrans VJ, Gralnick HR, Bjornson BH. NIH Conference. The idiopathic hypereosinophilic syndrome. *Ann Intern Med* 1982; 97: 78–92.

47 Dines DE. Chronic eosinophilic pneumonia. *Mayo Clin Proc* 1978; 53: 129–30.

48 Olson LC, Miller G, Hanshaw JB. Acute infectious lymphocytosis presenting as a pertussis-like illness: its association with adenovirus type 12. *Lancet* 1964; i: 200–1.

49 Anonymous. Lymphocytopoietic viruses. *N Engl J Med* 1968; 279: 432–3.

50 Mandal BK, Stokes KJ. Acute infectious lymphocytosis and enteroviruses. *Lancet* 1973; ii: 1392–3.

51 Nkrumah FK, Addy PAK. Acute infectious lymphocytosis. *Lancet* 1973; i: 1257–8.

52 Horwitz CA, Henle W, Henle G, Polesky H, Balfour HH, Siem RA, Borken S, Ward PCJ. Heterophil-negative infectious mononucleosis and mononucleosis-like illnesses. *Am J Med* 1977; 63: 947–57.

53 Rosenblatt JD, Plaeger-Marshall S, Giorgi JV, Swanson P, Chen ISY, Chin E, Wang HJ, Canavaggio M *et al.* A clinical, hematologic, and immunologic analysis of 21 HTLV-I infected intravenous drug users. *Blood* 1990; 76: 409–17.

54 Rogers L. The blood changes in plague. *J Pathol* 1905; 10: 291–5.

55 McDonald JC, MacLean JD, McDade JE. Imported rickettsial disease: clinical and epidemiologic features. *Am J Med* 1988; 85; 799–805.

56 Wilson ME, Brush AD, Meany MC. Murine typhus acquired during short-term urban travel. *Am J Med* 1989; 57: 233–4.

57 Bates I, Bedu-Addo G, Bevan DH, Rutherford TR. Use of immunoglobulin gene rearrangements to show clonal lymphoproliferation in hyper-reactive malarial splenomegaly. *Lancet* 1991; 337: 505–7.

58 Groom DA, Kunkel LA, Brynes RK, Parker JW, Johnson CS, Endres D. Transient stress lymphocytosis during crisis of sickle cell anaemia and emergency trauma and medical conditions. *Arch Pathol Lab Med* 1990; 114: 570–6.

59 Wentworth P, Salonen V, Pomeroy J. Transient stress lymphocytosis during crisis of sickle cell anaemia. *Arch Pathol Lab Med* 1991; 115: 211.

60 Chow K-C, Nacilla JQ, Witzig TE, Li C-Y. Is persistent polyclonal B lymphocytosis caused by Epstein–Barr virus? A study with polymerase chain reaction and *in situ* hybridization. *Am J Hematol* 1992; 41: 270–5.

61 Kerrigan DP, Castillo A, Foucar K, Townsend K, Neidhart J. Peripheral blood morphologic changes after high-dose antineoplastic chemotherapy and recombinant human granulocyte colony-stimulating factor administration. *Am J Clin Pathol* 1989; 92: 280–5.

62 Lascari AD. *Hematologic Manifestations of Childhood Diseases.* New York: Theme-Stratton, 1984.

63 Kapadia A, de Sousa M, Markenson AL, Miller DR,

Good RA, Gupta S. Lymphoid cell sets and serum immunoglobulins in patients with thalassaemia intermedia: relationship to serum iron and splenectomy. *Br J Haematol* 1980; 45, 405–16.

64 Marti GE, Ryan ET, Papadopoulos NM, Filling-Katz M, Barton N, Fleischer TA, Rick M, Gralnick HR. Polyclonal B-cell lymphocytosis and hypergammaglobulinaemia in patients with Gaucher's disease. *Am J Hematol* 1988; 29: 189–94.

65 Medeiros LJ, Bhagat SK, Naylor P, Fowler D, Jaffe E, Stetler-Stevenson M. Malignant thymoma associated with T-cell lymphocytosis. *Arch Pathol Lab Med* 1993; 117: 279–83.

66 Mariette X, Tsapis A, Oksenhendler E, Daniel M-T, d'Agay M-F, Berger R, Brouet J-C. Nodular lymphocyte predominance Hodgkin's disease featuring blood atypical polyclonal B-cell lymphocytosis. *Br J Haematol* 1993; 85: 813–15.

67 Cook PD, Osborn CD, Helbert BJ, Rappaport ES. Cleaved lymphocytes in pertussis. *Am J Clin Pathol* 1991; 96: 428.

68 Maldonado JE, Hanlon DG. Monocytosis: a current appraisal. *Mayo Clin Proc* 1965; 40: 248–59.

69 Glaser RM, Walker RI, Herion JC. The significance of hematologic abnormalities in patients with tuberculosis. *Arch Intern Med* 1970; 125: 691–5.

70 Dorfman DH, Glader JH. Congenital syphilis presenting in infants after the newborn period. *N Engl J Med* 1990; 323: 1299–302.

71 Barrett O'N. Monocytosis in malignant disease. *Ann Intern Med* 1970; 73: 991–2.

72 Schmitz LL, McClure JS, Letz CE, Dayton V, Weisdorf DJ, Parkin JL, Brunning RD. Morphologic and quantitative changes in blood and marrow cells following growth factor therapy. *Am J Clin Pathol* 1994; 101: 67–75.

73 Raska K, Raskova J, Shea SM, Frankel RM, Wood RH, Lifter J, Ghobrial I, Eisinger RP *et al.* T cell subsets and cellular immunity in end-stage renal disease. *Am J Med* 1983; 75: 734–40.

74 Pisani RJ, Witzig TE, Li CY, Morris MA, Thibodeau SN. Confirmation of lymphomatous pulmonary involvement by immunophenotypic and gene rearrangement analysis of bronchoalveolar lavage fluid. *Mayo Clin Proc* 1990; 65: 651–6.

75 Moake JL, Landry PR, Oren ME, Sayer BL, Heffner LT. Transient peripheral plasmacytosis. *Am J Clin Pathol* 1974; 62: 8–15.

76 Meade RH, Brandt L. Manifestations of Kawasaki disease in New England outbreak of 1980. *J Pediatr* 1982; 100: 558–62.

77 Feigert JM, Sweet DL, Coleman M, Variakojis D, Wisch N, Schulman J, Markowitz MH. Multicentric angiofollicular lymph node hyperplasia with peripheral neuropathy, pseudotumor cerebri, IgA dysproteinaemia, and thrombocytosis in women: a distinct syndrome. *Ann Intern Med* 1990; 113: 362–7.

78 Gherardi RK, Maleport D, Degos J-D. Castleman disease – POEMS syndrome overlap. *Ann Intern Med* 1991; 114: 520–1.

79 Weber J, Yang JC, Topalian SL, Parkinson DR, Schwartzentruber DS, Ettinghausen SE, Gunn H, Mixon A *et al.* Phase I trial of subcutaneous interleukin-6 in patients with advanced malignancies. *J Clin Oncol* 1993; 11: 499–506.

80 Halpérin DS, Wacker P, Lacourt G, Félix M, Babel J-F, Aapro M, Wyss M. Effects of recombinant human erythropoietin in infants with anemia of prematurity: a pilot study. *J Pediatr* 1990; 116: 779.

81 Ritchie JH, Fish MB, McMasters V, Grossman M. Edema and hemolytic anemia in premature infants. A vitamin E deficiency syndrome. *N Engl J Med* 1968; 279: 1185–90.

82 Pickering D, Cuddigan B. Infantile cortical hyperostosis associated with thrombocythaemia. *Lancet* 1969; ii: 464–5.

83 Burnstein Y, Rausen AR, Peterson CM. Duration of thrombocytosis in infants of polydrug (including methadone) users. *J Pediatr* 1982; 100: 506.

84 Schilling RF. Platelet millionaires. *Lancet* 1980; ii: 372–3.

85 Jones MJ, Pierre RV. The causes of extreme thrombocytosis. *Am J Clin Pathol* 1981; 76: 349.

86 Buss DH, Cashell AW, O'Connor ML, Richards F, Case LD. Occurrence, etiology, and clinical significance of extreme thrombocytosis: a study of 280 cases. *Am J Med* 1994; 96: 247–53.

87 Spigel SC, Mooney LR. Extreme thrombocytosis associated with malignancy. *Cancer* 1977; 39: 339–41.

88 Pearson HA, Lobel JS, Kocoshis SA, Naiman JL, Windmiller J, Lammi AT, Hoffman R, Marsh JC. A new syndrome of refractory sideroblastic anemia with vacuolation of marrow precursors and exocrine pancreatic dysfunction. *J Pediatr* 1979; 95: 976–84.

89 Niebrugge DJ, Benjamin DR, Christie D, Scott CR. Hereditary transcobalamin II deficiency presenting as red cell hypoplasia. *J Pediatr* 1982; 101: 732–5.

90 Baker RI, Manoharan A, de Luca E, Begley CG. Pure red cell aplasia of pregnancy: a distinct clinical entity. *Br J Haematol* 1993; 85: 619–22.

91 Volin L, Ruutu T. Pure red-cell aplasia of long duration after major ABO-incompatible bone marrow transplantation. *Acta Haematol* 1990; 84: 195–7.

92 Lau KS, White JC. Myelosclerosis associated with systemic lupus erythematosus in patients in West Malaysia. *J Clin Pathol* 1969; 22: 433–8.

93 Yetgin S, Ozsoylu S. Myeloid metaplasia in vitamin

D deficiency rickets. *Scand J Haematol* 1982; 28: 180–5.

94 Ravindranath Y, Paglia DE, Warrier I, Valentine W, Nakatani M, Brockway RA. Glucose phosphate isomerase deficiency as a cause of hydrops fetalis. *N Engl J Med* 1987; 316: 258–61.

95 Gray ES, Balch NJ, Kohler H, Thompson WD, Simson JG. Congenital leukaemia: an unusual cause of stillbirth. *Arch Dis Child* 1986; 61: 1001–6.

96 Letsky EA, Polycythaemia in the newborn infant. In: Hann IM, Gibson BES, Letsky EA, eds. *Fetal and Neonatal Haematology*. London: Baillière Tindall, 1991.

97 Parmley RT, Crist WM, Ragab AH, Boxer LA, Malluh A, Liu VK, Darby CP. Congenital dysgranulopoietic neutropenia: clinical, serologic, ultrastructural and *in vitro* proliferative characteristics. *Blood* 1980; 56: 465–75.

98 Wetzler M, Talpaz M, Kleinerman ES, King A, Huh YO, Gutterman JU, Kurzrock R. A new familial immunodeficiency disorder characterized by severe neutropenia, a defective marrow release mechanism, and hypogammaglobulinemia. *Am J Med* 1990; 89: 663–72.

99 Casadevall N, Croisille L, Auffray I, Tchernia G, Coulombel L. Age-related alterations in erythroid and granulopoietic progenitors in Diamond–Blackfan anaemia. *Br J Haematol* 1994; 87; 369–75.

100 Roe TF, Coates TD, Thomas DW, Miller JH, Gilsanz V. Treatment of chronic inflammatory bowel disease in glycogen storage disease type Ib with colony-stimulating factors. *N Engl J Med* 1992; 326: 1666–9.

101 Ino T, Sherwood G, Cutz E, Benson LN, Rose IV, Freedman RM. Dilated cardiomyopathy with neutropenia, short stature and abnormal carnitine metabolism. *J Pediatr* 1988; 113: 511–14.

102 Pullen RL, Stuart BM. Tularemia. *JAMA* 1945; 129: 495–500.

103 Sheehy TW, Hazlett D, Turk RE. Scrub typhus: a comparison of chloramphenical and tetracycline in its treatment. *Arch Intern Med* 1973; 132: 77–80.

104 Brettman LR, Lewin S, Holzman RS, Goldman WD, Marr JS, Kechijian P, Schinella R. Rickettsial pox: report of an outbreak and a contemporary review. *Medicine* 1981; 60: 363–72.

105 Goodwin RA, Shapiro JL, Thurman GH, Thurman SS, des Prez RM. Disseminated histoplasmosis: clinical and pathological correlations. *Medicine* 1980; 59: 1–33.

106 Bux J, Mueller-Eckhardt C. Autoimmune neutropenia. *Semin Hematol* 1992; 29: 45–53.

107 McClain K, Estrov Z, Chen H, Mahoney DH. Chronic neutropenia of childhood: frequent association with parvovirus infection and correlations with bone marrow culture studies. *Br J Haematol* 1993; 85: 57–62.

108 Cline MJ, Opelz G, Saxon A, Fahey JL, Golde DW. Autoimmune panleukopenia. *N Engl J Med* 1976; 295: 1489–93.

109 Levitt LJ, Ries CA, Greenberg PL. Pure white cell aplasia: antibody-mediated autoimmune inhibition of granulopoiesis. *N Engl J Med* 1983; 308: 1141–6.

110 Liu YK. Leukopenia in alcoholics. *Am J Med* 1973; 54: 605–10.

111 Cordano A, Placko RP, Graham GG. Hypocupremia and neutropenia in copper deficiency. *Blood* 1966; 28: 280–3.

112 Shoenfeld Y, Shaklai M, Ben-Baruch N, Hirschorn M, Pinkhas J. Neutropenia induced by hypercarotenaemia. *Lancet* 1982; i: 1245.

113 Rogers ZR, Bergstrom SK, Amylon MD, Buchanan GR, Glader BE. Reduced neutrophil counts in children with transient erythroblastopenia of childhood. *J Pediatr* 1989; 115: 746–8.

114 Koenig JM, Christensen RD. Incidence, neutrophil kinetics, and natural history of neonatal neutropenia associated with maternal hypertension. *N Engl J Med* 1989; 321: 557–62.

115 Engle WD, Rosenfeld CR. Neutropenia in high-risk neonates. *J Pediatr* 1984; 105: 982–6.

116 Zach TL, Steinhorn RH, Georgieff MK, Mills MM, Green TP. Leukopenia associated with extracorporeal membrane oxygenation in newborn infants. *J Pediatr* 1990; 116: 440–3.

117 Nakahate T, Spicer SS, Leary AG, Ogawa M, Franklin W, Goetzl EJ. Circulating eosinophil colony-forming cells in pure eosinophil aplasia. *Ann Intern Med* 1984; 101: 321–4.

118 Juhlin LL, Michaelsson G. A new syndrome characterized by absence of eosinophils and basophils. *Lancet* 1977; i: 1233–5.

119 Symmons DPM, Farr M, Salmon M and Bacon PA. Lymphopenia in rheumatoid arthritis. *J Roy Soc Med* 1989; 82: 462–3.

120 Budman DR, Steinberg AD. Hematologic aspects of systemic lupus erythematosus. *Ann Intern Med* 1977; 86: 220–9.

121 Daniele RP, Rowlands DT. Lymphocyte subpopulations in sarcoidosis: correlation with disease activity and duration. *Ann Intern Med* 1976; 85: 593–600.

122 Bynoe AG, Scott CS, Ford P, Roberts BE. Decreased T helper cells in the myelodysplastic syndromes. *Br J Haematol* 1983; 54: 97–102.

123 Bowers TK, Eckert E. Leukopenia in anorexia nervosa: lack of an increased risk of infection. *Arch Intern Med* 1978; 138: 1520–3.

124 Santos PC, Falcao RP. Decreased lymphocyte sub-

sets and K-cell activity in iron deficiency anemia. *Acta Haematol* 1990; 84: 118–21.

125 Robbins G, Brozovic B. Lymphocytopenia in regular platelet apheresis donors. *Br J Haematol* 1985; 61: 558–9.

126 Unkrig CJ, Schroder R, Scharf RE. Lorenzo's oil and thrombocytopenia. *N Engl J Med* 1994; 330: 577.

127 Hoffman R. Acquired pure amegakaryocytic thrombocytopenic purpura. *Semin Hematol* 1991; 28: 303–12.

128 Dickerman JD, Holbrook PR, Zinkham WH. Etiology and therapy of thrombocytopenia associated with sarcoidosis. *J Pediatr* 1972; 81: 758–64.

129 Wright JG. Severe thrombocytopenia secondary to asymptomatic cytomegalovirus infection in an immunocompetent host. *J Clin Pathol* 1992; 45: 1037–8.

130 Beattie RM. Mycoplasma and thrombocytopenia. *Arch Dis Child* 1993; 68: 250.

131 Castagnola E, Dufour C, Timitilli A, Giacchino R. Idiopathic thrombocytopenic purpura associated with scarlet fever. *Arch Dis Child* 1994; 70: 164.

132 Leissinger CA. Severe thrombocytopenia associated with cocaine abuse. *Ann Intern Med* 1990; 112: 708–10.

133 Hesseling PB. Onyalai. *Bailierè's Clin Haematol* 1992; 5: 457–73.

134 Schulman I, Pierce M, Lukens A, Currimbhoy Z. Studies on thrombopoiesis I. A factor in normal human plasma required for platelet production; chronic thrombocytopenia due to its deficiency. *Blood* 1960; 16: 943–57.

135 Upshaw JD. Congenital deficiency of a factor in normal plasma that reverses microangiopathic hemolysis and thrombocytopenia. *N Engl J Med* 1978; 298: 1350–2.

136 Turnbull A, Almeyda J. Idiopathic thrombocytopenic purpura and Kaposi's sarcoma. *Proc Roy Soc Med* 1970; 63: 603–5.

137 Auborg P. Lorenzo's oil and thrombocytopenia. *N Engl J Med* 1994; 330: 577.

138 O'Brien H, Amess JAL, Mollin JD. Recurrent thrombocytopenia, erythroid hypoplasia and sideroblastic anaemia associated with hypothermia. *Br J Haematol* 1982; 51: 451–6.

139 Willoughby MLN. *Paediatric Haematology*. Edinburgh: Churchill Livingstone, 1977.

140 Maurer HM, Fratkin M, McWilliams NB, Kirkpatrick D, Draper DW, Haggins JC, Hunter CR. Effects of phototherapy on platelet counts in low-birthweight infants and on platelet production and life span in rabbits. *Pediatrics* 1976; 57: 506–12.

141 Ballin A, Koren G, Kohelet D, Burger R, Greenwald M, Bryan AC, Zipursky A. Reduction in platelet counts induced by mechanical ventilation in the newborn infants. *J Pediatr* 1987; 111: 445–9.

142 Kurata Y, Nishioeda Y, Tsubakio T, Kitani T. Thrombocytopenia in Graves' disease: effect of T_3 on platelet kinetics. *Acta Haematol* 1980; 63: 185–90.

143 Paciucci PA, Mandeli J, Oleksowicz L, Ameglio F, Holland JF. Thrombocytopenia during immunotherapy with interleukin-2 by constant infusion. *Am J Med* 1990; 89: 308–12.

144 Pei SX, Chen XJ, Si Ren BZ, Liu YH, Cheng XS, Harris EM, Anand IS, Harris PC. Chronic mountain sickness in Tibet. *Q J Med* 1989; 71: 555–74.

145 Fischereder M, Jaffe JP. Thrombocytopenia following acute acetaminophen overdose. *Am J Hematol* 1994; 45: 258–9.

146 Press OW, Fingert H, Lott IT, Dickersin R. Pancytopenia in mannosidosis. *Arch Intern Med* 1983; 143: 1266–8.

147 Hricik DE, Hussain R. Pancytopenia and hepatosplenomegaly in oxalosis. *Arch Intern Med* 1984; 144: 167–8.

148 Kelleher JF, Yudkoff M, Hutchinson R, August CS, Cohn RM. The pancytopenia of isovaleric acidemia. *Pediatrics* 1980; 65: 1023–7.

149 Blatt J, Katerji A, Barmada M, Wenger SL, Penchansky L. Pancytopenia and vacuolation of marrow precursors associated with necrotizing encephalopathy. *Br J Haematol* 1994; 86: 207–9.

150 Resuke WH, Anderson C, Pastuszak WT, Conway SR, Firshein SI. Arsenic intoxication presenting as a myelodysplastic syndrome: a case report. *Am J Hematol* 1991; 36: 291–3.

151 Wiesneth M, Pflieger H, Frickhofen N, Heimpel H. Idiopathic combined immunocytopenia. *Br J Haematol* 1985; 61: 339–48.

152 Barrett AJ. Graft-versus-host disease: a review. *J Roy Soc Med* 1987; 80: 368–73.

153 Case records of the Massachusetts General Hospital. Case 33–1989. *N Engl J Med* 1989; 321: 454–63.

154 Millá F, Feliu E, Ribera JM, Juncà J, Flores A, Vidal J, Zarco MA, Masat T. Electron microscopic identification of parvovirus virions in erythroid and granulocytic-line cells in a patient with human parvovirus B19 induced pancytopenia. *Leuk Lymphoma* 1993; 10: 483–7.

155 Harkess JR. Ehrlichiosis: a causes of bone marrow hypoplasia in humans. *Am J Hematol* 1989; 30: 265–6.

156 Al-Eissa YA, Assuhaimi SA, Al-Fawaz IM, Higgy KF, Al-Nasser MN, Al-Mobaireek KF. Pancytopenia in children with brucellosis: clinical manifestations and bone marrow findings. *Acta Haematol* 1993; 89: 132–6.

157 Bilgrami S, Almeida GD, Quinn JJ, Tuck D, Bergstrom S, Dainiak N, Poliquin C, Ascensao JL.

Pancytopenia in allogeneic marrow transplant recipients: role of cytomegalovirus. *Br J Haematol* 1994; 887: 357–62.

158 Hoagland HC, Goldstein NP. Hematologic (cytopenic) manifestations of Wilson's disease (hepatolenticular degeneration). *Mayo Clin Proc* 1978; 53: 498–500.

159 Talansky AL, Schulman P, Vinciguerra VP, Margouleff D, Budman DR, Degman TJ. Pancytopenia complicating Graves' disease and drug-induced hypothyroidism (*sic*). *Arch Intern Med* 1981; 141: 544–5.

160 Ruocco L, Baldi N, Ceccone A, Marini A, Azzarà A, Ambrogi F, Grassi B. Severe pancytopenia due to copper deficiency. *Acta Haematol* 1986; 76: 224–6.

CHAPTER 7

Important Supplementary Tests

Peripheral blood cells can be used for many other tests which supplement the FBC and MGG-stained blood film. These include cytochemical tests, immunophenotyping, cytogenetic analysis, DNA analysis and ultrastructural examination. Only those which involve an element of interpreting or counting cells in a stained film are dealt with here, i.e., cytochemical techniques and some immunophenotyping techniques.

Cytochemical techniques

Some recommended techniques for cytochemical stains are given in Table 7.1. Reticulocyte counting and staining is dealt with in Chapter 2. The application of other cytochemical stains will be discussed in this chapter.

Heinz bodies

Heinz bodies are red cell inclusions composed of denatured haemoglobin. They can be seen as refractile bodies in dry unstained films viewed with the condenser lowered. They can be stained by a number of vital dyes including methyl violet, cresyl violet, new methylene blue, brilliant cresyl blue, brilliant green and rhodanile blue. Their characteristic shape and size (Fig. 7.1; see also Table 2.4) aid in their identification. Heinz bodies are not seen in normal subjects since they are removed by the spleen in a process known as 'pitting'. Small numbers are seen in the blood of splenectomized subjects. Larger numbers are found following exposure to oxidant drugs, particularly in subjects who are glucose-6-phosphate dehydrogenase deficient or who have been splenectomized, and in patients with an unstable haemoglobin who have been splenectomized. Patients with an unstable haemoglobin who have not been splenectomized may not show Heinz bodies but in some patients they form on prolonged *in vitro* incubation.

A stain for Heinz bodies is indicated when Heinz body-haemolytic anaemia is suspected. However, sometimes this diagnosis is readily evident from the clinical history and the MGG-stained film and the test is then redundant.

Haemoglobin H inclusions

Haemoglobin H (an abnormal haemoglobin with no α-chains but with a β-chain tetramer) is denatured and stained by the same vital dyes which stain reticulocytes. The characteristic regular 'golf ball' inclusions (Fig. 7.2a) take longer to appear than the reticulum of a reticulocyte. An incubation period of 2 hours is recommended. It is important that either new methylene blue or brilliant cresyl blue is used to demonstrate the characteristic inclusions. Methylene blue (which has been sold by manufacturers wrongly identified as new methylene blue) does not give the typical

Table 7.1 Some recommended methods for cytochemical stains

Procedure	Recommended method
Heinz body preparation	Rhodanile blue with 2 minutes incubation [1] or methyl violet
Haemoglobin H preparation	Brilliant cresyl blue with 2 hours incubation [1]
Haemoglobin F-containing cells	Acid elution [1]
Perls' reaction for iron	Potassium ferrocyanide [1]
Myeloperoxidase	*p*-phenylenediamine + catechol + H_2O_2 [2]*
Sudan black B (SBB)	SBB [1]*
Naphthol AS-D chloroacetate esterase (CAE)	Naphthol AS-D chloroacetate + hexazotized fuchsin [3] or fast blue BB [4] or corinth V*
α naphthyl acetate esterase	Naphthyl acetate + hexazotized pararosaniline [3] or fast blue RR*
Neutrophil alkaline phosphatase (NAP)	Naphthol AS-MX phosphate + fast blue RR*
Periodic acid–Schiff (PAS)	Periodic acid + Schiff's reagent [1]
Acid phosphatase and Tartrate-resistant acid phosphatase (TRAP)	Naphthol AS-BI phosphate + fast garnet GBC, with and without tartaric acid [5]

* Reagents suitable for these methods can be purchased from Sigma Diagnostics.

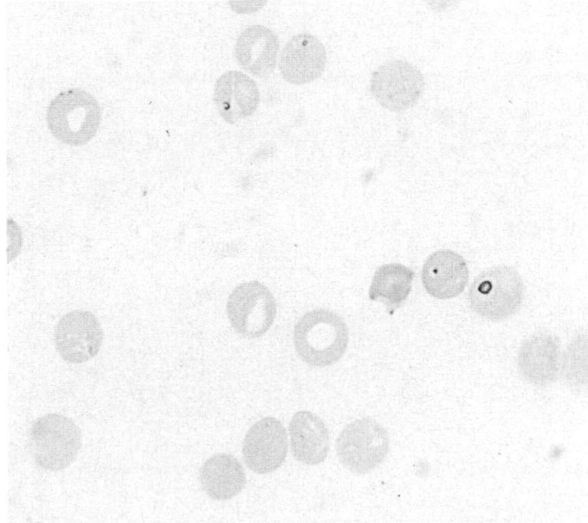

Fig. 7.1 A methyl violet preparation showing five Heinz bodies. The blood sample was from a patient who had been exposed to dapsone, an oxidant drug.

appearance [6]. Patients with haemoglobin H disease who have not been splenectomized show the characteristic golf-ball appearance whereas post-splenectomy patients have, in addition, preformed inclusions of haemoglobin H which are similar to Heinz bodies (Fig. 7.2b). Cells containing haemoglobin H are readily detected in patients with haemoglobin H disease in whom they may form the majority of cells. In patients with α-thalassaemia trait their frequency is of the order of one in 1000 cells (when two of the four α-genes are missing) or less (when one of the four α-genes is missing); even when a prolonged search is made they are not always detectable. Haemoglobin H inclusions are not found in the red cells of haematologically normal subjects; apparently similar cells may be seen, however, in very occasional cells in normal subjects so that a control normal sample should be incubated in parallel with the patient's sample.

The identification of haemoglobin H-containing cells is useful in the diagnosis of haemoglobin H disease. It is much less useful in the diagnosis of α-thalassaemia trait since the search is very time-consuming and false-negative results occur. When the diagnosis is important DNA analysis is to be preferred.

Haemoglobin F-containing cells

Haemoglobin F-containing cells are identified cytochemically by their resistance to haemoglobin elution in acid conditions (Fig. 7.3); the procedure is commonly referred to as a Kleihauer test from its originator, although Kleihauer's method is often modified. The test is useful for detecting fetal cells in the maternal circulation and thus for detecting and quantitating fetomaternal haemorrhage. It will also detect autologous cells containing appreciable quantities of haemoglobin F

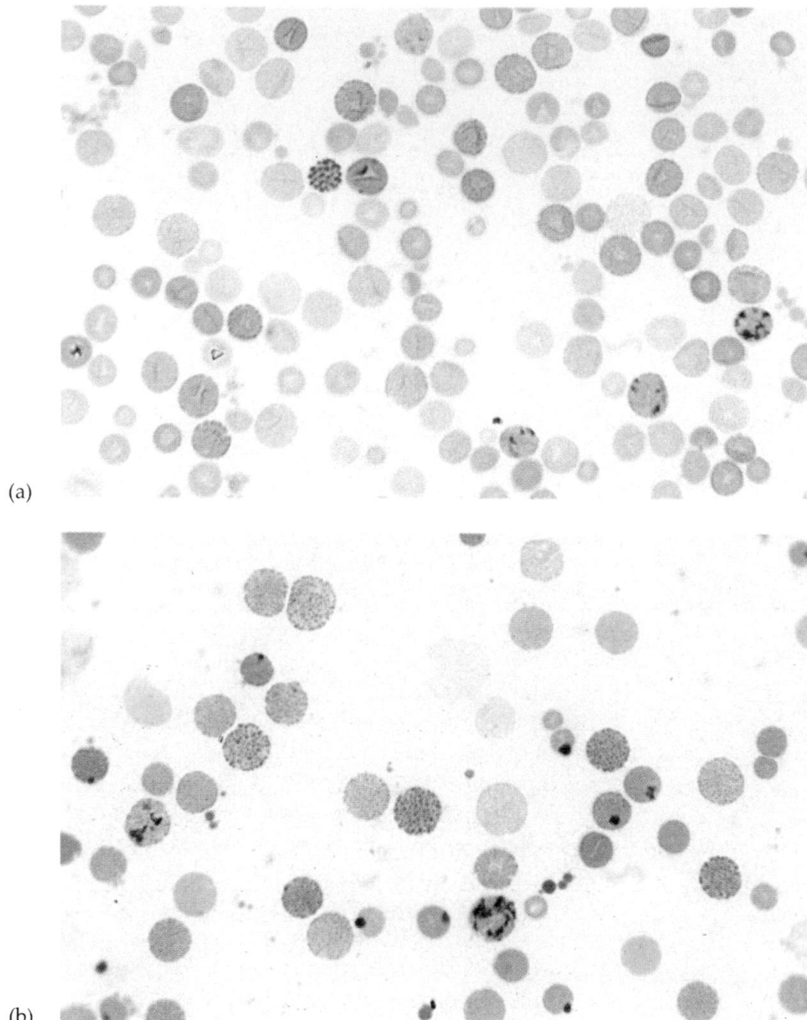

Fig. 7.2 Haemoglobin H preparations showing: (a) haemoglobin H-containing cells (containing multiple small pale blue inclusions) and reticulocytes (with a purple reticular network) in a patient with haemoglobin H disease); and (b) haemoglobin H-containing cells, a reticulocyte and Heinz bodies (large peripherally placed blue inclusions) in the blood of a patient with haemoglobin H disease who had been splenectomized.

such as may be seen in hereditary persistence of fetal haemoglobin and β-thalassaemia, and in some patients with thalassaemia major, β-thalassaemia trait, sickle cell disease, dyshaemopoietic states and various other conditions. The distribution of haemoglobin F in adult cells may be homogeneous (in some types of hereditary persistence of fetal haemoglobin) or heterogeneous (in other types of hereditary persistence of fetal haemoglobin and in other conditions). Both a positive and a negative control should be tested in parallel with the sample under investigation. A positive control can be prepared by mixing together adult and fetal cells.

Perls' reaction for iron

Perls' stain is based on a reaction between acid ferrocyanide and the ferric ion (Fe^{3+}) of haemosiderin to form ferric ferrocyanide which has an intense blue colour (Prussian blue). Ferritin, which is soluble, does not give a positive reaction. Perls' stain is most often performed on the bone marrow but it can be used to stain peripheral blood cells in order to detect sideroblasts and siderocytes.

On a Romanowsky-stained blood film, haemosiderin appears as small blue granules which are designated Pappenheimer bodies (see p. 65). On

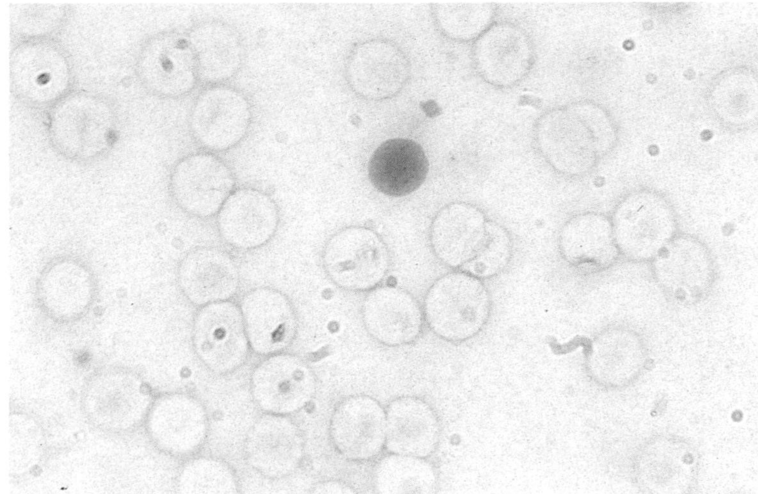

Fig. 7.3 Acid elution technique (Kleihauer test) for haemoglobin F-containing cells; the blood specimen was taken from a post-partum woman and shows that a fetomaternal haemorrhage had occurred. A single stained fetal cell is seen against a background of ghosts of maternal cells.

a Perls' stain they are referred to as siderotic granules and the cells containing them are designated siderocytes (Fig. 7.4a). Siderocytes are rarely detected in the blood of normal subjects; siderotic granules are present in reticulocytes newly released from the bone marrow, but disappear during maturation of the reticulocyte in the spleen, probably because the haemosiderin is utilized for further haemoglobin synthesis. When haematologically normal subjects are splenectomized, small numbers of siderocytes are seen in the blood. When red cells containing abnormally large or numerous siderotic granules are released from the bone marrow, as in sideroblastic anaemia or in thalassaemia major, many of the abnormal inclusions are 'pitted' by the spleen. Some remain detectable in the peripheral blood, both in reticulocytes and in mature red cells. If a patient with a defect of iron incorporation has been splenectomized or is hyposplenic for any reason, very numerous siderocytes are seen.

A sideroblast is a nucleated red blood cell which contains siderotic granules. Sideroblasts are normally present in the bone marrow, but since NRBC do not normally circulate, it is unusual to see them in the peripheral blood. When they do appear they may be morphologically normal, containing only one or a few fine granules, or abnormal with the granules being increased in number, size or both. Abnormal sideroblasts include ring sideroblasts in which a ring of siderotic granules is present adjacent to the nuclear membrane (Fig. 7.4b). When NRBC are present in the peripheral blood they can be stained with a Perls' stain to allow any siderotic granules present to be studied. Abnormal sideroblasts may be detected in the peripheral blood in sideroblastic anaemia, megaloblastic anaemia and thalassaemia major. They are seen in larger numbers when the spleen is absent or hypofunctional. Sideroblastic anaemia is usually diagnosed by bone marrow aspiration but strong support for the diagnosis is obtained if ring sideroblasts are detected in the peripheral blood, if necessary in a buffy coat preparation in which any NRBC are concentrated.

Cytochemical stains used in the diagnosis and classification of leukaemias

Cytochemical stains used in the diagnosis and classification of leukaemias can be applied to both the bone marrow and peripheral blood. Studies of peripheral blood cells are needed when bone marrow aspiration is difficult or impossible. In other circumstances, studies of peripheral blood and bone marrow are complementary. Cytochemical stains for neutrophil alkaline phosphatase are performed on the peripheral blood.

(a) 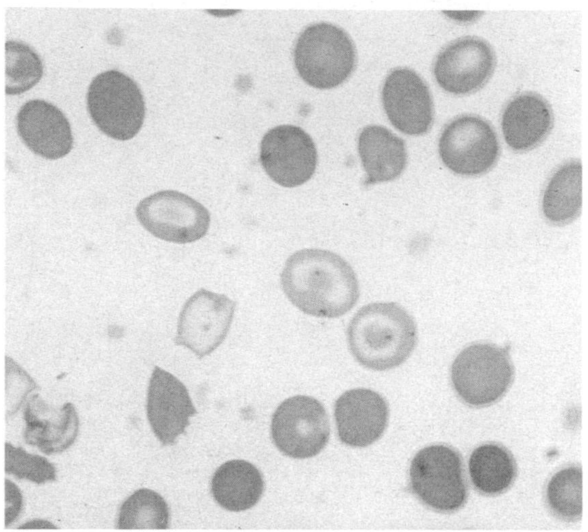 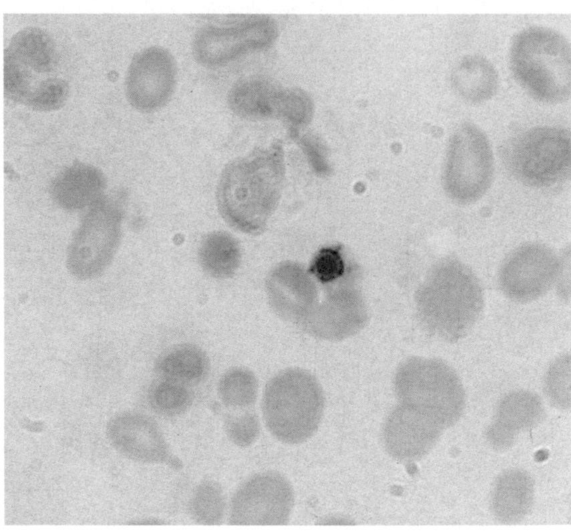 (b)

Fig. 7.4 Perls' stain showing: (a) siderocytes (cells containing fine blue dots) in the blood of a patient with thalassaemia major; and (b) a ring sideroblast in the blood of a patient with sideroblastic anaemia.

Table 7.2 Scoring NAP activity (after Kaplow [9]) 100 neutrophils are scored as shown

Score of cell	Percentage of cytoplasm occupied by precipitated dye	Size of granules	Intensity of staining	Cytoplasmic background
0	None	—	None	Colourless
1	<50	Small	Faint to moderate	Colourless to very pale blue
2	50–80	Small	Moderate to strong	Colourless to pale blue
3	80–100	Medium to large	Strong	Colourless to blue
4	100	Medium and large	Very strong	Not visible

Following the scoring of individual neutrophils the scores are summed to produce the final NAP score. This is most easily done by multiplying each score by the number of cells having that score and adding the results together.

Neutrophil alkaline phosphatase (NAP)

Mature neutrophils, but not eosinophils, have alkaline phosphatase in specific cytoplasmic organelles [7] which have been called phosphosomes. NAP has sometimes been referred to as leucocyte alkaline phosphatase (LAP) but the former designation is more accurate since it is the neutrophils which are assessed. A number of cytochemical stains can be used for demonstrating NAP activity. One suitable stain is that recommended by Ackerman [8] which permits grading of alkaline phosphatase activity as shown in Table 7.2 and Fig. 7.5 to give a NAP score which falls between 0 and 400. The normal range is dependent on the substrate used. With the above method it is of the order of 30–180. It is preferable for NAP scores to be determined on

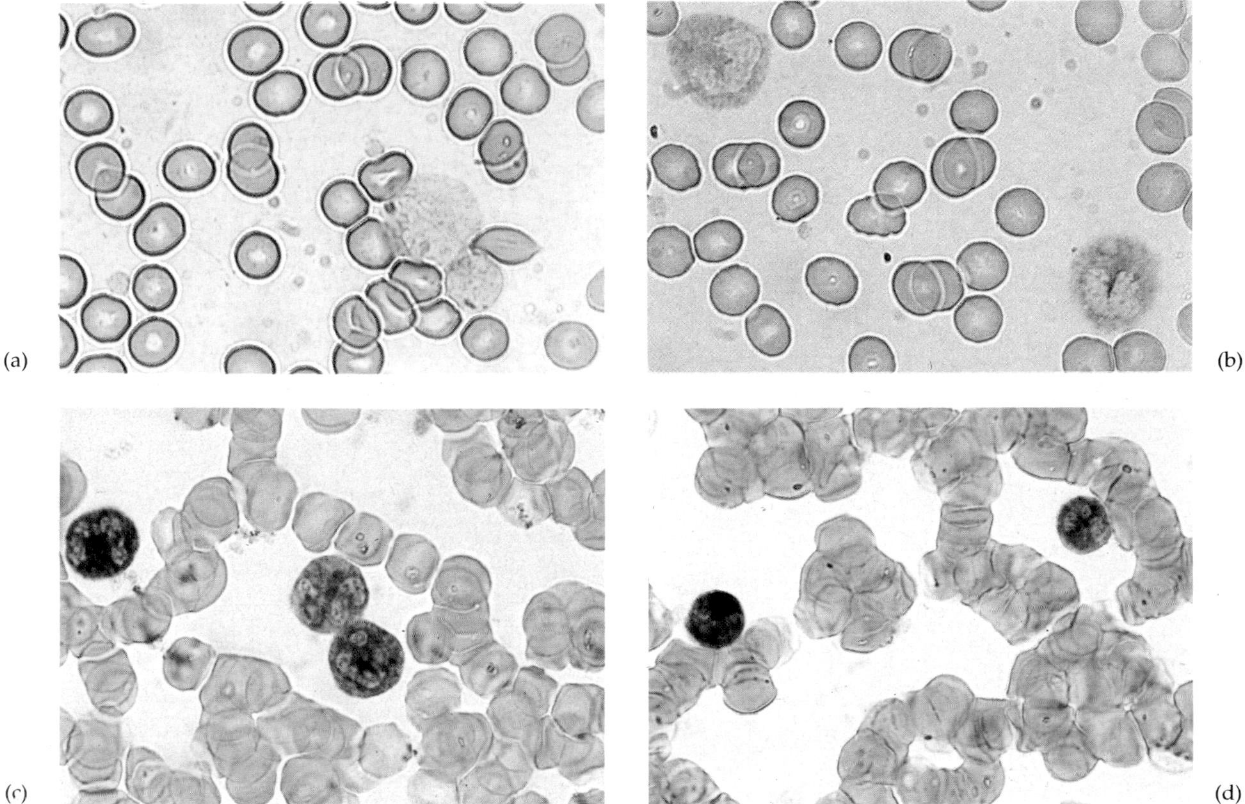

Fig. 7.5 NAP reaction (method of Ackerman [8]) showing cells with reactions graded 0 to 4: (a) neutrophil with a score of 0 plus a lymphocyte which is also negative; (b) two band cells with a score of 1; (c) two neutrophils with a score of 2 and one with a score of 3; and (d) one neutrophil with a score of 4 and one with a score of 2.

native or heparinized blood. The cytochemical reaction should be carried out within 8 hours of obtaining the blood specimen but, if this is not possible, the films can be fixed and stored, in the dark, at room temperature. EDTA-anticoagulated blood is not ideal as enzyme activity is inhibited; if it is used, the films should be made within 10–20 minutes of obtaining the blood, but even then there is some loss of activity. Low, normal and high controls should be stained with the patient's sample. A low control can be obtained from a patient with CGL, or prepared by immersing an appropriately fixed film of normal blood in boiling water for 1 minute. A high control can be obtained from a patient with infection or from a pregnant or post-partum woman or from a woman taking oral contraceptives. Positive and negative control films which have been appropriately fixed and wrapped in parafilm can be stored at −70°C for at least 1 year.

Some of the causes of high and low NAP scores are shown in Table 7.3. Neonates have very high NAP scores, usually exceeding 200. A fall to levels more typical of childhood occurs between 5 and 10 months of age [11]. Premature and low birthweight babies have lower scores than full-term babies. Children have higher NAP scores than adults with a gradual fall to adult levels occurring before puberty [12]. Women in the reproductive age range have higher NAP scores than men with the score varying with the menstrual cycle (Fig. 7.6). After the menopause, NAP scores of women approach those of men (Fig. 7.7) [12,13].

Table 7.3 Some causes of high and low NAP scores

High NAP	Low NAP
Cord blood and neonate	CGL
Mid-cycle in menstruating females	Paroxysmal nocturnal haemoglobinuria
Oral contraceptive intake	Some cases of infectious mononucleosis and other viral infections
Pregnancy and the post-partum period	Inherited hypophosphatasia (NAP absent)
Bacterial infection	
Inflammation	
Surgery and trauma	Lactoferrin deficiency [10]
Infarction	
Leukaemoid reactions	
Corticosteroids and ACTH administration	
Acute stress	
Some cases of AML, particularly acute monoblastic leukaemia	Some cases of AML, particularly when there is differentiation
Most cases of idiopathic myelofibrosis	Some cases of idiopathic myelofibrosis
Most cases of aplastic anaemia	Some cases of aplastic anaemia
Some cases of MDS	Some cases of MDS
Most cases of PRV	Juvenile CML
Carcinomatosis	
G-CSF and GM-CSF therapy	
ALL	
Hairy cell leukaemia	
Some cases of CLL	
Multiple myeloma	
Hodgkin's disease	
Down's syndrome	
Hepatic cirrhosis (particularly when decompensated)	

The NAP score is low in 95% of patients with CGL. The test is useful in distinguishing between CGL and other chronic myeloproliferative disorders which usually have a normal or elevated NAP score, and between CGL and reactive neutrophilia since the latter almost invariably has a high score. Patients with CGL may have a normal or elevated NAP during pregnancy, postoperatively (particularly following splenectomy), during bacterial infection, when the bone marrow is rendered hypoplastic by chemotherapy, and following the onset of transformation.

The NAP score may be of use in distinguishing between PRV, which usually has an elevated score, and secondary polycythaemia, in which the score is more likely to be normal.

Myeloperoxidase (MPO)

Peroxidases are enzymes which catalyse the oxidation of substrates by hydrogen peroxide. The granules of neutrophils and eosinophils contain peroxidases which are designated leucocyte peroxidase or myeloperoxidase. The demonstration of myeloperoxidase activity is useful in establishing and confirming the diagnosis of AML, since lymphoblasts are uniformly negative. Myeloperoxidase was initially demonstrated with benzidine or one of its derivatives as a substrate. A suitable non-carcinogenic substrate used in the method of Hanker [2] is *p*-phenylene diamine which produces a brownish-black reaction product. Myeloperoxidase is demonstrated in neutrophils and their precursors (Fig. 7.8), eosinophils and their precursors and the precursors of basophils. In neutrophils and eosinophils the primary granules have peroxidase activity and in eosinophils this is also true of secondary granules. Neutrophil and eosinophil peroxidases differ from each other, e.g., in their pH optima and in their sensitivity to inhibition by cyanide. Auer rods are peroxidase-positive. In the monocyte lineage, peroxidase activity is detectable at the promonocyte stage. Monocytes and promonocytes have fewer peroxidase-positive granules than neutrophils and their precursors. Inherited deficiency of neutrophil peroxidase is quite common. Deficiencies of eosinophil peroxidase and monocyte peroxidase also occur.

Sudan black B (SBB)

SBB (Fig. 7.9) has an affinity for polymorphonuclear and monocyte granules. In general, the intensity of a positive staining reaction parallels myeloperoxidase activity. SBB staining is slightly more sensitive than myeloperoxidase activity in the detection of myeloblasts. SBB stains the

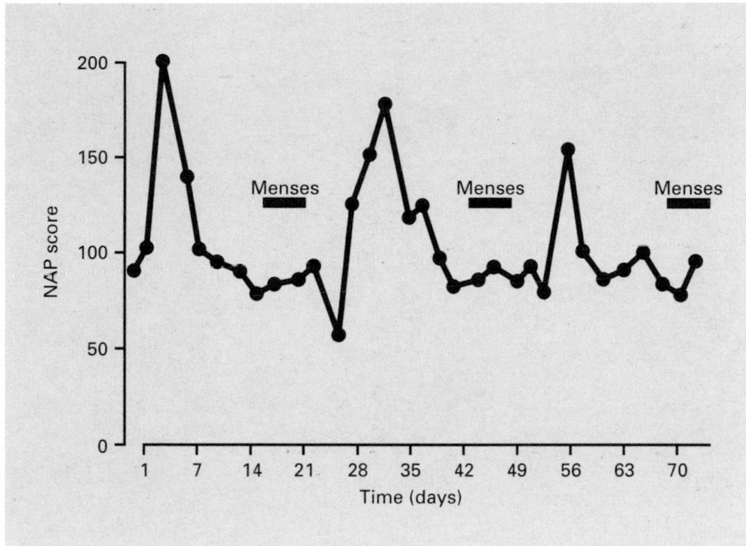

Fig. 7.6 Changes in NAP score during the menstrual cycle.

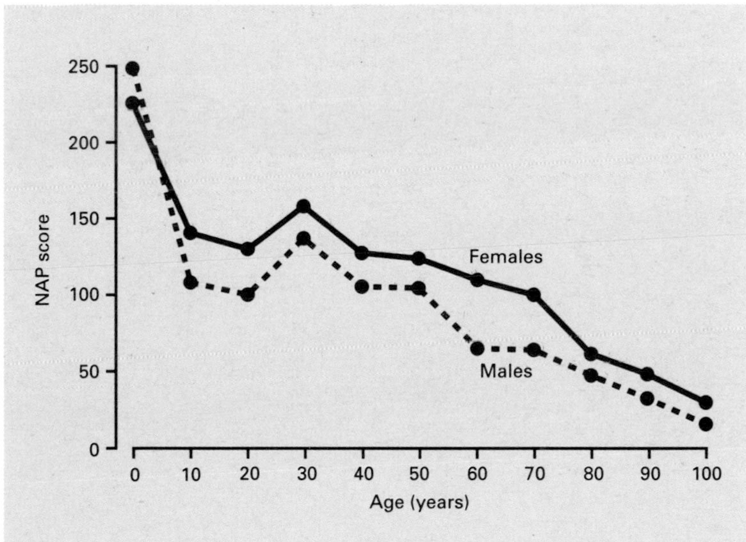

Fig. 7.7 Changes in NAP score with age in men and women. Data from Stavridis *et al.* [13].

granules of neutrophils (both the primary and the specific granules) and the specific granules of eosinophils and, to a variable extent, the specific granules of basophils. The staining of eosinophil granules may be peripheral with the central core remaining unstained. Auer rods are stained. Monoblasts are either negative or show a few small SBB-positive granules. Promonocytes and monocytes have a variable number of fine positively staining granules. In hereditary neutrophil, eosinophil and monocyte peroxidase deficiencies, the granules of cells of the deficient lineages are SBB-negative. Lymphoblasts can have occasional fine positive dots which may represent mitochondria [4]. Very rarely a stronger reaction is seen in the lymphoblasts of ALL [14] or in lymphoma cells of T or B lineage [15].

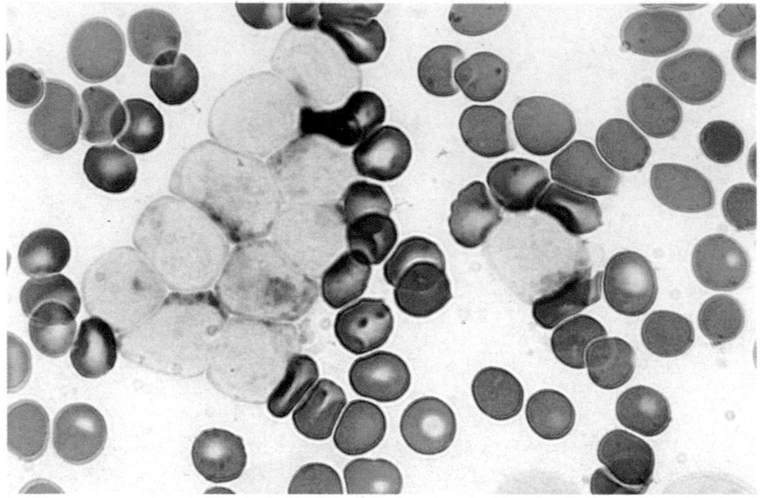

Fig. 7.8 Leukaemic blast cells stained by the Hanker technique [2] for myeloperoxidase showing a brownish-black deposit in the cytoplasm. This was a case of AML of FAB M2 category.

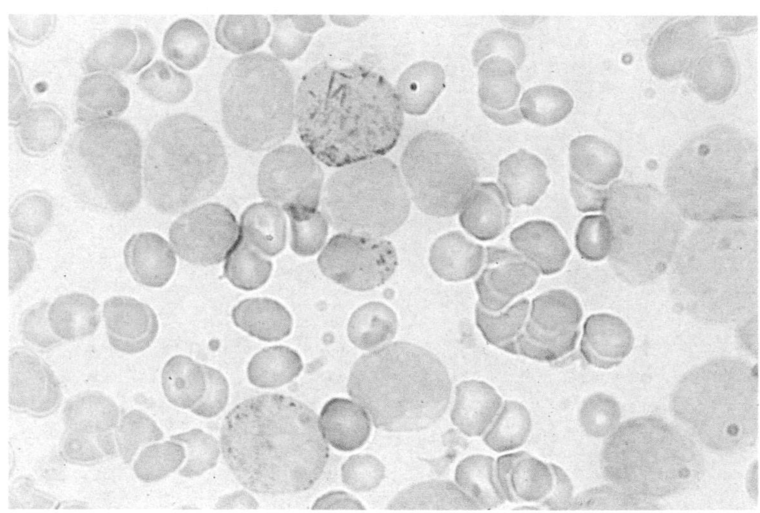

Fig. 7.9 Leukaemic blasts cells stained with SBB. One large blast cell contains both granules and Auer rods. Several other blasts contain granules. The cells of this case, which was AML of FAB M1, category had very few granules and only rare Auer rods visible on an MGG-stained film.

Naphthol AS-D chloroacetate esterase

Naphthol AS-D chloroacetate esterase ('chloroacetate esterase', CAE) activity is found in neutrophils and their precursors (Fig. 7.10) and in mast cells. Auer rods are positive. Normal eosinophils and basophils are negative but the eosinophils of certain types of eosinophil leukaemia may be positive. Monocytes are usually negative, but may show a weak reactivity. CAE is generally less sensitive than either MPO or SBB in the detection of myeloblasts, although occasional cases have been noted to be positive for CAE despite being MPO-negative [3,4].

'Non-specific' esterases

Esterase activity is common in haemopoietic cells. Nine isoenzymes have been demonstrated of which four are found in neutrophils and are responsible for their CAE activity. Five are found in monocytes and a variety of other cells and the

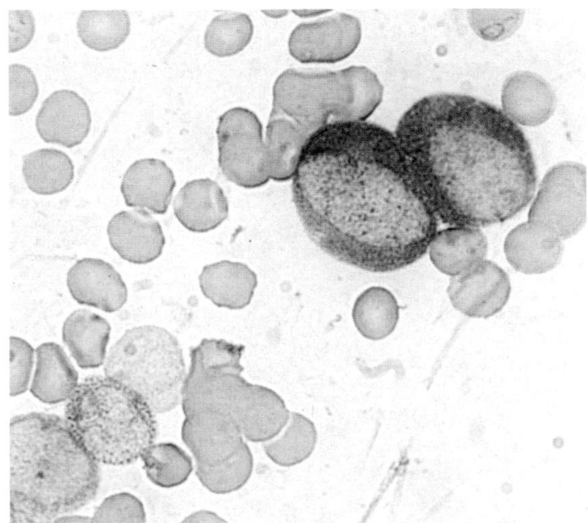

Fig. 7.10 Leukaemic blast cells stained for CAE activity, using Corinth V as the dye. This was a case of AML of FAB M2 category.

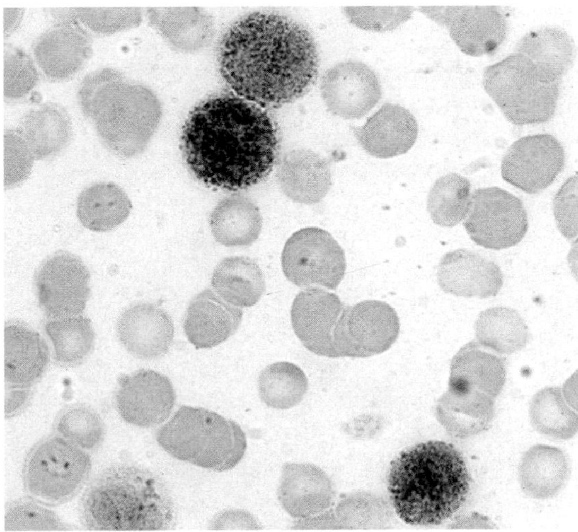

Fig. 7.11 Leukaemic blast cells stained for ANAE activity using fast RR as the dye. This was a case of AML of FAB M5 category.

esterase activity of these cells has been designated 'non-specific' esterase [4, 16]. Different isoenzymes are preferentially detected by different substrates and at different pHs. The most useful cytochemical reaction to detect the esterase activity of monocytes is α-naphthyl acetate esterase (ANAE) activity at acid pH (Fig. 7.11). α-Naphthyl butyrate esterase (ANBE) activity is quite similar. With ANAE, strongly positive reactions are given by monocytes and their precursors and by megakaryocytes and platelets. Weaker reactions are given by plasma cells. ANBE is more often negative with megakaryocytes and platelets than is ANAE. Monocyte and megakaryocyte non-specific esterase activity can also be detected as naphthol AS-D acetate esterase (NASDA esterase) activity or the very similar naphthol AS acetate esterase (NASA esterase). NASDA esterase is weakly positive in neutrophils and their precursors. It is therefore less suitable than ANAE for differentiating between the monocyte lineage and the neutrophil lineage; the specificity of the test can be improved by carrying out the reaction with and without fluoride since the monocyte and megakaryocyte enzymes are inhibited by fluoride whereas the neutrophil enzyme is fluoride-resistant. The ANAE activity of monocytes and megakaryocytes is also fluoride-sensitive, but ANAE permits a clearer distinction between monocytes and neutrophils and the addition of fluoride is not necessary. Non-specific esterase activity is often demonstrable in normal T lymphocytes and also in acute and chronic leukaemias of T lineage. With ANAE a characteristic dot positivity is often demonstrable in T-lineage ALL and T-prolymphocytic leukaemia; ANAE is superior to NASDA esterase in this regard [1] but this use of esterase cytochemistry is largely redundant since immunophenotyping is now widely available. The abnormal erythroblasts of erythroleukaemia or megaloblastic anaemia may also have non-specific esterase activity.

A combined reaction for ANAE and CAE activities permits both reactions to be studied on the one blood film and is useful in characterizing acute leukaemias.

Periodic acid–Schiff (PAS) reaction

PAS reaction stains a variety of carbohydrates including the glycogen which is often found in haemopoietic cells. The main clinical application of the stain is in the differential diagnosis of the acute leukaemias but its role has diminished considerably with the increasing use of immunophenotyping. Lymphoblasts of ALL are PAS-positive in the great majority of cases, this positivity often being in the form of coarse granules or large blocks on a clear background (Fig. 7.12). A negative PAS reaction is more often seen in T-lineage than in B-lineage (common) ALL. Myeloblasts and monoblasts may be PAS-negative or may have faint diffuse or granular positivity. Block positivity is rare in AML but it has been observed in basophil precursors, monoblasts, megakaryoblasts and erythroblasts.

Many other haemopoietic cells are PAS-positive but the reaction is rarely of diagnostic importance. The reaction has a limited application in the diagnosis of erythroleukaemias and megakaryoblastic leukaemia. Platelets, megakaryocytes and the more mature megakaryoblasts are positive. Megakaryoblasts may have PAS-positive granules within cytoplasmic blebs. Normal erythroblasts are PAS-negative. Strong, diffuse or block PAS positivity may be seen in erythroleukaemia. However, quite strong reactions, either diffuse or granular, may also be seen in thalassaemia major and iron deficiency, and weaker reactions in sideroblastic anaemia, severe haemolytic anaemia and a number of other disorders of erythropoiesis. Mature neutrophils have fine positive granules which appear to pack the cytoplasm whereas eosinophils and basophils have a positive cytoplasmic reaction contrasting with the negative granules. Most normal lymphocytes are PAS-negative. Lymphocytes containing PAS-positive granules become more numerous in reactive conditions, such as infectious mononucleosis and other viral infections, and in lymphoproliferative disorders such as CLL and non-Hodgkin's lymphoma. A circlet of PAS-positive granules surrounding the nucleus, likened to rosary beads, may be found in Sézary cells.

A PAS stain can be performed on a film which has been stained previously with a Romanowsky stain.

Acid phosphatase

Acid phosphatase activity is demonstrated by a variety of haemopoietic cells. The two main applications of this reaction are in the diagnosis of hairy cell leukaemia and in the diagnosis of T-lineage leukaemias, particularly T-lineage ALL.

Acid phosphatase activity is usually stronger in acute and chronic leukaemias of T lineage than in those of B lineage where it is often negative. T-lineage ALL often demonstrates focal positivity (Fig. 7.13) which is of some use in confirming this

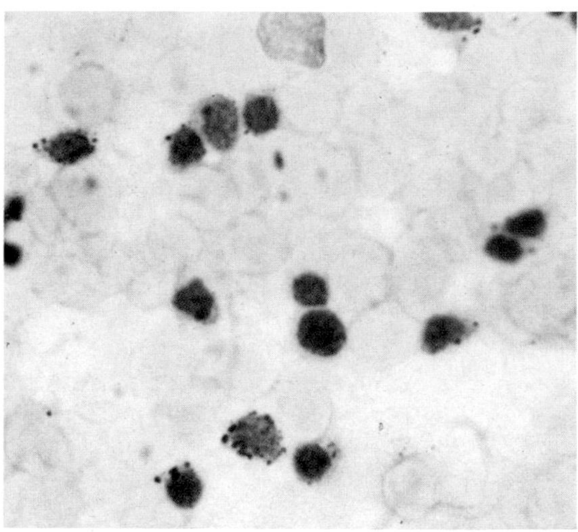

Fig. 7.12 PAS reaction showing block positivity in the blasts cells of a case of B-lineage ALL of FAB L1 category. Courtesy of Dr A. Eden.

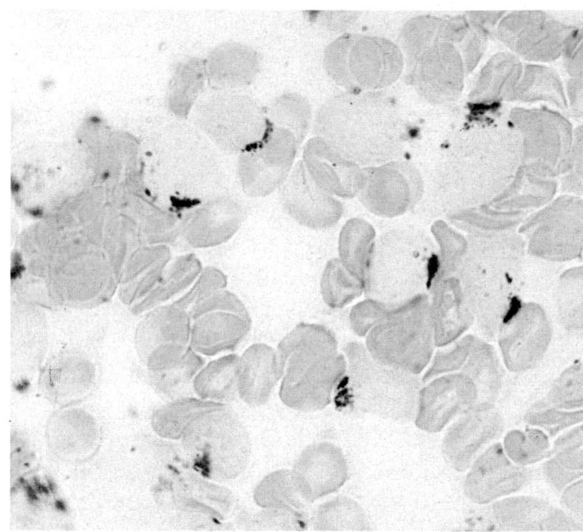

Fig. 7.13 Acid phosphatase stain by the method of Janckila [5] showing focal positivity in the blast cells of a patient with T-lineage ALL of FAB L2 category.

diagnosis. However, with the availability of immunophenotyping its importance has declined greatly. Acid phosphatase activity is also demonstrable in granulocytes and their precursors, in the monocyte lineage, and in platelets, megakaryocytes and the more mature megakaryoblasts. Auer rods are positive.

A number of isoenzymes of acid phosphatase are found in haemopoietic cells. That of hairy cells is characteristically tartrate resistant whereas that of other cells is sensitive to inhibition by tartrate. The demonstration of tartrate-resistant acid phosphatase (TRAP) activity is still important in the diagnosis of hairy cell leukaemia. It is present in the great majority of cases and is uncommon in other disorders; however TRAP positivity has also been reported in occasional cases of infectious mononucleosis, CLL, prolymphocytic leukaemia (PLL), non-Hodgkin's lymphoma and the Sézary's syndrome. The monocytes of patients with Gaucher's disease are also TRAP-positive but normal monocytes are not [17].

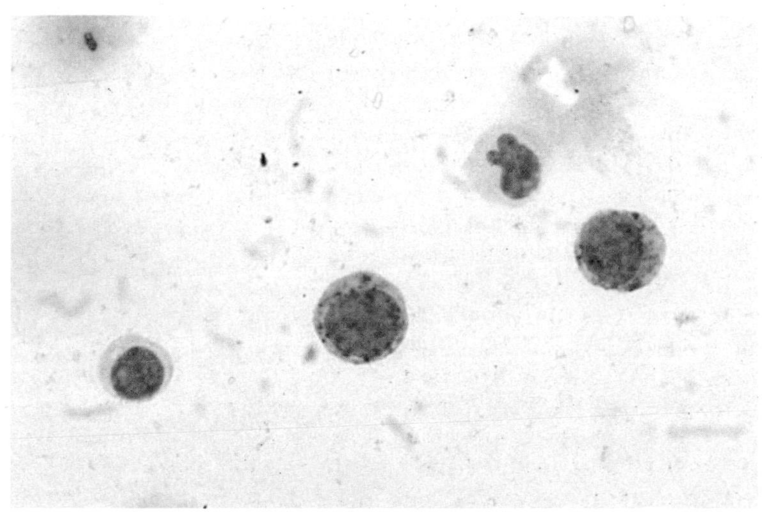

Fig. 7.14 Immunophenotyping using a monoclonal antibody to CD13 and the immunoperoxidase technique. The blast cells of this case gave negative reactions with MPO, SBB and CAE but were identified as myeloid (FAB M0 category) by the positivity with CD13 and negativity with monoclonal antibodies directed at lymphoid antigens. Courtesy of Professor D. Catovsky, London.

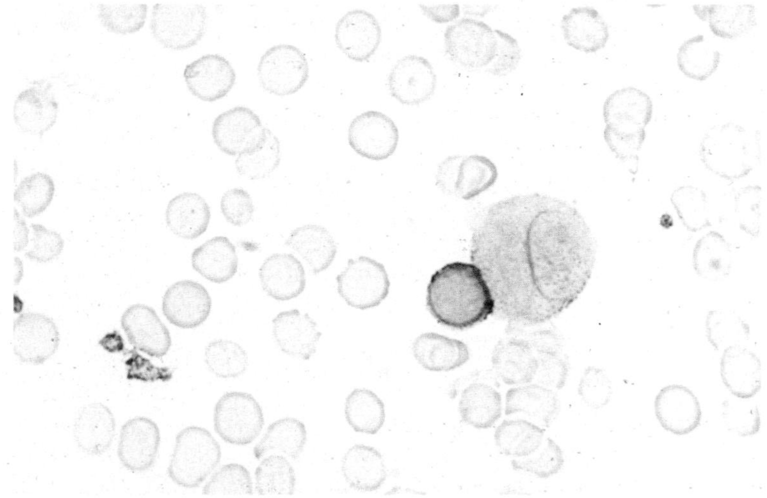

Fig. 7.15 Immunophenotyping using a monoclonal antibody to CD42 (antiplatelet glycoprotein Ib) and the alkaline phosphatase–anti-alkaline phosphatase (APAAP) technique. Positive reactions are given by two platelets, by a lymphocyte sized micromegakaryocyte and by a larger mononuclear megakaryocyte.

Immunophenotyping

Immunophenotyping of the neoplastic cells in leukaemia and lymphoma can be carried out with a panel of antibodies, mainly monoclonal antibodies, which detect antigens on the surface membrane or, if the cell is lightly fixed, cytoplasmic antigens [18,19]. With such panels, cells can be assigned to T-cell, B-cell or myeloid lineages. Certain specific antibodies can identify cells of erythroid and megakaryocyte lineages. The use of secondary panels of antibodies permits the establishment of characteristic profiles which are very useful in the identification of specific types of lymphoproliferative disorder.

Immunophenotyping is often performed on a flow cytometer using antibodies labelled with a fluorochrome. This is efficient if large numbers of specimens are being processed. Immunophenotyping can also be carried out on fixed cells on cytospin preparations, using antibodies which are detected by either an immunoperoxidase (Fig. 7.14) or an alkaline phosphatase–anti-alkaline phosphatase (APAAP) technique (Fig. 7.15). By these techniques surface membrane, cytoplasmic and nuclear antigens are readily detected. These techniques have some advantages over flow cytometry since the cytological features of positively staining cells can be appreciated.

References

1 Dacie JV, Lewis SM. *Practical Haematology*, 6th edn. Edinburgh: Churchill Livingstone, 1984.

2 Hanker JS, Yates PE, Metz CB, Rustioni A. A new, specific, sensitive and non-carcinogenic reagent for the demonstration of horseradish peroxidase. *Histochem J* 1977; 9: 789–92.

3 Yam LT, Li CY, Crosby WH. Cytochemical identification of monocytes and granulocytes. *Am J Clin Pathol* 1971; 55: 283–90.

4 Hayhoe FGJ, Quaglino D. *Haematological Cytochemistry*. Edinburgh: Churchill Livingstone, 1980.

5 Janckila A, Li C-Y, Lam K-W, Yam LT. The cytochemistry of tartrate-resistant acid phosphatase — technical considerations. *Am J Clin Pathol* 1978; 70: 45–55.

6 Gadson D, Hughes M, Dean A, Wickramasinghe SN. Morphology of redox-dye-treated HbH-containing red cells: confusion caused by wrongly-identified dyes. *Clin Lab Haematol* 1986; 8: 365–6.

7 Rustin GJS, Wilson PD, Peters TJ. Studies on the subcellular localization of human neutrophil alkaline phosphatase. *J Cell Sci* 1979; 36: 401–12.

8 Ackerman GA. Substituted naphthol AS phosphate derivatives for the localization of leukocyte alkaline phosphatase activity. *Lab Invest* 1962; 11: 563–7.

9 Kaplow LS. Leukocyte alkaline phosphatase cytochemistry: applications and methods. *Ann NY Acad Sci* 1968; 155: 911–47.

10 Breton-Gorius J, Mason DY, Buriot D, Vilde J-L, Griscelli C. Lactoferrin deficiency as a consequence of a lack of specific granules in neutrophils from patient with recurrent infections. *Am J Pathol* 1980; 99: 413–19.

11 O'Kell RT. Leukocyte alkaline phosphatase activity in the infant. *Ann NY Acad Sci* 1968; 155: 980–2.

12 Rosner F, Lee SL, Schultz FS, Gorfien PC. The regulation of leukocyte alkaline phosphatase. *Ann NY Acad Sci* 1968; 155: 902–10.

13 Stavridis J, Creatsas G, Lolis D, Traga G, Antonopoulos M, Kaskarelis D. Relationships between leucocyte alkaline phosphatase and nitroblue tetrazolium reduction activities in the peripheral blood polymorphonuclear leucocytes in normal individuals. *Br J Haematol* 1981; 47: 157–9.

14 Stein P, Peiper S, Butler D, Melvin S, Williams D, Stass S. Granular acute lymphoblastic leukaemia. *Am J Clin Pathol* 1983; 79: 426–30.

15 Savage RA, Fishleder J, Tubbs SR. Confirming myeloid differential. *Am J Clin Pathol* 1985; 80: 412.

16 Catovsky D. Leucocyte enzymes in leukaemia. In: S Roath, ed. *Topical Reviews in Haematology*, Vol. 1. Bristol: John Wright, 1980.

17 Beutler E. Gaucher disease. *Blood Rev* 1988; 2: 59–70.

18 General Haematology Task Force of BCSH. Immunophenotyping in the diagnosis of the acute leukaemias. *J Clin Pathol* 1994; 47: 777–81.

19 General Haematology Task Force of BCSH. Immunophenotyping in the diagnosis of the chronic lymphoproliferative disorders. *J Clin Pathol* 1994; 47: 871–5.

CHAPTER 8

Disorders of Red Cells and Platelets

Disorders of red cells

Disorders of red cells are most often divided into three broad categories, depending on whether the erythrocytes are (i) microcytic and hypochromic; (ii) normocytic and normochromic; or (iii) macrocytic. Red cell disorders can also be classified as congenital or acquired. Anaemia can be further categorized according to the mechanism, whether due predominantly to a failure of production or to shortened red cell survival, and if the latter whether it is caused by an intrinsic defect of the red cell or by extrinsic factors. In this chapter red cell disorders will be discussed in groups which relate mainly to the morphological features of the cells including their size and degree of haemoglobinization.

Hypochromic and microcytic anaemias and thalassaemias

Iron-deficiency anaemia

Iron deficiency develops when (i) iron intake is inadequate for needs; (ii) there is malabsorption of iron; (iii) there is increased loss of iron, usually consequent on blood loss; (iv) there is a combination of these factors; or, rarely, (v) there is sequestration of iron at an inaccessible site, as in idiopathic pulmonary haemosiderosis. Anaemia occurs when a lack of reticuloendothelial storage iron in the bone marrow and an inadequate rate of delivery of iron to the marrow leads to reduced synthesis of haem and therefore reduced production of haemoglobin and red blood cells.

Blood film and count

In iron deficiency, a normocytic normochromic anaemia with anisocytosis precedes the development of anisochromasia, hypochromia and microcytosis. Morphological changes are not usually marked until Hb falls below 10–11 g/dl when characteristic features appear (Fig. 8.1). Poikilocytes include elliptocytes, particularly very narrow elliptocytes which are often referred to as pencil cells. Occasional target cells can be present but they are not usually numerous, except in patients with haemoglobin C or S trait who sometimes develop target cells only when they become iron deficient. Basophilic stippling is infrequent. Polychromasia is sometimes present.

With most automated full blood counters the earliest evidence of iron deficiency is an increase in RDW. This is indicative of the anisocytosis which precedes anaemia. The next change observed is a fall in the Hb, RBC and PCV/Hct followed by a fall in the MCV and MCH. In early iron-deficiency anaemia, the RBC is occasionally elevated rather than decreased, particularly in children. With a Technicon H.1 series automated

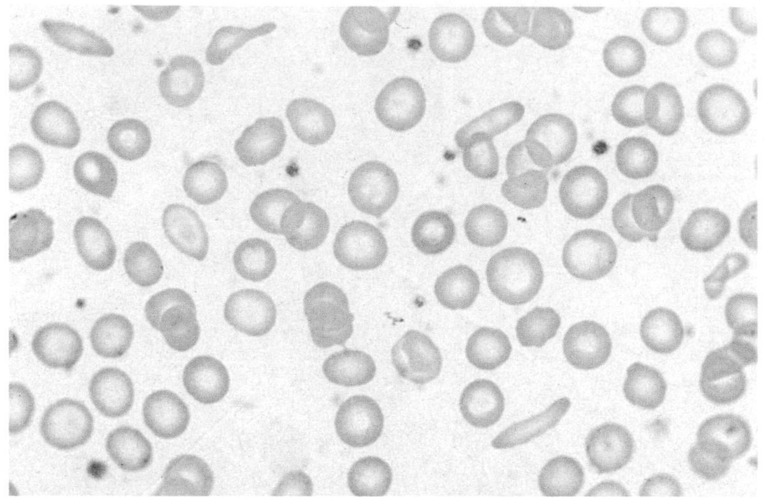

Fig. 8.1 The blood film of a patient with iron-deficiency anaemia showing anisocytosis, poikilocytosis (including elliptocytes), hypochromia and microcytosis. The blood count (Coulter S Plus IV) was: RBC $4.22 \times 10^9/l$, Hb 7 g/dl, Hct 0.29, MCV 67 fl, MCH 16.6 pg, MCHC 24.5 g/dl.

counter the appearance of a population of hypochromic cells and an increase in the HDW is the earliest change detected; a fall in the MCH and MCHC precedes any fall in the MCV [1]. A low MCHC is a sensitive indicator of iron deficiency when it is calculated from a microhaematocrit and the Hb or when it is measured by current Technicon instruments. When measured by impedance-based instruments (such as Coulter or Sysmex instruments) it is insensitive but more specific for iron deficiency. The reticulocyte percentage may be normal or elevated in iron deficiency anaemia, while the absolute reticulocyte count is normal or reduced.

Patients with iron deficiency not infrequently have an increased platelet count which may be consequent on the iron deficiency itself, blood loss or underlying malignant disease. In severe iron deficiency the platelet count is sometimes low. Leucopenia and thrombocytopenia occur in up to 10% of patients. Hypersegmented neutrophils are sometimes present and are not necessarily indicative of coexisting vitamin B_{12} or folate deficiency. In geographical regions where hookworm occurs, the observation of eosinophilia may suggest that this is the cause of the iron deficiency.

Differential diagnosis

The important differential diagnoses of iron-deficiency anaemia are thalassaemia trait and the anaemia of chronic disease. The blood film and count are of some use in distinguishing these disorders but specific tests are needed for a precise diagnosis. Prominent target cells and basophilic stippling favour thalassaemia trait whereas anisochromasia and pencil cells favour iron deficiency and increased rouleaux formation, background staining and other signs of inflammation suggest the anaemia of chronic disease. A high RBC and a low MCV despite a normal Hb are characteristic of thalassaemia trait but very similar red cell indices occur in patients with PRV who are iron deficient. The RDW is usually elevated in iron deficiency and most often normal in thalassaemia trait [2]. A low MCHC on the less sensitive impedance counters is strongly suggestive of iron deficiency since it is usually normal in thalassaemia trait and in the anaemia of chronic disease. Rare conditions which can cause a microcytic anaemia are listed in Table 3.1.

Further tests

In uncomplicated iron-deficiency anaemia, the diagnosis can be confirmed by either (i) a low serum ferritin; or (ii) a low serum iron coexisting with an increased transferrin concentration or serum iron binding capacity. It should be noted that a low serum iron by itself gives little useful information since it is found in both iron deficiency and anaemia of chronic disease. When iron deficiency and chronic inflammation coexist there may be no elevation in transferrin concentration and iron binding capacity, and serum ferritin may be in the lower part of the normal range rather than reduced. An elevated free erythrocyte protoporphyrin concentration is found in iron deficiency anaemia and in the anaemia of chronic disease but not in thalassaemia trait. In complicated cases the definitive test is the demonstration of absent bone marrow iron.

Anaemia of chronic disease

'Anaemia of chronic disease' is a term used to describe anaemia which is consequent on chronic infection or inflammation or, less often, on malignant disease and which is characterized by (i) low serum iron concentration and defective incorporation of iron into haemoglobin despite adequate bone marrow stores of iron; and (ii) a blunted erythropoietin response to anaemia.

Blood film and count

Anaemia of chronic disease, when mild, is normocytic and normochromic, but as it becomes more severe hypochromia and microcytosis develop (Fig. 8.2). In severe chronic inflammation the degree of microcytosis may be just as marked as in iron deficiency. The RDW has been reported to be normal in anaemia of chronic disease [2] but this has not been a consistent observation [3]. The absolute reticulocyte count is reduced. Associated features indicative of chronic inflammation may be present, e.g., neutrophilia, thrombocytosis, increased rouleaux formation and increased background staining.

Differential diagnosis

The differential diagnosis is with iron-deficiency anaemia (see above).

Further tests

Serum iron and serum transferrin or iron-binding capacity are reduced. Serum ferritin is increased, consequent on synthesis of apoferritin by inflammatory or neoplastic cells. Associated features indicative of chronic inflammation are useful in making the diagnosis. In addition to blood film features they commonly include elevated plasma viscosity and ESR, a reduced serum albumin concentration and an increased concentration of fibrinogen, α_2-macroglobulin and γ-globulins. It is not uncommon for a patient with anaemia of chronic disease due to malignancy or chronic inflammation to develop iron deficiency, usually as a consequence of gastrointestinal blood loss. It may be impossible to diagnose such a complex situation from the blood film and biochemical

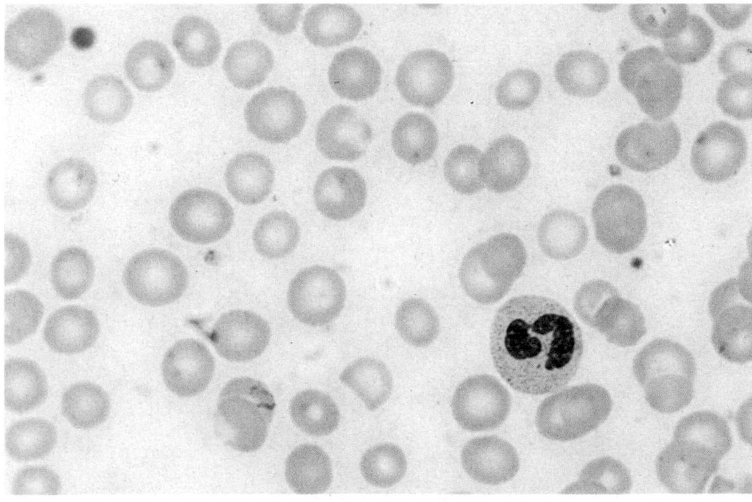

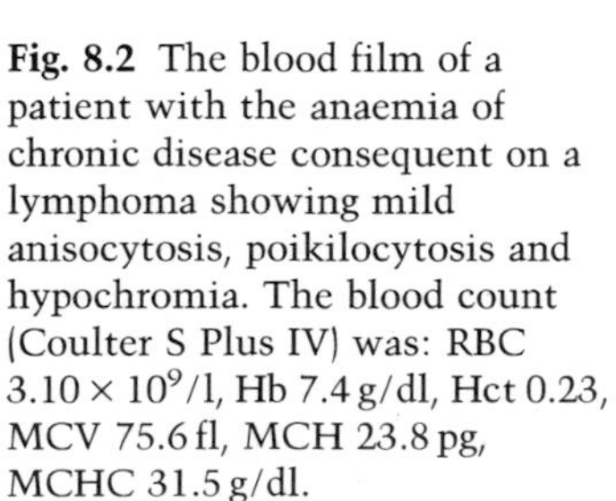

Fig. 8.2 The blood film of a patient with the anaemia of chronic disease consequent on a lymphoma showing mild anisocytosis, poikilocytosis and hypochromia. The blood count (Coulter S Plus IV) was: RBC 3.10×10^9/l, Hb 7.4 g/dl, Hct 0.23, MCV 75.6 fl, MCH 23.8 pg, MCHC 31.5 g/dl.

tests. A bone marrow aspiration will allow a correct appraisal.

β-thalassaemia trait

β-thalassaemia trait refers to heterozygosity for β-thalassaemia, an inherited condition in which a mutation in a β-globin gene or, less often, the deletion of a β-globin gene leads to a reduced rate of synthesis of β-globin chains. There is consequently a reduced rate of synthesis of haemoglobin. Compensatory erythroid hyperplasia leads to production of increased numbers of red cells of reduced size and haemoglobin content. The mutations giving rise to β-thalassaemia are very numerous and very heterogeneous. In some cases the abnormal gene leads to no β-chain production (β^0-thalassaemia) whereas in others the abnormal gene permits β-chain synthesis at a reduced rate (β^+-thalassaemia). Different mutations producing defects of varying severity are prevalent in different parts of the world.

β-thalassaemia trait occurs in virtually all ethnic groups although in white people of northern European origin it is very infrequent. It is common in Greece and Italy where the prevalence in some regions reaches 15–20%. There is a similar prevalence in Cyprus among both Greek and Turkish Cypriots. The prevalence in some parts of India, Thailand and other parts of South-East Asia reaches 5–10%. In black Americans the prevalence is about 0.5% and in West Indians it is about 1%.

Blood film and count

The majority of subjects with β-thalassaemia trait have a normal Hb; a minority are mildly anaemic, particularly during pregnancy or intercurrent infections. Anaemia is more common among Greeks and Italians than among black people. Despite the lack of anaemia, microcytosis is usually marked. The blood film (Figs 8.3 & 8.4) may or may not show hypochromia in addition to microcytosis. The haemoglobin concentration of cells usually appears very uniform, in contrast to the anisochromasia which is usual in iron deficiency. Poikilocytosis varies from trivial to marked. Target cells may be prominent but in some patients they are infrequent or absent. A few irregularly contracted cells are seen in some patients. Occasional patients have marked elliptocytosis but in general elliptocytes are not a feature. Basophilic stippling is quite common in Mediterranean subjects with β-thalassaemia trait but is less often seen in black and Oriental subjects. The reticulocyte percentage and absolute count are often somewhat elevated [4]. In uncomplicated cases the white cells and platelets are normal.

The red cell indices of β-thalassaemia trait are very characteristic and it is often easier to make a

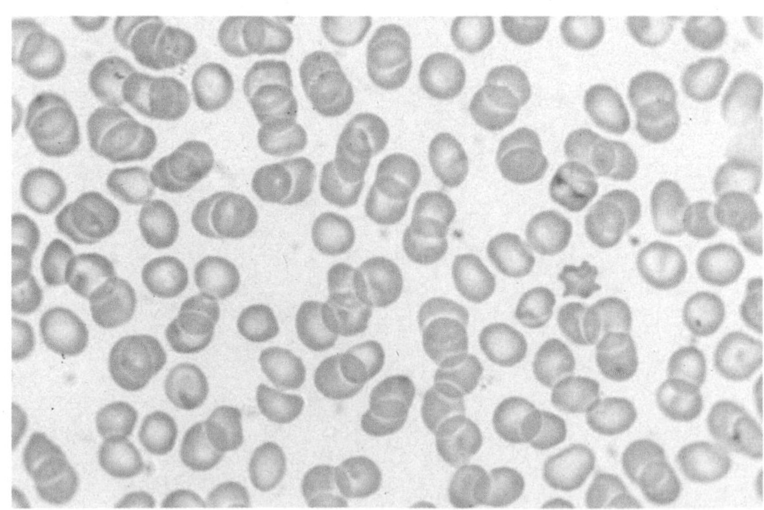

Fig. 8.3 The blood film of a healthy subject with β-thalassaemia trait showing minimal morphological abnormalities — microcytosis and mild poikilocytosis. The diagnosis could easily be missed without the red cell indices. The blood count (Coulter S Plus IV) was RBC 7.3×10^9/l, Hb 14.3 g/dl, Hct 0.43, MCV 59 fl, MCH 19.7 pg, MCHC 32.8 g/dl.

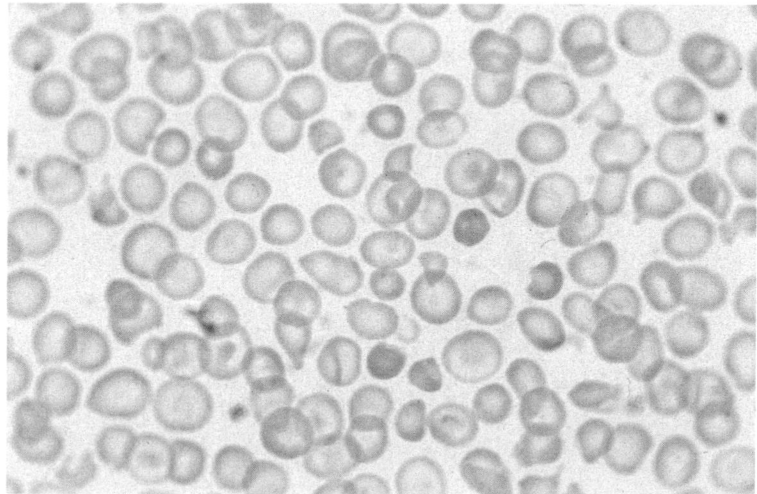

Fig. 8.4 The blood film of a healthy subject with β-thalassaemia trait showing more marked morphological abnormalities — anisocytosis, poikilocytosis, hypochromia, microcytosis, occasional target cells and several irregularly contracted cells. The blood count (Coulter S Plus IV) was: RBC 5.78×10^9/l, Hb 10.5 g/dl, Hct 0.32, MCV 56 fl, MCH 18.2 pg, MCHC 32.3 g/dl.

correct provisional diagnosis from the red cell indices than from the blood film. The Hb and PCV are normal or close to normal while the MCV and MCH are usually markedly reduced. The MCHC is normal when measured by impedance counters such as Sysmex and Coulter instruments but is often somewhat reduced when measured by Technicon H.1 series instruments. When the number of hypochromic cells and microcytic cells are measured independently the percentage of microcytes usually exceeds the percentage of hypochromic cells in thalassaemia trait whereas the reverse is found in iron deficiency [5]. The red cell cytogram characteristically has a 'comma' shape (Fig. 8.5). In contrast to iron deficiency, the RDW is usually normal [2] but when a patient with β-thalassaemia trait becomes anaemic the RDW tends to rise [2] so that this measurement is least useful when most needed. Other observers have often found the RDW to be elevated even in non-anaemic cases [3].

Diagnosis of thalassaemia trait is more difficult in pregnant patients for two reasons. (i) The red cell indices are less characteristic since haemodilution, which is a physiological effect of pregnancy, lowers the Hb, RBC and PCV; the Hb may fall as low as 5–6 g/dl [6]. The rise in MCV which occurs in pregnancy also contributes to the red cell indices being less characteristic than in a non-pregnant subject. (ii) Iron-deficiency anaemia has an increased incidence during pregnancy and when the two conditions coexist diagnosis is more complicated.

Differential diagnosis

The important differential diagnoses of β-thalassaemia trait are α-thalassaemia trait and iron-deficiency anaemia. Various formulae have been devised in an attempt to separate iron deficiency from β-thalassaemia trait (Table 8.1). Although such formulae may be useful in separating uncomplicated cases into the two diagnostic groups they are not generally applicable to pregnant women [13] or children and are not useful in patients who have both iron deficiency *and* thalassaemia trait, a not uncommon situation with patients from the Indian subcontinent. Although these formulae are useful in suggesting the most likely diagnosis there is little choice but to carry out specific diagnostic tests in circumstances where the diagnosis of thalassaemia trait is important, for example for genetic counselling in pregnant women when antenatal diagnosis is contemplated. In this situation either the MCV or the MCH can be used as a screening test with all patients whose test results fall below an arbitrary limit having haemoglobin electrophoresis performed. Occasional patients with mild variants of β-thalassaemia trait have only a very trivial reduction of the MCV and MCH and if such cases are to be identified it is necessary to test all

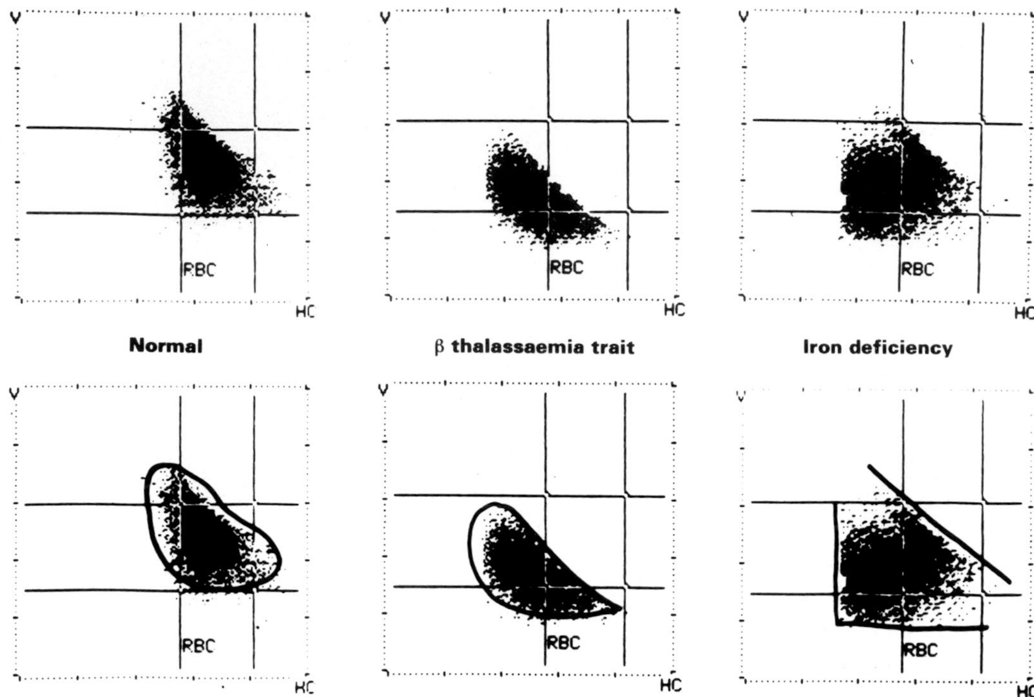

Fig. 8.5 Red cell cytograms from a Technicon H.2 counter showing the relationship between haemoglobinization (*x*-axis) and volume (*y*-axis) of individual red cells in a normal subject (left) and patients with β-thalassaemia trait (centre) and iron deficiency (right). The 'comma' shape of β-thalassaemia trait is apparent and has been emphasized by the sketched outlines of the cytograms in the lower series of scatter plots.

patients whose results fall below the lower limit of the reference range. Even this will not detect all cases since in some mild thalassaemic variants there is no apparent haematological defect in heterozygotes; such cases cannot be diagnosed from the blood film and indices. However, except when genetic counselling is being carried out in high incidence areas, it is generally necessary to have a cut-off point for further investigation which is at or below the lower limit of the reference range in order to avoid having a very high percentage of negative tests with a very low yield of positive diagnoses.

It is not possible on the basis of the blood film and count to distinguish β-thalassaemia trait from δβ- or γδβ-thalassaemia trait or from cases of α-thalassaemia trait in which two of the four α-genes are deleted. Cases of α-thalassaemia trait in which only one of the four α-genes is deleted have only minor haematological abnormalities and are less likely to be confused with β-thalassaemia trait. Occasional patients with a blood film and red cell indices suggestive of thalassaemia trait have either a highly unstable β-chain or an abnormal haemoglobin which is synthesized at a reduced rate. The commonest of the latter group is haemoglobin Lepore, consequent on a formation of a δ–β fusion gene. Haemoglobin E is also synthesized at a reduced rate and both heterozygosity and homozygosity for this abnormal haemoglobin can produce indices suggestive of thalassaemia trait. Sickle cell trait and haemoglobin C trait are also not infrequently associated with microcytosis.

The red cell indices in iron-deficient polycythaemia may be indistinguishable from those of thalassaemia trait but RDW is more likely to be elevated and there may be associated features which are useful in the differential diagnosis such as neutrophilia, basophilia, thrombocytosis

Table 8.1 Some formulae which have been recommended for distinguishing between β-thalassaemia trait and iron deficiency

Formula	Instrument	β-thalassaemia	Iron deficiency	Reference
$\frac{MCV}{RBC}$	Coulter	<13	>13	[7]
MCV − RBC − (Hb × 5) − constant*	Coulter	<0	>0	[8, 9]
$\frac{MCH}{RBC}$	Coulter	<3.8	>3.8	[10]
$\frac{MCV^2 \times MCH}{100}$	Coulter	<1530	>1530	[11]
RDW	Coulter	<14.6	>14.6	[3]
$\frac{MCV^2 \times RDW}{Hb \times 100}$	Coulter Sysmex E-5000 Technicon H.1 series	<65 <73 <73	>65 >73 >73	[12]
$\frac{\%\ microcytes}{\%\ hypochromic\ cells}$	Technicon H.1 series	>0.9	<0.9	[5]

* The constant is 3.4 with a plasma trapping correction [8] and 8.4 with no plasma trapping correction [9].

and the presence of giant platelets. The characteristic indices of thalassaemia can also be simulated by iron deficiency anaemia undergoing treatment. A marked elevation of the RDW (and HDW) or the detection of two cell populations on a blood film or on the graphical output of an automated counter suggests the correct diagnosis.

Anaemia of chronic disease can usually be readily distinguished from β-thalassaemia because of the greater degree of anaemia and retention of a normal MCV until significant anaemia has developed.

Further tests

Haemoglobin electrophoresis and demonstration of an increased percentage of haemoglobin A_2 are necessary for the definitive diagnosis of β-thalassaemia trait. Haemoglobin F is also elevated in one-third to one-half of patients but is less specific. δβ- or $^{G}\gamma(^{A}\gamma\delta\beta)^{0}$-thalassaemia trait is diagnosed when there are thalassaemic indices with a normal or low haemoglobin A_2 and an elevated haemoglobin F. Diagnosis of the rare cases of γδβ-thalassaemia trait requires DNA analysis. Haemoglobin Lepore trait is diagnosed when there are thalassaemic indices with a normal or reduced haemoglobin A_2 and with a minor abnormal haemoglobin having the same mobility as haemoglobin S at alkaline pH and the same mobility as haemoglobin A at acid pH. Haemoglobins E, C and S will also be detected on electrophoresis.

Because iron deficiency causes a reduction of the haemoglobin A_2 percentage some cases of mild β-thalassaemia trait may be missed if tests are done when the patient has a coexisting iron deficiency. Except in pregnant patients when immediate diagnosis is needed, it is better not to carry out electrophoresis in patients who appear to have uncomplicated iron deficiency, but rather to check that the FBC returns to normal after treatment.

β-*thalassaemia major*

β-thalassaemia major is an inherited disease consequent on homozygosity or compound heterozygosity for β-thalassaemia genes leading to a severe reduction or total lack of synthesis of β-globin chains. Consequently, there is an inability to synthesize adequate amounts of haemoglobin A. There is marked erythroid hyperplasia and ineffective haemopoiesis consequent on damage to developing erythroblasts by excess free α-chains. Clinical features are severe anaemia, hepatomegaly, splenomegaly and expansion of marrow-containing bones.

Blood film and count

Anaemia is severe with the Hb sometimes being as low as 2–3 g/dl. The blood film (Fig. 8.6) shows very marked anisocytosis and poikilocytosis with the poikilocytes including target cells, tear drop cells, elliptocytes, fragments and many cells of bizarre shape. Hypochromia is very striking but microcytosis is not always so obvious on the blood film since the cells are very flat and red cell diameter is thus greater than would be expected from the red cell size. Basophilic stippling and Pappenheimer bodies are present. Sometimes a minority of cells have inclusions with the same staining characteristics as haemoglobin; these represent precipitates of excess α-chains and are much more readily identified on a Heinz body preparation. NRBC are frequent. The circulating erythroblasts are micronormoblastic and show dyserythropoietic features, defective haemoglobinization and the presence of Pappenheimer bodies. There is often leucocytosis, consequent on neutrophilia and, in younger children, lymphocytosis. The platelet count may be normal or increased. In advanced disease with marked splenomegaly the platelet count falls.

Following splenectomy the TNCC, WBC and platelet count rise; the blood film is even more strikingly abnormal with many abnormal NRBC and numerous target cells, Pappenheimer bodies and Howell–Jolly bodies. Post-splenectomy, Heinz body preparations show ragged inclusions in 10–20% of cells; these represent α-chain precipitates and differ from the Heinz bodies consequent on oxidant stress in that they are not attached to the red cell membrane and are present in NRBC as well as mature erythrocytes [14]. Following splenectomy there is often an exaggerated lymphocytosis or neutrophilia in response to intercurrent infections.

When patients are adequately transfused the blood film is dimorphic with the percentage of the patient's own abnormal cells being low.

The blood count shows a severe microcytic anaemia with the MCV, MCH and MCHC being greatly reduced and the RDW and HDW being increased. The TNCC as measured on automated

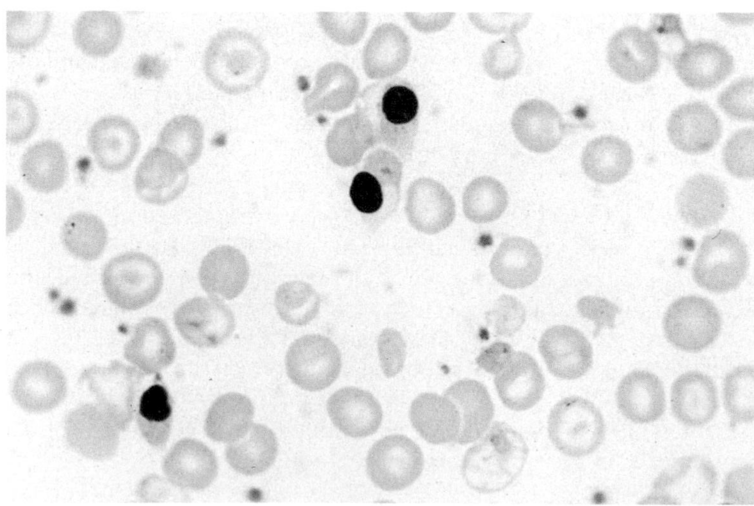

Fig. 8.6 The blood film of a patient with β-thalassaemia major who has been splenectomized and is receiving intermittent blood transfusions. The blood film is dimorphic with about two-thirds of the erythrocytes being donor cells. The patient's own red cells show marked anisocytosis, poikilocytosis and hypochromia. There are several target cells and three NRBC. Some cells contain Pappenheimer bodies and in two cells (a very hypochromic cell and a NRBC) there are inclusions which represent precipitated α-chains.

counters is greatly increased because of the presence of many NRBC; a true leucocytosis is also often present. The TNCC may be erroneous since, with many automated instruments, some but not all NRBC are included in the count.

Differential diagnosis

Thalassaemia intermedia is distinguished from thalassaemia major on clinical rather than haematological grounds. It is a genetically heterogeneous condition but is most often consequent on homozygosity or compound heterozygosity for mild β^+-thalassaemia genes. The Hb is usually above 7–8 g/dl and other peripheral blood features are also intermediate between those of thalassaemia major and thalassaemia trait. The compound heterozygous state for β-thalassaemia and haemoglobin E can also have haematological features which resemble those of thalassaemia major.

Further tests

Diagnosis requires haemoglobin electrophoresis which shows haemoglobins F and A_2 only when the genotype is β^0/β^0 and haemoglobins F and A_2 with a variable amount of haemoglobin A when the genotype is β^0/β^+ or β^+/β^+. Some cases of thalassaemia intermedia have a relatively high percentage of haemoglobin A while others have almost exclusively haemoglobin F. The compound heterozygous states for HbE and β-thalassaemia are distinguished from thalassaemia major by haemoglobin electrophoresis.

α-thalassaemia trait

Haematologically normal subjects have four α-genes. α-thalassaemia trait is consequent on deletion of either one or two of the four α-genes. The genotype $-\alpha/\alpha\alpha$ is designated α^+-thalassaemia or α-thalassaemia 2 trait. The genotype $--/\alpha\alpha$ is designated α^0-thalassaemia or α-thalassaemia 1 trait. The α-thalassaemia 1 phenotype can also be produced by heterozygosity for α^+-thalassaemia, i.e., $-\alpha/-\alpha$, or by a non-deletional α-thalassaemia trait, $\alpha^T\alpha/\alpha\alpha$. α-thalassaemia is common among many ethnic groups. A high incidence is found among various South-East Asian groups, particularly among Thais and Chinese, who have both the $-\alpha/\alpha\alpha$ and the $--/\alpha\alpha$ genotypes. Among black Americans 25–30% have $-\alpha/\alpha\alpha$ and 1–2% have $-\alpha/-\alpha$ [15]. In Jamaicans the prevalence is approximately 30 and 3%, respectively [97]. In Nigerians the prevalence is even higher with 35% having $-\alpha/\alpha\alpha$ and 8% $-\alpha/-\alpha$ [16]. $-\alpha/\alpha\alpha$ occurs in about 7% of Greeks [17] and is common in Cyprus and in some regions of Italy. On some Pacific islands the prevalence of α-thalassaemia 2 trait is as high as 85%.

Blood film and count

α-thalassaemia 1 trait produces haematological features similar to those of β-thalassaemia trait; basophilic stippling and target cells are often not very prominent (Fig. 8.7). α-thalassaemia 2 trait produces a lesser abnormality and there is often no discernible abnormality in the blood film.

The red cell indices of α-thalassaemia 1 trait are similar to those of β-thalassaemia trait. The indices in α-thalassaemia 2 trait overlap both with those of α-thalassaemia 1 trait and with the normal range.

Differential diagnosis

The differential diagnosis of α-thalassaemia trait is with β-thalassaemia trait and with iron deficiency. A similar haematological phenotype is also produced by several α-chain variant haemoglobins which are synthesized at a greatly reduced rate; the commonest of these is haemoglobin Constant Spring which is not uncommon in South-East Asia and is also found in the Caribbean area, around the Mediterranean, in the Middle East and in the Indian subcontinent. The blood film in haemoglobin Constant Spring trait often shows prominent basophilic stippling.

An α-thalassaemia phenotype can also result from certain rare, highly unstable α-chains variants which are largely degraded before haemoglobin can be formed.

Further tests

Haemoglobin electrophoresis is normal in α-

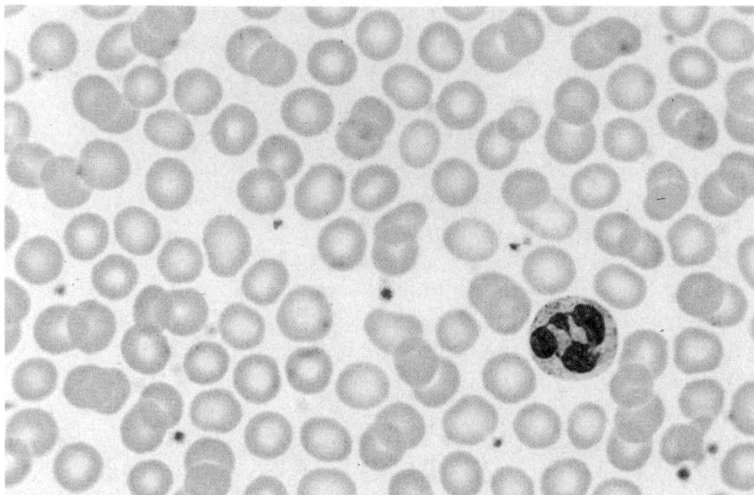

Fig. 8.7 The blood film of a healthy subject with α_1-thalassaemia trait showing microcytosis and mild hypochromia. The blood count (Coulter S) was: RBC 6.24 × 10^9/l, Hb 14.1 g/dl, Hct 0.45, MCV 72 fl, MCH 23 pg, MCHC 31.3 g/dl.

thalassaemia trait, except during the neonatal period when a low percentage of haemoglobin Bart's (γ_4) and haemoglobin H (β_4) may be detected. Haemoglobin Constant Spring can be detected electrophoretically although sometimes with difficulty since the percentage of the abnormal haemoglobin is usually low. In adults the diagnosis of α-thalassaemia trait should be suspected when a subject of an appropriate ethnic group who is not iron deficient has indices suggestive of thalassaemia trait with normal electrophoresis and a normal or low haemoglobin A_2 percentage. The demonstration of haemoglobin H inclusions in a very small percentage of red cells gives support for the diagnosis but this test is quite time-consuming and it may be negative, particularly in α-thalassaemia 2 trait. When diagnosis is important, as when genetic counselling is required in a patient of South-East Asian origin, DNA analysis is necessary.

Haemoglobin H disease

The lack of three of the four α-genes or a functionally similar disorder [6] causes haemoglobin H disease. This most often occurs in subjects of South-East Asian origin including Thais, Chinese and Indonesians but it is also seen in Greeks and Cypriots and less often in a variety of other ethnic groups. Clinical features are of a chronic haemolytic anaemia with hepatomegaly and splenomegaly.

Blood film and count

The diagnosis of haemoglobin H disease can usually be suspected from the blood film and red cell indices. There is anaemia of moderate degree; the Hb is typically 6–10 g/dl but it is lower during pregnancy, during intercurrent infections and following exposure to oxidant drugs. The blood film (Fig. 8.8) shows marked hypochromia, microcytosis and poikilocytosis, often including target cells, tear drop cells and fragments. Basophilic stippling and polychromasia are present. The reticulocyte percentage and absolute count are elevated.

The red cell indices show marked reduction of the MCV and MCH and reduction of the MCHC which are demonstrated by the red cell cytogram (Fig. 8.9). The RDW and HDW are elevated.

Differential diagnosis

The differential diagnosis of haemoglobin H disease is with β-thalassaemia, and with haemolytic and dyserythropoietic anaemias. The blood film and red cell indices are much more abnormal than in β-thalassaemia trait. The MCHC is reduced, irrespective of the method of measurement,

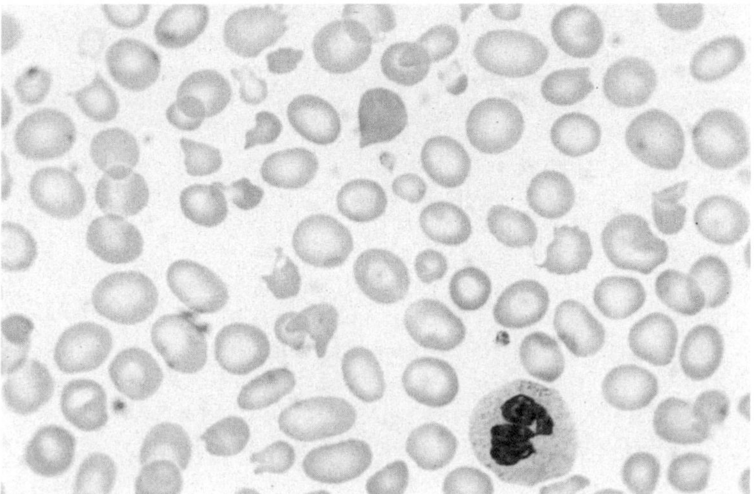

Fig. 8.8 The blood film of a patient with haemoglobin H disease showing anisocytosis, marked poikilocytosis, microcytosis and hypochromia. The blood count (Coulter S Plus IV) was: RBC 4.95×10^9/l, Hb 9.6 g/dl, Hct 0.30, MCV 60.5 fl, MCH 19.4 pg, MCHC 32.1 g/dl, RDW 25.7. The corresponding haemoglobin H preparation is shown in Fig. 7.2a.

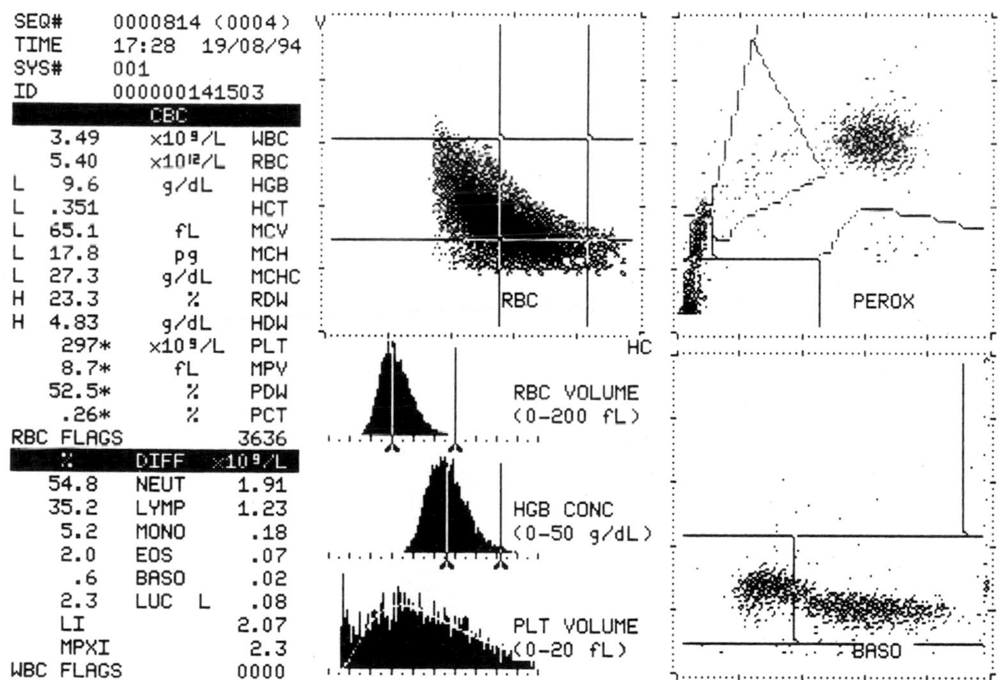

Fig. 8.9 Technicon H.2 scatter plots and histograms of a patient with haemoglobin H disease. The red cell cytogram and histograms show severe hypochromia and microcytosis. The white cell scatter plots are normal.

whereas in β-thalassaemia trait it is not reduced when measured by impedance counters but is reduced when measured by Technicon H.1 series instruments. The degree of haematological abnormality in β-thalassaemia intermedia may be similar; the elevated reticulocyte count and the usual lack of NRBC in haemoglobin H disease are useful in this differential diagnosis. Congenital dyserythropoietic anaemias and hereditary pyropoikilocytosis can show a similar degree of poikilocytosis to haemoglobin H disease but the former group of disorders have normocytic or macrocytic red cells and no reticulocytosis while the blood film in the latter condition shows specific types of poikilocyte such as microspherocytes and red cells with bud-like projections. Acquired haemoglobin H disease, which can be a manifestation of the myelodysplastic syndromes, should also be mentioned in the differential diagnosis of the inherited condition; it is differentiated by the age of onset, the lack of a relevant family history and the demonstration of other features of myelodysplasia (Fig. 8.10).

Further tests

The diagnosis is confirmed by the demonstration of haemoglobin H inclusions in red cells and by haemoglobin electrophoresis which shows 2–40% of haemoglobin H. Haemoglobin electrophoresis will also identify cases with both haemoglobin Constant Spring and haemoglobin H; such cases have the genotype $\alpha^{CS}\alpha/--$ which produces clinical and haematological features similar to haemoglobin H disease although often somewhat more severe.

Haemoglobin Bart's hydrops fetalis

Haemoglobin Bart's hydrops fetalis is a syndrome consequent on an absence of all four α-genes and a consequent total lack of α-chain synthesis. The result is severe anaemia and oedema causing stillbirth or early neonatal death.

Blood film and count

There is severe anaemia and the blood film (Fig. 8.11) shows striking hypochromia, microcytosis, poikilocytosis and the presence of NRBC.

Differential diagnosis

The differential diagnoses include other causes of severe anaemia in the fetus (see Table 6.18) and with other causes of hydrops fetalis.

Further tests

The diagnosis is confirmed by demonstration of α_1-thalassaemia trait in both parents and by haemoglobin electrophoresis which shows only haemoglobins Bart's, H and Portland.

Congenital sideroblastic anaemia

Congenital sideroblastic anaemia is a rare in-

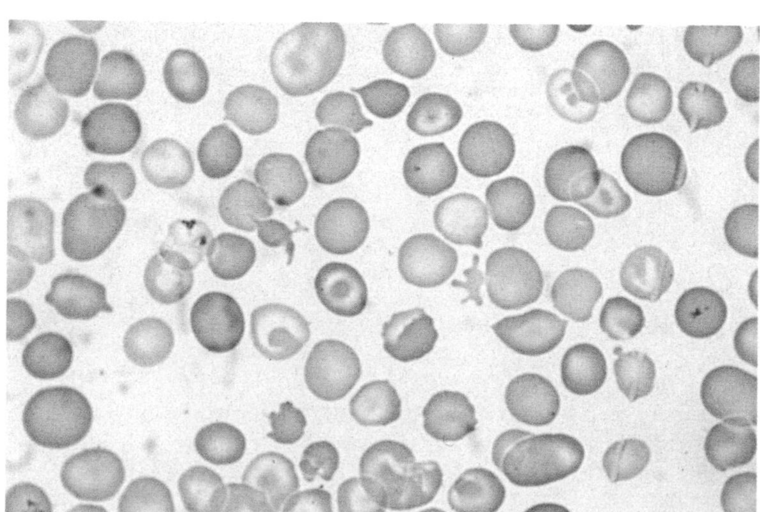

Fig. 8.10 The blood film of a patient with acquired haemoglobin H disease as part of a myelodysplastic syndrome showing anisocytosis, poikilocytosis, microcytosis and some hypochromic cells and target cells. One of the hypochromic cells contains Pappenheimer bodies. The blood count was WBC $9.2 \times 10^9/l$, Hb 10.2 g/dl, MCV 66 fl and platelet count $53 \times 10^9/l$. Courtesy of Dr A. Hendrick, South Shields.

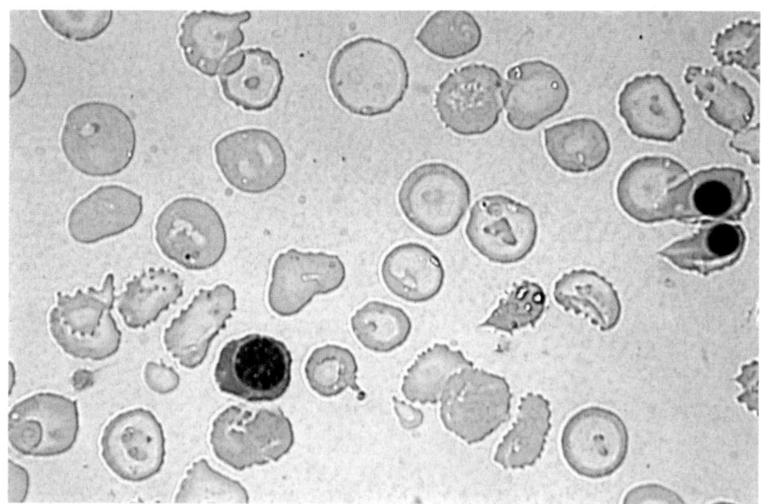

Fig. 8.11 The blood film of neonate with haemoglobin Bart's hydrops fetalis showing anisocytosis, poikilocytosis, many severely hypochromic cells and three NRBC. Courtesy of Professor Harry Smith, Brisbane.

herited condition which, in most families, has a sex-linked inheritance and is therefore largely confined to males. It results from a defect in haem synthesis and is characterized by hypochromia and microcytosis.

Blood film and count

The Hb ranges from 3–4 g/dl to almost normal. The blood film (Fig. 8.12) may be dimorphic or show uniform hypochromia and microcytosis. Occasionally, target cells and basophilic stippling are present. Poikilocytosis is sometimes marked and Pappenheimer bodies may be detectable. In older subjects, hypersplenism due to iron overload may cause mild leucopenia and thrombocytopenia.

The MCV and MCH are reduced and the MCHC is sometimes reduced. Red cell histograms and cytograms may show two populations of red cells.

Female carriers of congenital sideroblastic anaemia who are not themselves anaemic may have a minor population of hypochromic microcytic cells (Fig. 8.13).

Differential diagnosis

The differential diagnosis includes iron-deficiency anaemia and thalassaemia trait. Serum iron and ferritin are normal or elevated and haemoglobin electrophoresis and A_2 concentration are normal. There is usually no difficulty distinguishing between congenital and acquired sideroblastic anaemias since the latter are characterized by predominantly normocytic or macrocytic cells with only a small population of hypochromic microcytes.

Further tests

Diagnosis is by bone marrow aspiration which demonstrates ring sideroblasts. Biochemical assays of enzymes involved in haem synthesis will help to categorize cases further.

Lead poisoning

Excess lead interferes with haem synthesis and also causes haemolysis. Patients with significant haematological effects often have other symptoms and signs of lead poisoning such as constipation and a lead line on the gums.

Blood film and count

Anaemia is usually mild or moderate in severity. The blood film may show hypochromia and microcytosis or normocytic normochromic red cells with some polychromasia. Basophilic stippling is often prominent (Fig. 8.14). Pappenheimer bodies may also be present since lead causes sideroblastic erythropoiesis. The reticulocyte percentage and absolute count may be elevated.

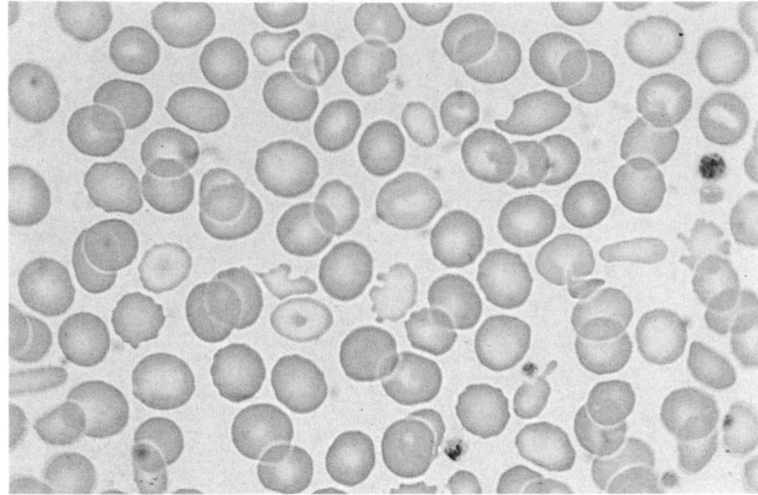

Fig. 8.12 A dimorphic blood film from a patient with congenital sideroblastic anaemia. There is a minor population of cells which are hypochromic and microcytic with a tendency to target cell formation; there is also poikilocytosis. The patient had previously responded to pyridoxine with a rise of Hb and was taking pyridoxine when this blood specimen was obtained.

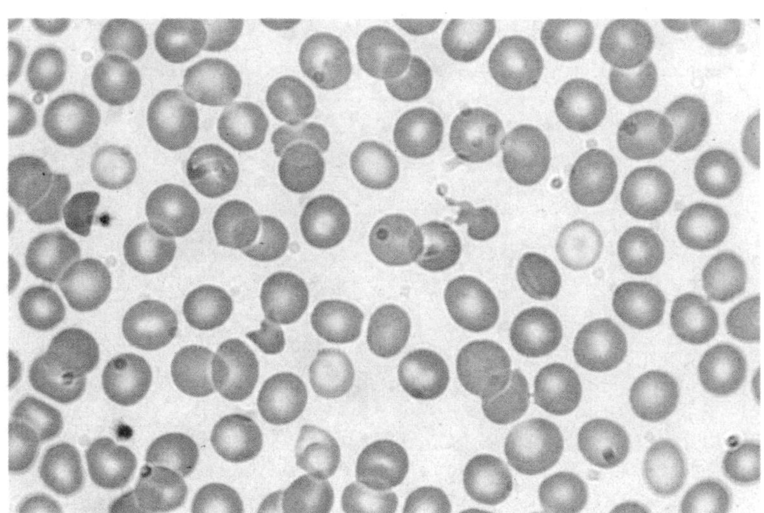

Fig. 8.13 Blood film obtained from a non-anaemic carrier of congenital sideroblastic anaemia, the daughter of a patient with moderately severe microcytic anaemia. The film is dimorphic, showing a minor population of hypochromic microcytes.

Red cell indices may be normal or there may be a reduction in the MCV, MCH and MCHC.

Differential diagnosis

The differential diagnosis includes other causes of hypochromic microcytic anaemia and also haemolytic anaemias, particularly that due to pyrimidine 5′ nucleotidase deficiency in which basophilic stippling is also prominent. It should be noted that lead poisoning and iron deficiency often coexist.

Further tests

Serum lead level is confirmatory.

Haemoglobinopathies

Haemoglobinopathies are inherited abnormalities of globin chain synthesis. Some haematologists use this term broadly to cover all such abnormalities, including the thalassaemias. Others classify disorders of globin chain synthesis as 'haemoglobinopathies' when there is a struc-

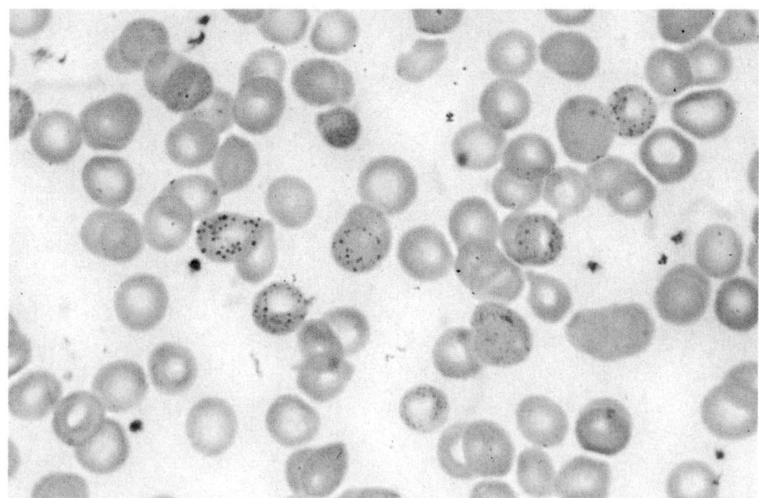

Fig. 8.14 The blood film of a patient with lead poisoning showing anisocytosis, hypochromia and prominent basophilic stippling. The blood count (Coulter S Plus IV) was: RBC $2.99 \times 10^9/l$, Hb 8.3 g/dl, Hct 0.25, MCV 85 fl, MCH 27.8 pg, MCHC 32.7 g/dl and reticulocyte count $281 \times 10^9/l$.

tural abnormality and as 'thalassaemias' when the principal abnormality is a reduced rate of synthesis of one of the globin chains. There is necessarily some overlap between 'haemoglobinopathies' and 'thalassaemias' since some abnormal haemoglobins (e.g., haemoglobin E) are synthesized at a reduced rate. Abnormal haemoglobins may also be formed in thalassaemias as a consequence of unbalanced chain synthesis (e.g., in haemoglobin H disease). Haemoglobinopathies and thalassaemias result from mutations in the genes for the α, β, γ and δ chains of haemoglobin. Mutations of α-genes produce abnormalities affecting haemoglobins A, A_2 and F. Mutations in β-genes affect haemoglobin A, mutations in γ-genes haemoglobin F, and mutations in δ genes haemoglobin A_2. Only mutations affecting α and β genes are important in adult life.

Sickle cell anaemia

Sickle cell anaemia is the disease caused by homozygozity for the β-chain variant haemoglobin, haemoglobin S or sickle cell haemoglobin. The genotype is β^S/β^S. The term 'sickle cell disease' is used more broadly than 'sickle cell anaemia' to include also other conditions which lead to red cell sickling such as sickle cell/β-thalassaemia.

Haemoglobin S is prone to polymerize in conditions of low oxygen tension causing the red cell to become sickle shaped and less deformable. The consequent obstruction of small blood vessels leads to tissue infarction which underlies the dominant clinical feature of the disease, the recurrent painful crises. Other clinical features are anaemia, which is partly caused by shortened red cell life span, and splenomegaly which is present only during childhood.

The β^S gene and therefore sickle cell anaemia have their greatest frequency in black people but the gene also occurs in Indian, Greek, Italian, Turkish, Cypriot, Spanish, Arabic and North African people and subjects from Central and South America.

Blood film and count

In sickle cell anaemia [18] the Hb is usually of the order of 7–8 g/dl, but with a range of 4–11 g/dl or even wider. Higher Hb levels are characteristic of Arabs with sickle cell anaemia. A typical blood film (Fig. 8.15a) shows anisocytosis, anisochromasia, sickle cells (Fig. 8.15b), boat-shaped cells (pointed at both ends but not crescent shaped), target cells, polychromasia, basophilic stippling, NRBC, sometimes occasional irregularly contracted cells and spherocytes and, once infancy is passed, the features of hyposplenism — Howell–Jolly bodies, Pappenheimer bodies and more numerous target cells but not acanthocytes. The reticulocyte count is usually 10–20%. The WBC,

(a)

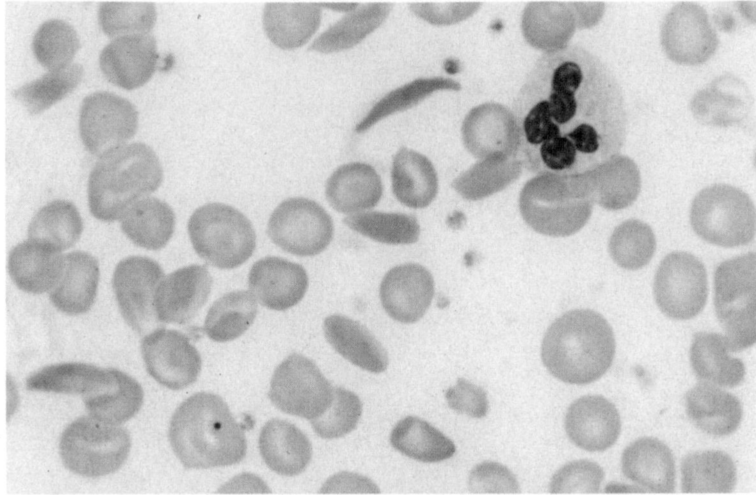

(b)

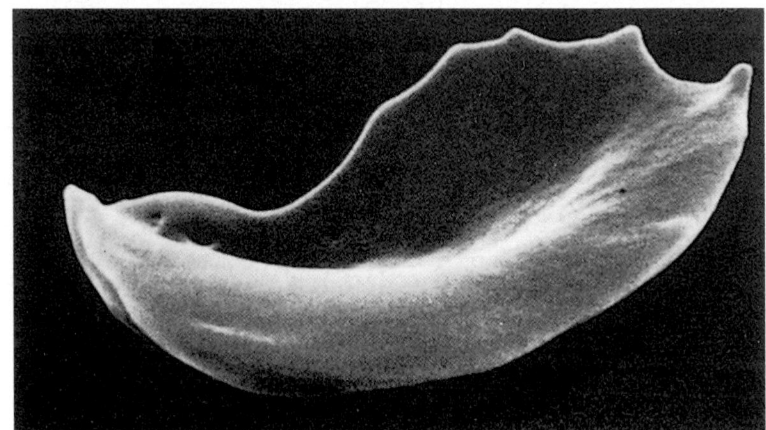

Fig. 8.15 (a) The blood film of a patient with sickle cell anaemia showing anisocytosis, poikilocytosis, one sickle cell, several boat-shaped cells and a cell containing a Howell–Jolly body. (b) Scanning electron micrograph of a sickle cell. From Bessis [96] with permission.

neutrophil count and platelet count are often somewhat elevated.

At birth, when only a small amount of haemoglobin S is present, the Hb, red cell indices and blood count are normal. Haematological abnormalities appear during the first year of life [19, 20]. The Hb falls below the normal range at 1–6 months of age. A few sickle cells and other features of sickle cell anaemia appear at 4–6 months of age; features of hyposplenism usually appear at 9–12 months of age but sometimes as early as 6 months. The features of hyposplenism appear at about the time that splenomegaly is detected. In early infancy hyposplenism is reversible by blood transfusion but later it is not. NRBC only become common after 12 months of age.

Some subjects, although homozygous for β^S, have a normal or near normal Hb and very few signs or symptoms of sickle cell anaemia; they are mainly Arabs with an unusually high percentage of haemoglobin F which is ameliorating the condition. In such subjects the morphological abnormalities may also be slight. When α-thalassaemia trait coexists with sickle cell anaemia there are subtle differences in the red cell indices, but only when groups of patients are considered. Individuals cannot be distinguished on haematological grounds. In a group with coexisting α-thalassaemia trait the mean Hb and RBC are higher, whereas the mean MCV, MCH, MCHC, reticulocyte count and degree of polychromasia and number of sickle cells are less.

During painful crises there is leucocytosis (with the WBC sometimes as high as $40-50 \times 10^9/l$), neutrophilia, a minor fall in the Hb, increasing polychromasia and a rise in the number of NRBC and the reticulocyte count. There is an increase in the number of sickle cells in the blood film but recognition of this requires careful counting and a knowledge of the baseline values for an individual patient.

Because of the shortened red cell survival, patients with sickle cell anaemia are prone to acute worsening of the anaemia when complicating conditions develop. The blood film and count may give some clues as to the cause of this. In acute splenic sequestration, which is largely confined to infants there is a very acute fall of the Hb and the platelet count also falls. Subsequently, there are increased numbers of NRBC, increasing polychromasia and an elevation of the reticulocyte count. In older subjects acute sequestration may involve the liver rather than the spleen. In bone marrow infarction the WBC and platelet count may fall, there are prominent leucoerythroblastic features and some circulating megakaryocytes may be seen. In parvovirus infection white cells and platelets are rarely affected; there is a disappearance of NRBC and polychromasia and the reticulocyte count is very low. During the recovery phase there is an outpouring of NRBC and a rise in WBC, neutrophil count and reticulocyte count. The suppression of reticulocyte production is usually less when other infections lead to the development of anaemia which has the characteristics of the anaemia of chronic disease. In megaloblastic anaemia due to folate deficiency, some circulating megaloblasts, macrocytes and hypersegmented neutrophils may be seen.

The blood count in sickle cell anaemia shows the Hb, RBC and PCV to be reduced. The MCV is normal or elevated but is not increased to a degree commensurate with the increase in the reticulocyte count [21]; this may be regarded as a relative microcytosis. The RDW and HDW are increased. Technicon H.1 series red cell cytograms (Fig. 8.16) show a population of dense cells representing irreversibly sickled cells and a population of hypodense cells representing reticulocytes. Although hyperdense cells are detected their percentage may be underestimated because irreversibly sickled cells are incapable of undergoing the sphering which should occur before measurement of red cell variables by these instruments [22]. Impedance counters fail to detect the increased MCHC of the most dense cells [22]. Further changes in red cell indices occur during, and sometimes 1–3 days before, painful crises [23]. The slight fall in the Hb and rise in the reticulocyte count are accompanied by further increases in the RDW and HDW. There is an increase in the MCHC and the percentage of abnormally dense cells.

Differential diagnosis

The differential diagnosis of sickle cell anaemia is mainly with sickle cell/haemoglobin C disease (see p. 216) and with sickle cell/β thalassaemia. Sickle cell/β^0-thalassaemia cannot be distinguished from sickle cell anaemia on haemoglobin electrophoresis since there is no haemoglobin A in either condition. The distinction is made on the basis of family studies and the lower MCV and MCH in the compound heterozygous state. Sickle cell/β^+-thalassaemia may show a less abnormal blood count and blood film than sickle cell anaemia, depending on the amount of haemoglobin A which is present; haemoglobin electrophoresis is diagnostic. Compound heterozygosity for haemoglobin S and hereditary persistence of fetal haemoglobin can be distinguished by the milder clinical and haematological phenotype, family studies and haemoglobin electrophoresis. Sickle cell trait should not be confused with sickle cell anaemia since the Hb is normal and there are no sickle cells in the blood film but heterozygotes for $HbS_{Antilles}$ may have sickle cells on routine blood films [24].

Further tests

Diagnosis requires a sickle solubility test and haemoglobin electrophoresis. Haemoglobin S predominates with smaller amounts of haemo-

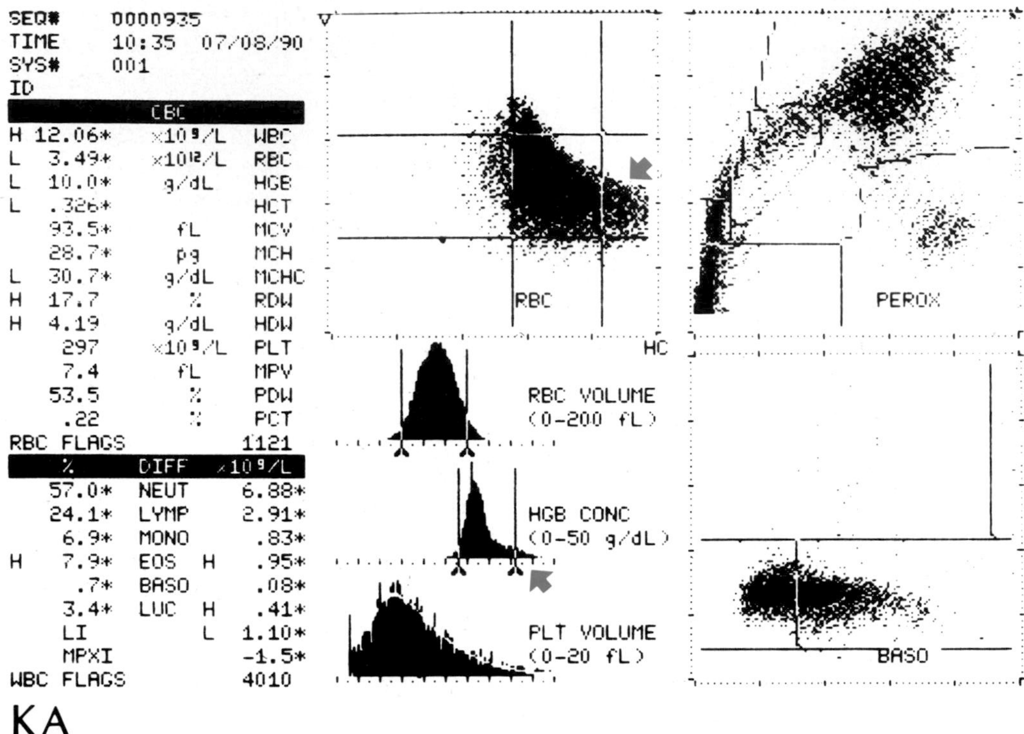

Fig. 8.16 Technicon H.1 red cell scatter plots and histograms of a patient with sickle cell anaemia; the presence of cells with an increased haemoglobin content is apparent on both the red cell cytogram and on the histogram of haemoglobin concentration.

globins F and A_2 and no haemoglobin A. Haemoglobin F varies from 2 to 15% and haemoglobin A_2 may be minimally elevated. It is desirable to perform haemoglobin electrophoresis at acid as well as alkaline pH to distinguish the compound heterozygous states S/D and S/G from sickle cell anaemia; D and G both move with S at alkaline pH but not at acid pH. In infants the percentage of haemoglobin S may be too low for the sickle solubility test to be positive and diagnosis then rests on electrophoresis at acid and alkaline pH.

Sickle cell trait

Sickle cell trait indicates heterozygosity for β^S so that both haemoglobin S and haemoglobin A are present. The genotype is β/β^S. Sickle cell trait does not generally interfere with health but is of genetic significance and is relevant if a patient is likely to become hypoxic.

Blood film and count

The blood film may be normal or show microcytosis or target cell formation. The blood count is either normal or shows reduction of the MCV and MCH. Reduction of the MCV is commoner in those with sickle cell trait than in other black people [25]. Although the microcytosis may be partly due to the slightly higher incidence of α-thalassaemia trait in subjects with sickle cell trait [26], this does not appear sufficient to explain the frequency of microcytosis; it appears that the β^S-gene must also make a contribution to the microcytosis.

Differential diagnosis

The main differential diagnosis is with other causes of microcytosis (Table 3.1) and with other causes of target cell formation (Table 3.7).

Further tests

The blood film and count must not be relied on for diagnosis. Diagnosis requires both haemoglobin electrophoresis (which shows S and A but with the percentage of A being greater than the percentage of S) and a sickle solubility test (which shows that the abnormal haemoglobin is haemoglobin S rather than another abnormal haemoglobin with the same mobility). Haemoglobin S is usually 25–45% of total haemoglobin. Diagnosis in the first 6 months of life, when the haemoglobin S percentage may be too low for a positive sickle solubility test, requires electrophoresis at acid and alkaline pH to confirm the nature of the variant haemoglobin.

Sickle cell/β-thalassaemia

Patients who are heterozygous for haemoglobin S and either β^0- or β^+-thalassaemia cannot be reliably distinguished from sickle cell anaemia on the basis of clinical features although those with β^S/β^+-thalassaemia tend to have milder disease and splenomegaly is more likely to persist beyond early childhood.

Blood film and count

The blood films and counts of compound heterozygotes for haemoglobin S and β-thalassaemia cannot be reliably distinguished from sickle cell anaemia, particularly sickle cell anaemia with coexisting α-thalassaemia trait, but as a group some differences are apparent. Those with β^S/β^0-thalassaemia show more microcytosis and hypochromia than is usual in sickle cell anaemia and Pappenheimer bodies may be more prominent (Fig. 8.17). Otherwise blood films are similar. The blood films of compound heterozygotes with β^S/β^+-thalassaemia generally show less marked abnormalities, depending on the levels of haemoglobin A and haemoglobin F; target cells are numerous but sickle cells are less frequent. When there is persistent splenomegaly leucopenia and thrombocytopenia can occur as a consequence of hypersplenism.

The blood counts in compound heterozygotes, particularly those with β^S/β^+-thalassaemia, as a group show a higher Hb, RBC and PCV and a lower MCV, MCH, MCHC, reticulocyte percentage and reticulocyte absolute count [27,28].

Differential diagnosis

The differential diagnosis is with sickle cell anaemia and sickle cell/haemoglobin C disease.

Further tests

The diagnosis of β^S/β^+-thalassaemia can be confirmed by haemoglobin electrophoresis which

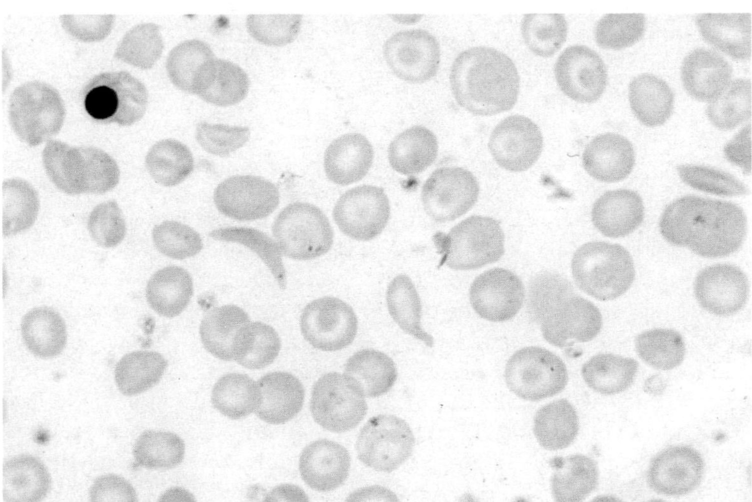

Fig. 8.17 The blood film of a patient with sickle cell/β^0-thalassaemia compound heterozygosity showing anisocytosis, poikilocytosis, one sickle cell, one boat-shaped cell and a NRBC. Many of the red cells contain Pappenheimer bodies.

demonstrates haemoglobins S and A but, in contrast to sickle cell trait, the S percentage is higher than the A percentage. Haemoglobin F may also be increased but does not usually exceed 10–15%. β^S/β^0-thalassaemia cannot be readily distinguished from sickle cell anaemia by haemoglobin electrophoresis since in neither condition is there any haemoglobin A. Diagnosis of cases with microcytosis and haemoglobins S and F requires family studies and, if necessary, DNA analysis.

Haemoglobin S/hereditary persistence of fetal haemoglobin (HPFH) compound heterozygosity

Patients with compound heterozygosity for haemoglobin S and pancellular HPFH, β^S/HPFH genotype, have a mild clinical condition in which painful crises are infrequent or absent.

Blood film and count

The haemoglobin is normal. Cells are normocytic and normochromic and features of hyposplenism are usually absent. There is anisocytosis, target cells are present and there are infrequent sickle cells.

The blood count is normal or shows very minor abnormalities.

Differential diagnosis

The differential diagnosis is with sickle cell anaemia and sickle cell/β-thalassaemia. The blood film shows much less abnormality than in either of the other conditions.

Further tests

Haemoglobin electrophoresis shows haemoglobin S and haemoglobin F. F constitutes 20–30% of total haemoglobin. The F percentage is higher than in S/β-thalassaemia compound heterozygotes who have haemoglobin F levels of less than 15%, usually less than 10%. The F percentage is also higher than in sickle cell anaemia in which levels of 0.5–15% are usual although some Arab patients with sickle cell anaemia and a hereditary ability to increase the haemoglobin F percentage in response to anaemia have intermediate levels.

Sickle cell/haemoglobin C disease

Haemoglobin C is a β-chain variant which originated in West Africa, west of the Niger river, and is also present in some West Indians and black Americans and, rarely, in other ethnic groups such as North Africans, Sicilian, Italians and Spaniards. Compound heterozygotes for haemoglobin S and haemoglobin C, genotype β^S/β^C, have a sickling disorder of very variable severity, ranging from virtually asymptomatic to a severity comparable with that of sickle cell anaemia. Splenomegaly is present in childhood and may persist into adult life.

Blood film and count

In sickle cell/haemoglobin C disease the Hb is higher than in sickle cell anaemia with little overlap, levels of 8–14 g/dl being seen in women and 8–17 g/dl in men [27]. Sickle cell/haemoglobin C disease can usually be distinguished from sickle cell anemia on the basis of the blood film (Fig. 8.18) although it may not always be possible to distinguish it from haemoglobin C disease [29]. There are few sickle cells and, in comparison with sickle cell anaemia, fewer NRBC, less polychromasia and less evidence of hyposplenism which tends to develop later in life. Target cells and boat-shaped cells are numerous. Irregularly contracted cells are more prominent and many patients have unusual poikilocytes which are specific to sickle cell/haemoglobin C disease; these resemble sickle cells in being dense and having some degree of curvature but they differ in that they have some straight edges or are angulated or branched [29,30]. Specific SC poikilocytes are sometimes present in large numbers but more often they are infrequent. Rare cells containing haemoglobin C crystals can also be found in a significant minority of patients.

A sudden fall in Hb may be due to superimposed megaloblastic anaemia, bone marrow necrosis or pure red cell aplasia. Megaloblastic anaemia and bone marrow necrosis are particularly likely during pregnancy. When these conditions are suspected as a complication of sickle cell/haemoglobin C disease, the same features should be sought as were described under sickle cell anaemia.

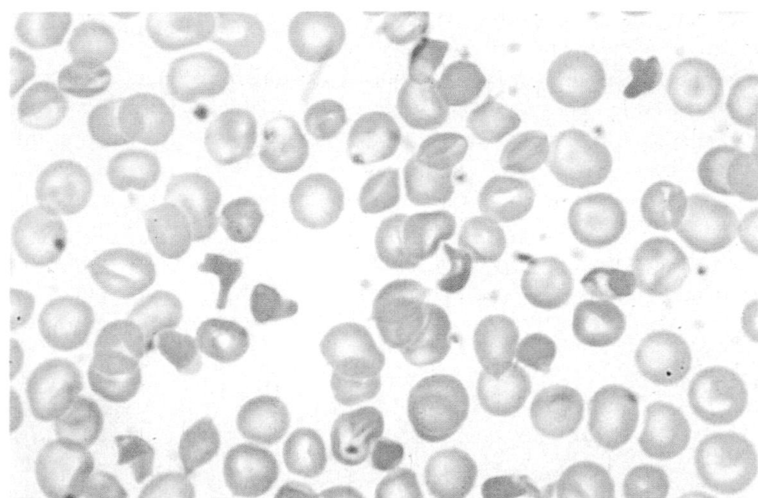

Fig. 8.18 The blood film of a patient with sickle cell/haemoglobin C compound heterozygosity showing numerous specific S/C poikilocytes.

The Hb, RBC and PCV are higher than in sickle cell anaemia. The MCV is generally lower and may be below the normal range, even in those who do not have coexisting thalassaemia trait [31]. The MCHC is higher than in sickle cell disease, often falling above the normal range, and red cell cytograms identify a population of hyperdense cells. The RDW and HDW are increased. The reticulocyte count is lower, averaging 3% in contrast with 10% in sickle cell anaemia [18].

Haemoglobin C disease

Homozygotes for haemoglobin C, genotype β^C/β^C, have chronic haemolysis and usually haemolytic anaemia. The spleen is enlarged and the incidence of gallstones is increased.

Blood film and count

There is usually a mild to moderate anaemia. The blood film generally shows large numbers of both target cells and irregularly contracted cells (Fig. 8.19). The latter cells resemble spherocytes but closer inspection shows that the majority are irregular in shape. Polychromasia and some NRBC may be noted. Some patients have hypochromia and microcytosis. Haemoglobin C crystals are uncommon but when present are sufficiently distinctive to confirm the presence of this haemoglobin. They are rhomboidal with parallel sides and triangular or obliquely sloping ends (see below). They are usually contained in a cell which appears otherwise to be empty of haemoglobin. A minority of patients have a lesser degree of blood film abnormality with smaller numbers of target cells and irregularly contracted cells.

The Hb, RBC and PCV are normal or mildly to moderately reduced. A marked reduction of MCV and MCH is common with the MCHC being increased [31]. The low MCV and MCH occur even in the absence of coexisting α-thalassaemia trait. The RDW and HDW are increased and red cell cytograms show a population of hyperdense cells. The reticulocyte count is increased.

Differential diagnosis

The differential diagnosis is with sickle cell/haemoglobin C disease and haemoglobin C/β-thalassaemia compound heterozygosity. The blood film of haemoglobin C trait is occasionally sufficiently abnormal to resemble that of milder cases of haemoglobin C disease.

Further tests

The diagnosis can usually be strongly suspected from the blood film but confirmation requires haemoglobin electrophoresis which shows haemoglobin C and small amounts of haemoglobin F. In microcytic cases family studies are needed

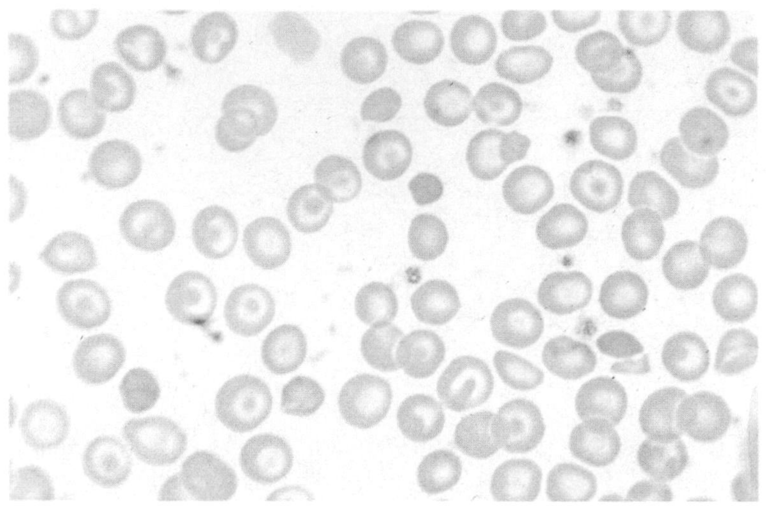

Fig. 8.19 The blood film of a patient with haemoglobin C disease showing a mixture of irregularly contracted cells and target cells.

to make the distinction from compound heterozygosity for haemoglobin C and β^0-thalassaemia.

Haemoglobin C trait

Haemoglobin C trait, genotype β/β^C, is an asymptomatic abnormality of no significance apart from the possibility of more severe disease in offspring.

Blood film and count

The haemoglobin is normal. The blood film (Fig. 8.20) may be normal or may show target cells, varying from occasional to frequent, or occasional irregularly contracted cells. Red cells are often hypochromic and microcytic, even in the absence of coexisting α-thalassaemia trait [31]. The reticulocyte count is normal. The blood count is either normal or shows a reduced MCV and MCH.

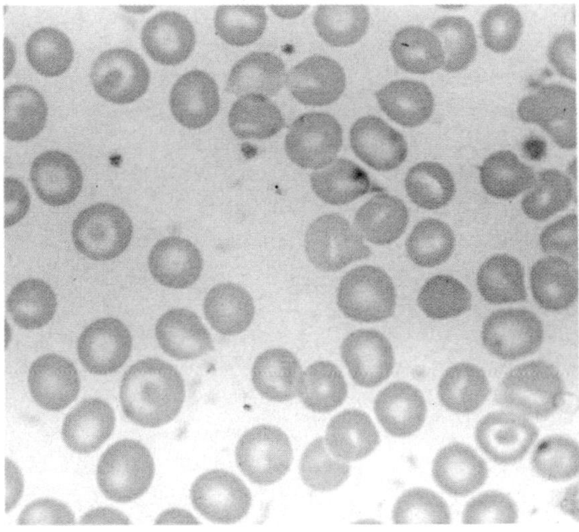

Fig. 8.20 The blood film of a patient with haemoglobin C trait showing several target cells.

Differential diagnosis

The differential diagnosis is with other causes of target cells (see Table 3.7) and sometimes with other causes of irregularly contracted cells (see Table 3.4).

Further tests

Since the blood film and blood count may be normal, haemoglobin electrophoresis is required to confirm or exclude haemoglobin C trait. Haemoglobin electrophoresis is therefore indicated if genetic counselling is required in West Africans, West Indians or black Americans, even when a negative sickle solubility test has excluded the presence of haemoglobin S.

Haemoglobin C/β-thalassaemia

The compound heterozygous state for haemoglobin C and β^0- or β^+-thalassaemia may be symptomatic because of anaemia.

Blood film and count

There is a moderate anaemia. The blood film (Fig. 8.21) shows microcytosis, hypochromia, target cells and irregularly contracted cells. Haemoglobin C crystals may be present. The blood count shows reduction of the Hb, RBC, PCV, MCV and MCH.

Differential diagnosis

The differential diagnosis is with haemoglobin C disease and various thalassaemic conditions.

Further tests

The diagnosis is dependent on haemoglobin electrophoresis, if necessary supplemented by family studies to distinguish haemoglobin C disease from haemoglobin C/β^0-thalassaemia.

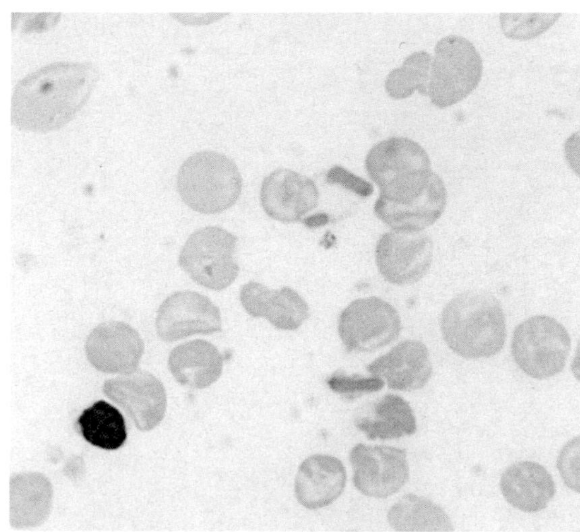

Fig. 8.21 The blood film of a patient with haemoglobin C/β^0-compound heterozygosity showing crystals of haemoglobin C within cells which otherwise appear empty of haemoglobin.

Haemoglobin E disease

Haemoglobin E is a β-chain variant which is common in Thailand, Myanmar, Laos, Cambodia, Vietnam and Malaysia and to a lesser extent in other countries in South-East Asia stretching from Indonesia to Nepal. It has a very low frequency in white and black people. Haemoglobin E disease, genotype β^E/β^E, is usually asymptomatic [32].

Blood film and count

There is a mild anaemia or a normal haemoglobin. The blood film (Fig. 8.22) shows hypochromia and microcytosis, a variable number of target cells and sometimes irregularly contracted cells. The reticulocyte count is usually normal. The blood count is often similar to that of β-thalassaemia trait with a mild anaemia or a normal Hb, elevated RBC and reduced MCV and MCH.

Differential diagnosis

The differential diagnosis is with haemoglobin E/β-thalassaemia compound heterozygosity, β thalassaemia trait and iron deficiency. Haemoglobin C disease would also be included in the differential diagnosis were it not for the fact that there is very little overlap between the ethnic groups in which these two haemoglobinopathies occur. Haemoglobin E/β^0-thalassaemia often has a greater degree of anaemia and microcytosis than does haemoglobin E disease and also more NRBC. Haemoglobin E/β^+-thalassaemia and the other conditions included in the differential diagnosis are excluded by haemoglobin electrophoresis.

Further tests

Diagnosis requires haemoglobin electrophoresis which shows mainly haemoglobin E with 5–10% haemoglobin F. Haemoglobin E has the same mobility as haemoglobin C at alkaline pH and the same mobility as haemoglobin A at acid pH.

Haemoglobin E trait

Haemoglobin E trait, genotype β/β^E, is a completely asymptomatic condition which is only of importance because of its potential genetic significance.

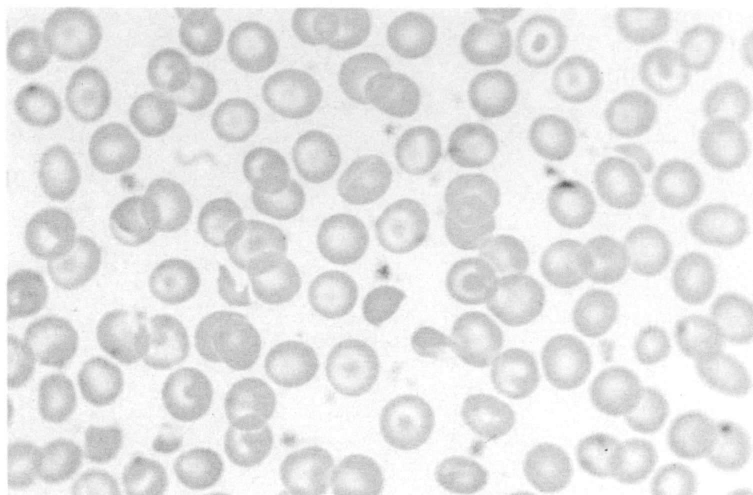

Fig. 8.22 The blood film of a patient with haemoglobin E disease showing hypochromia, microcytosis, target cells and occasional irregularly contracted cells and other poikilocytes. The blood count (Coulter S) was: RBC $6.84 \times 10^9/l$, Hb 11.9 g/dl, Hct 0.37, MCV 54 fl, MCH 17.4 pg, MCHC 26.7 g/dl.

Blood film and count

The blood film (Fig. 8.23) may be normal or show microcytosis or a few target or irregularly contracted cells.

The blood count may be normal or may show a minor reduction of MCV and MCH with a normal Hb.

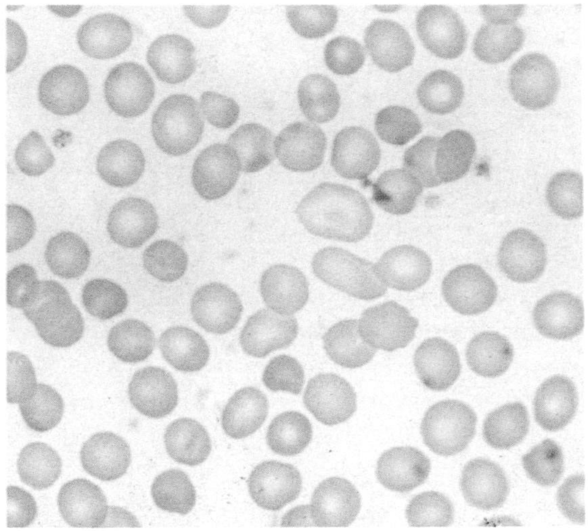

Fig. 8.23 The blood film of a patient with haemoglobin E trait showing hypochromia, microcytosis and occasional irregularly contracted cells. The blood count (Coulter S Plus IV) was: RBC $4.39 \times 10^9/l$, Hb 11 g/dl, Hct 0.32, MCV 74 fl, MCH 25.1 pg, MCHC 33.2 g/dl.

Differential diagnosis

The differential diagnosis is with mild iron deficiency or β-thalassaemia trait.

Further tests

Diagnosis is dependent on haemoglobin electrophoresis which shows haemoglobin E and haemoglobin A but with haemoglobin E being only about one-third of total haemoglobin because of its diminished rate of synthesis.

Haemoglobin E/β-thalassaemia

Haemoglobin E/β-thalassaemia compound heterozygosity, genotype β^E/β^0- or β^E/β^+-thalassaemia, is in general more severe than haemoglobin E disease. It occurs in South-East Asia and in India. Severity varies from a mild anaemia to a condition resembling thalassaemia intermedia or thalassaemia major with anaemia, hepatomegaly and splenomegaly.

Blood film and count

Anaemia is usually moderate with an Hb of

7–9 g/dl though it varies from 2 to 13 g/dl [33]. Marked hypochromia and microcytosis are usual. Red cells of some cases show basophilic stippling, anisocytosis and poikilocytosis. Poikilocytes may include target cells, keratocytes, tear drop cells, fragments and irregularly contracted cells. The reticulocyte percentage is increased and some NRBC may be present. The Hb, RBC, PCV, MCV and MCH are all reduced and often also the MCHC.

Complicating conditions which may affect the blood film and count are aplastic crisis, megaloblastic anaemia and hypersplenism.

Differential diagnosis

The differential diagnosis is with haemoglobin E disease and various thalassaemic conditions.

Further tests

Diagnosis is dependent on haemoglobin electrophoresis which may need to be supplemented by family studies. In haemoglobin E/β^0-thalassaemia electrophoresis shows haemoglobin E and haemoglobin F with F levels varying from less than 10% to well over 50%. In haemoglobin E/β^+-thalassaemia there is also haemoglobin A, usually constituting around 30% of total haemoglobin.

Unstable haemoglobins

Heterozygosity for an unstable haemoglobin produces mild, moderate or severe haemolytic anaemia, depending on the severity of the molecular defect. Haemolysis may be chronic or precipitated or aggravated by infection or exposure to oxidant drugs. The spleen is sometimes enlarged and patients may pass dark urine after episodes of haemolysis. Some unstable haemoglobins also have a high oxygen affinity and can therefore cause polycythaemia.

Blood film and count

The Hb varies from normal to markedly reduced, in cases with normal oxygen affinity, whereas the less common cases with a high affinity unstable haemoglobin may have an elevated Hb. In some patients the blood film is normal or shows only macrocytosis associated with an elevated reticulocyte count. In others there is anisocytosis, poikilocytosis, hypochromia, or variable numbers of irregularly contracted cells (Fig. 8.24), 'bite cells', basophilic stippling and polychromasia. During haemolytic crises features of hyposplenism may appear. Non-splenectomized subjects may be thrombocytopenic, sometimes to a degree which seems out of proportion to the expected degree of hypersplenism.

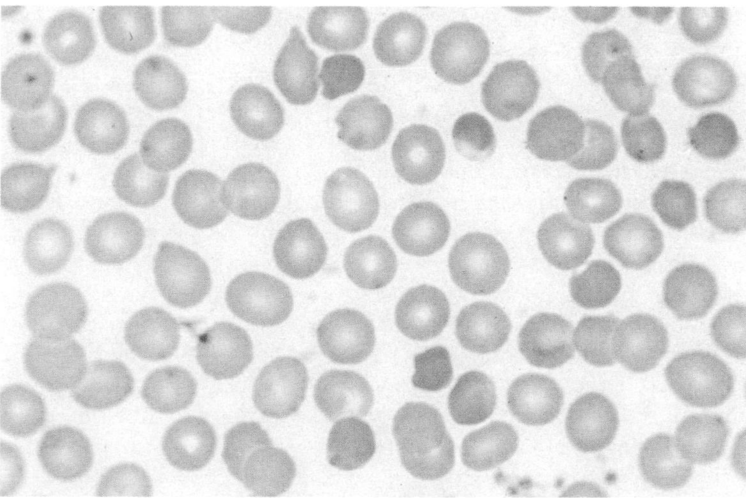

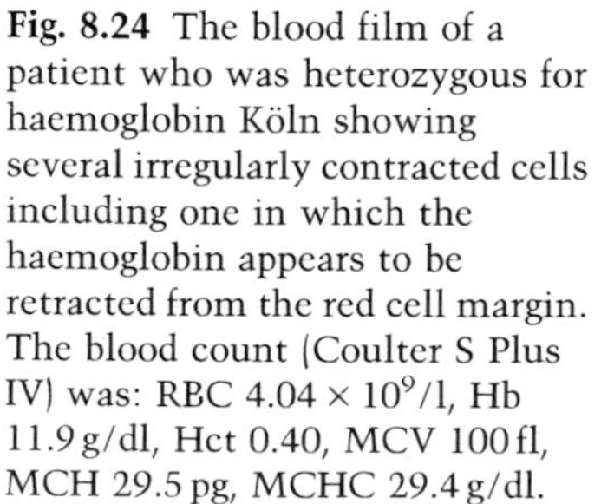

Fig. 8.24 The blood film of a patient who was heterozygous for haemoglobin Köln showing several irregularly contracted cells including one in which the haemoglobin appears to be retracted from the red cell margin. The blood count (Coulter S Plus IV) was: RBC 4.04×10^9/l, Hb 11.9 g/dl, Hct 0.40, MCV 100 fl, MCH 29.5 pg, MCHC 29.4 g/dl.

The FBC shows a reduced Hb, elevated MCV and RDW, and often reduced MCH and MCHC, the latter abnormalities as a consequence of removal of Heinz bodies by the spleen. In some cases a discrepancy has been noted between lowered MCH and MCHC and a lack of hypochromia in the blood film. This has been attributed to the fact that an unstable haemoglobin may lose some of its haem groups; the staining of red cells is attributable to their globin content whereas the biochemical measurement of Hb requires the presence of haem [34]. The reticulocyte count is elevated, sometimes out of proportion to the degree of anaemia. This occurs if an unstable haemoglobin also has an increased oxygen affinity.

Differential diagnosis

The differential diagnosis is with other causes of irregularly contracted cells and with other causes of haemolytic anaemia.

Further tests

Heinz bodies are detected following splenectomy and during haemolytic crises in some non-splenectomized patients. The definitive test is a test for an unstable haemoglobin such as a heat or isopropanol instability test. Haemoglobin electrophoresis should also be performed although it is not necessarily abnormal.

Macrocytic anaemias

Macrocytic anaemias result from abnormal erythropoiesis which may be either megaloblastic or macronormoblastic. Megaloblastic erythropoiesis is characterized by dyserythropoiesis, increased size of erythroid precursors and asynchronous maturation of nucleus and cytoplasm so that cytoplasmic maturation is in advance of nuclear maturation. Macronormoblastic anaemia is characterized by increased size of erythroid precursors with or without other features of dyserythropoiesis. The commonest causes of macrocytic anaemia are excess alcohol intake, liver disease, megaloblastic anaemia and the myelodysplastic syndromes.

Megaloblastic anaemia

Megaloblastic anaemia is usually consequent on deficiency of vitamin B_{12} or folic acid or on the administration of drugs which interfere with DNA synthesis (see Table 3.2). Certain rare congenital defects in the absorption, transport or metabolism of vitamin B_{12} or folic acid can also cause megaloblastic anaemia. Excess alcohol intake may be complicated by dietary folic acid deficiency but alcohol can produce macrocytosis even in the absence of folate deficiency; in these cases erythropoiesis may be macronormoblastic or mildly megaloblastic. Megaloblastic erythropoiesis can also occur in the myelodysplastic syndromes (see p. 285) and in erythroleukaemia.

Blood film and count

The haematological features of vitamin B_{12} and folate deficiency are indistinguishable. Characteristic blood film features (Figs 8.25 & 8.26) are anaemia, macrocytosis, anisocytosis, poikilocytosis (including the presence of oval macrocytes and tear drop cells) and neutrophil hypersegmentation. The macrocytes have increased thickness as well as diameter and central pallor is therefore lacking. There may also be occasional hypersegmented eosinophils, macropolycytes and basophilic stippling. As anaemia becomes more severe there is increasing anisocytosis and poikilocytosis with the appearance of microcytes and fragments. Small numbers of Howell–Jolly bodies and circulating megaloblasts and granulocyte precursors may appear. The WBC and platelet count fall with the development of moderate neutropenia and mild lymphopenia. There is usually no polychromasia despite severe anaemia and the reticulocyte count is low. When megaloblastic anaemia develops acutely there may be a sudden failure of bone marrow output of cells. There is pancytopenia with a normal MCV and with few or no macrocytes or hypersegmented neutrophils. Polychromasia is absent and the reticulocyte count is very low. Such 'megaloblastic arrest' is seen in acutely ill patients, often in association with pregnancy, surgery or sepsis. In patients with minimal haematological features of vitamin B_{12} or folic acid deficiency, e.g., some

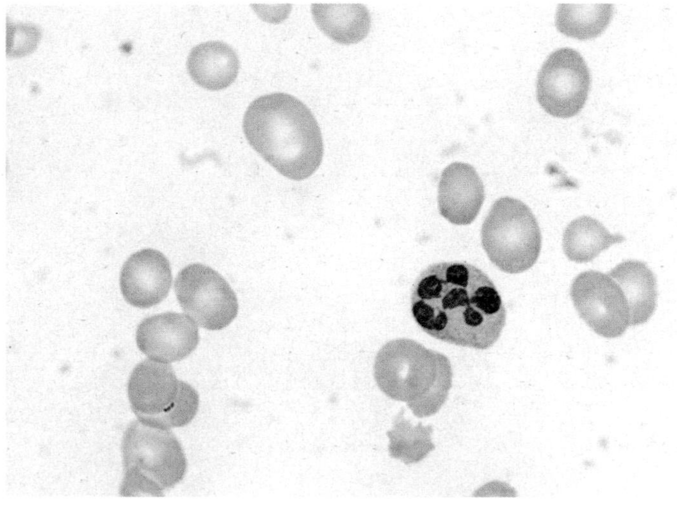

Fig. 8.25 The blood film of an elderly woman with both malabsorption of vitamin B_{12} and dietary deficiency of folic acid showing marked anisocytosis, macrocytosis, several oval macrocytes, a tear drop poikilocyte and a hypersegmented neutrophil. The blood count (Coulter S Plus IV) was: WBC $4.2 \times 10^9/l$, RBC $0.76 \times 10^9/l$, Hb 3.6 g/dl, Hct 0.10 MCV 133 fl, MCH 47.4 pg, MCHC 35.6 g/dl, platelet count $50 \times 10^9/l$.

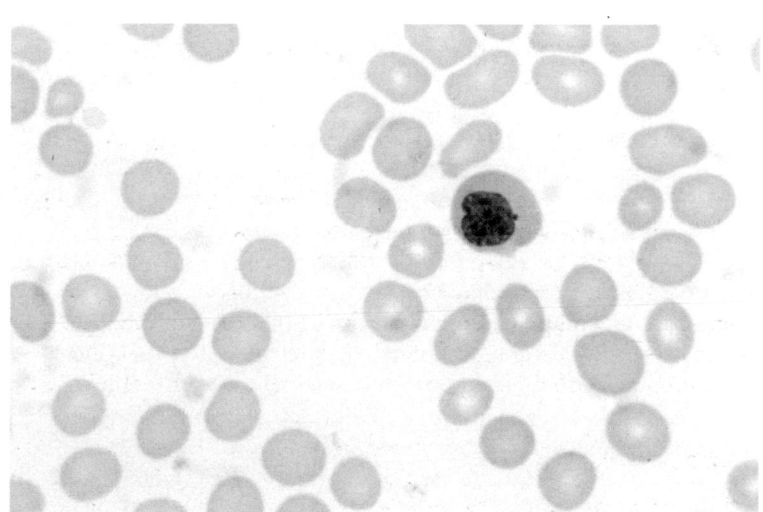

Fig. 8.26 The blood film of a patient with pernicious anaemia showing macrocytosis and a circulating megaloblast.

patients presenting with the neurological complications of vitamin B_{12} deficiency, the only haematological features may be occasional round or oval macrocytes and occasional hypersegmented neutrophils. Sometimes macrocytosis is associated with prominent features of hyposplenism, particularly with the presence of Pappenheimer bodies and with large and numerous Howell–Jolly bodies (Fig. 8.27); in a patient who has not had a splenectomy this suggests underlying coeliac disease with splenic atrophy as the cause of vitamin B_{12} or, more often, folate deficiency.

Megaloblastic anaemia consequent on folic acid antagonists such as methotrexate is indistinguishable from that due to vitamin B_{12} or folate deficiency but there are subtle differences when megaloblastosis is caused by other drugs which interfere more directly with DNA synthesis. When they are administered over a long period of time there may be striking macrocytosis with or without anaemia. Sometimes there is also

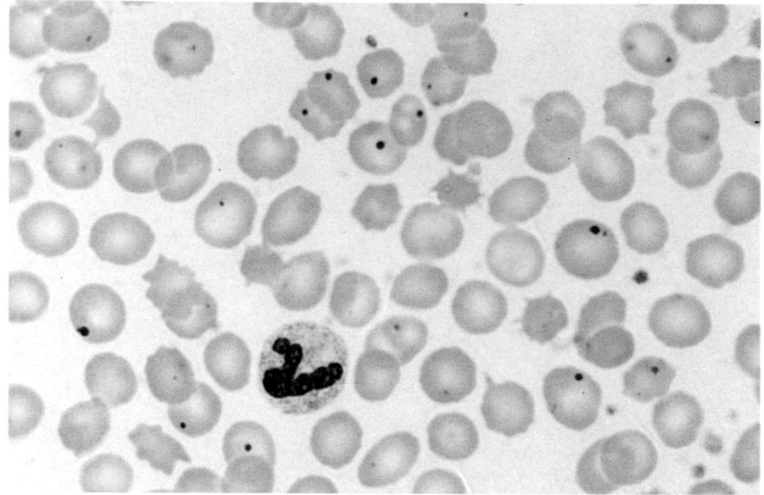

Fig. 8.27 The blood film of a splenectomized post-renal transplant patient with megaloblastic anaemia caused by azathioprine therapy showing macrocytosis, acanthocytes and prominent Howell–Jolly bodies.

stomatocytosis. Hypersegmented neutrophils are much less common than in the deficiency states.

When iron deficiency coexists with deficiency of either vitamin B_{12} or folic acid, blood film features are variable. There may be hypochromic microcytes in addition to macrocytes or the blood film features of iron deficiency may dominate with only the presence of hypersegmented neutrophils suggesting a possible double deficiency. Hypersegmented neutrophils may, however, be seen in uncomplicated iron deficiency and for other reasons (see p. 68). Iron deficiency is sometimes unmasked when vitamin B_{12} or folic acid treatment is given to a patient with megaloblastic anaemia and inadequate iron stores. Following an initial rise of Hb and the production of well haemoglobinized cells iron stores are exhausted, hypochromic microcytes are produced and the blood film becomes dimorphic. Thalassaemia trait, like iron deficiency, can prevent the development of macrocytosis in megaloblastic anaemia. The MCV may rise into the normal range rather than above it.

When effective treatment is given to a patient with megaloblastic anaemia there is a lag phase of a few days and then a rise in the WBC and platelet count, followed by the production of polychromatic macrocytes and then a rise in Hb. If the patient has been pancytopenic there may be a rebound thrombocytosis, often associated with left shift or a leucoerythroblastic blood film. Hypersegmented neutrophils persist in the blood for 5–7 days or even longer and in those who were cytopenic they may actually increase.

The blood count in megaloblastic anaemia shows reduction in the Hb, PCV and RBC. There is a parallel increase in the MCV and MCH. The MCHC is normal and the RDW increased. The increase in RDW precedes a rise in the MCV. As anaemia becomes more severe the presence of severe poikilocytosis with red cell fragmentation may lead to a paradoxical decrease of the MCV; the RDW is then very high. On Technicon instruments megaloblastic anaemia is associated with an increased HDW, an increased MPXI (indicating an increased mean peroxidase activity of neutrophils) and a reduction of the lobularity index (indicating an immature structure of nuclear chromatin) [35] (Fig. 8.28). On impedance counters the MPV remains relatively low when thrombocytopenia is caused by megaloblastic anaemia whereas it is increased when thrombocytopenia is consequent on decreased platelet lifespan [36].

The various methods of assessing neutrophil hypersegmentation are discussed on p. 68. In a study comparing B_{12} or folate-deficient patients who had megaloblastic erythropoiesis with patients who were not vitamin deficient the index proposed by Edwin was found to be the most sensitive indicator of megaloblastosis [35]. Next most sensitive was the percentage of neutrophils with at least five lobes. In equal third place were

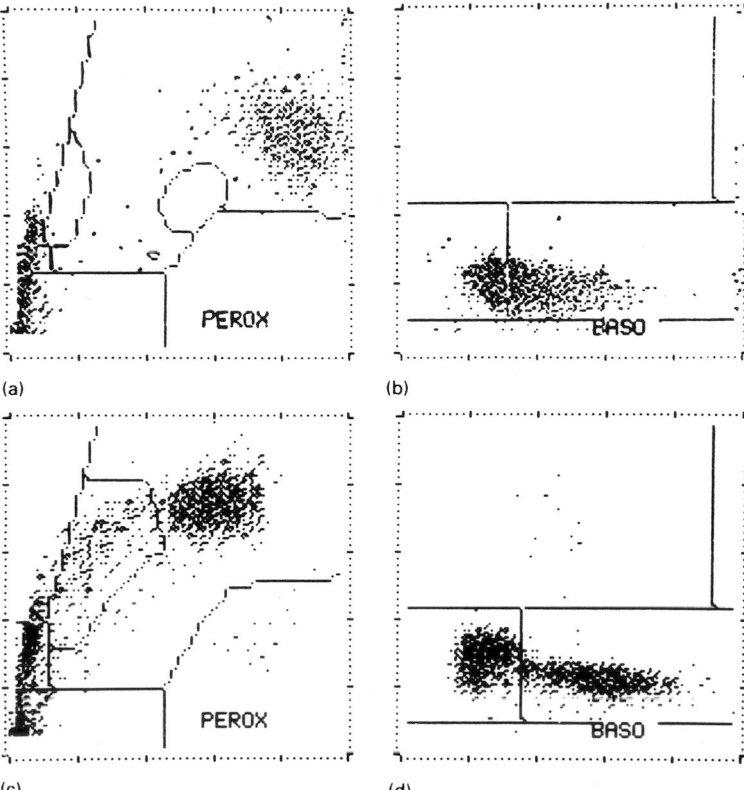

Fig. 8.28 Technicon H.1 scatter plots of the peroxidase channel and basophil/lobularity channels in a patient with megaloblastic anaemia (a, b) and a normal subject (c, d). In the peroxidase channel the neutrophil cluster is displaced to the right indicating a high peroxidase activity which is reflected in a high MPXI. In the basophil lobularity channel the abnormal chromatin structure of the neutrophils has led to a loss of the normal valley between the mononuclear cluster (left) and the granulocyte cluster (right) which is reflected in a low 'lobularity index'.

the mean lobe count (Arneth score), the presence of neutrophils with at least six lobes and an elevated MPXI on the Technicon H.1 counter.

Differential diagnosis

The differential diagnosis is with other causes of macrocytosis (see Table 3.2). An increased RDW [2] and increased MPXI [37] have been found of some use in separating megaloblastic anaemia from other causes of macrocytosis in which these parameters are less often abnormal. Blood film features are also useful. In macrocytosis due to liver disease and chronic alcohol abuse macrocytes are round rather than oval, hypersegmented neutrophils are absent and there may be other abnormalities (see below). In macrocytosis due to the myelodysplastic syndromes (see p. 285) there may be dysplastic neutrophils or a population of hypochromic microcytes consequent on sideroblastic erythropoiesis and in a minority there is thrombocytosis. In chronic haemolytic anaemia macrocytosis may be marked but polychromasia is usually apparent. The blood film features are very important in the identification of congenital dyserythropoietic anaemia as a cause of macrocytosis (see p. 254).

Further tests

The peripheral blood features of severe megaloblastic anaemia are so characteristic that the diagnosis is often obvious from the blood film and count. A bone marrow aspiration is confirmatory. Tests which are useful in distinguishing between vitamin B_{12} or folic acid deficiency are serum B_{12} and red cell folate assays and a test of B_{12} absorption (Schilling test). Tests for intrinsic factor antibodies are useful in confirming the diagnosis of pernicious anaemia, the commonest cause of vitamin B_{12} deficiency, and may obviate the need for a Schilling test. Parietal cell antibodies are also usually present in pernicious anaemia but are less specific than intrinsic factor antibodies.

Macrocytic anaemia associated with excess alcohol intake and liver disease

Both excess alcohol intake and chronic liver disease can cause macrocytic anaemia. The two aetiologies often coexist. Associated leucopenia and thrombocytopenia are common, caused either by the effect of alcohol on the bone marrow or by hypersplenism associated with chronic liver disease.

Blood film and count

The blood film shows macrocytosis with the macrocytes being predominantly round rather than oval. Anisocytosis and poikilocytosis are less than in megaloblastic anaemia and there may be associated target cells and stomatocytes. There may be leucopenia and thrombocytopenia but hypersegmented neutrophils are not present. In chronic liver disease rouleaux formation is increased as a consequence of increased concentration of immunoglobulins. Patients with acute alcoholic liver disease may also suffer from haemolytic anaemia with spherocytes (or, more likely, irregularly contracted cells) and associated hyperlipidaemia. Patients with advanced liver failure from any cause may suffer 'spur cell haemolytic anaemia', characterized by acanthocytosis.

The Hb, RBC and PCV are reduced. The MCV and MCH are increased. The MCHC is normal and the RDW is often normal.

Differential diagnosis

The differential diagnosis is mainly with megaloblastic anaemia, particularly that due to dietary folate deficiency in 'Skid Row' alcoholics.

Other tests

Red cell folate is normal or low. Serum B_{12} is increased as a consequence of release of transcobalamin II from the damaged liver. A normal bone marrow deoxyuridine suppression test is useful for excluding significant deficiency of vitamin B_{12} or folic acid in alcoholics with macrocytosis.

Haemolytic anaemias

Congenital haemolytic anaemias

Congenital haemolytic anaemias are usually consequent on inherited abnormalities of the red cell membrane, haemoglobin or red cell enzymes. Enzyme deficiencies are mainly those of the glycolytic pathway, which are concerned with the energy requirements of the cell, and those of the pentose shunt, which protect the cell from oxidant damage. Congenital haemolytic anaemias of these types persist throughout life. Congenital haemolytic anaemia can also be acquired *in utero*, e.g., haemolytic disease of the newborn caused by ABO or rhesus incompatibility, in which case it is a transient disorder. Haemolysis associated with abnormal haemoglobins has been discussed above (see pp. 216 and 221). Red cell membrane and enzyme abnormalities will be discussed here. The structure of the normal red cell membrane, which is a lipid bilayer supported by a cytoskeleton, has been discussed on p. 47.

Hereditary spherocytosis

Hereditary spherocytosis is a heterogeneous group of disorders, most of which show autosomal dominant inheritance. Hereditary spherocytosis occurs in various ethnic groups including white, black and Japanese subjects. The prevalence in white people is at least one in 5000. Most cases of the common autosomal dominant hereditary spherocytosis are associated with spectrin deficiency or a combined deficiency of spectrin and ankyrin [38,39]. Less commonly there is band 3 deficiency [39] or, in a minority of cases, a deficiency or abnormality of band 4.2. The uncommon autosomal recessive forms of hereditary spherocytosis have been associated with mutations of the α- or β-spectrin genes or the protein 4.2 gene. The mechanism of spherocytosis is that a deficiency of spectrin, either primary or secondary to an abnormality of ankyrin, leads to reduced density of the cytoskeleton and consequent instability of unsupported areas of the lipid bilayer. There is then loss of lipid as vesicles from the destabilized membrane, *in vitro* and probably *in vivo*, leading to spherocytosis. Abnormalities of band 3 are also associated with accelerated membrane loss and hence formation of spherocytes.

Blood film and count

Depending on the specific genetic abnormality, there may be either anaemia or compensated haemolysis. The blood film (Fig. 8.29) shows variable numbers of spherocytes and less easily recognized spherostomatocytes. There are also some cells with normal central pallor. Scanning electron microscopy has shown that generally only a minority of the cells are spherical, the majority being discocytes, stomatocytes or spherostomatocytes [40]. In mild cases of hereditary spherocytosis it is sometimes very difficult to be certain, on examining the blood film, whether or not spherocytes are present and confirmatory tests are needed. In severe cases there is obvious spherocytosis, polychromasia and polychromatic macrocytes and sometimes the presence of other poikilocytes. The reticulocyte percentage and absolute count are elevated. After splenectomy the usual post-splenectomy features are seen but target cells are not a feature; sphero-acanthocytes may be very numerous (Fig. 8.30). Ultrastructural studies show that splenectomy leads to disappearance of a minor population of microspherocytes [40].

Certain specific morphological features are associated with several uncommon mutations [39,41]: a mutant β-spectrin with defective binding to protein 4.1 is associated with spherocytes and acanthocytes; band 3 deficiency is associated with pincered or mushroom-shaped cells which are lost after splenectomy; band 4.2^{Nippon} is associated with stomatocytes, ovalocytes and sphero-ovalocytes in homozygotes; severe spectrin and ankyrin deficiency has irregular spherocytes, some of which resemble the cells of hereditary pyropoikilocytosis.

The blood count in hereditary spherocytosis shows a normal or reduced Hb and a normal MCV and MCH. With impedance counters the MCHC is towards the upper limit of normal or somewhat increased. With Technicon H.1 series counters the MCHC is increased in the majority of patients who also show an increased RDW and HDW and, on the histograms, a tail of microcytes and a tail of hyperchromic cells [42]. Red cell cytograms (Fig. 8.31) show a characteristic increase of hyperchromic or hyperdense cells and, if there is significant macrocytosis, an increase of hypochromic

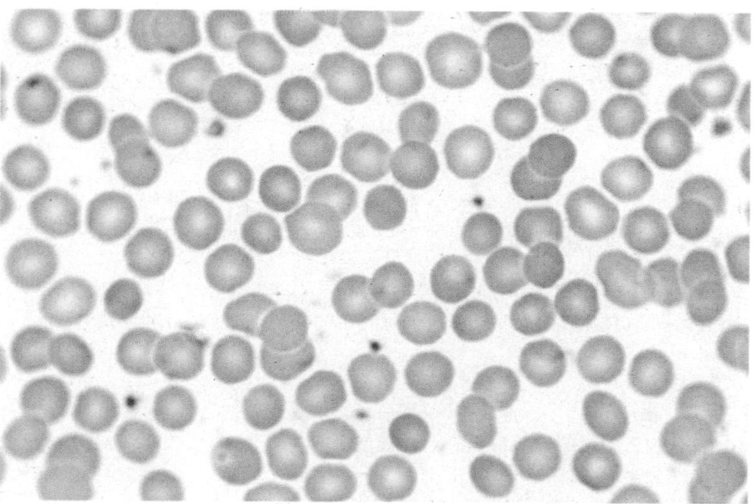

Fig. 8.29 The blood film of a patient with hereditary spherocytosis who had mild chronic haemolysis without anaemia showing moderately numerous spherocytes.

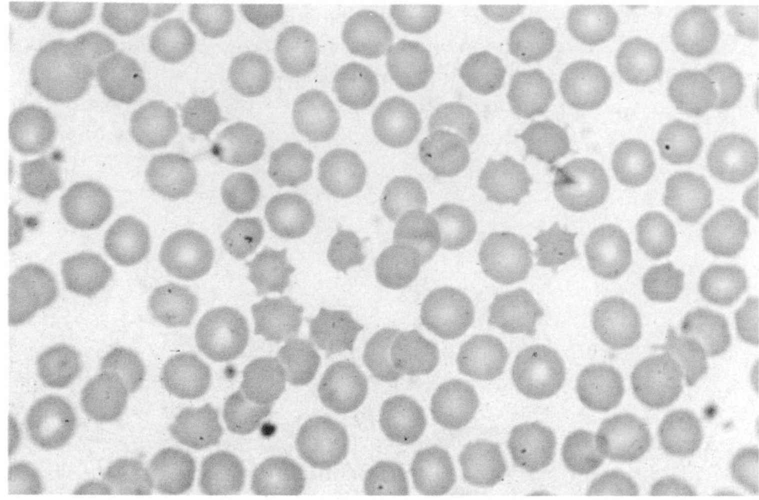

Fig. 8.30 The blood film of a patient with hereditary spherocytosis (the father of the patient shown in Fig. 8.29) who has been splenectomized, showing spheroacanthocytes.

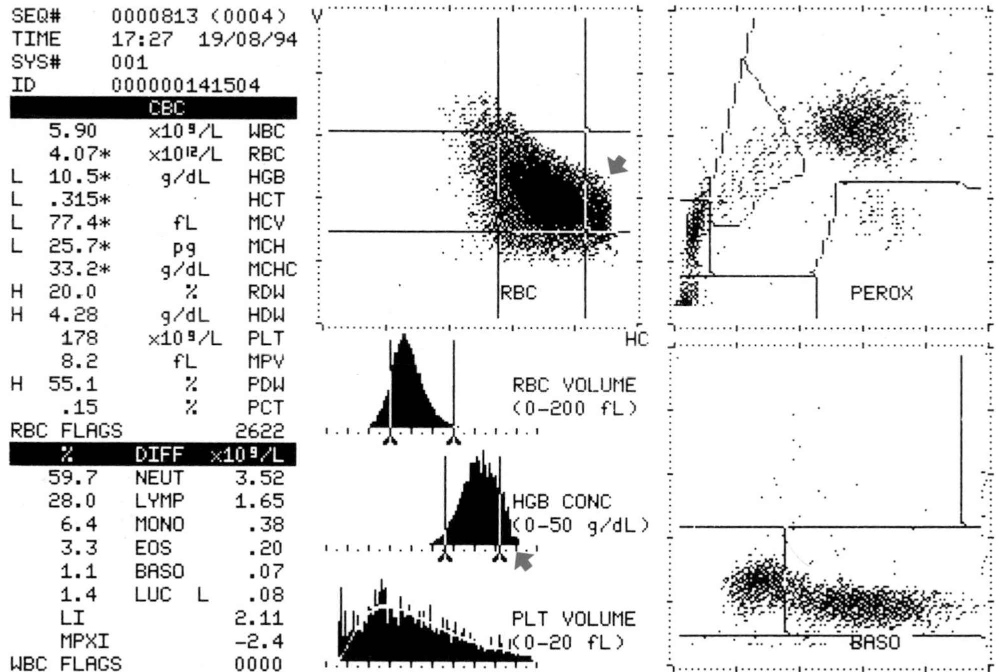

Fig. 8.31 Technicon H.2 scatter plots and histograms of a patient with hereditary spherocytosis. Both the red cell cytogram and the haemoglobin histogram show a large number of dense cells which are the spherocytes.

macrocytes. An increased percentage of hyperdense cells is not specific for spherocytosis but examination of the blood film allows spherocytes to be distinguished from other hyperdense cells such as sickle cells and irregularly contracted cells. Post-splenectomy the Hb rises, usually to normal, and the RDW and HDW usually return to normal. Microcytes are less consistently present but increased numbers of hyperchromic cells are usually still present [42].

Sudden worsening of anaemia in hereditary spherocytosis may be caused by: (i) megaloblastic anaemia consequent on folate deficiency; (ii) 'anaemia of chronic disease' developing during acute infection; or (iii) red cell aplasia induced by parvovirus infection. Because of the shortened red cell lifespan the anaemia develops acutely. In megaloblastic anaemia polychromasia is diminished in comparison with the stable state and some macrocytes, oval macrocytes and hypersegmented neutrophils are present (Fig. 8.32). In the anaemia of chronic disease, e.g., in association with acute infection, polychromasia also diminishes and red cells become less spherocytic, some developing central pallor. The blood film may be dimorphic (Fig. 8.33). If the patient is not known to suffer from hereditary spherocytosis the diagnosis may be difficult to make at this stage. In pure red cell aplasia cells remain spherocytic but polychromasia disappears and the reticulocyte count is close to zero. Previously undiagnosed hereditary spherocytosis may be unmasked by parvovirus infection and also by infectious mononucleosis which aggravates the haemolysis. Haemolytic episodes can also be induced by exercise or precipitated by pregnancy. Increased red cell breakdown in chronic haemolytic anaemias predisposes to gallstones; patients with hereditary spherocytosis thus have an increased likelihood of developing obstructive jaundice. When this occurs more lipid is taken up into the red cell membrane and consequently spherocytosis and haemolysis lessen. Iron deficiency is also associated with a reduction of spherocytosis and sometimes a dimorphic blood film.

Differential diagnosis

The main differential diagnosis is with warm autoimmune haemolytic anaemia (see p. 241). The blood films are often indistinguishable, and thus family history and a direct antiglobulin test are needed. Other causes of spherocytosis which may have to be considered in the differential diagnosis are shown in Table 3.3. Often the diagnosis is readily evident from the clinical history but laboratory features can help. In the mild, compensated haemolytic anaemia associated with the Rh null phenotype there are some stomatocytes as well as spherocytes and all Rh groups are lacking from red cell membranes. In Zieve's syndrome, an acute haemolytic anaemia associated with alcoholic liver disease, there are irregularly contracted cells as well as spherocytes. In *Clostridium welchii* sepsis the red cell membrane may be so damaged that numerous ghosts are seen. Further lysis occurring in the blood specimen *in vitro* can cause artefactual elevation of the MCH and MCHC.

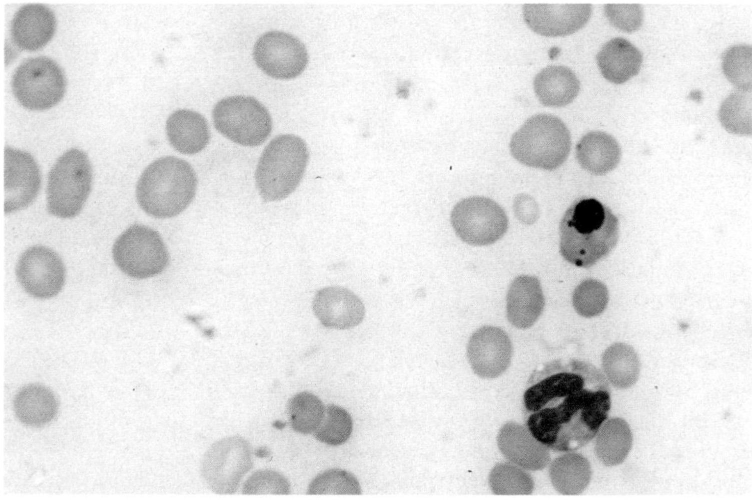

Fig. 8.32 The blood film of a patient with hereditary spherocytosis who has developed a megaloblastic anaemia consequent on inadequate dietary intake of folate in the face of increased requirements caused by chronic haemolysis. The film shows macrocytes, oval macrocytes, occasional spherocytes and a megaloblast containing Howell–Jolly bodies.

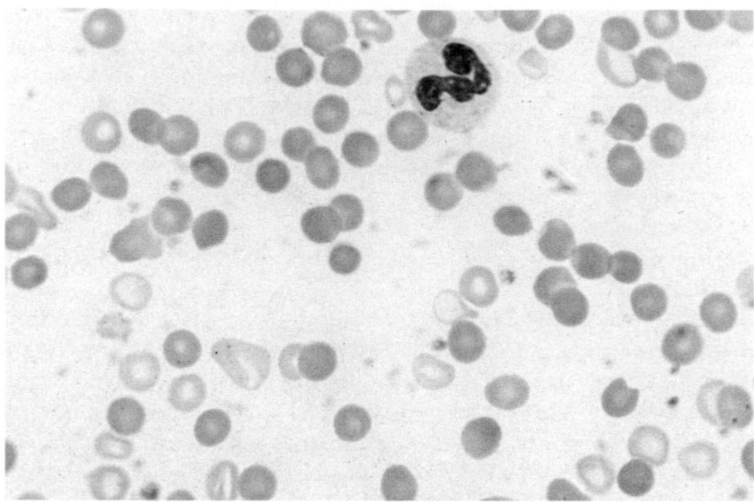

Fig. 8.33 The blood film of a patient with hereditary spherocytosis (the same patient as shown in Fig. 8.32) showing a superimposed anaemia of chronic disease caused by an intercurrent infection. Some cells have central pallor and are hypochromic and microcytic. The film is dimorphic.

In the neonatal period the differential diagnosis includes haemolytic disease of the newborn, particularly that due to ABO incompatibility (see p.245). It should, however, be noted that clinically evident ABO incompatibility is commoner in babies who are subsequently found to have hereditary spherocytosis.

Further tests

The direct antiglobulin test is negative. An osmotic fragility test confirms the presence of osmotically fragile cells but does not distinguish between hereditary spherocytosis and warm autoimmune haemolytic anaemia or other causes of spherocytosis. In mild cases, an osmotic fragility test after the incubation of red cells at 37°C for 24 hours may be necessary to demonstrate the presence of abnormal cells. In very mild cases the osmotic fragility may be normal, even after incubation. Post-splenectomy the osmotic fragility test remains abnormal but a small population of very fragile cells may have disappeared; this population probably represents very abnormal cells resulting from damage within the spleen. When an automated counter which detects hyperdense cells is available the need for an osmotic fragility test is much diminished. The definitive test for hereditary spherocytosis is quantification of spectrin and other proteins of the red cell membrane. Membrane spectrin is normal in autoimmune haemolytic anaemia.

Hereditary elliptocytosis

Hereditary elliptocytosis is a heterogeneous group of inherited conditions characterized by elliptocytic red cells. The presence of at least 25% elliptocytes or ovalocytes has been suggested as a diagnostic criterion. However, subjects with elliptogenic mutations can have from 0 to 100% elliptocytes so the selection of any cut-off point for diagnosis is arbitrary. Inheritance is usually autosomal dominant. Many ethnic groups are affected including black and white people, Chinese, Japanese and Indians. The incidence is highest in West Africans where the prevalence is at least six per 1000. Hereditary elliptocytosis results from a variety of genetic abnormalities which affect the integrity of the red cell cytoskeleton [39,41,43]. Most elliptogenic mutations affect the structure of α- or β-spectrin, causing either a truncated β-spectrin chain or a defect in either the α- or the β-chain near the sites which are involved in the self-assembly of the spectrin heterodimers into tetramers. As a result, the normal lattice of interconnected spectrin tetramers is disrupted. Less commonly, mutations affect either the transmembrane protein, glycophorin C or protein 4.1, which binds spectrin to glycophorin C.

Blood film and count

The severity of hereditary elliptocytosis is very variable, ranging from a morphological abnormality without any shortening of the red cell lifespan, through mild or moderate compensated haemolysis to severe intermittent or severe chronic haemolytic anaemia. The majority of cases, however, are not anaemic. The blood film (Fig. 8.34) shows predominantly elliptocytes or, in some patients with the same genetic defect, ovalocytes [43]. When there is anaemia there is also polychromasia; more severe cases sometimes have a variety of other poikilocytes including fragments and spherocytes. A variant with sphero-elliptocytes has been associated with a β-spectrin variant, spectrin Rouen [44]. Haemoglobinization of cells is normal. The reticulocyte count is normal or increased.

The Hb and red cell indices are usually normal. Cases with haemolytic anaemia have an increased RDW. Technicon H.1 series red cell cytograms are usually normal but in cases with haemolysis increased numbers of hyperdense cells may be detected.

In hereditary elliptocytosis there is considerable variation in the severity of the defect between individuals who have the same genotype; the phenotype in heterozygotes for some defects varies from an asymptomatic state with less than 2% elliptocytes to mild or moderately severe hereditary elliptocytosis [39,41,43]. In subjects with the same genotype there is a correlation between the degree of abnormality of red cell shape and the severity of haemolysis. However, the genotypes which most often cause severe haemolysis are not those in which the cells are most elliptocytic or in which the percentage of elliptocytes is highest [43]. Despite the variable expression, some generalizations can be made with regard to the usual phenotypic expression of different genetic abnormalities [39,41,43]. Glycophorin C deficiency causes no significant abnormality in heterozygotes while homozygotes have mild hereditary elliptocytosis. Protein 4.1 deficiency and several α-spectrin variants cause a minimal or mild abnormality in heterozygotes and severe hereditary elliptocytosis in homozygotes [41,45,46]. The most severe elliptogenic mutations generally cause the phenotype of hereditary elliptocytosis in heterozygotes while homozygotes and certain compound heterozygotes have the phenotype of hereditary pyropoikilocytosis (see below).

Exacerbations of haemolysis are sometimes seen during infections, in the post-partum period, or when the microcirculation is compromised, e.g., by splenomegaly, disseminated intravascular coagulation or TTP [39,43]. Patients with haemolysis severe enough to require splenectomy may thereafter have marked poikilocytosis, in addition to the usual post-splenectomy features; the poikilocytes include prominent spherocytes, microelliptocytes and fragments (Fig. 8.35).

In general, subjects with hereditary elliptocytosis have very few elliptocytes at birth. How-

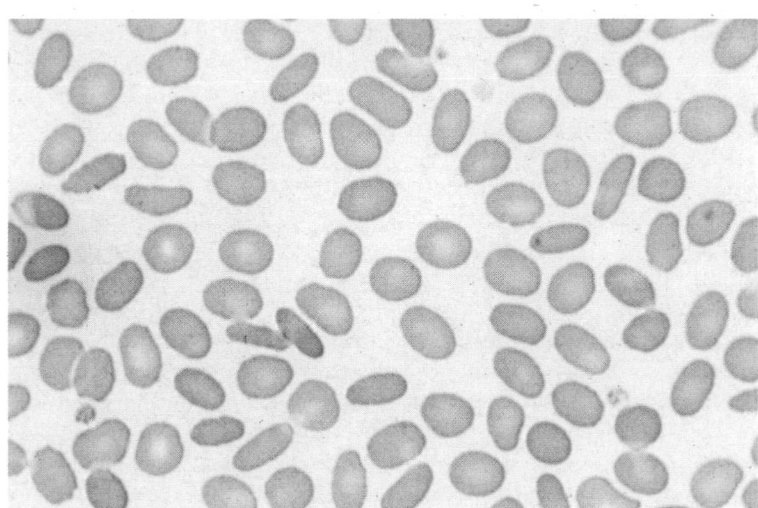

Fig. 8.34 The blood film of a patient with hereditary elliptocytosis showing elliptocytes and ovalocytes. The patient had a normal Hb and reticulocyte count.

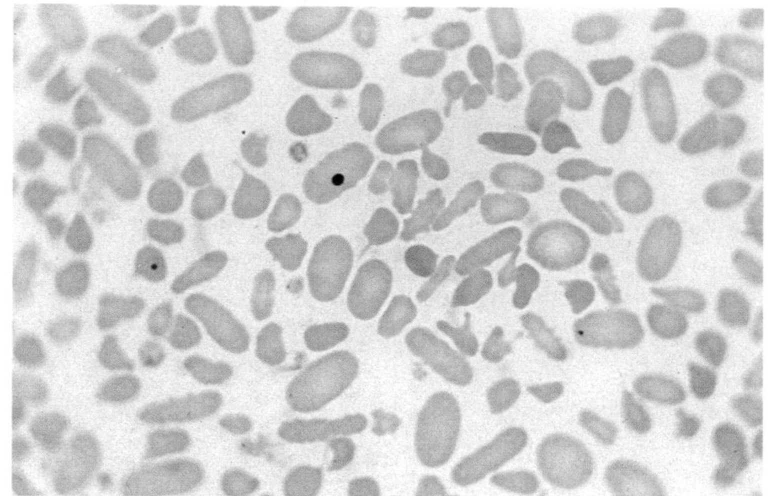

Fig. 8.35 The blood film of a patient with severe hereditary elliptocytosis who required splenectomy for haemolysis showing marked poikilocytosis with the poikilocytes including elliptocytes, ovalocytes and fragments. One ovalocyte contains a Howell–Jolly body. Courtesy of Dr Raina Liesner, London.

ever, some who in later life have typical hereditary elliptocytosis with only mild haemolysis may, in the neonatal period when haemoglobin F is high, have severe haemolysis and a blood film (Fig. 8.36) showing marked poikilocytosis with the presence not only of elliptocytes but also of fragments, irregularly contracted cells and microspherocytes [47,48].

Differential diagnosis

When the blood film shows a high proportion of elliptocytes or ovalocytes the diagnosis of hereditary elliptocytosis is very probable. Rare patients with developing myelofibrosis [49] or myelodysplastic syndromes [50] have shown similar numbers of elliptocytes. The differential diagnosis of cases of hereditary elliptocytosis with marked neonatal poikilocytosis is with hereditary pyropoikilocytosis. Follow-up beyond the neonatal period permits the two conditions to be distinguished.

Further tests

Osmotic fragility is normal except in those with severe haemolysis. Family studies are useful in confirming the inherited nature of the condition. A definitive diagnosis can be made by biochemical investigation of red cell membranes in a reference laboratory. Elliptocytosis associated with loss or mutation of the glycophorin C gene shows loss of the Gerbich red cell antigens, referred to as the Leach phenotype.

Hereditary pyropoikilocytosis

Hereditary pyropoikilocytosis is a heterogeneous group of inherited haemolytic anaemias characterized by recessive inheritance and bizarre poikilocytes including red cell fragments and microspherocytes. It has been described in white, black and Arab populations. The condition is defined by enhanced red cell fragmentation on *in vitro* heating which occurs at a lower temperature than with normal red cells. This feature is indicated in the name 'pyropoikilocytosis'. Hereditary elliptocytosis shows a similar but milder defect on heat exposure. Red cell membranes show two defects, a partial spectrin deficiency and a defect of self-assembly of spectrin dimers into tetramers, the latter as a result of an elliptogenic mutation. The underlying genetic defects are various [51]. There may be homozygosity or compound heterozygosity for a mutant spectrin which has a defect affecting dimer self-assembly and is also degraded rapidly. Alternatively, there may be compound heterozygosity for a mutant spectrin (α- or β-chain) and for a defect leading to a reduced rate of synthesis of α-spectrin. Parents of patients with hereditary pyropoikilocytosis may both have morphologically normal red cells or

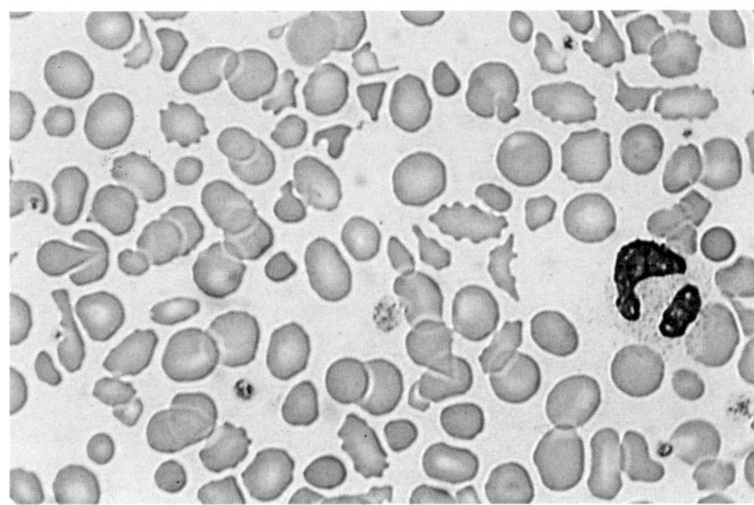

Fig. 8.36 The blood film of a neonate with hereditary elliptocytosis and neonatal poikilocytosis showing marked poikilocytosis with a mixture of elliptocytes and other poikilocytes. Courtesy of Dr Marilyn Treacy.

one or occasionally both parents may have typical hereditary elliptocytosis.

Blood film and count

There is anaemia and the blood film (Fig. 8.37) shows gross anisocytosis and poikilocytosis with the poikilocytes including microspherocytes, cells with bud-like projections and fragments; elliptocytes are a minor component. The reticulocyte count is increased. The Hb is reduced. The MCV and MCH are markedly reduced. The RDW and HDW are increased.

Differential diagnosis

In the neonatal period some cases of hereditary elliptocytosis resemble hereditary pyropoikilocytosis (see above). Haemoglobin H disease and the congenital dyserythropoietic anaemias also sometimes show a similar degree of poikilocytosis but they lack the microspherocytes and budding cells.

Further tests

Osmotic fragility is increased. The diagnosis is confirmed by demonstration of fragmentation on *in vitro* exposure to heat and by biochemical analysis of red cell membranes.

South-East Asian ovalocytosis

South-East Asian ovalocytosis, also sometimes referred to as hereditary ovalocytosis of Melanesians or stomatocytic elliptocytosis, is a distinct and homogeneous disorder which occurs in Melanesians in Papua and New Guinea, the Solomon and Torres Strait Islands, and in Malaysian aboriginals and the populations of Indonesia and the Philippines. Inheritance is autosomal dominant. In some of the affected ethnic groups as many as 20–30% of the population is affected [52]. The underlying genetic defect is a point mutation plus a deletion in the gene for band 3 which causes tight binding of band 3 to ankyrin and reduced lateral mobility and rigidity of the membrane.

Blood film and count

There is no anaemia. Red cells are round or oval and include stomatocytes. There is a minor population of macro-ovalocytes, many of which are stomatocytic (Fig. 8.38). Stomas may be longitudinal, transverse, V-shaped or Y-shaped or there may be two stomas per cell. The reticulocyte count is normal. The Hb, MCV, MCH and MCHC are normal.

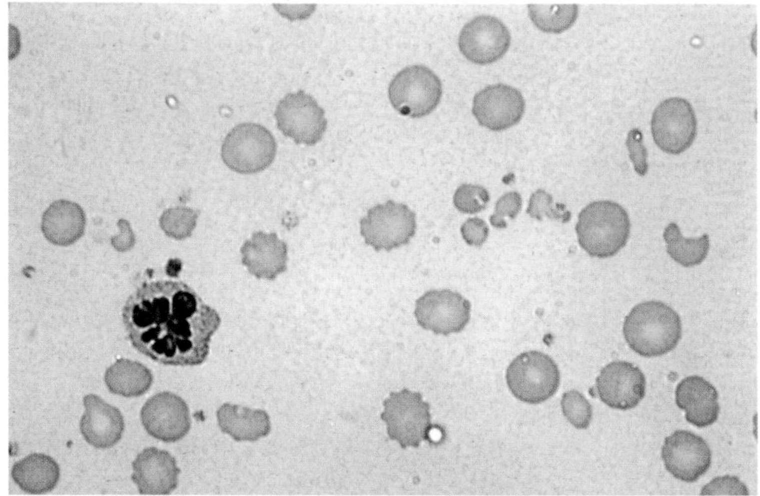

Fig. 8.37 The blood film of a patient with hereditary pyropoikilocytosis showing marked poikilocytosis. Courtesy of Professor Harry Smith.

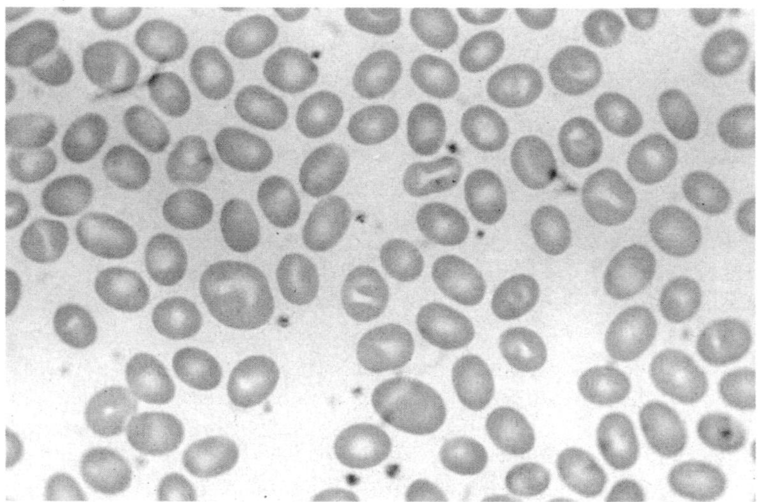

Fig. 8.38 The blood film of a patient with South-East Asian ovalocytosis showing several macro-ovalocytes one of which has a Y-shaped stoma and the other an eccentric transverse stoma. Many of the smaller cells are either stomatocytes, ovalocytes or stomato-ovalocytes.

Differential diagnosis

The blood film is so distinctive that as long as the characteristic features are known it is unlikely to be confused with any other condition.

Further tests

The blood film is pathognomonic so that further tests are unnecessary. There is reduced expression of many red cell antigens including D so that subjects may type as D^U [53].

Hereditary stomatocytosis

Hereditary stomatocytosis is a heterogeneous group of rare inherited haemolytic anaemias characterized by stomatocytes in blood films. Inheritance is usually autosomal dominant. In the majority of cases there is an abnormality of cation flux, increased intracellular sodium and decreased intracellular potassium. In at least some cases this is attributable to a defect of band 7.2 of the erythrocyte membrane [54]. Cells are swollen which has led to an alternative designation of 'hydrocytosis'. In a minority of cases there is no abnormality of cation flux; some but not all of these cases have an abnormality of membrane lipids such as an increase of phosphatidylcholine [55].

Blood film and count

Haemolysis may be compensated or there may be anaemia which is mild, moderate or severe. The blood film shows a variable number of stomatocytes, usually 10–30% (Fig. 8.39). In some variants there are also target cells [56].

In cases with an abnormality of cation flux there is an increased MCV and decreased MCHC. Red cell cytograms show increased normochromic and, in particular, hypochromic macrocytes. The HDW is increased.

Differential diagnosis

The differential diagnosis is with other inherited conditions characterized by stomatocytes and with the much more frequent cases of acquired stomatocytosis (see p. 63). Rh null disease has many characteristics in common with hereditary stomatocytosis. Blood films show similar numbers of stomatocytes together with a few spherocytes. Cation flux is abnormal. There is a mild haemolytic anaemia or well-compensated haemolysis. The demonstration of a total lack of Rh antigens allows the diagnosis to be made. Stomatocytosis has also been described in a significant minority of Mediterranean immigrants to Australia. Some patients are anaemic and there is an association with large platelets in half the cases. Strong familial clustering suggests that this is an inherited condition [57].

Further tests

Cases consequent on an abnormality of cation flux show increased osmotic fragility. Some of these cases show pseudohyperkalaemia consequent on leakage of potassium from cells if there is delay in processing blood specimens. Blood grouping is indicated to exclude Rh null disease.

Hereditary xerocytosis

Hereditary xerocytosis, also referred to as the dehydrated variant of hereditary stomatocytosis or desiccytosis, is a rare inherited haemolytic anaemia characterized by increased cation flux, normal or increased cellular cation content and loss of red cell water. Inheritance is autosomal dominant with variable penetrance.

Blood film and count

Some patients are anaemic and some have compensated haemolysis. The blood film (Fig. 8.40)

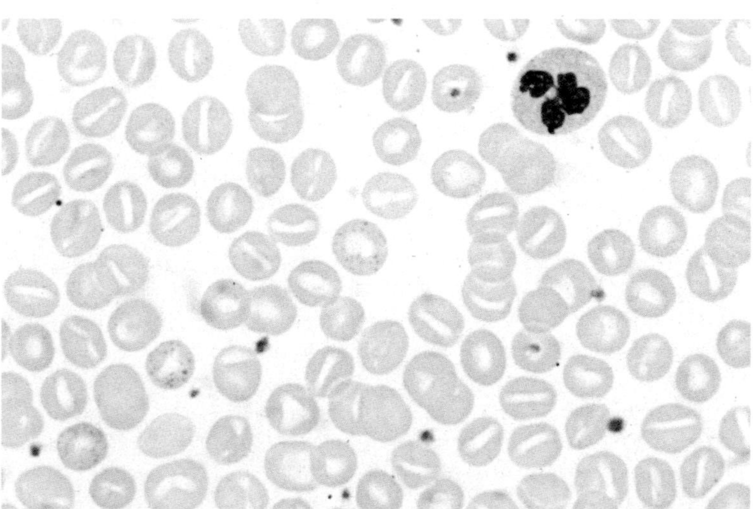

Fig. 8.39 The blood film of a patient with hereditary stomatocytosis showing basophilic stippling and numerous stomatocytes [54]. Courtesy of Dr Carol Barton.

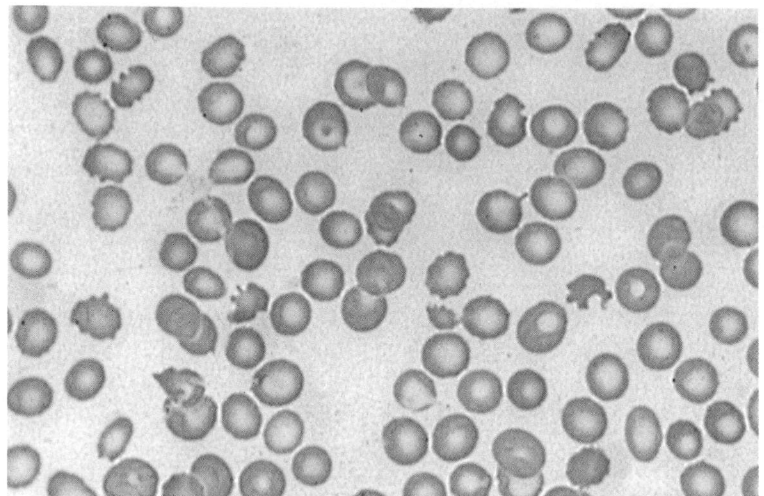

Fig. 8.40 The blood film of a patient with hereditary xerocytosis showing target cells, poikilocytes and several cells with haemoglobin distributed unevenly in the cell or 'puddled'. Courtesy of Dr J.L.L. Vives Corrons, Barcelona.

shows target cells, sometimes a small number of stomatocytes, echinocytes, irregularly contracted cells and cells with the haemoglobin apparently puddled at the periphery or on one or two edges of the cell [58]. There is polychromasia and the reticulocyte count is increased. Stomatocytes may be more prominent on wet preparations.

The MCV is normal or low and the MCHC may be slightly or moderately elevated. The RDW and HDW are increased. The H.1 Technicon series red cell cytogram may show a population of hyperdense cells.

Differential diagnosis

The differential diagnosis is with other causes of haemolytic anaemia, particularly those conditions which usually have some stomatocytes or target cells.

Further tests

The osmotic fragility is decreased although there may be a small tail of fragile cells. The demonstration of a population of cells with an increased MCHC is diagnostically useful. Patients may exhibit pseudohyperkalaemia if there is delay in measuring plasma potassium; this is consequent on loss of potassium from the cell.

Glucose-6-phosphate dehydrogenase (G6PD) deficiency

G6PD is an enzyme of the pentose shunt pathway which protects the erythrocyte from oxidant damage. G6PD deficiency is common in many ethnic groups including many Africans, Afro-Caribbeans and black Americans and populations around the Mediterranean basin, the Middle-East, the Indian subcontinent, South-East Asia and Papua and New Guinea. The gene for G6PD is on the X chromosome so that most cases of G6PD deficiency are in hemizygous males. However, in populations with a high incidence of mutant genes deficiency also occurs in homozygous females. In parts of Greece and the Middle-East the incidence in males is as high as 35–40%. Depending on the severity of the defect, G6PD deficiency may present as neonatal jaundice, congenital non-spherocytic haemolytic anaemia or intermittent haemolysis triggered by oxidant stress such as that caused by intercurrent infection, by eating broad beans (fava beans) or by exposure to naphthalene or oxidant drugs.

Blood film and count

When there is chronic haemolytic anaemia due to severe G6PD deficiency the blood film (Fig. 8.41) may show anisocytosis, poikilocytosis, basophilic

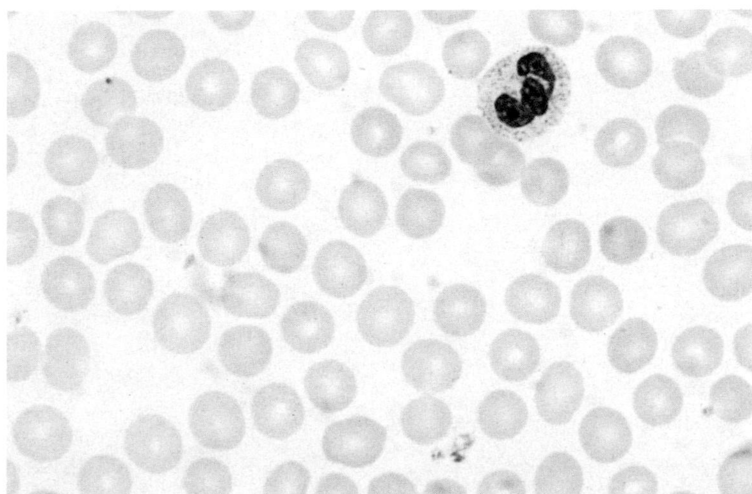

Fig. 8.41 The blood film of a patient with congenital non-spherocytic haemolytic anaemia caused by G6PD deficiency showing macrocytosis and slight polychromasia. Courtesy of Professor Lucio Luzzatto, New York.

stippling, macrocytosis and polychromasia without any specific diagnostic features. In less severe G6PD deficiency the blood film is normal except during haemolytic episodes. When such an episode occurs the morphological abnormalities are very characteristic (Figs 8.42 & 8.43). There are irregularly contracted cells, some of which have small protrusions caused by the presence of Heinz bodies. Some cells, often designated 'bite cells', have an irregular gap in their outline, probably caused by removal of Heinz bodies by the spleen. In other cells, often called hemighosts, the haemoglobin appears to have retracted to form a dense mass occupying half the cell while the rest of the cell appears empty. When haemolysis is very acute a few complete ghosts may be present. At the height of a haemolytic episode there is a leucocytosis and the features of hyposplenism can appear as a consequence of reticulo-endothelial overload. In the few days following an episode of oxidant stress there may be a further fall in the Hb as damaged cells are cleared by the spleen. Subsequently, polychromatic macrocytes appear. Patients with chronic non-spherocytic haemolytic anaemia caused by G6PD deficiency can have their haemolysis exacerbated by infection or other oxidant stress.

G6PD deficient patients with chronic non-spherocytic haemolytic anaemia have a reduced Hb, RBC and PCV and an increased MCV and MCH. Those with episodic haemolysis have a reduced Hb, RBC and PCV during attacks together with an increased RDW, a population of cells with an increased haemoglobin concentration and, if haemolysis is very acute, an increased MCHC. When recovery starts there is a further increase in the RDW and an increase in the MCV, MCH and HDW.

Differential diagnosis

In the neonatal period the differential diagnosis is with other causes of neonatal jaundice, particularly with haemolytic disease of the newborn with an immune basis. In cases with chronic haemolysis the differential diagnosis is with other causes of congenital non-spherocytic haemolytic anaemia (see below). In patients with intermittent haemolysis the differential diagnosis is with the other much less common defects of the pentose shunt and with haemolytic anaemia due to exposure to oxidant drugs or chemicals in a patient with no underlying enzyme deficiency (see p. 250); when there is oxidant damage to red cells the blood films are indistinguishable whether or not there is an underlying enzyme defect. To a lesser extent other causes of irregularly contracted cells, such as unstable haemoglobins, should be included in the differential diagnosis (see p. 221).

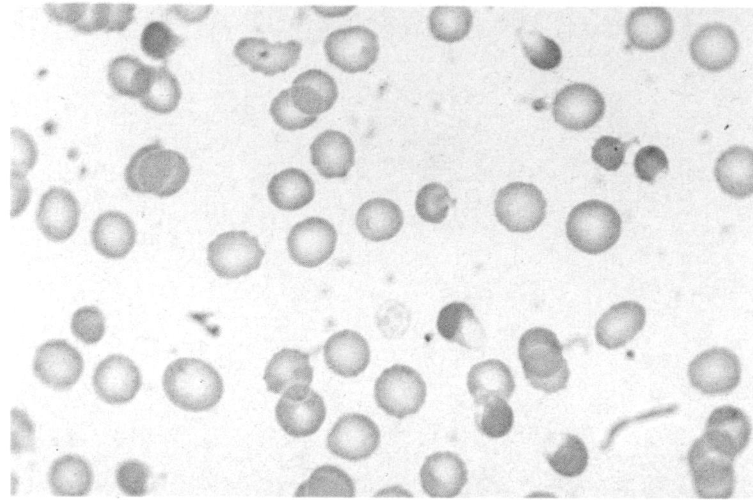

Fig. 8.42 The blood film of an Afro-Caribbean child with G6PD deficiency who had suffered an episode of acute haemolysis showing anaemia, irregularly contracted cells, a hemighost, a complete ghost, and a cell with a protrusion attributable to a Heinz body; the Heinz body preparation was positive.

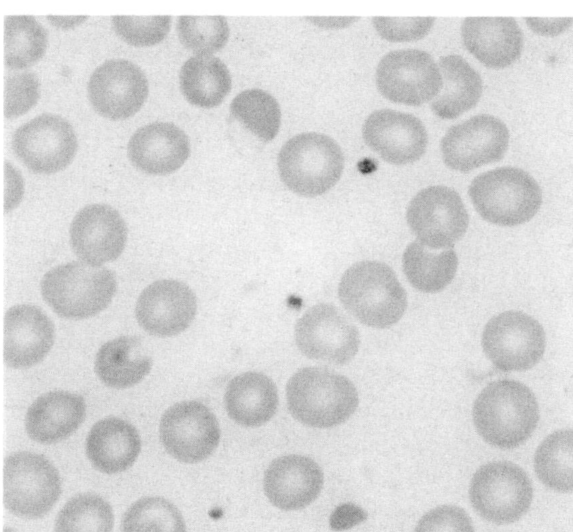

Fig. 8.43 The blood film of a patient with acute haemolysis associated with G6PD deficiency showing a 'bite cell' and a cell with haemoglobin retracted from the cell margin.

Further tests

Diagnosis can be based on screening tests for G6PD deficiency or on assay. Screening tests are very suitable for population surveys. During haemolytic episodes the high reticulocyte count can cause screening tests and sometimes even assays to be normal. This is particularly so in black people who can have relatively high G6PD levels in reticulocytes. If G6PD deficiency is suspected and the assay is normal it should be repeated after the reticulocyte count has returned to normal.

Congenital non-spherocytic haemolytic anaemias consequent on enzyme deficiencies

A variety of inherited congenital haemolytic anaemias consequent on a red cell enzyme deficiency have no characteristic abnormality of red cell shape and are grouped together under the designation 'congenital non-spherocytic haemolytic anaemia'. They should be suspected when there is either neonatal jaundice associated with haemolysis or chronic haemolysis in older children or adults. The underlying defect may be in the glycolytic pathway, pentose shunt (including some cases of G6PD deficiency; see above) or enzymes involved in nucleotide metabolism. Their inheritance and associated clinical features are summarized in Table 8.2. These conditions are all rare or very rare. The commonest is pyruvate kinase deficiency which has a prevalence of less than one in 10 000. Deficiencies of a single enzyme are heterogeneous; the mutations differ and they occur in a variety of ethnic groups spread over a wide geographical area. Most enzyme deficiencies show an autosomal recessive inheritance with affected individuals being homozygotes or, more often, compound heterozygotes. Excep-

Table 8.2 Clinical features and inheritance of enzyme deficiencies causing congenital non-spherocytic anaemias [59,60]

Enzyme	Frequency	Inheritance	Associated features
Glycolytic pathway			
Hexokinase	Rare	AR*	Multiple congenital abnormalities; latent diabetes mellitus or psychomotor retardation in some cases
Glucose phosphate isomerase	Third most common	Usually AR	Occasionally myopathy; two cases of mental retardation
Phosphofructokinase†	Rare	AR	Myopathy (type VII glycogen storage disease) in some cases
Aldolase	Very rare (three cases in two kindreds)	AR	Mental retardation, multiple congenital abnormalities, type VI glycogen storage disease in one of two kindreds
Triosephosphate isomerase	Rare	AR	Progressive neurological and cardiac dysfunction
Phosphoglycerate kinase	Rare	X-linked recessive	No associated defect *or* exercise-induced rhabdomyolysis *or* mental retardation and progressive neurological dysfunction
Enolase	Very rare	?AD	
Pyruvate kinase	Most common of this rare group of disorders	AR	
Nucleotide metabolism			
Adenylate kinase	Rare	AR	Mental retardation [61]
Pyrimidine 5′ nucleotidase	Rare	AR	
Adenosine deaminase excess	Rare	AD	
Hexose monophosphate shunt			
Glucose-6-phosphate dehydrogenase	Similar frequency to pyruvate kinase deficiency	X-linked	Neonatal jaundice
Glutathione synthetase	Rare	AR	Metabolic acidoses with 5-oxoprolinuria in some cases
γ-glutamyl cysteine synthetase	Rare	AR	Spinocerebellar disease and aminoaciduria

* AD in two families with unusual morphological features.
† Can be associated with haemolytic anaemia, compensated haemolysis or mild polycythaemia.
AD, autosomal dominant; AR, autosomal recessive.

tions are phosphoglycerate kinase and G6PD deficiency which have a sex-linked recessive inheritance, enolase deficiency which is probably autosomal dominant, and the very rare haemolytic anaemia associated with adenosine deaminase excess which is autosomal dominant. Heterozygotes do not suffer haemolysis with the exception of some female heterozygotes for phosphoglycerate kinase deficiency [60].

Blood film and count

There is chronic anaemia which may be exacerbated by intercurrent infections. The blood film (Fig. 8.44) usually shows non-specific features such as anisocytosis, macrocytosis, polychromasia and basophilic stippling. Sometimes there are echinocytes or other poikilocytes, usually in small numbers. Echinocytes have been noted in some cases of triose phosphate isomerase deficiency (Fig. 8.45), aldolase deficiency [62] and phosphoglycerate kinase deficiency [63]. Small numbers of irregularly contracted cells have been noted in triose phosphate isomerase deficiency [64] and stomatocytes in glucose phosphate isomerase deficiency [65]. Pyruvate kinase deficiency may be associated with occasional ovalocytes and elliptocytes and rare spiculated cells. It has been postulated that the spiculated cells are adenosine triphosphate (ATP)-depleted erythrocytes at the end of their lifespan. Enolase deficiency is unusual in that in the two reported kindreds it has been associated with the presence of spherocytes [60]. Only in pyrimidine 5′ nucleotidase deficiency is the blood film distinctive. In this condition there is very prominent basophilic stippling (Fig. 8.46), best seen when the blood film is made from heparinized or non-anticoagulated blood rather than from EDTA-anticoagulated blood. The reticulocyte count is increased in non-spherocytic haemolytic anaemia. Some cases also have leucopenia consequent on hypersplenism.

After splenectomy, the Hb rises by 1–3 g/dl and the MCV and MCH may rise. If there is a poor response to splenectomy thrombocytosis may be very marked. After splenectomy for pyruvate kinase deficiency some but not all cases have very frequent spiculated cells, resembling acanthocytes or abnormal echinocytes (Fig. 8.47) [66]; there may be improvement in haemolysis but a paradoxical rise in the reticulocyte count to 40–70%, the likely explanation being that prior to splenectomy some highly defective newly produced cells were removed rapidly by the spleen but in its absence they are surviving.

Differential diagnosis

The differential diagnosis includes congenital haemolytic anaemias due to membrane abnormalities but with only minor morphological

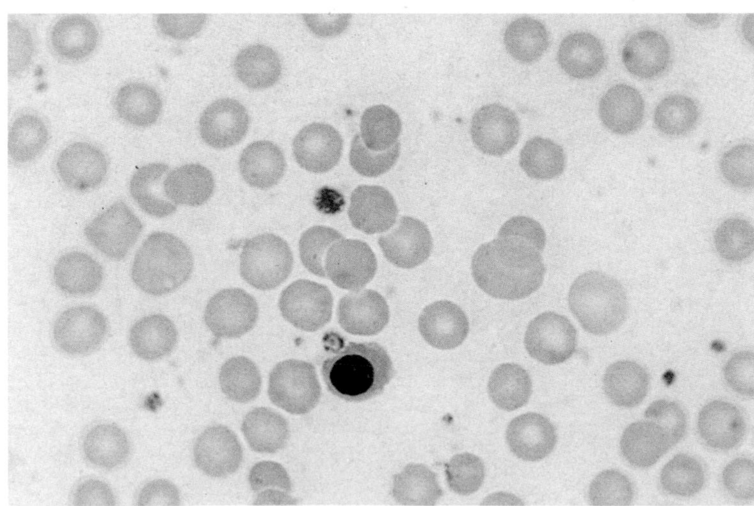

Fig. 8.44 The blood film of a patient with pyruvate kinase deficiency showing anisocytosis, macrocytosis, polychromasia and an NRBC.

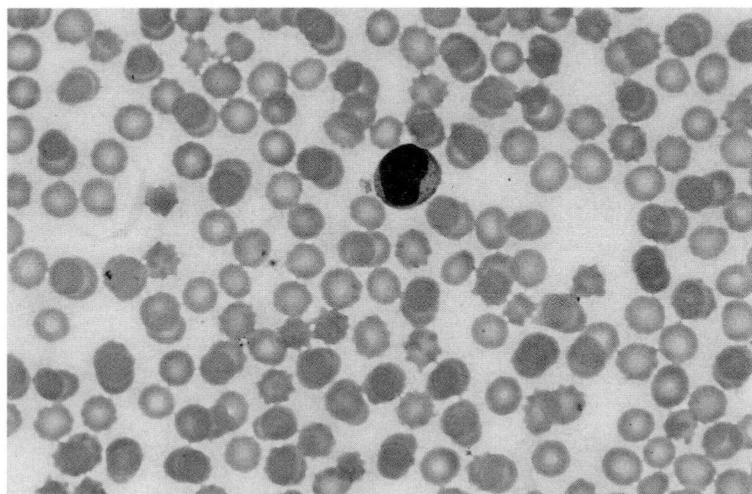

Fig. 8.45 The blood film of a patient with triose phosphate isomerase deficiency showing echinocytosis. Courtesy of Dr J.L.L. Vives Corrons.

abnormalities such as congenital xerocytosis and some cases of congenital stomatocytosis. Congenital erythropoietic porphyria also causes chronic haemolysis with or without anaemia. The differential diagnosis of pyrimidine 5′ nucleotidase deficiency includes haemolytic anaemia due to lead poisoning in which there is an acquired deficiency of the same enzyme and consequently prominent basophilic stippling. In cases presenting beyond the neonatal period Wilson's disease, congenital erythropoietic porphyria and acquired haemolytic anaemias also enter into the differential diagnosis. Wilson's disease can cause acute haemolysis with minimal morphological abnormalities in advance of any obvious evidence of liver disease.

Further tests

The demonstration of normal osmotic fragility with or without increased autohaemolysis is consistent with a red cell enzyme deficiency. However, definitive diagnosis requires biochemical assays which can generally only be performed in a reference laboratory. Congenital erythropoietic porphyria can be confirmed by demonstrating fluorescence in a proportion of erythrocytes and in the nuclei of any circulating erythroblasts when the blood is examined under ultraviolet light.

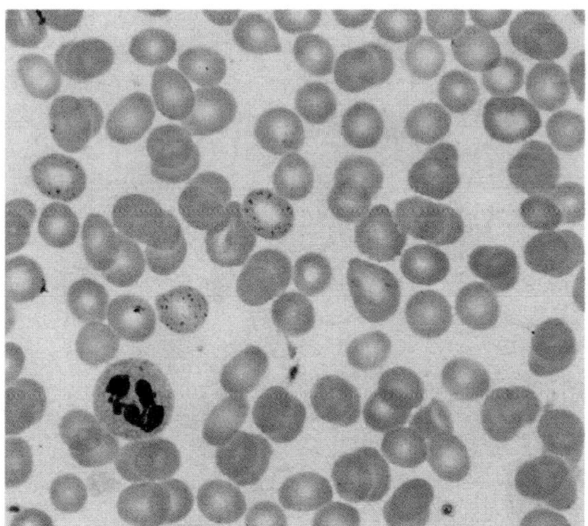

Fig. 8.46 The blood film of a patient with pyrimidine 5′ nucleotidase deficiency showing prominent basophilic stippling. Courtesy of Dr J.L.L. Vives Corrons.

Acquired haemolytic anaemias

Acquired haemolytic anaemias with an immune mechanism

Warm autoimmune haemolytic anaemia

Most cases of autoimmune haemolytic anaemia are caused by warm-acting antibodies, usually

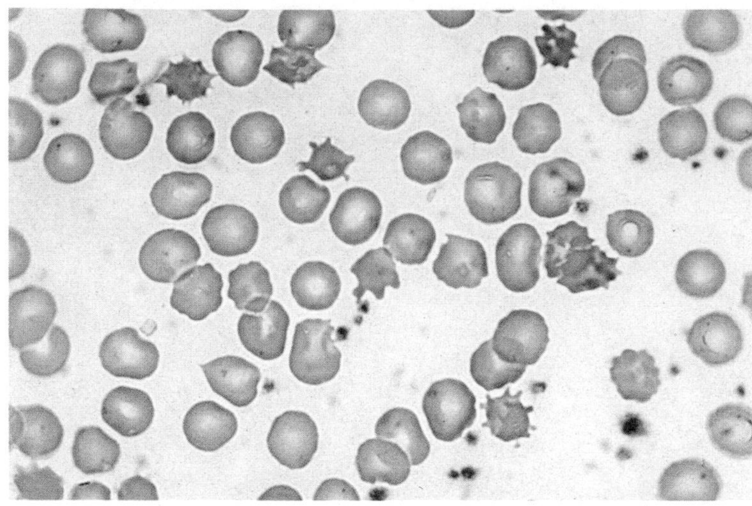

Fig. 8.47 The blood film of a patient with pyruvate kinase deficiency who has been splenectomized showing macrocytosis and acanthocytosis.

IgG, which are directed at red cell membrane antigens. The phagocytic cells of the spleen, and to a lesser extent the liver, remove both whole cells and parts of the red cell membrane to which immunoglobulin and sometimes also complement have been bound. Removal of pieces of the red cell membrane leads to spherocyte formation. Autoimmune haemolytic anaemia may be primary, one feature of an autoimmune disease such as systemic lupus erythematosus, secondary to other diseases such as CLL or lymphoma or, rarely, it may have been induced by a drug, in the past most often α-methyl dopa but occasionally levodopa, mefenamic acid or other drugs.

Blood film and count

The blood film (Fig. 8.48) shows spherocytosis and sometimes also polychromasia and polychromatic macrocytes. In severe cases granulocyte precursors and NRBC are present and there may be features of hyposplenism consequent on reticuloendothelial overload. In occasional patients tear drop poikilocytes have been prominent and have disappeared after splenectomy [67]. Some patients have an associated immune thrombocytopenia, the combination being referred to as Evans' syndrome. The blood film may show features of an underlying disease such as CLL, large granular lymphocyte leukaemia, non-Hodgkin's lymphoma or angioimmunoblastic lymphadenopathy.

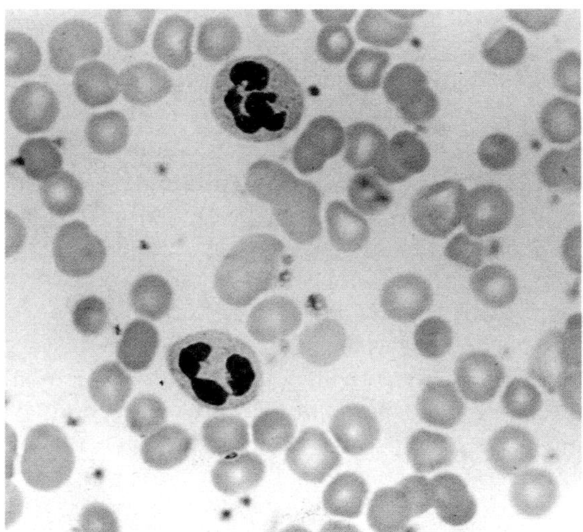

Fig. 8.48 The blood film of a patient with autoimmune haemolytic anaemia showing spherocytes and polychromatic macrocytes.

The Hb, RBC and Hct are reduced. The MCH and MCV may be normal or elevated. The MCHC is elevated when measured by an instrument which is sensitive to changes in this variable. The RDW and HDW are increased. The reticulocyte count is increased. Technicon H.1 series instruments indicate the presence of hyperchromia. The red cell cytogram is not distinguishable from that of hereditary spherocytosis but, because haemolysis is often more severe, there may be a prominent population of hypochromic and normochromic macrocytes which represent reticulocytes and other young red cells (Fig. 8.49).

Differential diagnoses

The differential diagnosis is with hereditary spherocytosis and with other causes of immune haemolytic anaemia. Occasionally, there are specific blood film features which suggest immune haemolysis, such as small red cell agglutinates, red cell phagocytosis by monocytes, rosetting of red cells around neutrophils [68] or thrombocytopenia. More often the peripheral blood features are indistinguishable from those of hereditary spherocytosis. Other immune haemolytic anaemias which can also be confused with autoimmune haemolytic anaemia if sufficient weight is not given to the clinical history are: (i) drug-induced immune haemolytic anaemia; (ii) delayed transfusion reactions following transfusion of incompatible red cells; and (iii) immune haemolysis following transfusion of incompatible plasma, high dose intravenous immunoglobulin or other blood products containing immunoglobulin such as factor VIII or IX concentrates. Immune haemolysis can also follow transplantation of ABO incompatible bone marrow.

In delayed transfusion reactions examination of a blood film permits a diagnosis since only transfused cells are affected and the film is dimorphic (see Fig. 3.23). When ABO incompatible plasma or immunoglobulin is transfused the spherocytosis is generalized so the film appearances do not differ from those of autoimmune haemolytic anaemia. Spherocytosis may persist for weeks [69] so that confusion with autoimmune haemolytic anaemia is possible. Immediate transfusion reactions are unlikely to be confused with autoimmune haemolysis since most of the donor cells are destroyed and spherocytosis is not prominent.

Chronic haemolytic anaemia mediated by a cold agglutinin (see below) can usually be readily distinguished from warm autoimmune haemolytic anaemia on the blood film. The blood film of acute cold antibody haemolytic anaemia is more

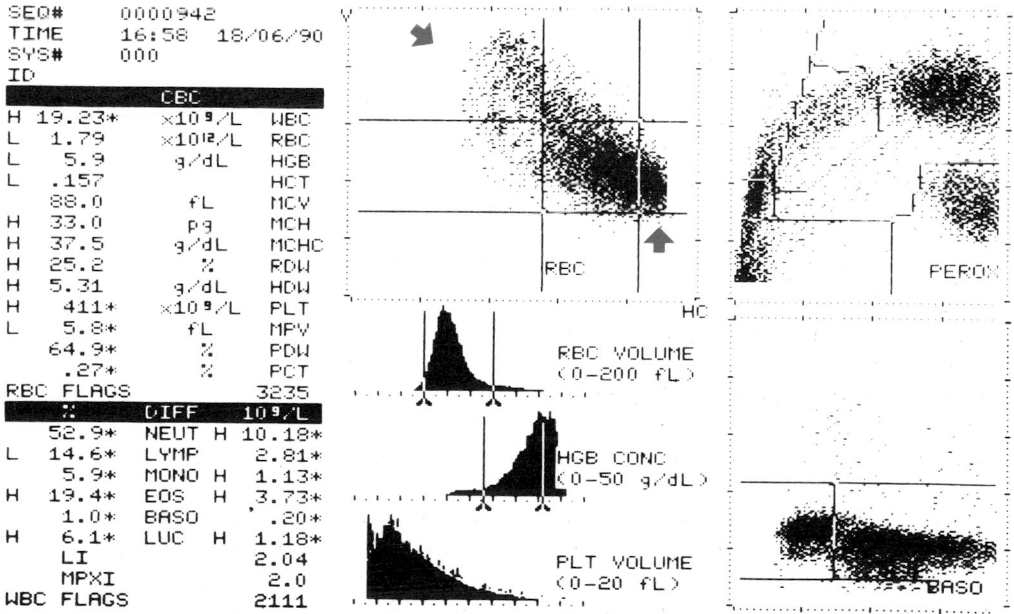

Fig. 8.49 Technicon H.2 red cell histograms and cytogram from a patient with autoimmune haemolytic anaemia showing dense cells which are spherocytes and hypochromic macrocytes which are mainly reticulocytes. There is also eosinophilia evident from the peroxidase channel.

likely to cause confusion but, in comparison with warm autoimmune haemolytic anaemia, red cell agglutinates are more prominent and spherocytes are not so numerous.

Drug-induced immune haemolytic anaemias (see below) can sometimes cause confusion since some spherocytes are present but consideration of the history should suggest the correct diagnosis.

Further tests

A positive direct antiglobulin test (Coombs' test) is critical in distinguishing autoimmune haemolytic anaemia from hereditary spherocytosis. There may also be free autoantibody in the plasma, detected by an indirect antiglobulin test. Some patients have other autoantibodies such as anti-DNA antibodies or antinuclear factor. An osmotic fragility test is positive in both hereditary spherocytosis and in autoimmune haemolytic anaemia so is not of use in distinguishing between these two conditions.

Cold antibody-induced haemolytic anaemia

Haemolysis may be induced by autoantibodies which have maximal activity at low temperatures. Cold antibodies are often IgM antibodies which can cause both red cell agglutination and complement-mediated haemolysis. Clinical features may be mainly due to haemolysis or mainly due to red cell agglutination in small peripheral vessels following exposure to cold. Cold antibody production may be an acute phenomenon when polyclonal antibodies are produced following infections such as infectious mononucleosis or Mycoplasma infection. In these cases acute haemolysis is the dominant clinical feature. Cold antibody production can also be chronic, when a clone of neoplastic lymphocytes produces a monoclonal cold agglutinin, the syndrome being known as cold haemagglutinin disease. The dominant clinical features are those of peripheral cyanosis and ischaemia following cold exposure but there may also be some haemolysis and features, such as lymphadenopathy, suggestive of a lymphoproliferative disease.

Cold antibodies produced following infections such as measles and other viral infections can also cause a distinct clinical syndrome known as paroxysmal cold haemoglobinuria. These antibodies are usually non-agglutinating IgG antibodies with anti-P specificity.

Blood film and count

In acute cold antibody-induced haemolytic anaemia the peripheral blood (Fig. 8.50) shows red cell agglutinates, variable numbers of spherocytes and, subsequently, polychromasia and the presence of polychromatic macrocytes. Erythrophagocytosis is occasionally present. Variable numbers of atypical lymphocytes are present when haemolysis is caused by infectious mononucleosis and, less often, when it is caused by other infections. In chronic cold agglutinin disease the dominant peripheral blood feature is red cell agglutination which may be massive (see Fig. 3.2). Some cases also have lymphocytosis and plasmacytoid lymphocytes may be present. In paroxysmal cold haemoglobinuria most of the antibody-damaged cells are rapidly lysed and the peripheral blood shows only anaemia and a few spherocytes. There may be erythrophagocytosis and associated features such as leucopenia, neutropenia, eosinopenia, monocytopenia and a lesser degree of lymphopenia [70].

The presence of a cold agglutinin is often first suspected from the automated FBC as the red cell agglutinates cause a factitious elevation in the MCV, MCH and MCHC with impedance counters such as Coulter counters and, to a lesser extent, with light-scattering counters like the Technicon H.1 series. Histograms and cytograms may show two populations of red cells, the apparent macrocytes being red cell agglutinates. The presence of a cold agglutinin is easily verified by warming the blood specimen and repeating the FBC.

Differential diagnosis

The differential diagnosis is with other causes of acute haemolysis, spherocytosis and red cell agglutination.

Further tests

Confirmation that haemolysis or ischaemia is caused by a cold haemagglutinin is by a direct antiglobulin test which is positive for complement but not IgG and by the detection of a cold agglut-

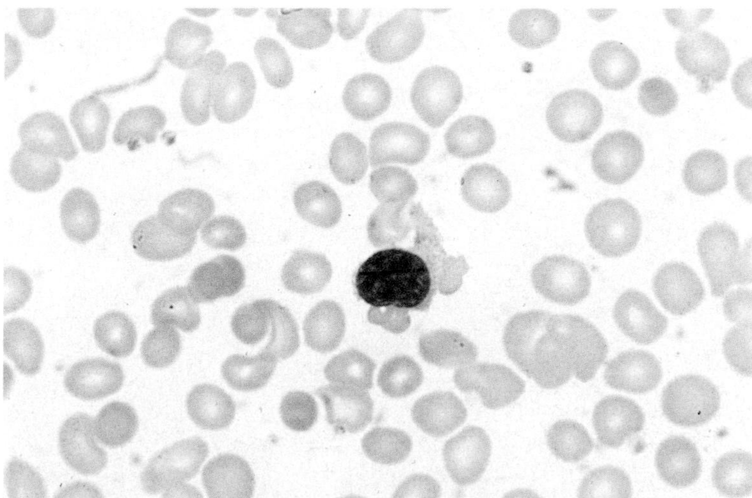

Fig. 8.50 The blood film of a patient with acute haemolytic anaemia caused by anti-i autoantibodies occurring as a complication of infectious mononucleosis. There are several spherocytes, a single small agglutinate and an atypical lymphocyte.

inin. This is usually IgM. It most often has anti-I specificity and less often anti-i or other specificity. In Mycoplasma infections anti-I specificity is usual and in infectious mononucleosis anti-i. Cold agglutinins are not uncommon in healthy subjects but in patients with relevant clinical features they are present at a high titre and/or have a wide thermal amplitude. The diagnosis of paroxysmal cold haemoglobinuria is confirmed by demonstration of the Donath–Landsteiner antibody, usually anti-P, which causes biphasic haemolysis, i.e., haemolysis on rewarming a previously chilled blood sample.

Drug-induced immune haemolytic anaemia

Drugs are now a rare but important cause of haemolytic anaemia. Antibodies are produced which damage red cells only in the presence of the drug. Haemolysis is acute and severe when the red cell is an 'innocent bystander', damaged by drug–antibody complexes. When the antibody is directed at a drug bound to the red cell membrane ('hapten mechanism'), as in penicillin-induced haemolysis, haemolysis is usually less acute and less severe.

Blood film and count

In drug-induced haemolysis of the 'innocent bystander' type the blood film usually shows only the features of anaemia and spherocytes are rare. In penicillin-induced haemolytic anaemia there may be moderate numbers of spherocytes.

Differential diagnosis

The differential diagnosis is with other causes of acute haemolysis and other causes of spherocytosis.

Further tests

Suspected drug-induced haemolysis can be confirmed serologically. With penicillin-induced haemolysis the direct antiglobulin test is positive in the absence of the drug and the patient's serum immunoglobulins bind to penicillin-coated cells. When there is haemolysis with an innocent-bystander mechanism the anti-globulin test is usually positive as complement is bound to the red cells. Serological tests using normal red cells, the patient's serum and the causative drug are positive.

Haemolytic disease of the newborn

IgG maternal alloantibodies cross the placenta and those with specificity for antigens on fetal red cells can cause hydrops fetalis and haemolytic disease of the newborn. The commonest form of haemolytic disease of the newborn is now that caused by anti-A or -B antibodies. Rhesus haemolytic disease of the newborn, caused by anti-D or

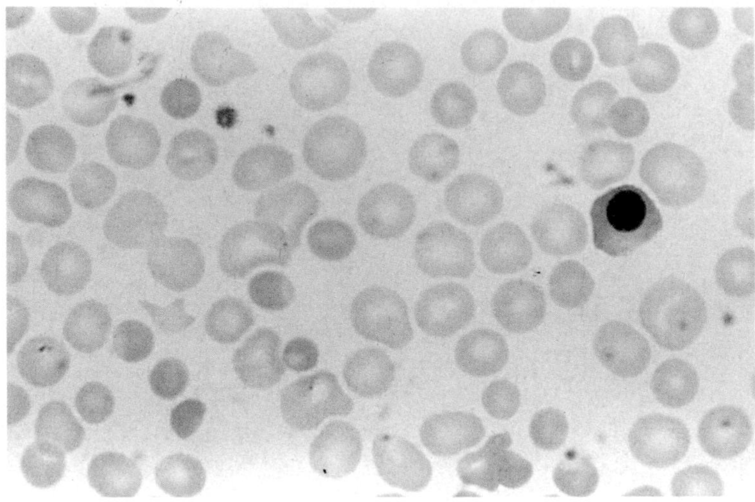

Fig. 8.51 The blood film of a baby with ABO haemolytic disease of the newborn showing marked spherocytosis and an NRBC.

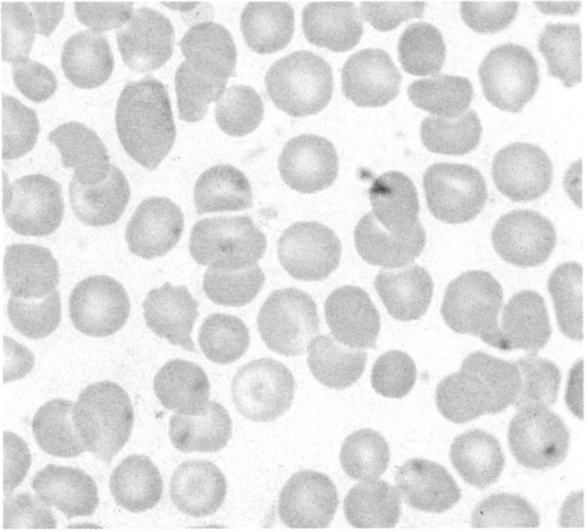

Fig. 8.52 The blood film of a baby with rhesus haemolytic disease of the newborn showing that the degree of spherocytosis is much less than that which is seen in ABO haemolytic disease of the newborn (see Fig. 8.51).

other rhesus antibodies, is now the second most common cause. Occasionally, haemolytic disease of the newborn is caused by antibodies of other systems such as Kell.

Blood film and count

Anaemia varies from mild to severe. The blood film in ABO haemolytic disease of the newborn shows prominent spherocytosis (Fig. 8.51) whereas in rhesus haemolytic disease of the newborn the degree of spherocytosis is much less (Fig. 8.52). There may be associated neutropenia and thrombocytopenia [71]. Since the blood films of normal neonates show some spherocytes, mild cases of rhesus haemolytic disease may not be readily diagnosed from the blood film.

Differential diagnosis

The differential diagnosis is with hereditary spherocytosis.

Further tests. The diagnosis is confirmed by a positive direct antiglobulin test in the baby and detection of an IgG antibody in maternal serum with specificity against a fetal red cell antigen.

Non-immune acquired haemolytic anaemias

Microangiopathic and related haemolytic anaemias

The term microangiopathic haemolytic anaemia refers to haemolytic anaemia caused by red cell fragmentation consequent on endothelial damage, fibrin deposition in capillaries or both. Causes are multiple (Table 8.3). In childhood the commonest cause is enteric infection, most often by a

Table 8.3 Some causes of red cell fragmentation

Microangiopathic haemolytic anaemia
Epidemic or sporadic haemolytic uraemic syndrome, thrombotic thrombocytopenic purpura and related thrombotic microangiopathies
following infection by *Shigella*, verotoxin-producing *Escherichia coli*, *Campylobacter jejuni*, other bacteria, viruses (including HIV) or fungi [72–75] or vaccination (influenza, polio, measles, smallpox, triple antigen or typhoid–paratyphoid) [76]
familial haemolytic uraemic syndrome
associated with pregnancy, oral contraceptive intake or the post-partum state
toxicity of mitomycin C, bleomycin, other chemotherapeutic agents, cyclosporin A, penicillin, penicillamine [74]; quinine hypersensitivity [77]
Other pathological processes involving small vessels in the kidney (with or without extrarenal vascular lesions)
pregnancy-associated hypertension
malignant hypertension
renal cortical necrosis
microscopic polyarteritis nodosa
acute glomerulonephritis
renal involvement by systemic lupus erythematosus
renal involvement by systemic sclerosis (scleroderma) [78]
Wegener's granulomatosis
renal irradiation
rejection of transplanted kidney
Diabetic angiopathy [79]
Systemic amyloidosis
Disseminated intravascular coagulation (including that associated with malignant disease, aortic aneurysm and renal vein thrombosis)
Therapeutic defibrination (occasionally)
Disseminated carcinoma (particularly mucin-secreting carcinoma, particularly carcinoma of the stomach)
Congenital [80,81]
Associated with congenital cobalamin C defect [82]
Following arteriography [83]
Reaction to bee sting [74]
Bone marrow transplantation
Thymoma-associated (one case) [84]

Associated with vascular malformations and other large vessel lesions
Haemangioma
Haemangioendothelioma of the liver
Haemangioendotheliosarcoma
Plexiform pulmonary lesions of pulmonary hypertension
Plexiform pulmonary lesions of cirrhosis [85]
Giant cell arteritis [86]

Mechanical fragmentation
Prosthetic valves (aortic more than mitral, much more common when there is regurgitation around a valve)
Homograft, xenograft (porcine) and fascia lata autograft valves (less likely than with prosthetic valves)
Prosthetic patches
Severe aortic stenosis (very uncommon)
Severe mitral valve disease and following valvuloplasty for mitral valve disease (rare)
Aortic coarctation (rare)
Use of subclavian dialysis catheters [87]

Extracorporeal circulation (associated with thrombosis in the apparatus) [87] ***and long-term extracorporeal membrane oxygenation in neonates*** [88]

verocytotoxin-secreting *Escherichia coli*. In adults the commonest causes are probably pregnancy-associated hypertension and carcinoma. A similar haemolytic anaemia can occur with large vessel or valvular lesions and with prosthetic cardiac valves. In some of these instances there is thrombosis on an abnormal surface and in others there is red cell damage consequent on turbulent flow or on mechanical damage of red cells by components of a malfunctioning prosthetic valve.

Blood film and count

The blood film shows microspherocytes, keratocytes and other schistocytes and often polychromasia and polychromatic macrocytes. When there is associated platelet consumption, thrombocytopenia and large platelets are apparent. In the post-diarrhoeal haemolytic uraemic syndrome of childhood there is often leucocytosis and neutrophilia, the severity of which correlates

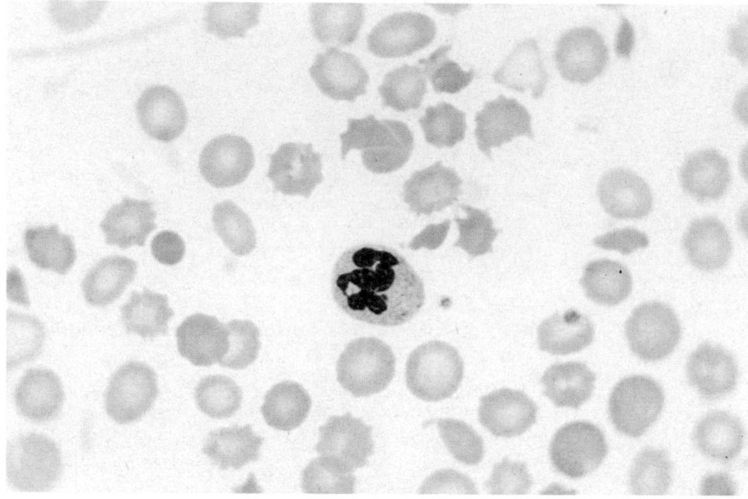

Fig. 8.53 The blood film of an adult patient at the onset of haemolytic uraemic syndrome showing both fragments and echinocytes. Courtesy of Dr Ayed Eden.

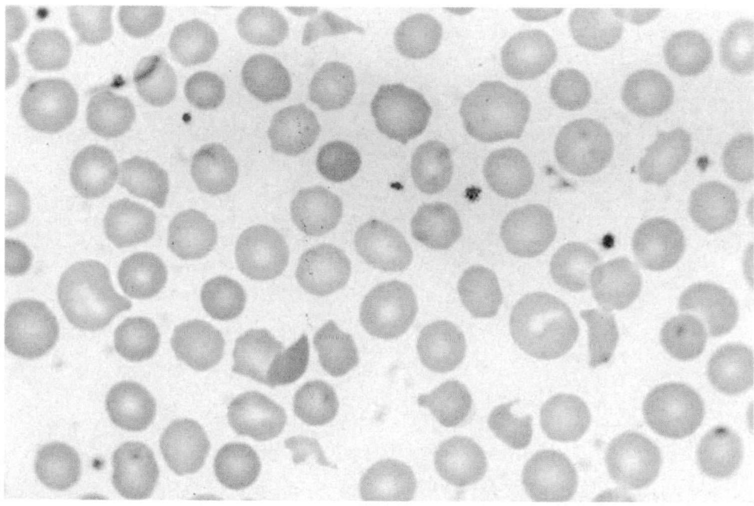

Fig. 8.54 The blood film of an adult with the haemolytic uraemic syndrome showing fragments, several spherocytes and several polychromatic macrocytes.

with associated renal damage. Occasionally at presentation, there is also marked echinocytosis, probably indicative of damage to the red cell membrane by the toxin which is causing the haemolysis (Fig. 8.53). In microangiopathic haemolytic anaemia there is often associated thrombocytopenia but otherwise the blood films of microangiopathic haemolytic anaemia (Fig. 8.54) and of haemolytic anaemia caused by large vessel or valvular diseases or prostheses (Fig. 8.55) cannot be readily distinguished. Haemolysis in the microangiopathic and mechanical haemolytic anaemias is intravascular and when it is severe and chronic the consequent haemoglobinuria can lead to complicating iron deficiency, the features of which are then apparent on the blood film (Fig. 8.56).

The FBC shows a reduced Hb, increased RDW and sometimes an increased MCV and HDW (consequent on reticulocytosis) or a low platelet count with an increased MPV. There may be 'flagging' indicating the presence of both microcytes and macrocytes. If there are large numbers of schistocytes there may be 'flagging' indicating poor

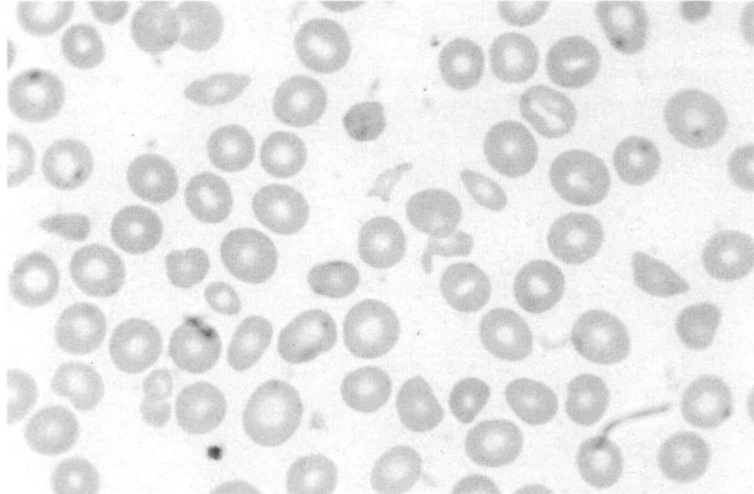

Fig. 8.55 The blood film of a patient with mechanical haemolytic anaemia due to a defective prosthetic mitral valve showing numerous fragments.

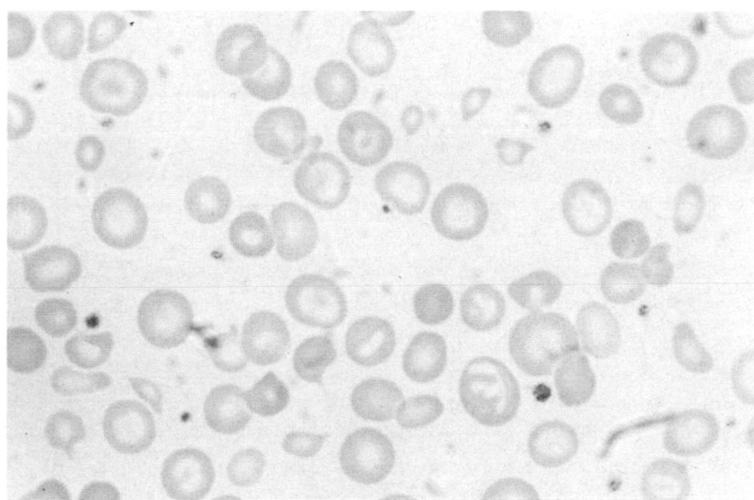

Fig. 8.56 The blood film of an Afro-Caribbean patient with iron deficiency as a complication of mechanical haemolysis from a defective prosthetic valve. There are fragments, hypochromia, microcytosis, and one target cell. The patient also had haemoglobin C trait.

separation of red cells and platelets and the possibility of factitious elevation of the platelet count. Red cell histograms and cytograms (Fig. 8.57) may show hyperchromic cells, normochromic and hyperchromic microcytes and hypochromic macrocytes.

Differential diagnosis

The blood film of microangiopathic and related haemolytic anaemias is distinctive and usually there is no diagnostic difficulty.

Further tests

Bilirubin and lactic acid dehydrogenase estimations and a reticulocyte count are useful in assessing the severity of the haemolysis. In cases with chronic mild haemolysis and few fragments the detection of haemosiderin in urinary sediment is useful in demonstrating that intravascular haemolysis has occurred.

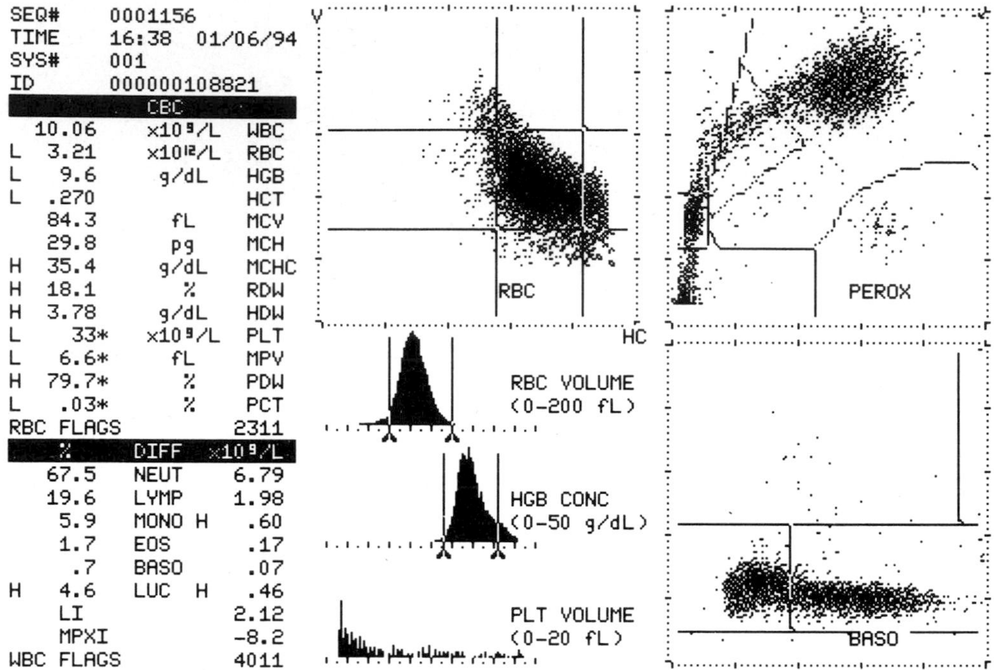

Fig. 8.57 Technicon H.2 red cell and platelet histograms and cytograms from a patient with microangiopathic haemolytic anaemia. There are many hyperchromatic cells which are spherocytes and microspherocytes and microcytic cells which are other fragments. The platelet histogram illustrates that in this patient the platelet count was very low.

Oxidant-induced haemolytic anaemia

Exposure to sufficiently potent oxidants, either drugs or chemicals, can cause haemolytic anaemia even in individuals in whom G6PD and other enzymes of the pentose shunt are normal. Neonates, especially premature neonates, are particularly susceptible to oxidant-induced haemolysis. Oxidants can cause acquired methaemoglobinaemia, consequent on oxidation of haemoglobin, and acute or chronic haemolytic anaemia consequent on oxidation both of haemoglobin and of membrane components. When haemolysis is acute, oxidized haemoglobin precipitates as Heinz bodies, hence the name 'Heinz-body haemolytic anaemia'. Heinz bodies are cleared by the spleen but when haemolysis is acute they may be detected in circulating red cells.

Oxidant-induced haemolysis is most often caused by drugs, particularly dapsone and salazopyrine. It can also be consequent on nitrate contamination of drinking water or on accidental or deliberate exposure to agricultural and industrial chemicals.

Blood film and count

When the haemolysis is acute the blood film (Fig. 8.58) is similar to that of G6PD deficiency during acute haemolytic episodes. When haemolysis is milder and more chronic there are variable numbers of irregularly contracted cells and possibly also macrocytosis and polychromatic macrocytes.

Differential diagnosis

The differential diagnosis is with G6PD deficiency and with unstable haemoglobins and other causes of irregularly contracted cells.

Further tests

The diagnosis can usually be made from the clinical history and the blood film. A Heinz body

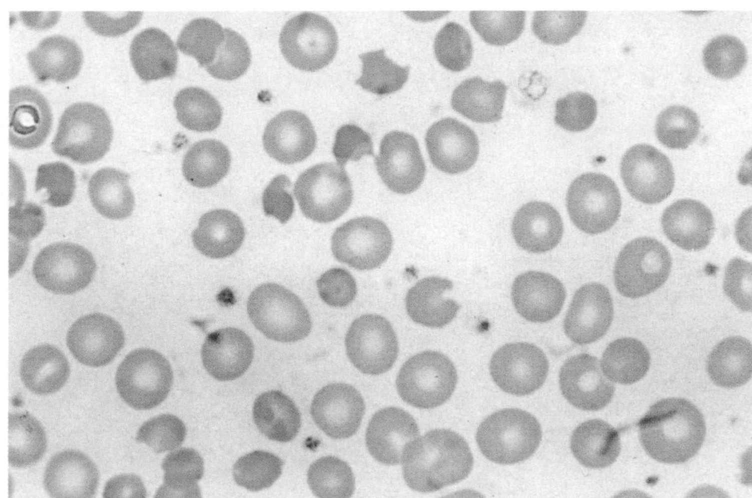

Fig. 8.58 The blood film of a patient taking dapsone for a skin condition showing macrocytosis, irregularly contracted cells and several bite cells.

preparation is positive in acute cases. In some patients it may be necessary to confirm that the G6PD activity is normal after the episode of haemolysis has passed.

OTHER ACQUIRED HAEMOLYTIC ANAEMIAS

Other acquired haemolytic anaemias are uncommon and the aetiology is often suggested by the clinical setting.

Renal disease

Red cell survival is usually reduced in acute renal failure. The features of a microangiopathic haemolytic anaemia are commonly present. Reduced red cell survival is one of the mechanisms, although not the principal one, in anaemia of chronic renal failure. Small numbers of keratocytes and other fragments may be present.

Liver disease

Liver disease is associated with several haemolytic syndromes. In Zieve's syndrome there is acute alcoholic liver disease associated with hyperlipidaemia and acute haemolysis. Zieve [89] and others [90] have described the abnormal cells as 'spherocytes' and in one case Zieve suspected an inherited haemolytic anaemia. However, illustrations have shown irregularly contracted cells [90] and these are sometimes prominent (Fig. 8.59). A distinct syndrome initially called 'spur cell haemolytic anaemia' which is characterized by numerous acanthocytes (Fig. 8.60) is caused by liver failure of any aetiology.

Wilson's disease

Wilson's disease can cause both acute haemolytic anaemia with no morphological abnormality and an acute Heinz body haemolytic anaemia consequent on sudden release of copper from a gravely damaged liver (Fig. 8.61). It is important to think of previously undiagnosed Wilson's disease when an acute haemolytic anaemia is unexplained since this may be the presenting feature of a condition which is fatal if left untreated.

Bacterial and parasitic infections

Bartonellosis, malaria and babesiosis characteristically cause haemolytic anaemia. Bacterial and viral infections can be associated with microangiopathic haemolytic anaemia. Clostridial toxins can cause a severe spherocytic haemolytic anaemia. Bacterial infections can also alter red cell membrane antigens to cause T activation. Anti-T antibodies in the plasma can then bind to red cells causing spherocytosis and haemolysis. This has been observed with infection by

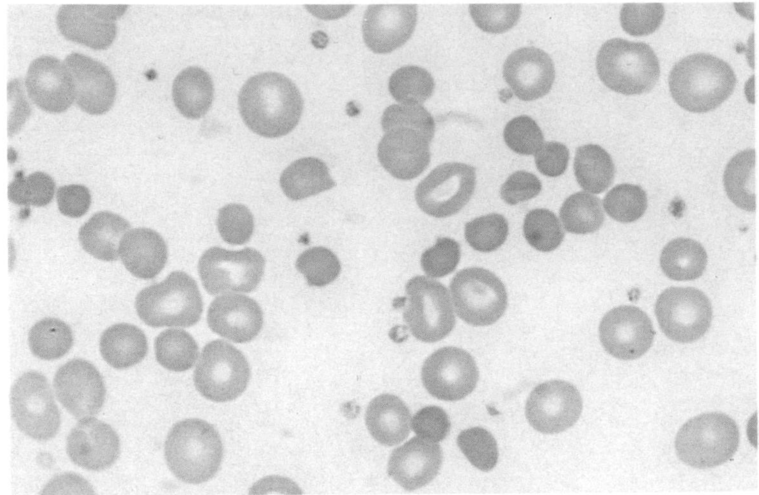

Fig. 8.59 The blood film of a patient with Zieve's syndrome as a complication of acute alcoholic liver disease showing irregularly contracted cells and polychromatic macrocytes.

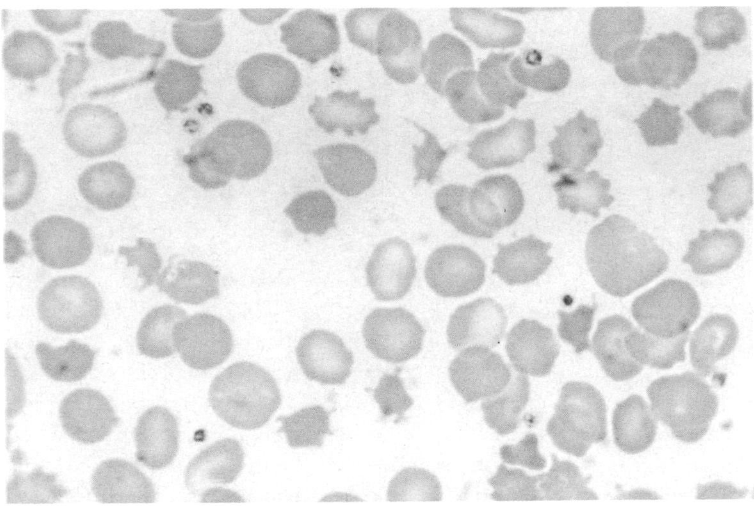

Fig. 8.60 The blood film in a patient with terminal liver disease of unknown aetiology showing numerous acanthocytes ('spur cell' haemolytic anaemia).

Staphylococcus aureus, *Escherichia coli* and pneumococcus and in necrotizing enteritis caused by *Clostridium perfringens*. Acute haemolysis can follow transfusion of normal blood which contains anti-T antibodies and this type of haemolysis can therefore be confused with other types of haemolytic transfusion reaction [91].

Snake and insect bites

Bites of a number of snakes (Fig. 8.62) and insects can cause an acute spherocytic haemolytic anaemia, sometimes with associated disseminated intravascular haemolytic anaemia and thrombocytopenia. Sometimes red cell fragments are the most prominent feature.

March haemoglobinuria

March haemoglobinuria describes haemolytic anaemia observed in soldiers on forced marches. Although haemolysis is mechanical, consequent on damage of red cells in blood vessels in the feet, it is rare for any fragments or other specific features

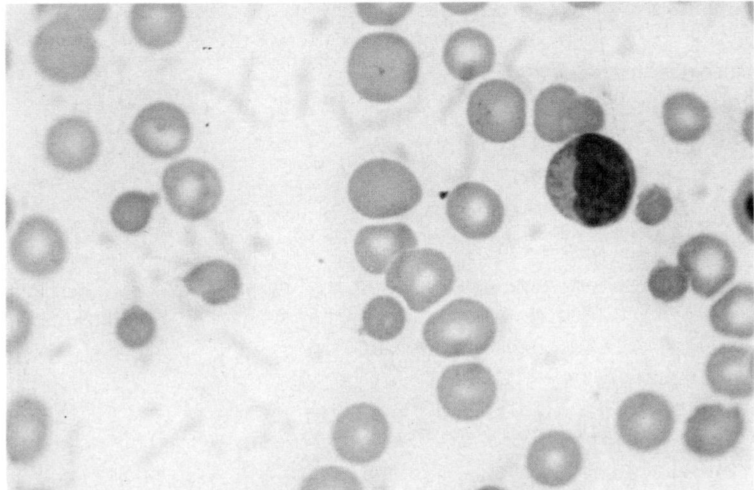

Fig. 8.61 The blood film in a patient with terminal liver disease as a complication of Wilson's disease showing irregularly contracted cells and polychromatic macrocytes.

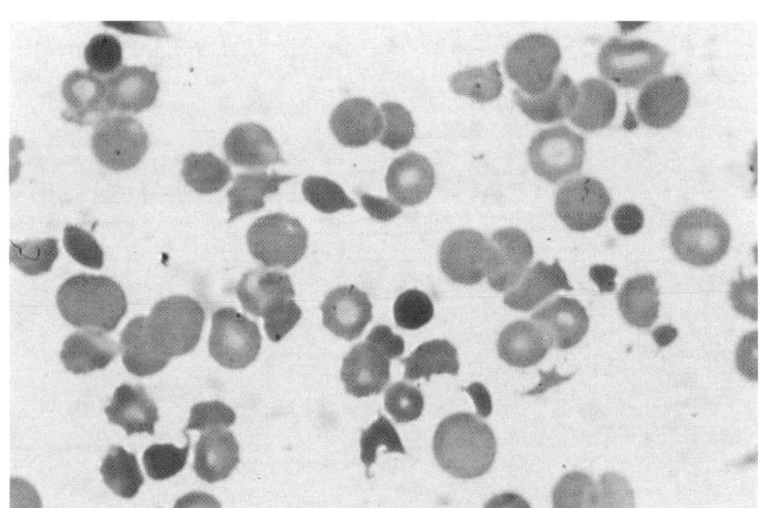

Fig. 8.62 The blood film of a Sri Lankan patient who had suffered a viper bite showing fragments and microspherocytes. Courtesy of Dr Sudharma Vidyatilake, Colombo.

to be observed. A similar type of haemolysis can be induced by jogging on hard surfaces, karate and drumming with the hands. These conditions should be sought by specific questioning whenever there is mild unexplained anaemia in an apparently fit, usually young, person. (There may be factors other than haemolysis operating in some cases of exercise-induced anaemia, e.g., exercise-induced gastrointestinal haemorrhage.)

Paroxysmal nocturnal haemoglobinuria (PNH)

PNH is a clonal haemopoietic stem cell disorder in which red cells with a membrane defect are abnormally sensitive to complement-induced lysis. Some but not all patients give a history of nocturnal haemolysis, i.e., of the first urine specimen passed in the morning being red. There are no specific blood film features but PNH should be considered when there is a haemolytic anaemia associated with leucopenia or thrombocytopenia.

A Ham test for lysis of red cells following exposure to acidified serum should be performed when this diagnosis is suspected.

Dyserythropoietic anaemias

Congenital dyserythropoietic anaemias (CDA)

CDAs are inherited defects characterized by ineffective and dysplastic erythropoiesis, anaemia and marked poikilocytosis. There are three well-characterized types, the features of which are summarized in Table 8.4. There are also cases which appear to conform to these types but have a different inheritance and therefore presumably a different underlying defect. There are autosomal dominant cases resembling type I and autosomal recessive cases resembling type III. In addition there are individual cases or families with distinctive features. In most cases the underlying abnormality is not understood. Some cases have other associated congenital abnormalities.

Blood film and count

In a minority of cases the anaemia is severe. Usually it is mild or moderate. Some cases are macrocytic and others are normocytic. Cells show marked anisocytosis and striking poikilocytosis (Figs 8.63 & 8.64). Haemoglobinization is generally normal but some cells may be poorly haemoglobinized. The absolute reticulocyte count is normal. In addition to type I, II and III CDA, variants have been described with microcytosis attributable to sideroblastic erythropoiesis [93] and with prominent ovalocytosis [94]. Some cases have had circulating NRBC which become very numerous after splenectomy [95]. The RDW and HDW are increased, the RDW markedly so, and this is reflected in the red cell cytograms and histograms (Fig. 8.65).

Differential diagnosis

The differential diagnosis includes haemolytic anaemias with marked morphological abnormalities, particularly hereditary poikilocytosis and haemoglobin H disease. In both these conditions the reticulocyte count is elevated and in haemoglobin H disease there is hypochromia and microcytosis. Cases presenting beyond childhood need to be distinguished from the myelodysplastic syndromes and other conditions causing acquired dyserythropoiesis. Cases of CDA usually lack significant dysplastic features in non-erythroid lineages.

Further tests

Diagnosis requires bone marrow examination and, in the case of type II CDA, the demonstration

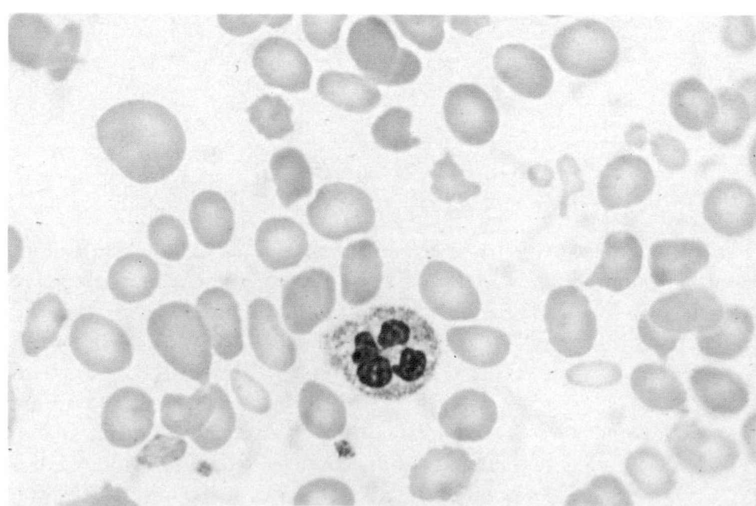

Fig. 8.63 The blood film of a patient with type I congenital dyserythropoietic anaemia showing marked anisocytosis, poikilocytosis and some macrocytes.

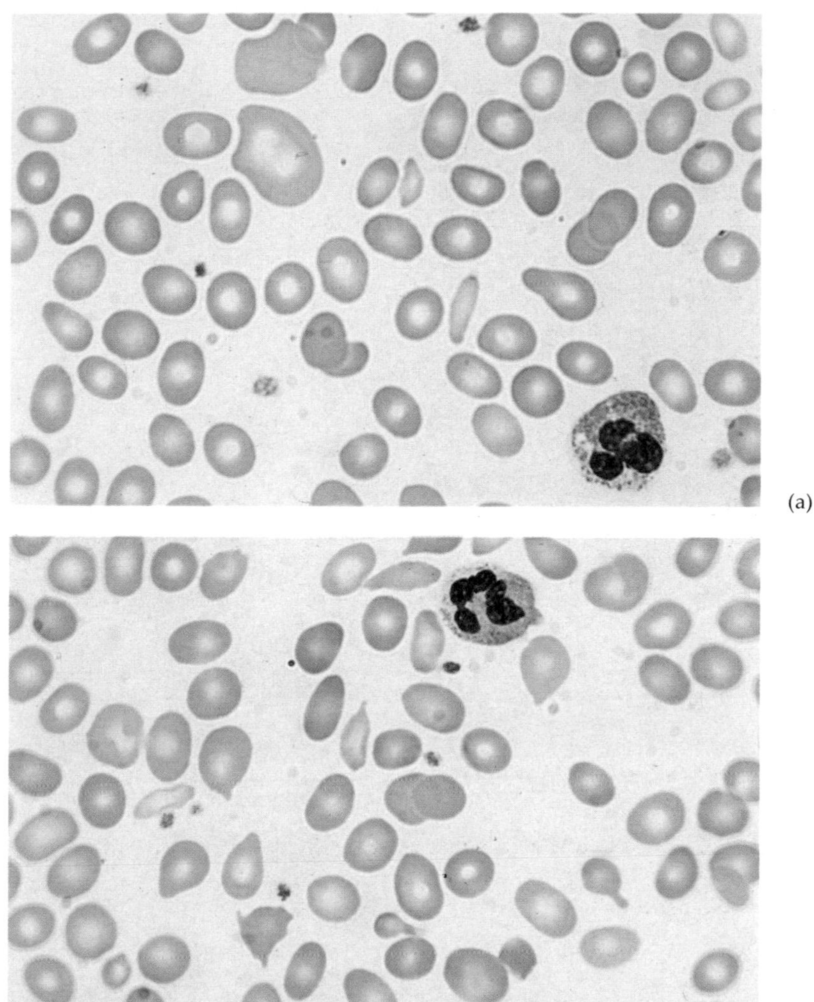

Fig. 8.64 (a, b) The blood film of a patient with type III congenital dyserythropoietic anaemia showing anisocytosis and poikilocytosis. Courtesy of Professor S.N. Wickramasinghe, London.

of a positive acid lysis (Ham) test. However, a provisional diagnosis can be made from peripheral blood examination alone.

Acquired dyserythropoietic anaemias

Dyserythropoiesis as an acquired phenomenon can be secondary to severe protein–calorie malnutrition, HIV infection or exposure to drugs (such as cytotoxic drugs) or to toxic substances (such as alcohol or arsenic). It can also be a manifestation of one of the myelodysplastic syndromes (see p. 285) or of other haemopoietic neoplasms.

Blood film and count

Red cells may show anisocytosis, poikilocytosis, macrocytosis or basophilic stippling and there may be a population of hypochromic microcytes. Neutrophils may show hypogranularity and defects of nuclear lobulation. The FBC may show anaemia, neutropenia or thrombocytopenia. Red cell histograms and cytograms may show an increased MCV, RDW and HDW.

Differential diagnosis

The differential diagnosis is with congenital

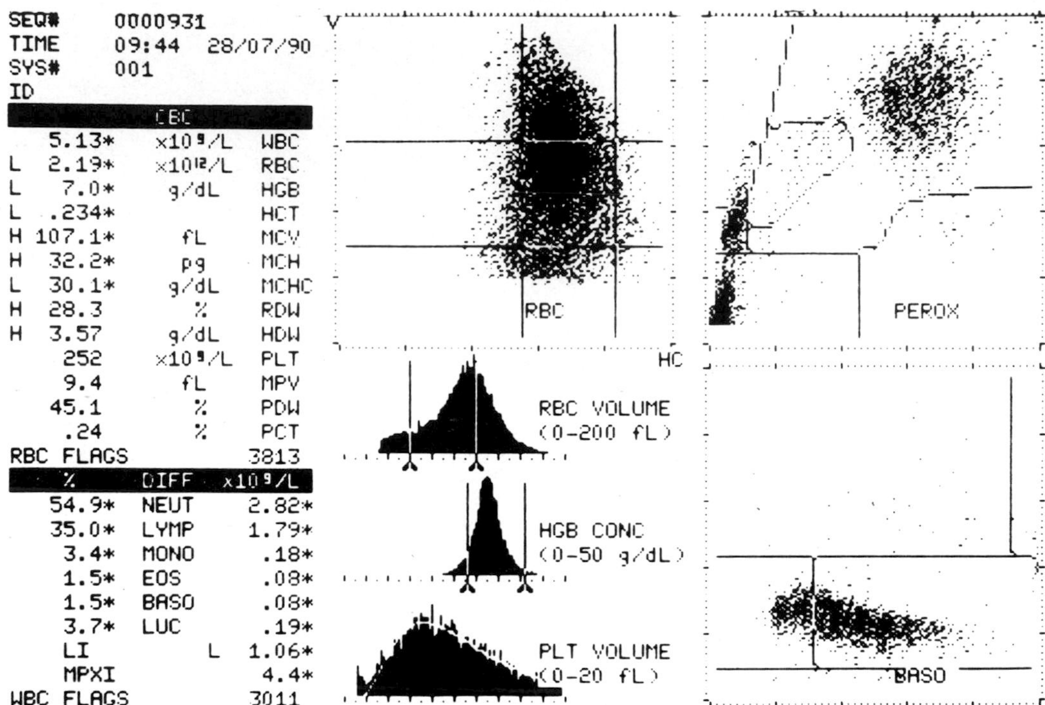

Fig. 8.65 Technicon H.2 red cell histograms and cytograms from a patient with type I congenital dyserythropoietic anaemia (same patient as in Fig. 8.63) showing a marked variation in red cell size (as reflected in the RDW) and a lesser degree of variation in red cell haemoglobinization (as reflected in the HDW).

Table 8.4 Inheritance pattern and morphological features of the congenital dyserythropoietic anaemias

Type	Inheritance	Red cell size	Other blood film features
Type I	AR	Macrocytic	Oval macrocytes, marked anisocytosis, marked poikilocytosis, basophilic stippling, irregularly contracted cells, polychromasia
Type II (Hempas)	AR	Normocytic	Moderate anisocytosis, moderate poikilocytosis including 'pincer cells' [92] and irregularly contracted cells, some NRBC, polychromasia
Type III	AD	Normocytic or slightly macrocytic	Marked anisocytosis, marked poikilocytosis including fragments and irregularly contracted cells, basophilic stippling, polychromasia

Hempas, hereditary erythroid multinuclearity with positive acidified-serum lysis test.

dyserythropoietic anaemias and with other causes of anaemia and cytopenia.

Further tests

Which further tests are indicated is dependent on the clinical setting and the specific cytological abnormalities present.

Polycythaemic rubra vera (PRV)

PRV, also known as primary proliferative polycythaemia, is a myeloproliferative disorder in which there is increased production of red cells and sometimes also of granulocytes and platelets. The term 'essential erythrocytosis' is used to refer to cases with unexplained polycythaemia but without clear evidence of a myeloproliferative disorder. Some of these patients subsequently develop features of PRV. PRV is largely a disease of the middle-aged and elderly population, although occasional cases are seen in younger adults and very rare cases in children. Common clinical features are those resulting from the hyperviscosity of the polycythaemic blood, such as cerebrovascular accidents and peripheral gangrene, and those indicative of the myeloproliferative disorder, such as hepatomegaly, splenomegaly and itch.

PRV may eventually enter a 'burnt-out' phase or may be complicated by the development of myelofibrosis or AML.

Blood film and count

The peripheral blood film in polycythaemia of any aetiology shows a 'packed film' appearance since the viscosity of the blood means that the film of blood is not spread as thinly as normal (Fig. 8.66). The WBC, neutrophil and basophil counts are increased in the majority of cases. Monocyte and eosinophil counts are much less often increased. Platelet count is elevated in about two-thirds of cases and platelet size is increased. Red cells may be normocytic and normochromic or, if hyperplastic erythropoiesis has led to exhaustion of iron stores, they may be hypochromic and microcytic. If complicating iron deficiency occurs there may be anaemia (Fig. 8.67) but the underlying polycythaemia is revealed if the patient is given iron. Less often PRV is masked by complicating vitamin B_{12} or folate deficiency.

The FBC usually shows an elevated RBC, Hb and PCV and normal or reduced MCV and MCH. The platelet count may be increased. The MPV is raised in relation to the platelet count. In PRV complicated by iron deficiency the red cell indices are very similar to those of thalassaemia trait but the MCHC is reduced and the RDW is increased.

Differential diagnosis

The differential diagnosis is with other causes of polycythaemia (see Table 6.1). Neutrophilia, basophilia, thrombocytosis, giant platelets and

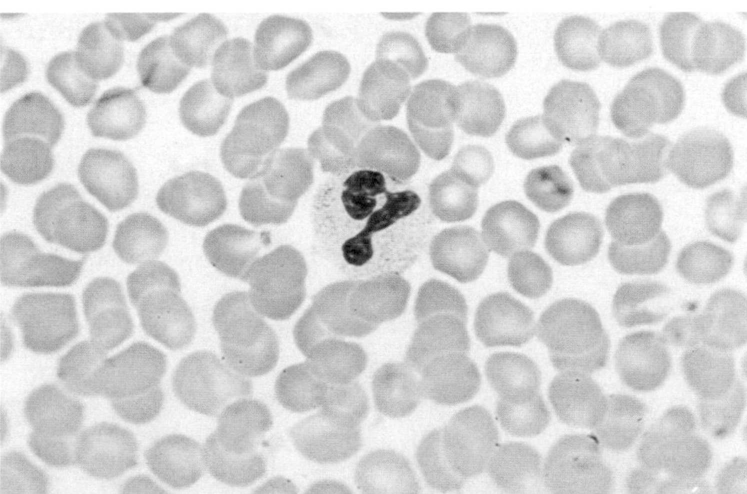

Fig. 8.66 A 'packed film' consequent on post-transplant polycythaemia. The Hb was 20 g/dl and the PCV 0.59. The MCV was increased to 114 fl as a consequence of azathioprone therapy.

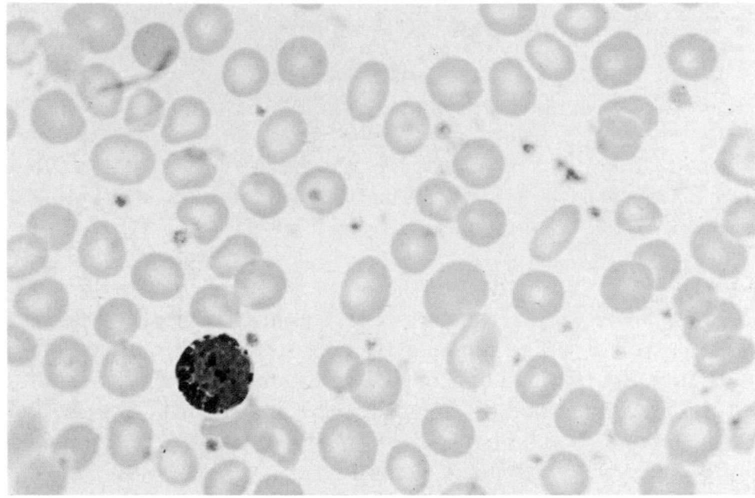

Fig. 8.67 The blood film of a patient with PRV complicated by iron deficiency, showing anaemia and thrombocytosis and some hypochromic and microcytic cells. There was an increased basophil count and there is one basophil in the field. FBC (Coulter S Plus IV) was WBC 6.7×10^9/l, RBC 4.38×10^{12}/l, Hb 10.6 g/dl, PCV 0.33, MCV 75 fl, MCH 24.2 pg, MCHC 32.3 g/dl, RDW 24.9, platelet count 1056×10^9/l.

an elevated MPV favour a diagnosis of PRV. Basophilia is particularly useful in the differential diagnosis since it is not seen in secondary polycythaemia.

Further tests

Polycythaemia should be confirmed by obtaining a repeat blood specimen without use of a tourniquet before proceeding to further investigations. Determination of total red cell and plasma volume by radioisotopic dilution studies excludes pseudopolycythaemia. A bone marrow aspirate and trephine biopsy are useful to confirm a myeloproliferative disorder. The NAP score is often increased and is much less likely to be increased in secondary polycythaemia. Tests which are useful to exclude commoner causes of secondary polycythaemia are blood gas estimations and radiological investigation of the kidneys.

Disorders of platelets

Congenital thrombocytopenias

Congenital thrombocytopenia may be inherited or due to a pathological process, e.g., infection or exposure to a toxic substance, occurring during intra-uterine life. It may be caused by failure of production or increased consumption or destruction of platelets. Babies who have been exposed to teratogenic substances or have an inherited condition causing thrombocytopenia may have other congenital abnormalities as seen, for example, in the thrombocytopenia with absent radii syndrome.

Blood film and count

The peripheral blood film may show platelets which are small, normal in size or large. Small platelets are uncommon but are seen in the Wiskott–Aldrich syndrome (see Fig. 3.109). Platelets of normal size are seen when there is bone marrow or megakaryocytic hypoplasia. Large platelets are common in various inherited causes of thrombocytopenia, e.g., Bernard–Soulier syndrome (Fig. 8.68) and May–Hegglin anomaly (see Fig. 3.61). The platelets usually show normal granulation but in the rare grey platelet syndrome they appear agranular or hypogranular (Fig. 8.69). Neutrophils should be examined for abnormal inclusions which are present not only in the May–Hegglin anomaly but in several other rare inherited causes of thrombocytopenia. In Down's syndrome the blood film should be examined for features of transient abnormal myelopoiesis (see p. 284) which may cause thrombocytopenia. Rarely, the blood film may show features of congenital leukaemia.

The platelet count is low but when a large

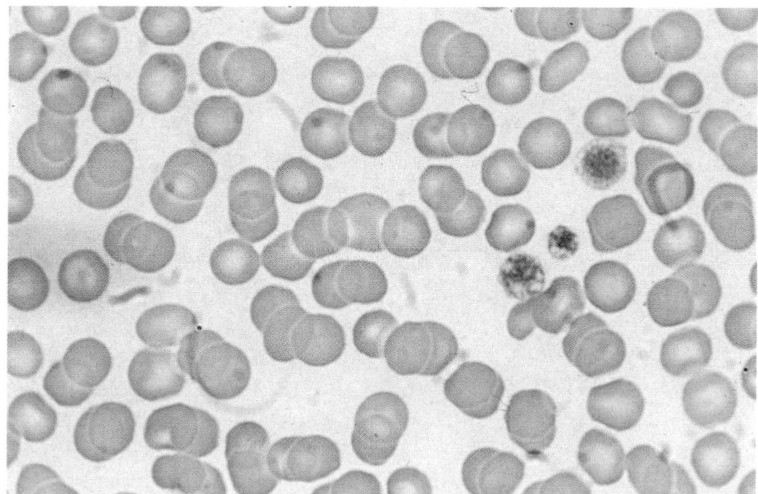

Fig. 8.68 The blood film of a patient with the Bernard–Soulier syndrome showing thrombocytopenia and three giant platelets.

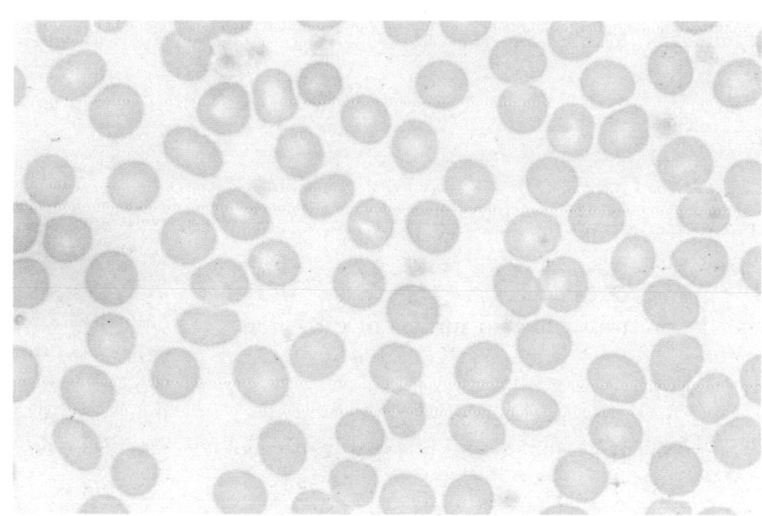

Fig. 8.69 The blood film of a patient with the grey platelet syndrome showing six agranular platelets.

proportion of platelets are very large the count on an automated instrument may be an underestimate of the true count. Depending on the aetiology of the thrombocytopenia, the MPV may be low, normal or high.

Differential diagnosis

The differential diagnosis includes all the causes of congenital thrombocytopenia listed in Table 6.24.

Further tests

Whether further tests are needed and the choice of any further tests depends on the aetiology which is suspected on the basis of the clinical features, blood film and count. Useful tests may include cytogenetic analysis, bone marrow examination, testing of the mother's serum for antiplatelet antibodies, platelet function studies and examination of platelet membrane antigens by immunological techniques. Investigation of other family members may be useful.

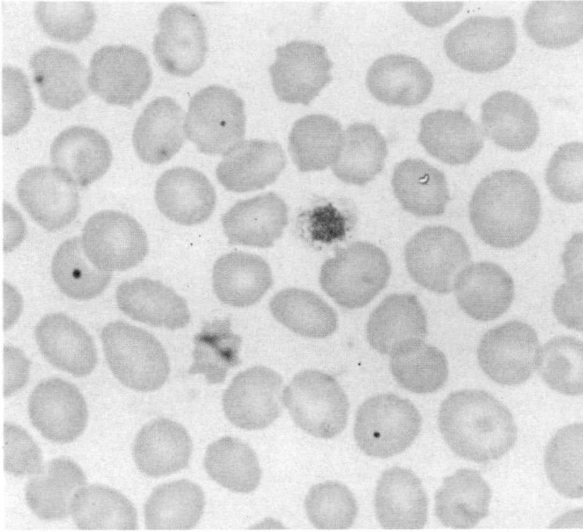

Fig. 8.70 The blood film of a patient with ITP post-splenectomy showing thrombocytopenia, a single giant platelet and Howell–Jolly bodies.

Autoimmune (idiopathic) thrombocytopenic purpura (ITP)

Autoimmune or 'idiopathic' thrombocytopenic purpura is an acquired condition in which platelet survival is reduced by the presence of platelet-directed autoantibodies.

Blood film and count

The blood film shows thrombocytopenia and, unless the onset is very acute, increased platelet size (Fig. 8.70). Usually other cell lineages are normal but occasionally there is associated autoimmune haemolytic anaemia or evidence of an underlying causative condition such as CLL, lymphoma or large granular lymphocyte leukaemia.

The platelet count is reduced and unless the onset is very acute the MPV is increased.

Differential diagnosis

The differential diagnosis includes HIV infection which may present initially with features resembling ITP. Cytomegalovirus infection, infectious mononucleosis and other viral infections can also present with severe thrombocytopenia as the major manifestation. Thrombocytopenia following rubella and other viral infections, drug-induced thrombocytopenia and TTP can also be confused with ITP.

Further tests

Before any other investigations are performed the blood film must be examined to confirm thrombocytopenia and, unless the patient has obvious petechiae or purpura, the thrombocytopenia must be confirmed on a second carefully taken blood specimen. The blood film should also be examined for spherocytes, red cell fragments, polychromasia, atypical lymphocytes or lymphoma cells. Other tests which are indicated depend on the diagnosis suspected on the basis of the clinical features and the blood film examination. For example, if ITP seems the most likely diagnosis a bone marrow examination is indicated to confirm that megakaryocyte numbers are normal or increased and to exclude other conditions. Tests for antinuclear antibodies and DNA binding should also be carried out since ITP may be the initial presentation of systemic lupus erythematosus. If, however, atypical lymphocytes are detected, a Paul–Bunnell test for infectious mononucleosis and specific serology for cytomegalovirus may be useful; and if HIV infection appears clinically likely a specific test for HIV infection should be considered. If red cell fragments are present, investigations relevant to TTP should be initiated.

Thrombotic thrombocytopenic purpura (TTP)

TTP is a systemic disorder of unknown cause in which microthrombi in multiple organs lead to platelet consumption and renal and cerebral manifestations. The thrombocytopenia may lead to haemorrhage.

Blood film and count

The blood film shows the features of a microangiopathic haemolytic anaemia (fragments and polychromasia) together with thrombocytopenia with platelet anisocytosis. The RDW, MPV and PDW may be increased.

Differential diagnosis

The differential diagnosis includes other causes of red cell fragmentation, particularly those which may also cause thrombocytopenia.

Further tests

A biopsy confirmation of capillary thrombi confirms the diagnosis.

Essential thrombocythaemia

Essential thrombocythaemia is a myeloproliferative disorder characterized by increased platelet production. It is predominantly a disease of the middle-aged and elderly population but cases also occur in young adults and even in children. Clinical features are either caused directly by the thrombocytosis or reflect the abnormal proliferation of myeloid cells. They include microvascular obstruction, bleeding and, less often, splenomegaly and itch. An increasing proportion of patients are being diagnosed at a presymptomatic stage as a consequence of the increasing use of automated blood cell counters.

Essential thrombocythaemia terminates, uncommonly, in myelofibrosis and, rarely, in AML.

Blood film and count

The diagnosis is not usually made unless the platelet count is at least $600 \times 10^9/l$ and in many cases it is in excess of $1000 \times 10^9/l$. The blood film shows increased platelet anisocytosis and usually a large number of giant platelets (Fig. 8.71). Some of the platelets may be hypogranular. Neutrophilia is present in about one-third of patients. The basophil count is often elevated but does not usually exceed 3%. A basophil count of more than 5% suggests that the patient may be Philadelphia positive. Occasional NRBC and immature granulocytes may be present. There may be features of iron deficiency as a consequence of bleeding. Rarely, there are features of hyposplenism following earlier splenic infarction.

The platelet count, MPV and PDW are elevated whereas in reactive thrombocytosis the MPV and PDW are not usually increased. Splenectomy or hyposplenism can, however, cause thrombocytosis with an increased MPV and PDW.

Differential diagnosis

The differential diagnosis is with other causes of thrombocytosis (see Table 6.13). The conditions which may cause reactive thrombocytosis without clear clinical features suggesting the underlying disease include occult neoplasms and

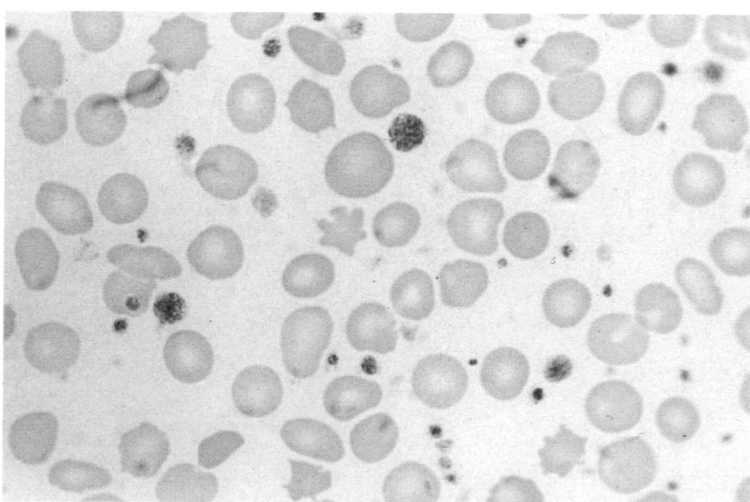

Fig. 8.71 The blood film of a patient with essential thrombocythaemia showing thrombocytosis with platelet anisocytosis and giant platelets. There is also red cell anisocytosis and poikilocytosis.

connective tissue disorders. In iron deficient patients uncomplicated iron deficiency should be included in the differential diagnosis since iron deficiency alone can cause a platelet count of $600 \times 10^9/l$ or even higher. Patients with iron deficiency may also have an occult neoplasm, occult haemorrhage or both as a cause of thrombocytosis. It can also be difficult or impossible to distinguish iron deficient PRV from essential thrombocythaemia with iron deficiency but this distinction is not clinically important since satisfactory treatment does not require that the two conditions be distinguished.

Further tests

A bone marrow aspirate and trephine biopsy may provide evidence of a myeloproliferative disorder. It should be noted, however, that iron deficiency alone can cause thrombocytosis, marked erythroid hyperplasia and quite a marked increase in megakaryocytes so that the diagnosis of essential thrombocythaemia should be made with caution in iron deficient patients. Sometimes a trial of therapy is necessary to make the distinction. The NAP score is low in a minority of patients, elevated in some and normal in the majority. Cytogenetic analysis can be useful if it is not clear that the patient has a myeloproliferative disorder. Cytogenetic investigations are also indicated if there are atypical disease characteristics — such as myelodysplastic features, blast cells or a markedly elevated basophil count — which suggest either Philadelphia-positivity or another unfavourable karyotype which may influence management. The NAP score is not useful in differentiating Philadelphia-positive and Philadelphia-negative cases. Various laboratory tests such as an elevated plasma fibrinogen or an elevated ESR can provide indirect evidence of an occult neoplasm or connective tissue disorder as a cause of thrombocytosis.

References

1 Patton WN, Cave RJ, Harris RI. A study of changes in red cell volume and haemoglobin concentration during phlebotomy induced iron deficiency and iron repletion using the Technicon H1. *Clin Lab Haematol* 1991; 13: 153–61.

2 Bessman JD, Gilmer PR, Gardner FH. Improved classification of the anemias by MCV and RDW. *Am J Clin Pathol* 1983; 80: 322–6.

3 Marsh WL, Bishop JW, Darcy TP. Evaluation of red cell volume distribution width (RDW). *Hematol Pathol* 1987; 1: 117–23.

4 Mazza U, Saglio G, Cappio FC, Camaschella C, Neretto G, Gallo E. Clinical and haematological data in 254 cases of beta-thalassaemia trait in Italy. *Br J Haematol* 1976; 33: 91–9.

5 d'Onofrio G, Zini G, Ricerca BM, Mancini S, Mango G. Automated measurement of red blood cell microcytosis and hypochromia in iron deficiency and β-thalassaemia trait. *Arch Pathol Lab Med* 1992; 116: 84–9.

6 Weatherall DJ, Clegg JB. *The Thalassaemia Syndromes*. Oxford: Blackwell Scientific Publications, 1981.

7 Mentzer WC. Differentiation of iron deficiency from thalassaemia trait. *Lancet* 1973; i: 882.

8 England JM, Fraser PM. Differentiation of iron deficiency from thalassaemia trait by routine blood count. *Lancet* 1973; i: 449–52.

9 England JM, Bain BJ, Fraser PM. Differentiation of iron deficiency from thalassaemia trait. *Lancet* 1973; i: 1514.

10 Srivastava PC. Differentiation of thalassaemia minor from iron deficiency. *Lancet* 1973; ii: 154–5.

11 Shine I, Lal S. A strategy to detect β thalassaemia trait. *Lancet* 1977; i: 692–4.

12 Green R, King R. A new red cell discriminant incorporating volume dispersion for differentiating iron deficiency anemia from thalassemia minor. *Blood Cells* 1989; 15: 481–95.

13 Bain BJ. Screening of antenatal patients in a multiethnic community for β-thalassaemia trait. *J Clin Pathol* 1988; 41: 481–5.

14 Polliack A, Rachmilewitz EA. Ultrastructural studies in β-thalassaemia major. *Br J Haematol* 1983; 24: 319–26.

15 Dozy AM, Kan YW, Embury SH, Mentzer WC, Wang WC, Lubin B, Davis JR, Koenig HM. α-globin gene organization in blacks precludes the severe form of α-thalassaemia. *Nature* 1979; 280, 605–7.

16 Falusi AG, Esan GJF, Ayyub H, Higgs DR. Alpha-thalassaemia in Nigerian: its interaction with sickle-cell disease. *Eur J Haematol* 1987; 38: 370–5.

17 Tzotzos S, Kavavakis E, Metaxotou-Mavromati A, Kattamis C. The molecular basis of haemoglobin H disease in Greece. *Br J Haematol* 1986; 63: 263–71.

18 Serjeant GR. *The Clinical Features of Sickle Cell Disease*. Amsterdam: North Holland Publishing Company, 1974.

19 Davis LR. Changing blood picture in sickle cell anaemia from shortly after birth to adolescence. *J Clin Pathol* 1976; 29: 898–901.

20 Serjeant GR, Grandison Y, Lowrie Y, Mason K,

Phillips J, Serjeant BE, Vaidya S. The development of haematological changes in homozygous sickle cell disease: a cohort study from birth to 6 years. *Br J Haematol* 1981; 48: 533–43.

21 Glader BE, Propper RD, Buchanan GR. Microcytosis associated with sickle cell anemia. *Am J Clin Pathol* 1979; 72: 63–4.

22 Mohandas N, Kim YR, Tycko DH, Orlik J, Wyatt J, Groner W. Accurate and independent measurement of volume and hemoglobin concentration of individual red cells by laser light scattering. *Blood* 1986; 68: 506–13.

23 Ballard SK, Smith ED. Red blood cell changes during the evolution of the sickle cell painful crisis. *Blood* 1992; 79: 2154–63.

24 Monplaisir N, Merault G, Poyart C, Rhoda CT, Craescu CT, Vidaud M, Galacteros F, Blouquit Y *et al.* Hb-S-Antilles ($\alpha_2\beta_2$Glu Val, 23Val Ile): a new variant with lower solubility than Hb S and producing sickle cell disease in heterozygotes. *Acta Haematol* 1987; 78: 222.

25 Sheehan RG, Frenkel EP. Influence of hemoglobin phenotype on the mean erythrocyte volume. *Acta Haematol* 1983; 69: 260–5.

26 Mears JG, Lachman HM, Labie D, Nagel RL. Alpha-thalassaemia trait is related to prolonged survival in sickle cell anemia. *Blood* 1983; 62: 286–90.

27 Serjeant GR, Serjeant BE. A comparison of erythrocyte characteristics in sickle cell syndromes in Jamaica. *Br J Haematol* 1972; 23: 205–13.

28 Serjeant GR, Sommereux A, Stevenson M, Mason K, Serjeant BE. Comparison of sickle cell-β^0 thalassaemia with homozygous sickle cell disease. *Br J Haematol* 1979; 41: 83–93.

29 Bain BJ. Blood film features of sickle cell-haemoglobin C disease. *Br J Haematol* 1992; 83: 516–18.

30 Diggs LW, Bell A. Intraerythrocytic hemoglobin crystals in sickle cell-hemoglobin C disease. *Blood* 1965; 25: 218–23.

31 Ballas SK, Larner J, Smith ED, Surrey S, Schwartz E, Rappaport EF. The xerocytosis of SC disease. *Blood* 1987; 69: 124–30.

32 Lachant NA. Hemoglobin E: an emerging hemoglobinopathy in the United States. *Am J Hematol* 1987; 25: 449–62.

33 Bunyaratvej A, Sahaphong S, Bhamarapravati N, Wasi P. Quantitative changes in red blood cell shapes in relation to clinical features in β-thalassemia/HbE disease. *Am J Clin Pathol* 1985; 83: 555–9.

34 Rieder RF, Bradley TB. Hemoglobin Gun Hill: an unstable protein associated with chronic hemolysis. *Blood* 1968; 32: 355–69.

35 Taylor C, Bain BJ. Technicon H.1 automated white cell parameters in the dignosis of megaloblastic erythropoiesis. *Eur J Haematol* 1991; 46: 248–9.

36 Bessman JD, Williams LJ, Gilmer PR. Platelet size in health and hematologic disease. *Am J Clin Pathol* 1982; 78: 150–3.

37 Bain BJ, Taylor C. L'uso dei parametri leucocitari automatizzati nella diagnosi dell'anemia megaloblastica. Atti del V Incontro del Club Utilizzatori Sistemi Ematologici Bayer-Technicon, Montecatini Terme, Giugno, 1991.

38 Savvides P, Shalev O, John KM, Lux SE. Combined spectrin and ankyrin deficiency is common in autosomal dominant hereditary spherocytosis. *Blood* 1992; 82: 2953–60.

39 Palek J, Jarolim P. Clinical expression and laboratory detection of red blood cell membrane protein mutations. *Semin Hematol* 1993; 30: 249–83.

40 Sugihara T, Miyashima K, Yawata Y. Disappearance of microspherocytes in peripheral circulation and normalization of decreased lipids in plasma and in red cells of patients with hereditary spherocytosis after splenectomy. *Am J Hematol* 1984; 17: 129–39.

41 Palek J, Sahr K. Mutations of the red blood cell membrane proteins: from clinical evaluation to detection of the underlying genetic defect. *Blood* 1992; 80: 308–30.

42 Pati AR, Patten WN, Harris RI. The use of the Technicon H1 in the diagnosis of hereditary spherocytosis. *Clin Lab Haematol* 1989; 11: 27–30.

43 Lecomte MC, Garbarz M, Gautero H, Bournier A, Galand C, Boivin P, Dhermy D. Molecular basis of clinical and morphological heterogeneity in hereditary elliptocytosis (HE) with spectrin I variants. *Br J Haematol* 1993; 85: 584–95.

44 Lecomte MC, Gautero H, Bournier O, Galand C, Lahary A, Vannier JP, Garbarz M *et al.* Elliptocytosis-associated spectrin Rouen ($\beta^{220/218}$) has a truncated but still phosphorylatable β chain. *Br J Haematol* 1992; 80: 242–50.

45 Conboy JG, Mohandas N, Tchernia G, Kan YW. Molecular basis of hereditary elliptocytosis due to protein 4.1 deficiency. *N Engl J Med* 1986; 315: 680–5.

46 Alloisio N, Morlé L, Pothier B, Roux A-F, Maréchal J, Ducluzeau M-T, Benhadji-Zouaoui Z, Delaunay J. Spectrin Oran ($\alpha^{II/21}$), a new spectrin variant concerning the αII domain and causing severe elliptocytosis in the homozygous state. *Blood* 1988; 71: 1039–47.

47 Austin RF, Desforges JF. Hereditary elliptocytosis: an unusual presentation of hemolysis in the newborn associated with transient morphologic abnormalities. *Pediatrics* 1969; 44: 189–200.

48 Coetzer T, Lawler J, Prchal JT, Palek J. Molecular determinants of clinical expression of hereditary elliptocytosis and pyropoikilocytosis. *Blood* 1987; 70: 766–72.

49 Djaldetti M, Cohen A, Hart J. Elliptocytosis preceding myelofibrosis in a patient with polycythemia

vera. *Acta Haematol* 1982; 72: 26–8.
50 Rummens JL, Verfaillie C, Criel A, Hidajat M, Vanhoof A, van den Berghe H, Louwagie A. Elliptocytosis and schistocytosis in myelodysplasia: report of two cases. *Acta Haematol* 1986; 75: 174–7.
51 Palek J, Lambert S. Genetics of the red cell membrane skeleton. *Semin Hematol* 1990; 27: 290–332.
52 Liu S-C, Zhai S, Palek J, Golan DE, Amato D, Hassan K, Nurse GT, Babona D. Molecular defect of the Band 3 protein in Southeast Asian ovalocytosis. *N Engl J Med* 1990; 323: 1530–8.
53 Booth PB, Serjeantson S, Woodfield DG, Amato D. Selective depression of blood group antigens associated with hereditary ovalocytosis among Melanesians. *Vox Sang* 1977; 32: 99–110.
54 Stewart GW, Hepworth-Jones BE, Keen JN, Dash BCJ, Argent AC, Casimir CM. Isolation of cDNA coding for a ubiquitous membrane protein deficient in high Na^+, low K^+ stomatocytic erythrocytes. *Blood* 1992; 79: 1593–661.
55 Kanzaki A, Yawata Y. Hereditary stomatocytosis: phenotypic expression of sodium transport and band 7 peptides in 44 cases. *Br J Haematol* 1992; 82: 133–41.
56 Otsuka A, Sugihara T, Yawata Y. No beneficial effect of splenectomy in hereditary high red cell membrane phosphatidylcholine hemolytic anemia: clinical and membrane studies in 20 patients. *Am J Hematol* 1990; 34: 8–14.
57 Jackson JM, Stanley ML, Crawford IG, Barr AL, Hilton HB. The problem of Mediterranean stomatocytosis. *Aust N Z J Med* 1978; 8: 216–17.
58 Vives Corrons JL, Besson I, Merino A, Monteagudo J, Reverter JC, Aguilar JL, Enrich C. Occurrence of hereditary leaky red cell syndrome and partial coagulation factor VII deficiency in a Spanish family. *Acta Haematol* 1991; 86: 194–9.
59 Fujii H, Miwa S. Recent progress in the molecular genetic analysis of erythroenzymopathy. *Am J Hematol* 1990; 34: 301–10.
60 Tanaka KR, Zerez CR. Red cell enzymopathies of the glycolytic pathway. *Semin Hematol* 1990; 27: 165–85.
61 Toren A, Brok-Simoni F, Ben-Bassat I, Holtzman F, Mandel M, Neumann Y, Ramot B, Rechavi G *et al.* Congenital haemolytic anaemia associated with adenylate kinase deficiency. *Br J Haematol* 1994; 87: 376–80.
62 Miwa S, Fujii H, Tani K, Takahashi K, Takegawa S, Fujinami N, Sakurai M, Kubo M *et al.* Two cases of red cell aldolase deficiency associated with hereditary hemolytic anemia in a Japanese family. *Am J Hematol* 1981; 11: 425–37.
63 Feo CJ, Tchernia G, Subtil E, Leblond PF. Observations of echinocytosis in eight patients: a phase contrast and SEM study. *Br J Haematol* 1978; 40: 519–26.
64 Valentine WN, Schneider AS, Baughan MA. Hereditary hemolytic anemia with triosephosphate isomerase deficiency. Studies in kindreds with coexisting sickle cell trait and erythrocyte glucose-6-phosphate dehydrogenase deficiency. *Am J Med* 1966; 41: 27–41.
65 Vives Corrons JL, Carrera A, Triginer J, Kahn A, Rozman C. Anemia hemolitica por déficit congénito en fosfohexosaisomerasa – descripcíon de una nueva variante (PHI Barcelon) con estomatocitosis y disminución de la resistencia osmotica eritrocitaria. *Sangre* 1974; 20: 197–206.
66 Leblond PF, Lyonnais J, Delage J-M. Erythrocyte populations in pyruvate kinase deficiency anaemias following splenectomy. *Br J Haematol* 1978; 39: 55–61.
67 Farolino DL, Rustagi PK, Currie MS, Doeblin TD, Logue GL. Teardrop-shaped red cells in autoimmune hemolytic anemia. *Am J Hematol* 1986; 21: 415–18.
68 Pettit JE, Scott J, Hussein S. EDTA dependent red cell neutrophil rosetting in autoimmune haemolytic anaemia. *J Clin Pathol* 1976; 29: 345–6.
69 Ervin DM, Christian RM, Young LE. Dangerous universal donors. *Blood* 1950; 5: 553–67.
70 Jordan WS, Prouty RL, Heinle RW, Dingle JH. The mechanism of hemolysis in paroxysmal cold hemoglobinuria. *Blood* 1952; 7: 387–403.
71 Koenig JM, Christensen RD. Neutropenia and thrombocytopenia in infants with Rh hemolytic disease. *J Pediatr* 1989; 114: 625–31.
72 Riggs SA, Wray NP, Waddell CC, Rossen RD, Gyorkey F. Thrombotic thrombocytopenic purpura complicating Legionnaires' disease. *Arch Intern Med* 1982; 142: 2275–80.
73 Turner RC, Chaplinski TJ, Adams HG. Rocky Mountain spotted fever presenting as thrombotic thrombocytopenic purpura. *Am J Med* 1986; 81: 153–7.
74 Kwaan HC. Miscellaneous secondary thrombotic microangiopathy. *Semin Hematol* 1987; 24: 141–7.
75 Nishiura T, Miyazaki Y, Oritani K, Tominaga N, Tomiyama Y, Katagiri S, Kanayama Y, Yonezawa T *et al. Aspergillus* vegetative endocarditis complicated with schizocytic hemolytic anemia in a patient with acute lymphocytic leukemia. *Acta Haematol* 1986; 76: 60–2.
76 Brown RC, Blecher TE, French EA, Toghill PJ. Thrombotic thrombocytopenic purpura after influenza vaccination. *Br Med J* 1973; ii: 303.
77 Maguire RB, Stroncek DF, Campbell AC. Recurrent pancytopenia, coagulopathy, and renal failure associated with multiple quinine-dependent antibodies. *Ann Intern Med* 1993; 119: 215–17.
78 Salyer WR, Salyer DC, Heptinstall RH. Scleroderma and microangiopathic hemolytic anemia. *Ann Intern Med* 1973; 78: 895–7.

79 Brunning RD, Jacob HS, Brenckman WD, Jimenez-Pasqau F, Goetz FC. Fragmentation hemolysis in patients with severe diabetic angiopathy. *Br J Haematol* 1976; 34: 283–9.

80 Schulman I, Pierce M, Lukens A, Currimbhoy Z. Studies on thrombopoiesis I. A factor in normal human plasma required for platelet production, chronic thrombocytopenia due to its deficiency. *Blood* 1960; 16: 943–57.

81 Upshaw JD. Congenital deficiency of a factor in normal plasma that reverses microangiopathic hemolysis and thrombocytopenia. *N Engl J Med* 1978; 298: 1350–2.

82 Geraghty MT, Perlman EJ, Martin LS, Hayflick SJ, Casella JF, Rosenblatt DS, Valle D. Cobalamin C defect associated with hemolytic-uremic syndrome. *J Pediatr* 1992; 120: 934–7.

83 Fairley S, Ihle BU. Thrombotic microangiopathy and acute renal failure associated with arteriography. *Br Med J* 1986; 293: 922–3.

84 Rauch AE, Tartaglia AP, Kaufman B, Kausel H. RBC fragmentation and thymoma. *Arch Intern Med* 1984; 144: 1280–2.

85 Paré PD, Chan-Yan C, Wass H, Hooper R, Hogg JC. Portal and pulmonary hypertension with microangiopathic hemolytic anemia. *Am J Med* 1983; 74: 1093–6.

86 Zauber NP, Echikson AB. Giant cell arteritis and microangiopathic hemolytic anemia. *Am J Med* 1982; 73: 928–30.

87 Nand S, Bansal VK, Kozeny G, Vertuno L, Remlinger KA, Jordan JV. Red cell fragmentation syndrome with the use of subclavian hemodialysis catheters. *Arch Intern Med* 1985; 145: 1421–3.

88 Steinhorn RH, Isham-Schopt B, Smith C, Green TP. Hemolysis during long-term extracorporeal membrane oxygenation. *J Pediatr* 1989; 115: 625–30.

89 Zieve L. Jaundice, hyperlipidemia and hemolytic anemia: a heretofore unrecognized syndrome associated with alcoholic fatty liver and cirrhosis. *Ann Intern Med* 1958; 48: 471–96.

90 Melrose WD, Bell PA, Jupe DML, Baikie MJ. Alcohol-associated haemolysis in Zieve's syndrome: a clinical and laboratory study of five cases. *Clin Lab Haematol* 1990; 12: 159–69.

91 Placzek MM, Gorst DW. T activation haemolysis and death after blood transfusion. *Arch Dis Child* 1987; 62: 743–4.

92 McCann SR, Firth R, Murray N, Temperley IJ. Congenital dyserythropoietic anaemia type II (HEMPAS): a family study. *J Clin Pathol* 1980; 33: 1197–201.

93 Brien WF, Mant MJ, Etches WS. Variant congenital dyserythropoietic anaemia with ringed sideroblasts. *Clin Lab Haematol* 1985; 7: 231–7.

94 Jankovic M, Sansone G, Conter V, Iolascon A, Masera G. Atypical hereditary ovalocytosis associated with dyserythropoietic anemia. *Acta Haematol* 1993; 89: 35–7.

95 Bethlenfalvay NC, Hadnagy CS, Heimpel H. Unclassified type of congenital dyserythropoietic anaemia (CDA) with prominent peripheral erythroblastosis. *Br J Haematol* 1985; 60: 541–50.

96 Bessis M. *Living Blood Cells and their Ultrastructure*. Berlin: Springer-Verlag, 1973.

97 Serjeant GR, Serjeant BE, Forbes M, Hages RJ, Higgs DR, Lehmann H. Haemoglobin gene frequencies in the Jamaican population: a study of 100,000 newborns. *Br J Haematol* 1986; 64: 253–62.

CHAPTER 9

Disorders of White Cells

Acquired disorders primarily involving white cells may be either reactive to a primary non-haematological disease or neoplastic. Neoplastic disorders result from the clonal proliferation of a haemopoietic stem cell, either myeloid or lymphoid, which has undergone mutation. Numerical changes in white cells are summarized in Chapter 6. Here the typical peripheral blood changes in non-haematological diseases are described, followed by the characteristic features of haematological neoplasms.

Reactive changes in white cells

Bacterial infection

Acute and chronic bacterial infection

Blood film and count

In an adult, the usual response to a bacterial infection is a neutrophil leucocytosis with a left shift, toxic granulation, Döhle bodies and, when infection is severe, cytoplasmic vacuolation (Fig. 9.1). Occasionally, bacteria are seen within neutrophils (see p. 108). In severe infections there may be myelocytes, promyelocytes and even a few blast cells in the peripheral blood. The lymphocyte and eosinophil counts are reduced. A rise in the monocyte count occurs later than the rise in the neutrophil count. During recovery there is a rise in the eosinophil count, sometimes to above normal. If infection persists a normocytic normochromic anaemia develops and, if the infection becomes chronic, red cells may become hypochromic and microcytic. There is an increase in rouleaux formation and in background staining. The platelet count is often elevated during acute or severe chronic infection but is sometimes reduced. Sometimes bacterial infections are associated with pancytopenia as a consequence of haemophagocytosis.

In overwhelming sepsis, particularly in alcoholics and neonates, infection can be associated with paradoxical leucopenia and neutropenia. A left shift and toxic changes nevertheless occur. Neutropenia in the course of infections which more often cause neutrophilia may be consequent on increased margination of neutrophils, impaired granulopoiesis, or migration of peripheral blood neutrophils to tissues at a faster rate than they can be replenished by an inadequate bone marrow reserve. In some studies in neonates, an increased proportion of band cells has been found more useful than neutrophilia in identifying infected infants (see p. 68).

Although neutrophilia is the characteristic response to bacterial infection, this is not invariable. Certain infections are characterized by either a normal WBC or even leucopenia and neutropenia, e.g. typhoid fever, brucellosis and rickettsial infections. Lymphocytosis is characteristic

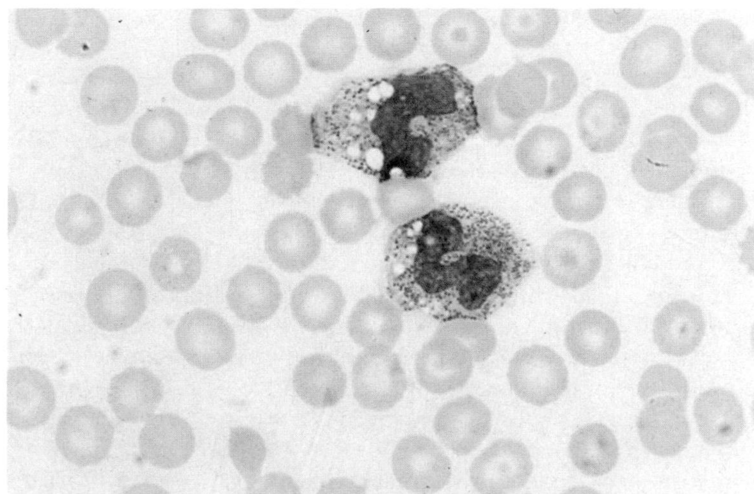

Fig. 9.1 Peripheral blood film in reactive neutrophilia; both cells are band forms showing vacuolation and marked toxic granulation.

of pertussis (whooping cough). Infants and young children sometimes also respond to other bacterial infections with lymphocytosis rather than neutrophilia.

In addition to the elevated WBC, automated instruments may indicate a left shift, the presence of immature granulocytes or increased peroxidase activity of neutrophils.

Differential diagnosis

The differential diagnosis of neutrophil changes suggestive of infection is with other causes of neutrophilia (see p. 160). Toxic granulation and Döhle bodies are not specific for infection, being seen also in pregnancy, inflammatory and autoimmune diseases, following administration of cytokines and when there is tissue damage or death, e.g., consequent on surgery, trauma or infarction. The presence of neutrophil vacuolation is more specific for infection, very commonly indicating septicaemia [1]. The observation of bacteria within neutrophils in a film made without delay (see p. 108) may indicate colonization of an indwelling venous line (if the blood specimen is obtained directly from the line) but otherwise is specific for bacteraemia. However, this finding is rare.

In the neonatal period, neutrophilia may be caused not only by infection but also by hypoxia or stressful labour, intrapartum oxytocin administration, maternal fever or seizures, neonatal hypoglycaemia and haemolytic disease of the newborn [2] (see p. 164). Even crying can cause an increase in WBC and the proportion of band cells [3].

Further tests

Characteristic peripheral blood features are often present in bacterial infection but, since they are neither specific nor invariably present, a definitive diagnosis necessitates consideration of clinical features and specific bacteriological tests. In patients with known bacterial infection the neutrophil count can be used to monitor the progress of the disease.

Tuberculosis

The haematological manifestations of tuberculosis are protean, although some of the abnormalities attributed to tuberculosis in the past are likely to have been caused by the coexistence of tuberculosis and a disease such as hairy cell leukaemia or idiopathic myelofibrosis.

Blood film and count

Pulmonary tuberculosis causes a normocytic normochromic anaemia with increased rouleaux formation and an increased ESR. When the disease is severe, leucocytosis and neutrophilia are common [4]. Lymphocytosis is present in about one-quarter of patients and lymphopenia in one-fifth. Although monocytosis has been regarded as characteristic of tuberculosis it is present in only about one-quarter of patients while about one-half have monocytopenia. Thrombocytosis is common. Automated blood counts show a low Hb, normal or reduced MCV and increased RDW.

Patients with miliary tuberculosis [5] are usually anaemic. In contrast to acute pulmonary tuberculosis, leucocytosis is uncommon and leucopenia is common. Monocytosis occurs in about one-quarter of patients. Lymphopenia is usual. A minority of patients have pancytopenia (which is sometimes consequent on haemophagocytosis).

Differential diagnosis

The haematological manifestations of tuberculosis are so variable that many infective, inflammatory and neoplastic conditions enter into the differential diagnoses.

Further tests

Bone marrow aspiration and trephine biopsy can be useful in the diagnosis of miliary tuberculosis.

Viral infections

Infectious mononucleosis

Infectious mononucleosis is an acute clinicopathological syndrome consequent on primary infection by EBV. It is predominantly a disease of adolescents and young adults. Common clinical features are fever, pharyngitis, lymphadenopathy (hence the common designation 'glandular fever'), splenomegaly and hepatitis. Haematologically, the disease is characterized by 'atypical mononuclear cells' or 'atypical lymphocytes' which are mainly activated T lymphocytes produced as part of the immunological response to EBV-infected B lymphocytes.

Blood film and count

There is lymphocytosis and usually leucocytosis consequent on the presence of atypical lymphocytes. Some patients are thrombocytopenic and a minority are anaemic. Atypical lymphocytes are highly pleomorphic (Fig. 9.2). Many are large, with diameters up to 15–30 μm, and have abundant strongly basophilic cytoplasm. Some have large central nucleoli and resemble immunoblasts (i.e., they have the same cytological features as lymphocytes stimulated *in vitro* by mitogens); others resemble the blasts of ALL. Nuclei can be round, oval, reniform, lobulated or, occasionally, clover-leaf shaped. The chromatin pattern may be diffuse or partly condensed. The cytoplasm may be vacuolated, foamy or (occasionally) granulated, and moderately or strongly basophilic. Cytoplasmic basophilia may be generalized or confined to the cytoplasmic margins. When the atypical cells have contact with other cells the cytoplasmic margins sometimes appear scalloped (Fig. 9.2b). Some cells have a hand-mirror conformation. Binucleate cells and mitotic figures may be seen. Some plasmacytoid lymphocytes and plasma cells may be present and large granular lymphocytes may be increased. The abnormal cells can have cytochemical abnormalities such as block-positivity on a PAS stain (usually a feature of ALL) and TRAP activity (usually a feature of hairy cell leukaemia). However, cytochemistry is not recommended in the diagnosis of infectious mononucleosis.

Changes in other cell lines are quite common although they tend to be overshadowed by the abnormalities in the lymphocytes. In one series 10% of patients had neutrophil counts of less than $1 \times 10^9/l$ [6]. Occasionally, neutropenia is very severe [7]. Neutrophilia can also occur. Neutrophils sometimes show toxic granulation, left shift and Döhle bodies; despite these changes the NAP score is usually reduced. Reduction of the eosinophil count is usual; during recovery there is eosinophilia. Thrombocytopenia is not uncommon, the platelet count being less than $150 \times 10^9/l$ in about one-third of patients. Severe thrombocytopenia which sometimes occurs is likely to be due to immune destruction of platelets. Haemolytic anaemia due to a cold antibody can occur and the blood film then shows red cell agglutination, some spherocytes and, later, the development of polychromasia. A larger number

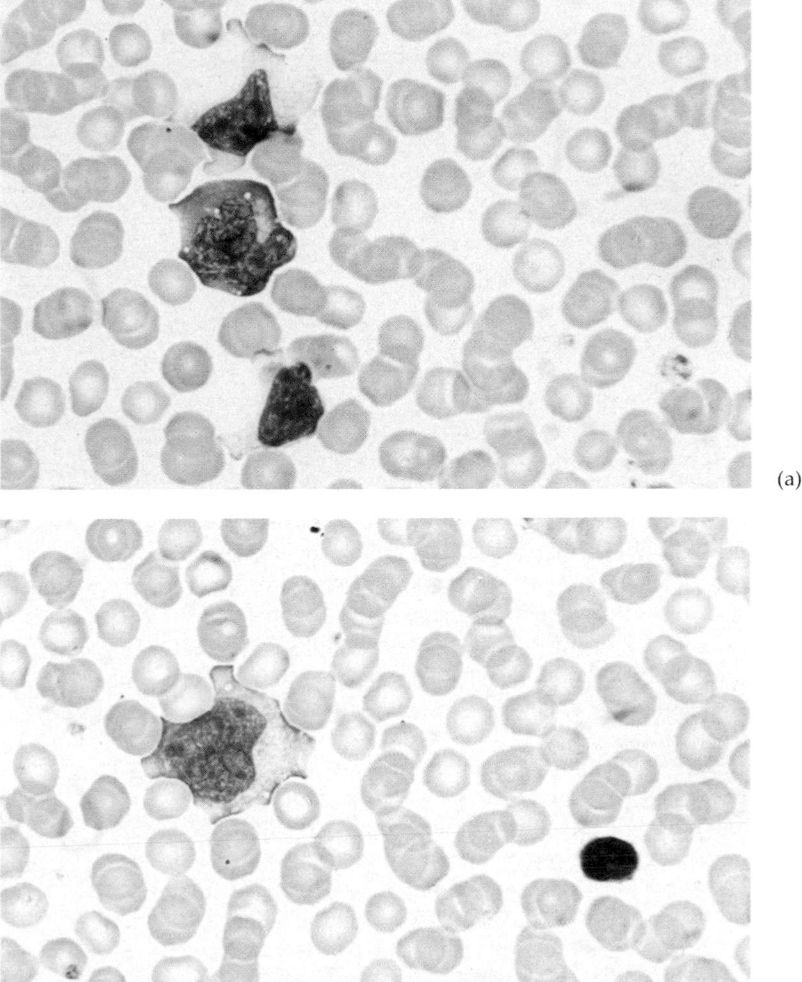

Fig. 9.2 Peripheral blood film in infectious mononucleosis showing atypical lymphocytes (atypical mononuclear cells): (a) pleomorphic cells, with plentiful cytoplasm; the largest cell has moderately basophilic vacuolated cytoplasm and a lobulated nucleus containing a nucleolus; and (b) a normal small lymphocyte and an atypical lymphocyte with voluminous cytoplasm and scalloped edges.

of patients show some red cell agglutination without overt haemolysis. Subjects with hereditary spherocytosis appear to be particularly prone to haemolysis during infectious mononucleosis. Some patients develop severe cytopenias consequent on virus-triggered haemophagocytosis. Aplastic anaemia is a rare complication, developing 1–6 weeks after presentation.

Not all patients with primary infection by EBV have the clinicopathological features of infectious mononucleosis. Young children have a greater degree of lymphocytosis and a lower percentage of atypical lymphocytes than older children but the absolute count of atypical lymphocytes is similar in children under and over 4 years of age [8]. In older patients the degree of lymphocytosis and the percentage of atypical lymphocytes may be less than is usually observed in adolescents and young adults [9]. Rare patients with infectious mononucleosis have severe lymphopenia [10]. This is associated with severe disease and a worse prognosis.

Automated counters usually 'flag' the presence of atypical lymphocytes. Depending on the instrument, there may be an increase in 'mononuclear cells' or 'LUC' or a factitious increase in 'basophils'.

Differential diagnosis

The differential diagnosis of infectious mononucleosis is with other causes of atypical lymphocytes (Table 9.1) and, to a lesser extent, with ALL and non-Hodgkin's lymphoma.

Further tests

The finding of a blood film suggestive of infectious mononucleosis is an indication to test for a heterophile antibody which agglutinates sheep or horse red cells and differs from heterophile antibodies in other conditions in that it is absorbed by ox red cells but not by guinea pig kidney. Rapid slide tests for heterophile antibodies are sensitive and very convenient with a false positive rate of 1–2%. Specific test for antibodies to EBV are too complex and expensive to be of use for routine diagnostic purposes. At presentation, 60% of patients with infectious mononucleosis have a positive heterophile antibody test and up to 90% become positive if closely followed. In adolescents and adults 'heterophil-negative infectious mononucleosis' most often represent cytomegalovirus infection (70% of cases in one series [20]) but a minority (16% in the same series) can be demonstrated by specific serological tests to be due to primary infection with EBV. Well below one-half of infants with primary EBV infection have heterophile antibodies [8] so that in this age group EBV infection is the commonest cause of heterophil-negative infectious mononucleosis. Serological tests for toxoplasmosis should also be performed in patients with heterophil antibody-negative infectious mononucleosis and in high-risk groups testing for HIV (see below) should be considered.

Table 9.1 Some causes of atypical lymphocytes

Viral infections: infectious mononucleosis (EBV), cytomegalovirus infection,* infectious hepatitis (hepatitis A),* measles (rubeola), German measles (rubella), echovirus infection, adenovirus infection,* chickenpox (varicella) and herpes zoster, herpes simplex infection, human herpes virus 6 infection* [11], influenza, mumps, lymphocytic meningitis (lymphocytic choriomeningitis virus infection), HIV infection, HTLV-I infection

Bacterial infections: brucellosis, tuberculosis, syphilis, rickettsial infections* including tick typhus (*Rickettsia conorii*), scrub typhus (*Rickettsia tsutsugamushi*), murine typhus (*Rickettsia typhi*) [12,13], Ehrlichia infections including Sennetsu fever (Japan) and ehrlichiosis (USA) [14], *Mycoplasma pneumoniae* infection

Protozoan infections: toxoplasmosis,* malaria, babesiosis

Immunizations

Serum sickness (rarely)

Hypersensitivity to drugs* such as para-aminosalicylic acid, sulphasalizine, sodium phenytoin, mesantoin, dapsone, phenothiazines, streptokinase [15]

Angioimmunoblastic lymphadenopathy [16]

Systemic lupus erythematosus [17]

Sarcoidosis [18]

Graft-versus-host disease

Graft rejection

Hodgkin's disease

Kawasaki's syndrome [19]

* Conditions which can be associated with sufficiently large numbers of atypical lymphocytes to be confused with infectious mononucleosis.

HIV infection

HIV infection causes an acute illness at the time of seroconversion followed by a phase of latent infection before the manifestations of chronic infection appear.

Blood film and count

The acute illness can resemble infectious mononucleosis both clinically and haematologically. Following recovery from the acute phase the infected person is haematologically normal, often for many years.

Chronic infection is associated with a progressive decline in the lymphocyte count, particularly a decline in the number of CD4-positive lymphocytes, with an associated progressive decline in immune function. Once the declining immune function has led to the development of certain specified infective or neoplastic conditions the patient is said to be suffering from AIDS. Isolated thrombocytopenia consequent on immune destruction of platelets can be a relatively early occurrence. Thrombocytopenia in HIV infection can also be due to a syndrome resembling TTP. Reactive lymphocytosis consequent on intercurrent infections can initially mask the progressive decline in CD4-positive lymphocytes. Intercurrent infection can also be associated with toxic changes in neutrophils or with severe pancytopenia consequent on virus-associated haemophagocytosis. Minor reactive changes in lymphocytes are common even when the patient does not have any evident infection. In the final stages of the disease there is a progressive decline in the Hb, neutrophil count and platelet count. The anaemia is normocytic or mildly macrocytic and normochromic. Neutropenia is associated with dysplastic changes in neutrophils (see p. 81).

Patients with HIV infection are also prone to iatrogenic haematological complications, most often macrocytosis and pancytopenia caused by zidovudine therapy or oxidant-induced haemolytic anaemia caused by dapsone therapy.

In patients with chronic HIV infection the automated count with Technicon H.1 series counters can show increased peroxidase activity of neutrophils and a reduction of nuclear density seen as a reduced lobularity index. Both these features are indicative of dysplastic granulopoiesis.

Differential diagnosis

Depending on the stage of the disease and the specific haematological features, the differential diagnoses can include infectious mononucleosis and other viral infections, ITP and TTP. It is important to think of the possibility of HIV infection and consider performing specific serological tests in patients participating in high-risk activities who present with these haematological features. HIV infection is part of the differential diagnosis of chronic red cell aplasia since immune deficiency can lead to failure to eliminate the parvovirus. Late in the disease, confusion with the myelodysplastic syndromes and other causes of bone marrow failure can occur.

Further tests

Diagnosis is customarily by serological detection of antibodies to HIV. If there is chronic red cell aplasia in an HIV-positive patient serological tests for parvovirus should be supplemented by tests for parvovirus DNA since there may be a failure of specific antibody production.

Other viral infections

Viral infections may be acute or chronic. They cause a variety of effects on blood cells.

Blood film and count

Acute viral infections are associated with transient haematological abnormalities, most often lymphocytosis with reactive changes in lymphocytes. With some viruses these changes can be sufficiently severe to simulate infectious mononucleosis (see Table 9.1). Other acute viral infections are associated with neutrophilia (see Table 6.3). The eosinophil count is reduced during acute infection and rises during recovery. Thrombocytopenia, as a consequence of platelet consumption, can occur during active viral infection. In the case of the viral haemorrhagic fevers, disseminated intravascular coagulation can cause severe thrombocytopenia. During recovery from some viral infections, e.g., rubella, there may be thrombocytopenia consequent on interaction of immune complexes with platelets. Acute haemolysis caused by the Donath–Landsteiner (anti-P) antibody can follow viral infections, e.g., measles, and acute haemolysis consequent on a cold agglutinin (anti-I or anti-i) can occur during other viral infections. Parvovirus infection in normal subjects causes acute, transient red cell aplasia associated with a slight fall in Hb and the disappearance of reticulocytes and therefore a lack of polychromasia. In some patients there is associated neutropenia or thrombocytopenia. In patients with a shortened red cell lifespan, more severe but transient anaemia occurs.

The effects of chronic viral infection vary with the virus. There may be an increase of large granular lymphocytes. In chronic infection with HTLV-I, there may be lymphocytosis with occasional atypical lymphocytes including some with clover-leaf nuclei (Fig. 9.3). Immunologically incompetent subjects, e.g., with HIV infection or iatrogenic immunosuppression, can develop chronic parvovirus infection which causes chronic red cell aplasia. Viral hepatitis, particularly non-A, non-B, non-C hepatitis [21], can be followed by aplastic anaemia. Patients with chronic infection by any of the hepatitis viruses can develop haematological abnormalities consequent on chronic liver disease and hypersplenism.

Differential diagnosis

The differential diagnosis of the haematological effects of viral infection is complex, since the abnormalities caused are very variable. The differential diagnoses include the various conditions which can cause lymphocytosis, atypical lymphocytes and thrombocytopenia.

Further tests

Tests for heterophile antibodies and serological tests for specific viruses should be performed when clinically appropriate.

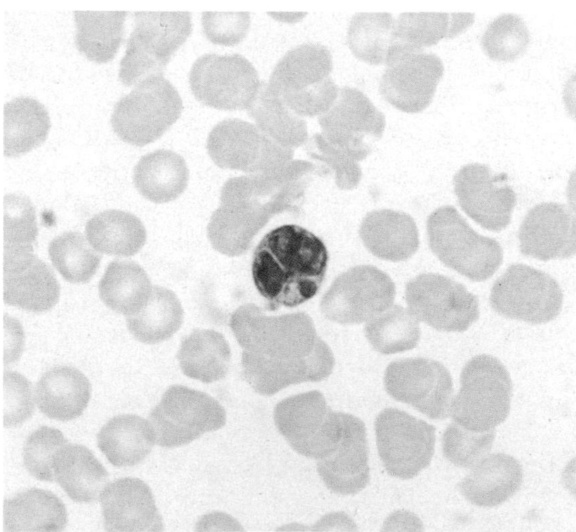

Fig. 9.3 Peripheral blood film of a healthy carrier of the HTLV-I virus showing a lymphocyte with a flower-shaped nucleus.

Idiopathic hypereosinophilic syndrome (HES)

The term 'idiopathic HES' is used to describe a probably heterogeneous group of conditions characterized by persistent unexplained eosinophilia and tissue damage (e.g., involving the heart and nervous system) attributable to the release of eosinophil granule contents. The condition is much commoner in males. Cases are arbitrarily classified as idiopathic HES when the eosinophil count is in excess of $1.5 \times 10^9/l$, when unexplained eosinophilia persists for at least 6 months and when there is associated tissue damage [22]. Some cases appear to be attributable to an abnormality, sometimes clonal, of T lymphocytes with eosinophilia provoked by lymphokines [23]. Other cases may represent a myeloproliferative disorder with predominant eosinophil differentiation.

Blood film and count

There is a moderate or marked eosinophilia. Eosinophils often show marked degranulation and vacuolation including even completely agranular eosinophils (Fig. 9.4). Granules are often smaller than normal. Eosinophil nuclei may be hyperlobated, hypolobated or ring-shaped. Other haematological features can include anaemia, anisocytosis, poikilocytosis (including tear drop poikilocytes), a leucoerythroblastic blood film, basophilia, thrombocytopenia, thrombocytosis, neutrophilia and the presence of neutrophils with heavy rather basophilic granules (see Fig. 3.55). The latter abnormality may be so marked that the abnormal neutrophils are confused with basophils. A true increase in basophils can also occur [22].

Eosinophil degranulation is usually more marked in HES than in reactive eosinophilia. The number of degranulated cells is also of prognostic significance. If more than $1 \times 10^9/l$ degranulated cells are present it is likely that cardiac damage is already present or will occur [24].

Differential diagnosis

Idiopathic HES is a diagnosis of exclusion. Many of the characteristic features are not specific.

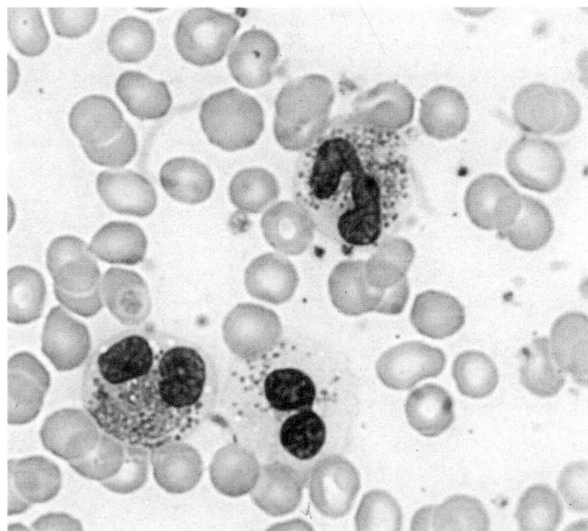

Fig. 9.4 Peripheral blood film from a patient with idiopathic HES; the three eosinophils show various degrees of degranulation.

Tissue damage from the release of eosinophil granule contents can also occur both in reactive eosinophilia (see p. 162) and in eosinophilic leukaemia. Degranulation and vacuolation of eosinophils can also be marked both in eosinophil leukaemia and in severe reactive eosinophilia. Peripheral blood features indistinguishable from idiopathic HES can occur in some patients who are subsequently found to have systemic mastocytosis [25], ALL or lymphoma. Making a distinction between idiopathic HES and chronic eosinophilic leukaemia (see p. 277) at the onset of the disease can be difficult or even impossible.

Further tests

Bone marrow aspiration, a trephine biopsy and cytogenetic analysis are indicated since detection of increased blast cells or a clonal cytogenetic abnormality permits the diagnosis of eosinophilic leukaemia. Systemic mastocytosis or a lymphoma may also be diagnosed on the bone marrow aspirate or trephine biopsy.

Cases without specific features which identify them as 'leukaemia' are best classified as idiopathic HES. However, in some such patients subsequent transformation to AML provides evidence that the condition was neoplastic from the beginning.

Leukaemoid reactions

A leukaemoid reaction is a haematological abnormality which simulates leukaemia and thus may be confused with it, but which is, in fact, reactive to some other disease. In a leukaemoid reaction the abnormalities reverse when the underlying condition is corrected. In many of the early reports of leukaemoid reactions, the patient did not recover from the primary disease and correction of the haematological abnormality did not occur. In such cases, it is difficult to be sure that the patient did not have leukaemia coexisting with some other disease. This is so in many of the early reports of an apparent leukaemoid reaction with tuberculosis. Transient abnormal myelopoiesis in neonates with Down's syndrome (see p. 284) should not be described as a leukaemoid reaction. It is a neoplastic condition and is more correctly regarded as a spontaneously remitting leukaemia [26]. Leukaemoid reactions may be myeloid or lymphoid.

Myeloid leukaemoid reactions

Leukaemoid reactions rarely simulate CGL since the characteristic spectrum of changes (see p. 287) is virtually never seen in reactive conditions. The differences are summarized in Table 9.2. The myeloid leukaemias which are most likely to be simulated by a leukaemoid reaction are AML, atypical Philadelphia-negative CML, CMML and neutrophilic leukaemia. Causes of myeloid leukaemoid reactions (Fig. 9.5) include any strong stimulus to bone marrow activity such as severe bacterial infection (particularly if complicated by megaloblastic anaemia, alcohol-induced bone marrow damage or prior agranulocytosis), carcinoma or other malignant disease (with or without bone marrow metastases) and tuberculosis. Leukaemoid reactions in neonates may result from congenital syphilis [27] and in infants may be consequent on the syndrome of thrombocytopenia with absent radii, particularly if complicated by haemorrhage [28].

Useful features in making the distinction

Table 9.2 Some features which may be useful in distinguishing CGL from reactive neutrophilia

Feature	Reactive neutrophilia	CGL
WBC	Rarely > $60 \times 10^9/l$	Usually 20–500 × $10^9/l$ or higher
Left shift	May be moderate or marked; if slight in relation to neutrophilia supports reactive neutrophilia	Proportional to WBC; may be marked
White cell morphology	Toxic granulation, neutrophil vacuolation and Döhle bodies may be present	Toxic changes not present
Absolute eosinophil count	Usually reduced	Usually elevated; eosinophil myelocytes may be present
Absolute basophil count	Usually reduced	Almost invariably elevated; basophil myelocytes may be present
Absolute monocyte count	May be elevated	Usually moderately elevated
Erythropoiesis	Anaemia may be present; usually normocytic and normochromic but if hypochromic and microcytic supports a reactive neutrophilia; rouleaux may be present	Anaemia may be present; normocytic and normochromic
Platelet count	Thrombocytosis or thrombocytopenia may occur; if there is a reactive thrombocytosis the platelets are usually small	The platelet count is usually normal or high; giant platelets may be present; platelets are large, even in the presence of thrombocytosis; megakaryocytes may be present
NAP score	Usually elevated	Almost always reduced

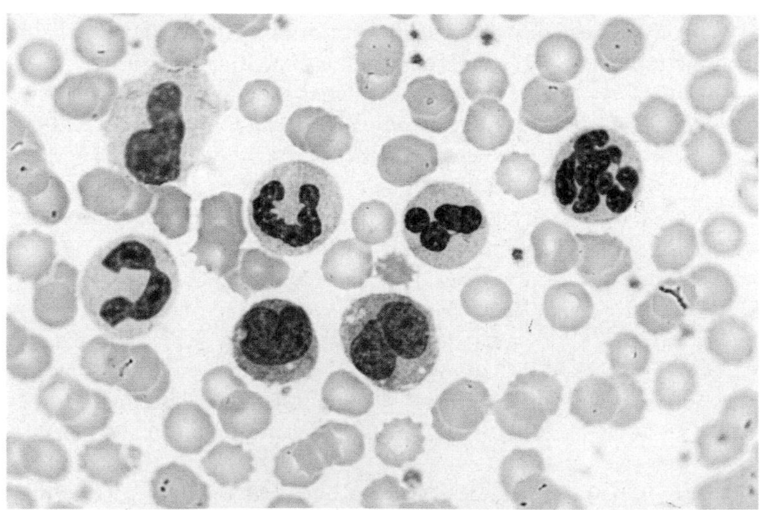

Fig. 9.5 Peripheral blood film of a patient with a leukaemoid reaction consequent on severe post-operative sepsis due to a Gram-negative organism. WBC was $92 \times 10^9/l$ with a neutrophil count of $74 \times 10^9/l$ and a monocyte count of $16 \times 10^9/l$; the film shows a band form, a macropolycyte and monocytes with increased cytoplasmic basophilia.

between leukaemia and a leukaemoid reaction include toxic changes, such as toxic granulation and vacuolation, and a preponderance of more mature cells (in a leukaemoid reaction) and hypogranular neutrophils and the presence of a disproportionate number of myeloblasts (in many leukaemias). A low NAP score is strongly in favour of a diagnosis of leukaemia since it is almost invariably raised in leukaemoid reactions. If Auer rods are seen in blast cells, a confident diagnosis of leukaemia or myelodysplastic syndrome can be made.

If clinical and haematological features do not permit the distinction between leukaemia and a leukaemoid reaction then bone marrow aspiration with cytogenetic analysis and microscopy and culture for *Mycobacterium tuberculosis* are indicated.

Lymphoid leukaemoid reactions

The blood film of whooping cough (Fig. 9.6) and of infectious lymphocytosis may simulate CLL but, since the clinical features and the age range of the two diseases are totally different, no problem occurs in practice. CLL has also been misdiagnosed in patients with post-splenectomy lymphocytosis. Knowledge of the high levels the lymphocyte count may reach post-splenectomy, and careful examination of the peripheral blood film for post-splenectomy features will avoid this problem. Post-splenectomy lymphocytosis can also simulate large granular lymphocyte leukaemia since the dominant cell may be a large granular lymphocyte (Fig. 9.7). Lymphocytosis associated with cigarette smoking can also be confused with CLL or non-Hodgkin's lymphoma. Knowledge of this syndrome and detection of the characteristic cytological features (see p. 91) allows a distinction to be made.

ALL can be simulated by infectious mononucleosis and other viral infections which cause atypical lymphocytes to appear in the blood, and by tuberculosis and congenital syphilis. When there is diagnostic uncertainty a bone marrow aspirate and immunophenotyping may be required.

Haematological neoplasms

Acute myeloid leukaemia (AML)

AML is a disease resulting from proliferation of a clone of myeloid stem cells which show defective maturation. Disease manifestations are those consequent on the cell proliferation, such as hepatomegaly and splenomegaly, and those consequent on replacement of normal bone marrow, such as anaemia and bleeding. The neoplastic clone is usually derived from a multipotent

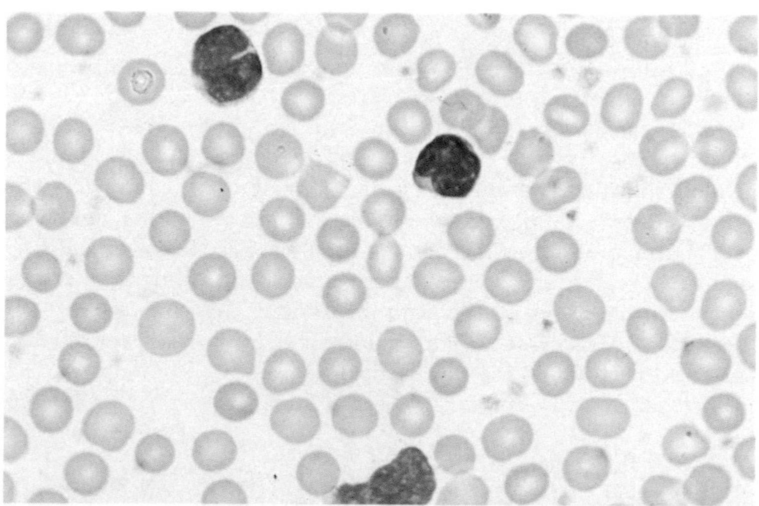

Fig. 9.6 Peripheral blood film of a child with whooping cough showing a cleft lymphocyte, a lymphocyte of normal morphology and a smear cell.

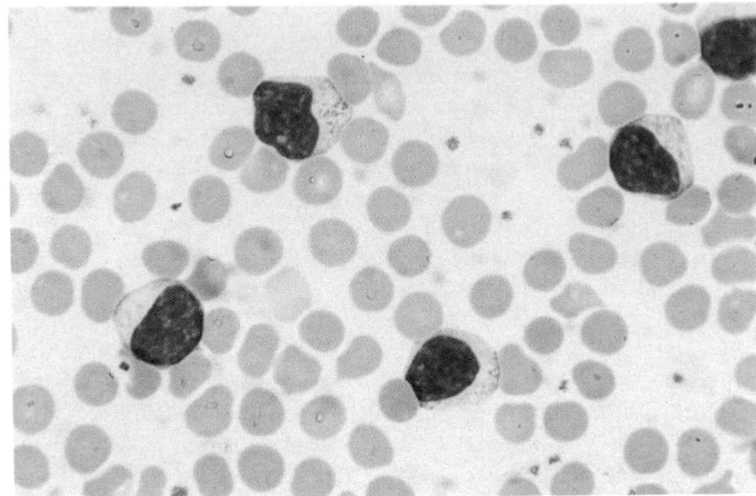

Fig. 9.7 Peripheral blood film following splenectomy for hereditary spherocytosis. WBC was $29.3 \times 10^9/l$ and the lymphocyte count $24 \times 10^9/l$. The lymphocytes were predominantly large granular lymphocytes. Courtesy of Dr J. Houghton, Salford.

myeloid stem cell but in some cases it may be derived either from a lineage-committed progenitor or a pluripotent lymphoid–myeloid stem cell.

Blood film and count

The majority of patients have leukaemic blast cells in the peripheral blood. These may be myeloblasts, monoblasts, megakaryoblasts or a mixed population. There may be some maturing cells, most often promyelocytes. In some patients an abnormal promyelocyte is the dominant cell. Most patients are neutropenic but in some types of AML there is differentiation of the leukaemic clone with consequent neutrophilia or, less often, eosinophilia. Rarely, there is an increase in basophils. Most patients have a normocytic normochromic anaemia or, if there has been preceding myelodysplastic syndrome (see below), a macrocytic anaemia. Most patients are thrombocytopenic but in a minority there is a normal platelet count or even thrombocytosis. Peripheral blood cells may show dysplastic features similar to those of the myelodysplastic syndromes. In a minority of patients, there is cytopenia, usually pancytopenia, without any circulating immature cells.

AML is further classified on the basis of peripheral blood and bone marrow features. The most generally accepted classification is that of the FAB cooperative group [29–33]. This classification is summarized in Table 9.3 and is illustrated in Figs 9.8–9.17.

Differential diagnosis

The differential diagnoses are mainly with ALL, the transformation of CGL and other myeloproliferative disorders, myelodysplastic syndrome and other causes of bone marrow failure such as aplastic anaemia. Occasionally, it is necessary to distinguish between acute leukaemia and a leukaemoid reaction (see p. 273).

Further tests

When AML is suspected, a bone marrow aspiration is indicated, together with cytochemistry to confirm granulocytic or monocytic differentiation and cytogenetic analysis to give information on prognosis. The most useful cytochemical reactions are myeloperoxidase or SBB to confirm granulocyte differentiation and a 'non-specific' esterase reaction, such as ANAE, to confirm monocytic differentiation. A positive CAE reaction confirms neutrophilic differentiation and can be combined with ANAE (combined esterase) for the easy identification of acute myelomonocytic (M4) leukemia. When there is

Table 9.3 The French-American-British (FAB) classification of AML. The criteria given apply to the bone marrow unless stated otherwise

M1 *(AML without maturation)* Blasts ≥90% of NEC; ≥3% of blasts positive for peroxidase or SBB; monocytic component ≤10% of NEC; granulocytic component ≤10% of NEC	***M5****(acute monocytic/monoblastic leukaemia)*
M2 *(AML with granulocytic maturation)* Blasts 30–89% of NEC; granulocytic component >10% of NEC; monocytic component <20% of NEC	***M5a*** *(without maturation or acute monoblastic leukaemia)* Monocytic component ≥80% of NEC; monoblasts ≥80% monocytic component
M3 and M3 variant Characteristic morphology	***M5b*** *(with maturation or acute monocytic leukaemia)* Monocytic component ≥80% of NEC; monoblasts <80% of monocytic component
M4 *(Acute myelomonocytic leukaemia)* Blasts ≥30% of NEC; granulocytic component (including myeloblasts) ≥20% of NEC	***M6*** *(erythroleukaemia)* Erythroblasts ≥50%; blasts ≥30% of NEC
AND	***M7*** *(megakaryoblastic leukaemia)* Blasts demonstrated to be megakaryoblasts, for example by ultrastructural cytochemistry showing the presence of platelet peroxidase or by immunological cell marker studies showing the presence of platelet antigens
EITHER BM monocytic component ≥20% of NEC and PB monocyte count ≥5 × 10^9/l OR BM monocytic component ≥20% of NEC and lysozyme elevated* OR BM monocytic component ≥20% of NEC and cytochemical confirmation of monocyte component in BM† OR BM resembling M2 but PB monocyte count ≥5 × 10^9/l and lysozyme elevated OR BM resembling M2 but PB monocyte count ≥5 × 10^9/l and cytochemical demonstration of monocytic component in BM	***M0*** *(AML with minimal evidence of myeloid differentiation)* Peroxidase and SBB positive in <3% of blasts but blasts demonstrated to be myeloid by immunophenotyping

BM, bone marrow, NEC, non-erythroid cells; PB, peripheral blood.
* Lysozyme in serum or urine elevated threefold compared with normal.
† Positive for NASA esterase activity, with activity being inhibited by fluoride.

no cytological or cytochemical evidence of myeloid differentiation, immunophenotypic analysis is essential to distinguish AML with minimal evidence of myeloid differentiation (M0 AML) from ALL [32].

Eosinophilic leukaemia

Eosinophilia can be a feature of AML and is usual in CML. AML with eosinophilia falls into the FAB M2 or M4 categories and is referred to as M2

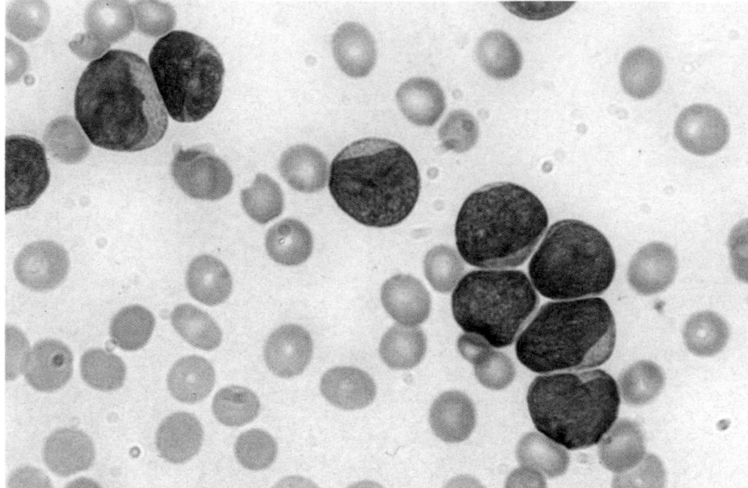

Fig. 9.8 Peripheral blood film in M1 AML (acute myeloblastic leukaemia without maturation). The blast cells have a fine chromatin pattern; they resemble lymphoblasts in having small nucleoli and a high nucleo-cytoplasmic ratio; in this patient only occasional blast cells had fine azurophilic granules but myeloperoxidase, SBB and CAE were positive in a high percentage of cells.

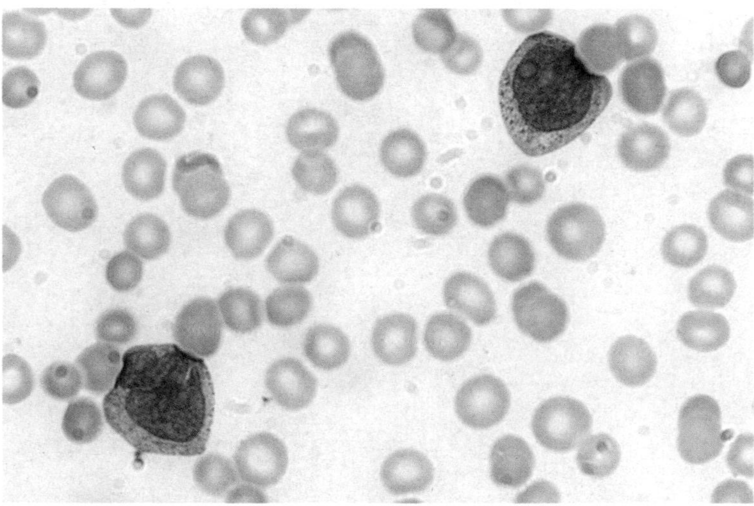

Fig. 9.9 Peripheral blood film in M2 AML (AML with maturation) showing leukaemic cells which are maturing beyond the blast stage. Both cells are promyelocytes, one with a nucleus of abnormal shape. Differentiation in M2 AML can be neutrophilic, eosinophilic, basophilic or any combination of these.

Eo or M4Eo AML. There are also cases of leukaemia in which the leukaemic cells are almost exclusively mature eosinophils or both mature and immature cells of eosinophil lineage. These cases are referred to as eosinophilic leukaemia. The prognosis is variable and is related to the percentage of blast cells. Patients with eosinophilic leukaemia can have tissue damage consequent on the release of eosinophil granule contents.

Blood film and count

The blood film (Fig. 9.18) shows mature eosinophils and sometimes also blast cells, promyelocytes and eosinophil myelocytes. The mature eosinophils often show hypogranularity, vacuolation and hypolobulation. Eosinophils and eosinophil myelocytes may contain some granules with basophilic staining characteristics. Blast cells, and occasionally maturing cells, may contain Auer rods. Anaemia and thrombocyto-

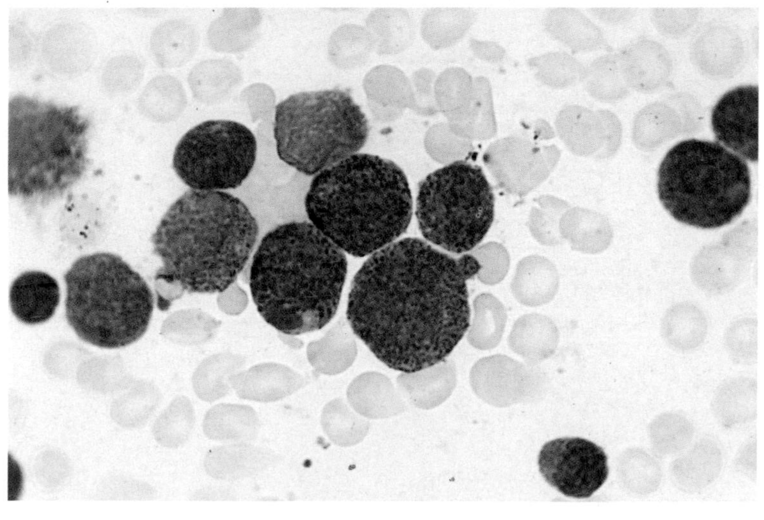
(a)

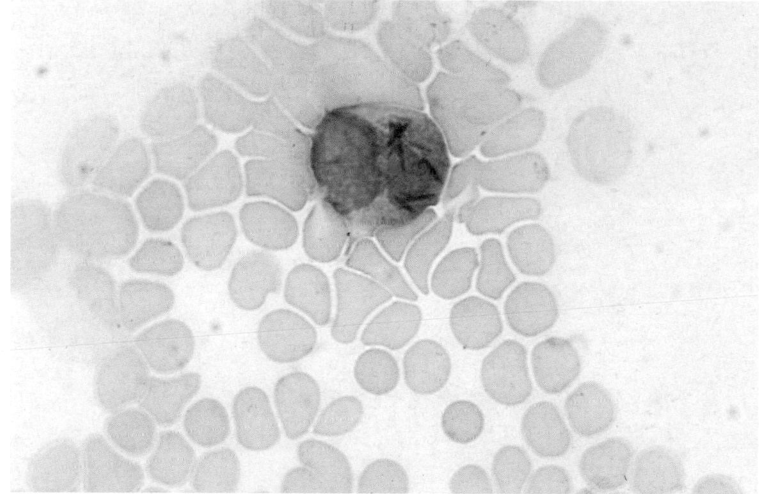
(b)

Fig. 9.10 Peripheral blood films of two patients with M3 AML (acute hypergranular promyelocytic leukaemia) showing: (a) hypergranular promyelocytes, one of which has a giant granule; and (b) a promyelocyte with few granules but stacks of Auer rods.

penia are common. Some patients, particularly those whose leukaemic clone is Philadelphia-positive, have an increased basophil count. Neutrophils often show heavy granulation.

Differential diagnosis

The differential diagnoses are with reactive eosinophilia (see pp. 162–5) and with idiopathic HES (see p. 272). ALL with reactive eosinophilia (Fig. 9.19) also enters into the differential diagnosis.

Further tests

Bone marrow aspiration and cytogenetic analysis are indicated. The bone marrow should be specifically examined for increased blast cells (either myeloblasts or lymphoblasts), lymphoma cells and abnormal mast cells. If there is doubt as to the diagnosis, a trephine biopsy should also be performed since the features of lymphoma or systemic mastocytosis may be revealed. The diagnosis of eosinophilic leukaemia is readily established in those cases in which there is a significant

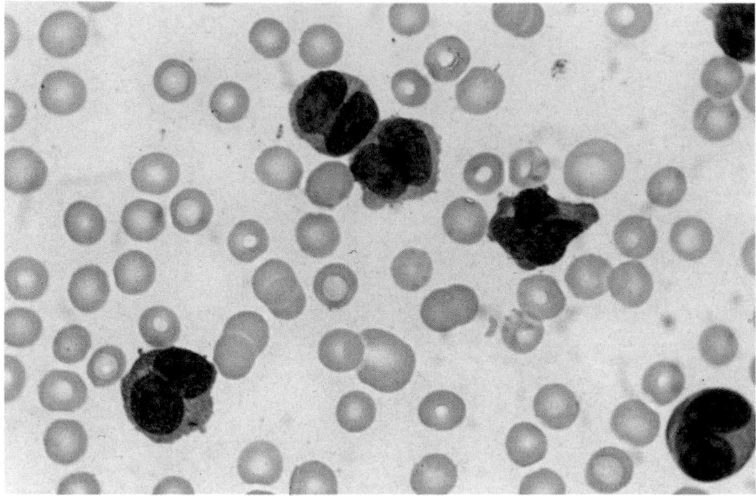

Fig. 9.11 Peripheral blood film in M3 variant AML (hypogranular or microgranular variant of promyelocytic leukaemia) showing characteristic bilobed cells; only occasional cells have granules visible by light microscopy but despite this there was strong cytoplasmic positivity with SBB, myeloperoxidase and CAE.

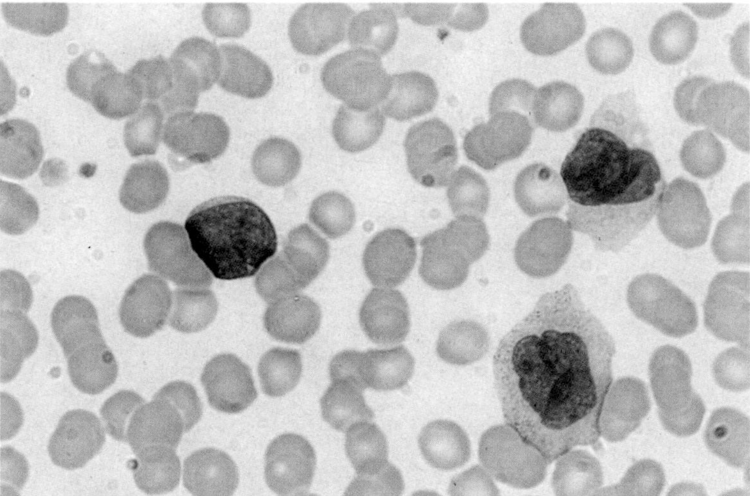

Fig. 9.12 Peripheral blood film of a patient with M4 AML (acute myelomonocytic leukaemia) showing one myeloblast and two monoblasts; the monoblasts are large with a lobulated nucleus, a fine lacy chromatin pattern, several nucleoli and voluminous finely granulated cytoplasm whereas the myeloblast is smaller with a higher nucleo–cytoplasmic ratio. In M4 AML the granulocytic differentiation may be neutrophilic, eosinophilic (see Fig. 9.13) or basophilic.

increase in blast cells and other immature cells, dysplasia of other lineages, a clonal cytogenetic abnormality or other evidence of clonality. A history of preceding myelodysplastic syndrome or the presence of soft tissue tumours composed of immature granulocytic cells also confirms the diagnosis. In cases with predominantly mature eosinophils the diagnosis can be difficult to establish. The presence of marked morphological abnormalities confined to eosinophils is *not* useful in diagnosis since such abnormalities can be seen also in reactive eosinophilia, systemic mastocytosis and idiopathic HES. In some cases, which cannot initially be distinguished from idiopathic HES, only subsequent evolution of the disease confirms the leukaemic nature.

Cases which are found to have the Philadelphia chromosome are best classified as variants of CGL and treated accordingly.

Mast cell leukaemia

Mast cell leukaemia is a rare disease which may occur *de novo* or as a complication of systemic

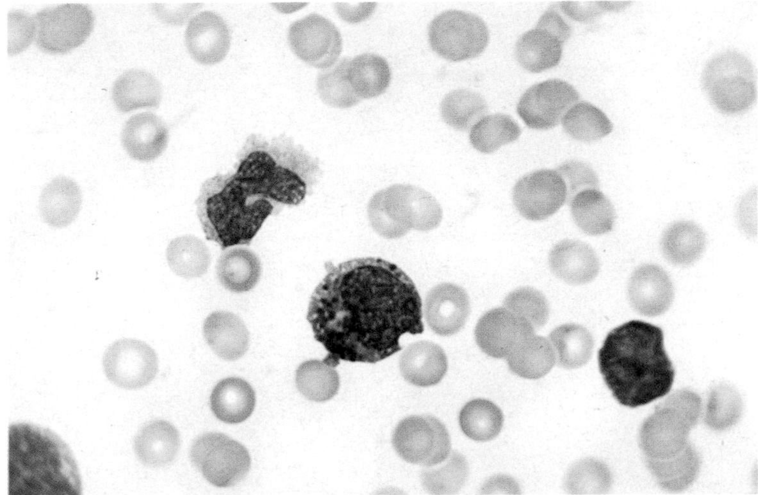

Fig. 9.13 Peripheral blood film in M4 Eo AML (acute myelomonocytic leukaemia with eosinophilia) showing a myeloblast, a monocyte and an eosinophil myelocyte in which some granules have basophilic staining characteristics. Courtesy of Dr D. Swirsky, London.

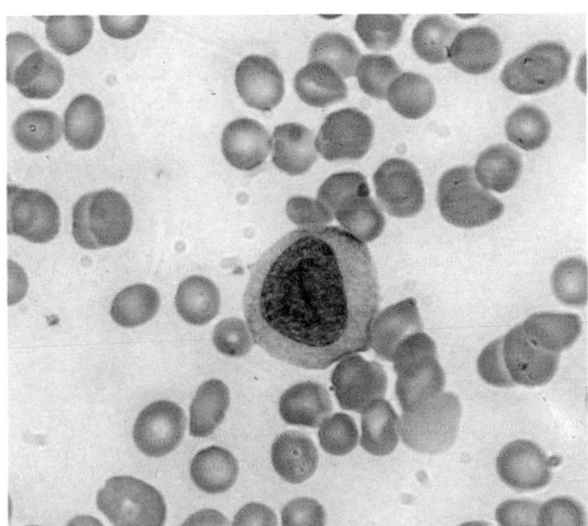

Fig. 9.14 Peripheral blood film in M5a AML (acute monoblastic leukaemia) showing a monoblast with a non-lobulated nucleus and a vesicular nucleolus. Monoblasts are usually strongly positive for non-specific esterase reactions, such as ANAE, and may have a few myeloperoxidase and SBB-positive granules.

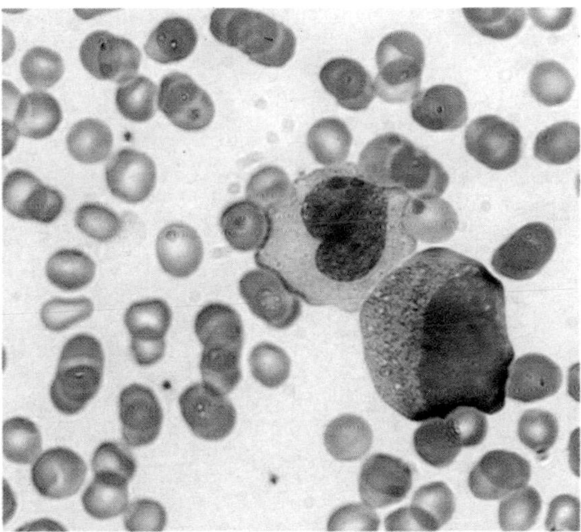

Fig. 9.15 Peripheral blood film in M5b AML (acute monocytic leukaemia) showing one promonocyte and one monocyte; the promonocyte has moderately basophilic cytoplasm which is granulated and vacuolated; promonocytes are positive with SBB, myeloperoxidase and non-specific esterase reactions.

mastocytosis. A mast cell leukaemia or mixed mast cell/basophil leukaemia can also occur as a terminal phase of CGL [34]. Since the mast cell is derived from a haemopoietic stem cell, mast cell leukaemia should be regarded as a variant of AML. It should be noted, however, that the majority of cases of acute leukaemia supervening in systemic mastocytosis are not mast cell leukaemia but other types of AML.

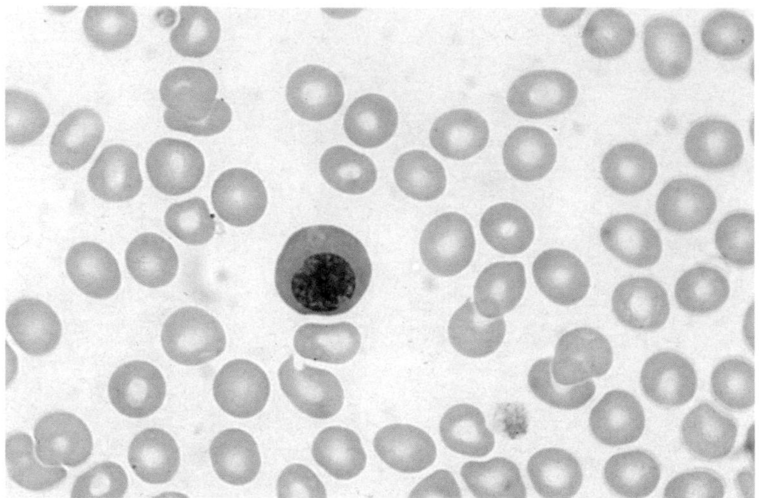

Fig. 9.16 Peripheral blood film in M6 AML (acute erythroleukaemia) showing a circulating NRBC which is megaloblastic.

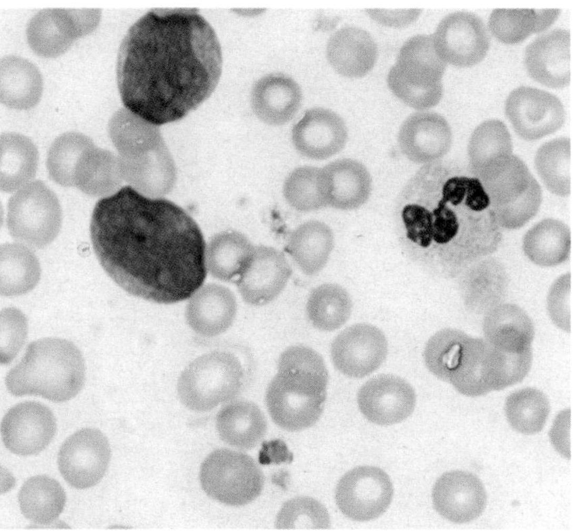

Fig. 9.17 Peripheral blood film in M7 AML (acute megakaryoblastic leukaemia) showing a neutrophil and two blast cells; the blasts have no cytological features which permit their identification as megakaryoblasts but they expressed platelet-associated antigen detectable on immunophenotyping; the giant hypogranular platelet adjacent to the neutrophil is the only clue that this leukaemia may be of megakaryocyte lineage.

Blood film and count

Normal mast cells have a small oval nucleus which is not obscured by the purple granules which pack the cytoplasm (see Fig. 3.106). In mast cell leukaemia (Fig. 9.20), some neoplastic cells may resemble normal mast cells, while others have larger nuclei or nuclei which are bilobed or multilobed. Granules vary in colour from red to dark purple and may or may not obscure the nucleus. They may fuse into homogeneous masses. Less mature cells may have scanty granules and a nucleus which is oval or kidney-shaped with nucleoli [35,36].

Differential diagnosis

The differential diagnosis is with other leukaemias with hypergranular neoplastic cells, specifically hypergranular promyelocytic leukaemia (M3 AML) and basophilic leukaemia. The presence of Auer rods suggest a diagnosis of M3 AML.

Further tests

Bone marrow aspiration and cytochemistry (Table 9.4) are useful in confirming the diagnosis. Mast cells can also be distinguished from basophils by electron microscopy which shows basophils to have granules which are either of a uniform consistency or finely particulate whereas mast cell granules are heterogeneous and contain whorled, scrolled, lamellate and crystalline structures.

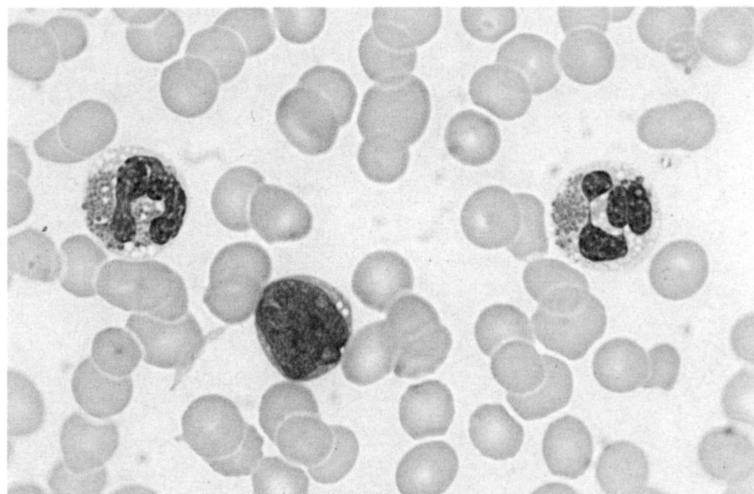

Fig. 9.18 Peripheral blood film in eosinophilic leukaemia showing a blast cell and two vacuolated and partly degranulated eosinophils.

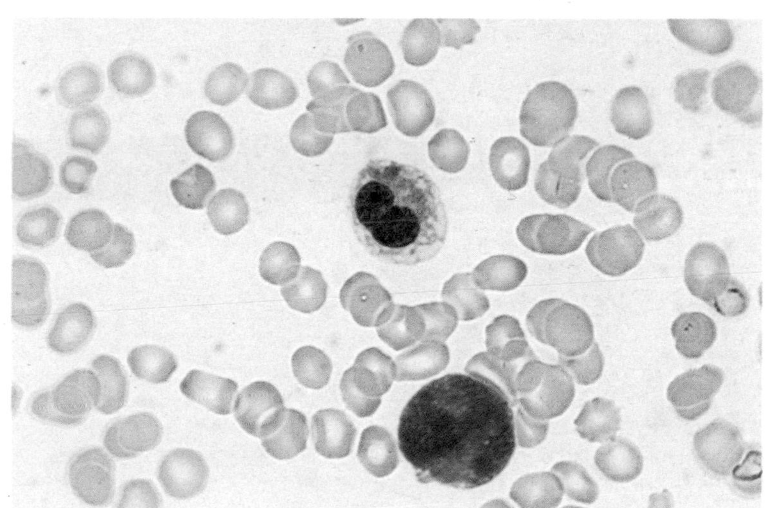

Fig. 9.19 Peripheral blood film of a patient with ALL with reactive eosinophilia showing a lymphoblast and a partially degranulated hypolobulated eosinophil.

Acute myelofibrosis

Acute myelofibrosis is a specific clinicopathological presentation of AML, mainly acute megakaryoblastic leukaemia (M7 AML), consequent on bone marrow fibrosis which is reactive to the leukaemic infiltration. Clinical features result from anaemia and cytopenia. There is no splenomegaly.

Blood film and count

The blood film shows pancytopenia and sometimes occasional blasts. There is little poikilocytosis.

Differential diagnosis

The differential diagnosis is with aplastic anaemia and other causes of pancytopenia and to a lesser extent with other presentations of AML.

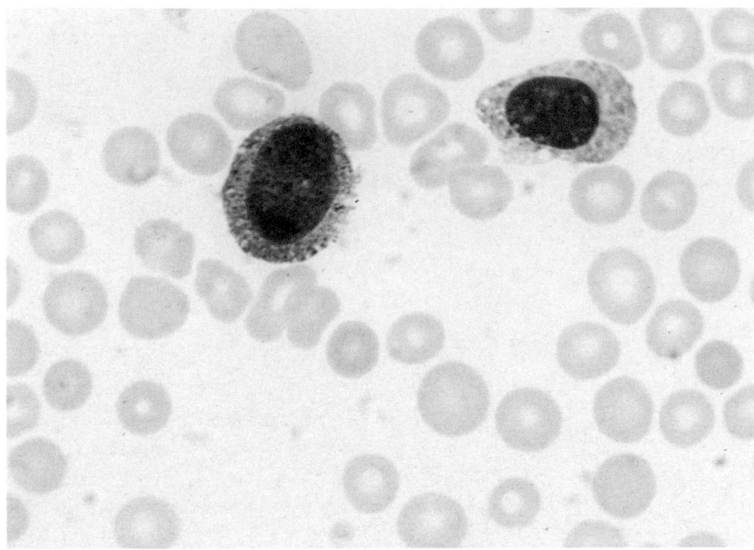

Fig. 9.20 Peripheral blood film of a patient with acute mast cell leukaemia showing two mast cells. Courtesy of Miss Desley Scott and Dr Ian Bunce, Brisbane.

Table 9.4 Some cytochemical tests useful in distinguishing between basophils, mast cells and hypergranular promyelocytes

	Basophiloblast	Basophil	Mast cell	Hypergranular promyelocyte
Myeloperoxidase	−	− or +*	−	+++
SBB	−	− or +	− or +	+++
CAE	−	− †	+++	+++
toluidine blue (metachromatic staining)	− or +	+++	+++	−

−, negative; +, weakly positive; +++, strongly positive.
* Positive in basophil promyelocytes to metamyelocytes.
† Positive in basophil promyelocytes to metamyelocytes and may be positive in leukaemic basophils [37].

Further tests

Bone marrow aspiration is often unsuccessful or yields an undiagnostic specimen so that bone marrow trephine biopsy is essential for diagnosis.

Transient abnormal haemopoiesis of Down's syndrome

Transient abnormal myelopoiesis or transient myeloproliferative disorder of Down's syndrome occurs in neonates (and during intra-uterine life). Cytogenetic and molecular evidence suggests that this disorder is actually spontaneously remitting AML, often acute megakaryoblastic leukaemia [38]. Remission occurs within a few weeks but, in a significant percentage of affected infants, AML develops at 1–2 years of age.

Blood film and count

The blood film cannot be distinguished from that

of AML. The WBC may be moderately to greatly elevated with a high percentage of blast cells. There may be anaemia and thrombocytopenia.

Differential diagnosis

The differential diagnosis is with other cases of congenital leukaemia.

Further tests

Cytogenetic analysis is indicated in order to both confirm Down's syndrome by demonstration of trisomy 21 and to exclude cytogenetic abnormalities which may be associated with other cases of congenital leukaemias. There are no laboratory investigations which will distinguish transient abnormal myelopoiesis from AML. This is achieved only by being aware of this disorder and observing its clinical course.

The myelodysplastic syndromes (MDS)

The MDS are a morphologically heterogeneous group of conditions which are consequent on proliferation of a clone of neoplastic haemopoietic cells showing abnormalities of proliferation and maturation. Haemopoiesis is functionally ineffective and morphologically dysplastic. The MDS are potentially preleukaemic although some patients die from complications of cytopenia without evolution to AML. They may arise *de novo* or following exposure to mutagenic agents such as ionizing radiation, benzene and anti-cancer agents including alkylating agents. The FAB group have categorized the myelodysplastic syndromes, as shown in Table 9.5.

Blood count and film

The peripheral blood film usually shows features suggesting the diagnosis (Figs 9.21–9.23). Most patients are anaemic with red cells being normo-

Table 9.5 The FAB classification of the myelodysplastic syndromes

Category	Peripheral blood		Bone marrow
Refractory anaemia or refractory cytopenia*	Anaemia,* blasts ≤ 1% monocytes ≤ 1 × 10⁹/l	AND	Blasts < 5%, ringed sideroblasts ≤ 15% of erythroblasts
Refractory anaemia with ringed sideroblasts	Anaemia, blasts ≤ 1% monocytes ≤ 1 × 10⁹/l	AND	Blasts <5%, ringed sideroblasts > 15% of erythroblasts
Refractory anaemia with excess of blasts (RAEB)	Anaemia, monocytes ≤ 1 × 10⁹/l; Blasts > 1% BUT Blasts < 5%	OR / AND	Blasts ≥ 5% / Blasts ≤ 20%
Chronic myelomonocytic leukaemia (CMML)	Monocyte count > 1 × 10⁹/l, granulocytes often increased, blasts < 5%		Blasts up to 20% promonocytes often increased
Refractory anaemia with excess of blasts in transformation (RAEB-T)	Blasts ≥ 5% OR Auer rods in blasts in blood or marrow	OR	Blasts > 20% BUT Blasts <30%

* Or in the case of refractory cytopenia either neutropenia or thrombocytopenia.

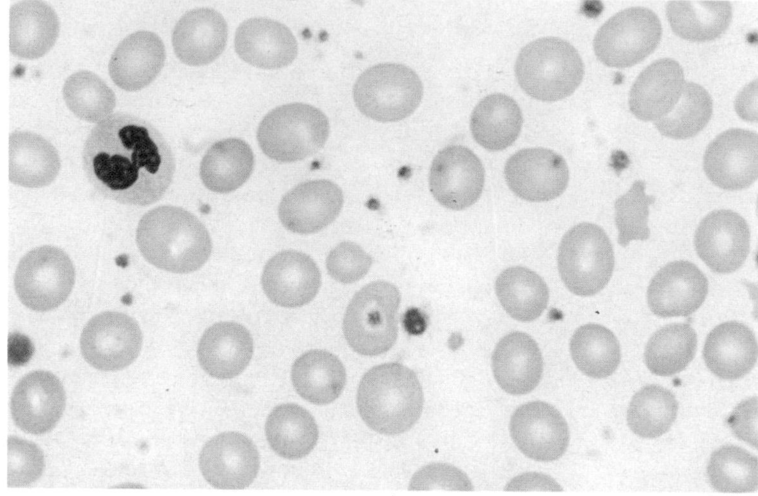

Fig. 9.21 Peripheral blood film of a patient with myelodysplastic syndrome (refractory anaemia) showing anisocytosis, macrocytosis and one poikilocyte; the neutrophil is hypogranular.

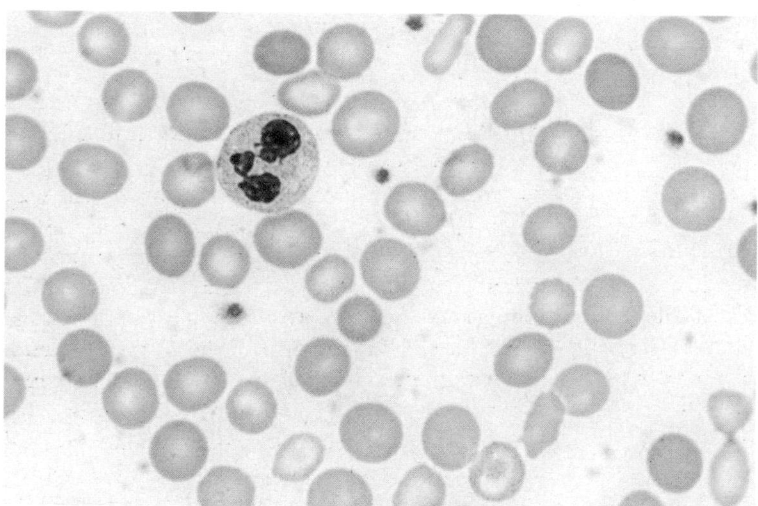

Fig. 9.22 Peripheral blood film of a patient with myelodysplastic syndrome (refractory anaemia with ring sideroblasts) showing one target cell and several hypochromic microcytes; the remainder of the erythrocytes are normochromic cells which are either normocytic or macrocytic; MCV was 103 fl.

chromic and either normocytic or macrocytic. In patients with sideroblastic erythropoiesis there is a minor population of hypochromic microcytes and Pappenheimer bodies are present. Red cells may also show anisocytosis, poikilocytosis and basophilic stippling. There may be leucocytosis or leucopenia. Leucocytosis is usually attributable to monocytosis, sometimes with associated neutrophilia. An increase of eosinophils or basophils is very uncommon. Blast cells may be present and they may contain Auer rods. There may be occasional promyelocytes, myelocytes or NRBC. Neutrophils commonly show dysplastic features, particularly hypogranularity (Fig. 9.23) and the acquired Pelger–Hüet anomaly (see Fig. 3.50). The platelet count is often reduced but in a minority of patients it is increased. Platelets may show dysplastic features such as large size and hypogranularity.

Differential diagnosis

The differential diagnosis is with other causes of macrocytic anaemia and cytopenia, with AML

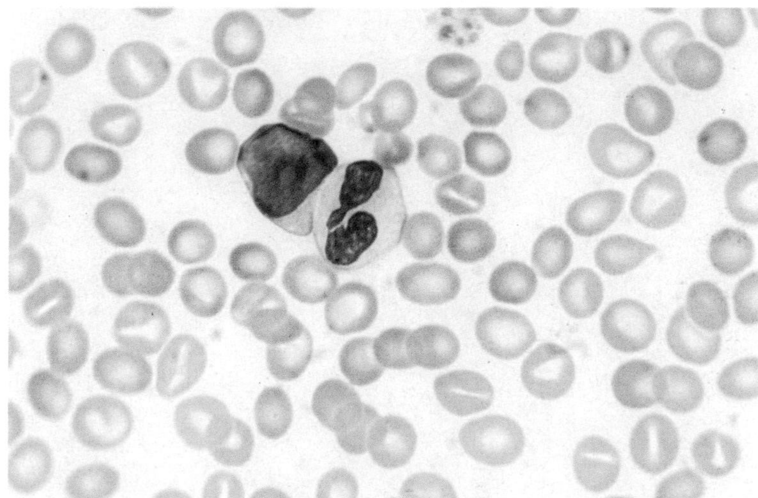

Fig. 9.23 Peripheral blood film of a patient with myelodysplastic syndrome (refractory anaemia with excess of blasts) showing a myeloblast and a hypogranular neutrophil; the red cells show anisocytosis and poikilocytosis including tear drop cells and stomatocytes.

and with non-neoplastic conditions causing dysplasia such as HIV infection and the direct rather than long-term effects of the administration of anti-cancer drugs.

Further tests

Bone marrow aspiration with cytochemical stains (Perls' stain and either myeloperoxidase or SBB stain) is often necessary for diagnosis and is always necessary for further classification (see Table 9.5) and for determining prognosis. When cytological evidence is insufficient for a firm diagnosis, cytogenetic analysis or other investigations to establish clonality of haemopoietic cells may be useful.

Chronic myeloid leukaemias (CMLs)

CMLs differ from AML in that there is effective maturation with production of granulocytes. About 95% of cases of CML are the specific entity referred to as CGL. Other less common CMLs are atypical CML, juvenile CML and neutrophilic leukaemia. CMML is usually classified with the myelodysplastic syndromes but could equally well be regarded as a CML.

Chronic granulocytic leukaemia (CGL)

CGL is a disease of adults characterized clinically by anaemia, splenomegaly and hepatomegaly.

Blood film and count

The WBC is elevated, often markedly so. The differential count (Fig. 9.24) [39] and blood film (Fig. 9.25) are very characteristic with myelocytes and neutrophils being the most frequent cells. In patients with a very high WBC the blast cells may be as high as 15% but nevertheless blasts remain less frequent than promyelocytes and promyelocytes less frequent than myelocytes. There is an increase in the absolute basophil count in almost every case and an increase in the absolute eosinophil count in about 80% of cases. Some eosinophils may have a proportion of granules with basophilic staining characteristics. Monocytes are increased, but not in proportion to neutrophils. Some NRBC are present. Dysplastic features are minor. The platelet count is usually normal or increased but in a minority of cases it is decreased. Platelet size is increased. Circulating megakaryocytes, mainly almost bare nuclei, are sometimes present.

Occasional patients with CGL have striking cyclical changes in WBC with a periodicity of 50–70 days, and with the WBC varying from frankly leukaemic levels to almost normal. All myeloid cells participate in the cycles.

A minority of patients have bone marrow fibrosis at presentation and the typical peripheral blood features of myelofibrosis are then superimposed on the features of CGL.

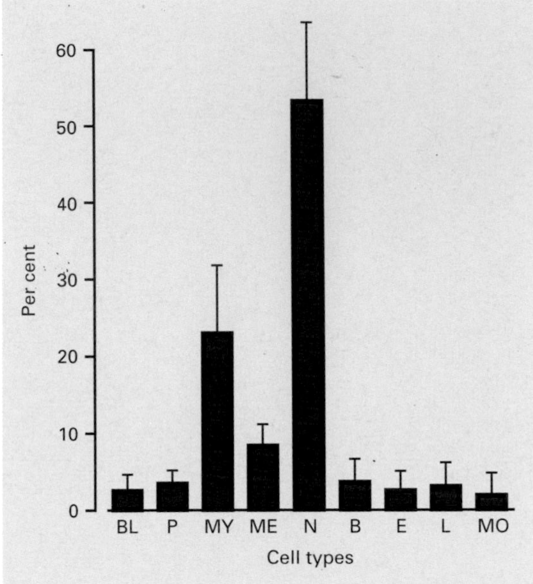

Fig. 9.24 A diagrammatic representation of the typical differential count in CGL based on 1500 cell differential counts in 50 patients with Philadelphia-positive CGL [39]. BL, blasts; P, promyelocytes; MY, myelocytes; ME, metamyelocytes; N, neutrophils; B, basophils; E, eosinophils; L, lymphocytes; MO, monocytes.

Most patients with CGL present with symptoms and well-established disease. Occasional patients who have developed the disease while being monitored haematologically have allowed the early stages of the disease to be defined. The first detectable peripheral blood features are an increase in the basophil count, thrombocytosis and a low NAP score. Following this, the neutrophil count and the WBC rise and small numbers of immature cells appear. With the progressive rise of WBC which follows, the percentage of immature cells steadily increases.

CGL terminates in myelofibrosis or in blast transformation (see below), often preceded by an accelerated phase.

Differential diagnosis

The differential diagnosis is with reactive neutrophilia and with other CMLs. Features useful in distinguishing CGL from reactive neutrophilia are shown in Table 9.2 but in practice diagnostic difficulty only rises in early cases of CGL.

Further tests

Cytogenetic analysis is indicated to confirm the diagnosis. The great majority of cases of CGL are associated with the presence of the Philadelphia chromosome, an abbreviated chromosome 22 resulting from a t(9;22) (q34;q11) translocation. A minority of cases of CGL which are Philadelphia-negative and lack the classical microscopically detectable translocation nevertheless have a related DNA rearrangement (BCR-ABL rearrangement). Such cases, which are clinically and haematologically indistinguishable from the Philadelphia-positive cases, should be classified as Philadelphia-negative CGL.

NAP score is reduced in more than 90% of cases of chronic phase CGL but its importance in diagnosis has decreased with the more ready availability of cytogenetic and molecular analysis.

Atypical chronic myeloid leukaemia (atypical CML)

Atypical CML has the same clinical features as CGL.

Blood film and count

Patients are anaemic and have a moderate to marked elevation in the WBC. On average, patients with atypical CML present with a lower Hb and a lower WBC than patients with CGL. Peripheral blood features (Fig. 9.26) differ from CGL in that monocytosis and thrombocytopenia are more common while basophilia and eosinophilia are less common. Granulocyte precursors are present. Dysplastic features are common.

Atypical CML may terminate in blast transformation.

Differential diagnosis

The differential diagnosis is with other types of CML and occasionally with leukaemoid reactions.

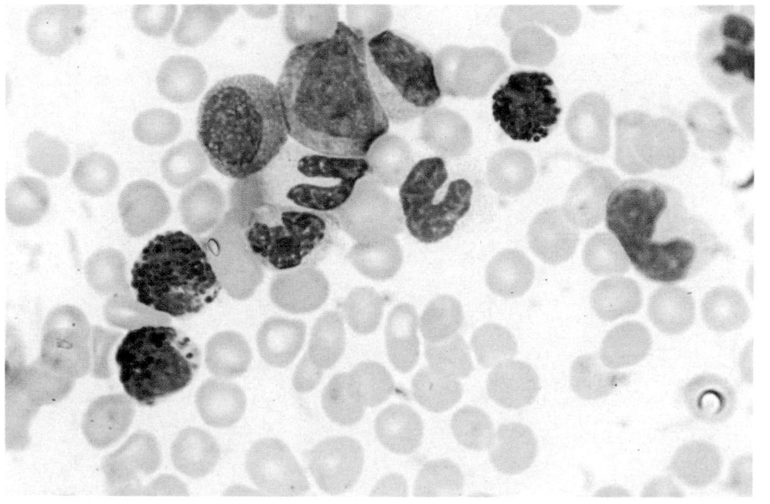

(a)

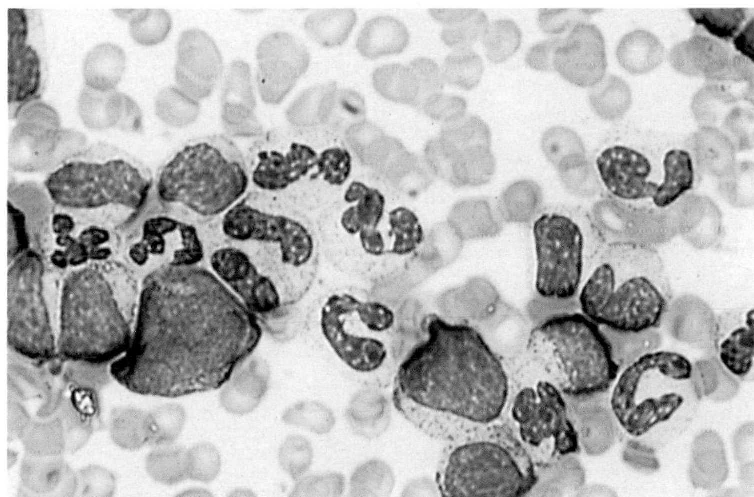

(b)

Fig. 9.25 Peripheral blood film in Philadelphia-positive CGL showing: (a) a promyelocyte, an eosinophil myelocyte, three basophils and a number of neutrophils and band forms; and (b) a promyelocyte, several myelocytes, neutrophil band forms and neutrophils; the presence of a binucleate neutrophil is relatively uncommon.

Further tests

Bone marrow aspiration and cytogenetic analysis may be useful in diagnosis. The Philadelphia chromosome is not detected but other clonal cytogenetic abnormalities may be present. NAP score is low in the majority of patients but elevated in a minority.

Chronic myelomonocytic leukaemia (CMML)

CMML is a disease of the elderly population characterized by anaemia, hepatosplenomegaly and, occasionally, tissue infiltration by leukaemic monocytes.

Blood film and count

The blood film (Fig. 9.27) shows monocytosis and most cases also have anaemia and neutrophilia. As defined by the FAB group (see Table 9.5), the monocyte count must be greater than $1 \times 10^9/l$. The monocytes may be somewhat immature with cytoplasmic basophilia or nucleoli. Granulocyte precursors may be present but they are usually less than 5% of white cells whereas in atypical

(a)

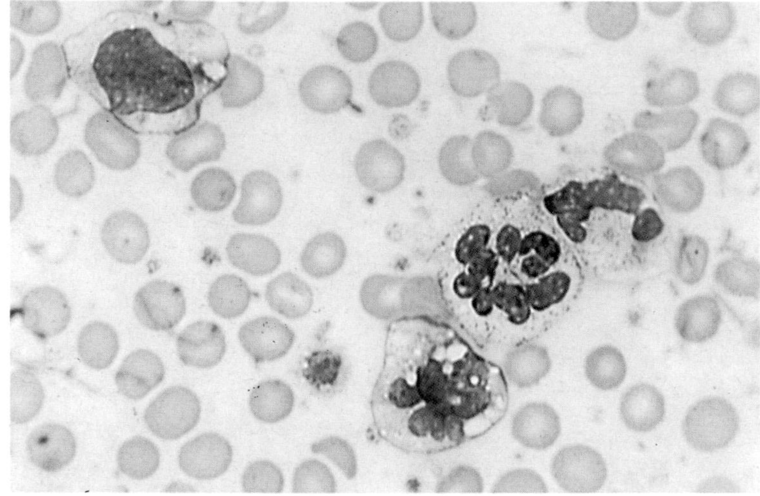

(b)

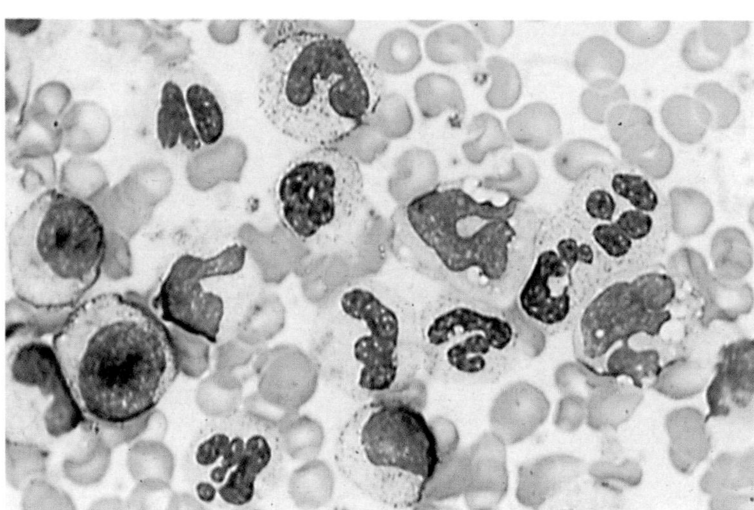

Fig. 9.26 Peripheral blood film in atypical CML showing: (a) a normal neutrophil, a macropolycyte, a monocyte and a somewhat immature monocyte; there is one large platelet (b) numerous neutrophils, band forms, monocytes and hypogranular myelocytes.

CML there are significant numbers of immature granulocytes, often over 15% and almost always over 5%. Basophilia and eosinophilia are quite uncommon. Dysplastic features in other lineages are often but not invariably present.

CMML may terminate by evolving into AML.

Differential diagnosis

The differential diagnosis is with other types of CML, other categories of myelodysplastic syndromes and reactive conditions.

Further tests

Bone marrow aspiration and cytogenetic analysis are useful in diagnosis. The Philadelphia chromosome is not detected but other clonal cytogenetic abnormalities may be present.

Juvenile chronic myeloid leukaemia (juvenile CML)

Children may develop typical Philadelphia-positive CGL although it is rare before adolescence. Children below the age of 5 years may also develop

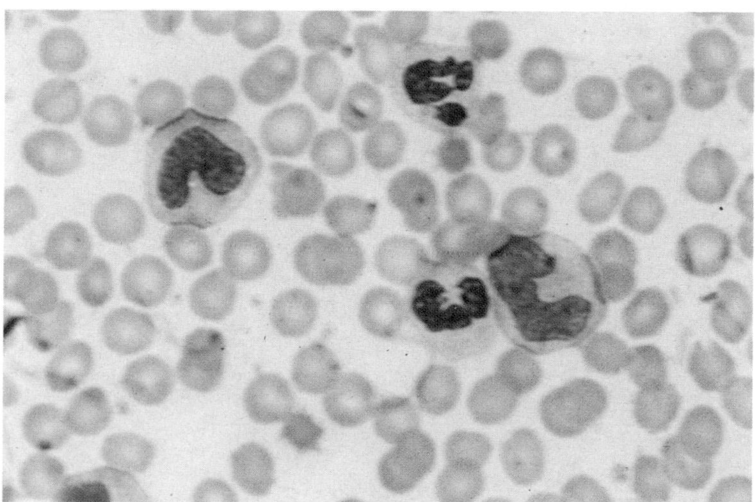

Fig. 9.27 Peripheral blood film in CMML showing two neutrophils and two monocytes; there are also several acanthocytes and a tear drop poikilocyte.

a distinctive, Philadelphia-negative condition known as juvenile CML. Clinical features are anaemia and splenomegaly and sometimes hepatomegaly and lymphadenopathy.

Blood film and count

The blood count shows anaemia, neutrophilia and monocytosis. In comparison with CGL, the WBC is usually lower and myelocytes are less frequent, while monocytosis, thrombocytopenia and circulating NRBC are common features. Monocytosis is particularly important in diagnosis since it is almost always present. Dysplastic features are present (Fig. 9.28). A high blast count, large numbers of NRBC and a low platelet count are indicative of a worse prognosis [40].

The disease may terminate in acute transformation.

Differential diagnosis

The differential diagnosis is with MDS and the childhood monosomy 7 syndrome. Monocytosis is often a feature of myelodysplastic syndrome in childhood. The childhood monosomy 7 syndrome has both myelodysplastic and myeloproliferative features.

Further tests

Bone marrow aspiration and cytogenetic analysis are indicated. NAP score may be high, normal or low. Commonly associated abnormalities include features associated with fetal haemopoiesis, specifically high haemoglobin F, low haemoglobin A_2 and red cell carbonic anhydrase, reduced expression of the red cell I antigen and increased expression of the red cell i antigen. These features are not associated with the childhood monosomy 7 syndrome or with MDS. Immunoglobulin concentration may be increased.

Neutrophilic leukaemia

Neutrophilic leukaemia is a rare condition characterized clinically by anaemia, splenomegaly and sometimes hepatomegaly.

Blood film

There is anaemia and a marked neutrophilia with very few circulating immature cells (Fig. 9.29). The WBC is usually of the order of $40-70 \times 10^9/l$. There is no basophilia, eosinophilia or monocytosis. Neutrophils may have both toxic granulation and Döhle bodies [41]. Ring neutrophils are relatively common [42]. Some cases have also had

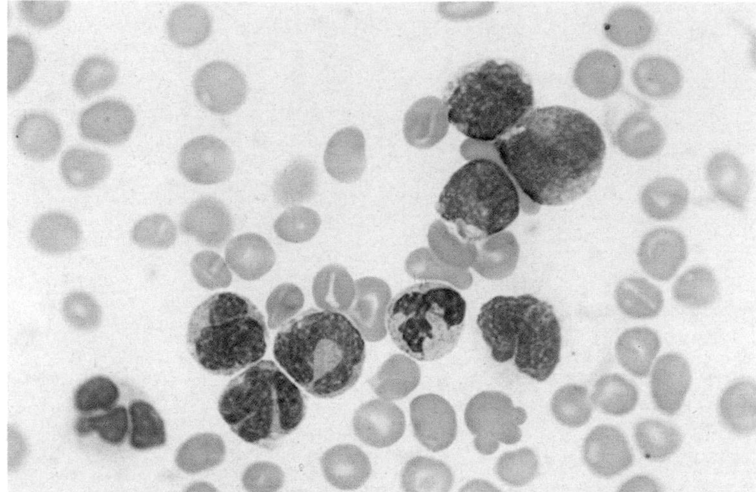

Fig. 9.28 Peripheral blood film in juvenile CML showing several neutrophils, a blast, a promyelocyte and several very dysplastic cells which may be of monocyte lineage. Courtesy of Dr O. Oakhill and Dr G.R. Standen, Bristol. The patient was a child of 6 months with hepatosplenomegaly, WBC 94×10^9/l, Hb 10.2 g/dl, platelet count 28×10^9/l, NAP score 10 and haemoglobin F concentration 11%.

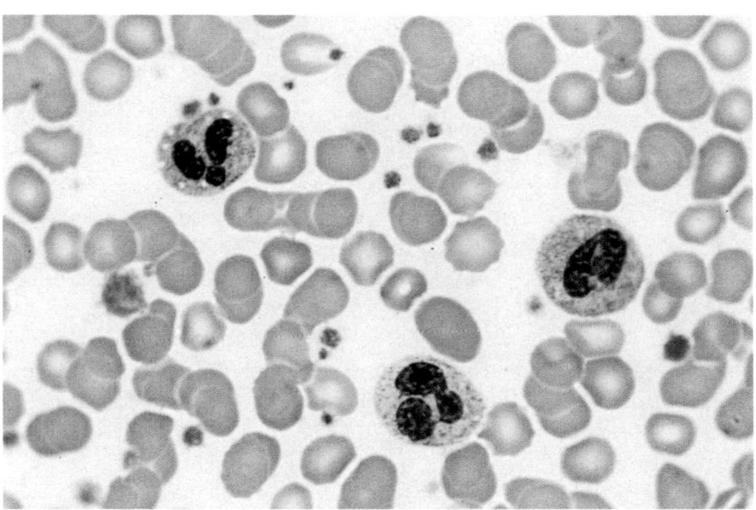

Fig. 9.29 Peripheral blood film in chronic neutrophilic leukaemia. The neutrophils show 'toxic' granulation and vacuolation. One giant platelet is present. Other neutrophils showed Döhle bodies and macropolycytes were present.

marked dysplastic features [43]. The disease may terminate in acute transformation.

Differential diagnosis

The differential diagnosis is with reactive neutrophilia and with other chronic leukaemias and myeloproliferative disorders.

Further tests

Bone marrow aspiration and cytogenetic analysis are indicated. NAP score is usually high. When no clonal cytogenetic abnormality is present, a period of observation may be necessary to make the distinction from reactive neutrophilia.

Chronic granulocytic leukaemia (CGL) in accelerated phase and transformation

In the majority of patients with CGL a chronic phase which lasts for weeks, months or years is followed by blast transformation. This is sometimes preceded by an accelerated phase. Clinical features of disease evolution are pallor and bruising, increasing hepatomegaly and splenomegaly, lymphadenopathy or, less often, soft tissue tumours and refractoriness to treatment.

Blood film and count

During the accelerated phase there may be anaemia, leucocytosis, thrombocytopenia, thrombocytosis, a rising basophil count, an increasing blast cell percentage and the appearance of dysplastic features (Table 9.6). Blast transformation may occur without any warning or be preceded by an accelerated phase. It is lymphoblastic in about one-quarter of cases and myeloid or mixed lymphoblastic and myeloid in the remainder (Table 9.7). Myeloid transformation is often megakaryoblastic or mixed myeloblastic/megakaryoblastic. A patient who remits from one blast crisis (e.g., lymphoblastic) may subsequently suffer a second blast crisis with cells of different lineage (e.g., megakaryoblastic).

Differential diagnosis

Patients may present already in blast transformation in which case the differential diagnosis is with acute leukaemia. Otherwise the likely diagnosis is readily evident from the clinical and haematological features.

Further tests

Bone marrow aspiration is indicated unless there are large numbers of blasts in the peripheral blood. Cytogenetic analysis is indicated since cytogenetic evolution often precedes or occurs simultaneously with the development of acceleration or acute transformation. Immunophenotyping of blast cells is indicated since there is more likelihood of a response to treatment in lymphoblastic transformation.

Chronic idiopathic myelofibrosis

Chronic idiopathic myelofibrosis or myelofibrosis with myeloid metaplasia is a haematological neoplasm characterized by extramedullary haemopoiesis together with bone marrow fibrosis

Table 9.6 Some haematological abnormalities which may be detected during the accelerated phase of CGL

Red cells and precursors
Anaemia (including that due to red cell aplasia in which reticulocytes are very infrequent or absent), macrocytosis, marked poikilocytosis (may be consequent on bone marrow fibrosis), vacuolated erythroblasts (PAS-positive), hypochromia and microcytosis

White cells and precursors
Refractory leucocytosis, increasing basophil count, disappearance of eosinophilia, increasing monocytosis, acquired Pelger–Hüet anomaly of neutrophils or eosinophils, hypogranular neutrophils, pseudo-Chediak–Higashi anomaly (giant granules) of neutrophils and precursors, binuclearity and other dysplastic features of neutrophil precursors, increasing blast cell percentage with decreasing percentage of more mature cells, Auer rods in blast cells

Platelets and megakaryocytes
Thrombocytopenia, thrombocytosis, micromegakaryocytes, bare megakaryocyte nuclei

General
Pancytopenia (may be consequent on refractory splenomegaly or, rarely, bone marrow necrosis)

Table 9.7 Types of transformation which can occur in CGL

Myeloblastic transformation
Lymphoblastic transformation
Megakaryocytic transformation (with micromegakaryocytes and thrombocytosis)
Megakaryoblastic transformation
Erythroblastic transformation [44] and acquired sideroblastic erythropoiesis
Monoblastic transformation [45]
Basophil blast transformation [46]
Mast cell and mixed basophil/mast cell transformation [34]
Eosinophil blast transformation [47]
Hypergranular promyelocytic transformation [48]
Transformations with various mixtures of cell types
Acute myelofibrosis

which is reactive to the underlying proliferation of myeloid cells.

Blood film and count

The blood film is leucoerythroblastic and shows anisocytosis and poikilocytosis, particularly the presence of tear drop poikilocytes (Fig. 9.30). In the early stages of the disease there may be leucocytosis and thrombocytosis. Later in the course there is pancytopenia. Often there are some giant platelets and occasional circulating micromegakaryocytes or megakaryocyte nuclei.

Differential diagnosis

The differential diagnosis is with other causes of a leucoerythroblastic blood film and with other causes of pancytopenia (see Tables 6.17 and 6.25).

Further tests

A bone marrow trephine biopsy is required for diagnosis. Cytogenetic analysis can be useful, particularly to exclude the presence of the Philadelphia chromosome. A clonal cytogenetic abnormality is sometimes demonstrated.

Acute lymphoblastic leukaemia (ALL)

ALL is most common in children under 10 years of age but there is a second peak in incidence in middle-aged and elderly adults. Clinical features are those due to leukaemic cell proliferation, such as hepatosplenomegaly and lymphadenopathy, and those which are an indirect consequence of bone marrow infiltration, such as pallor and bruising. ALL may be of T or B lineage.

Blood film and count

Some cases present with anaemia and thrombocytopenia without any circulating leukaemic cells. Others have variable numbers of lymphoblasts in the peripheral blood with the WBC sometimes being greatly elevated. ALL has been categorized by the FAB group [29] as L1, L2 and L3. In L1 ALL (Fig. 9.31) the blast cells are small to medium in size and are fairly uniform in appearance. Larger cells have diffuse chromatin and sometimes small nucleoli whereas the smaller blasts have no visible nucleolus and show some chromatin condensation. Cytoplasm is scanty and weakly to moderately basophilic. There may be a few cytoplasmic vacuoles. In L2 ALL (Fig. 9.32) the blasts are larger and more pleomorphic with more irregular nuclei, more prominent nucleoli and more abundant cytoplasm. Cytoplasm is weakly to strongly basophilic and may contain some vacuoles. L3 ALL (Fig. 9.33) is characterized by moderately intense cytoplasmic basophilia and variable but usually heavy cytoplasmic vacuolation.

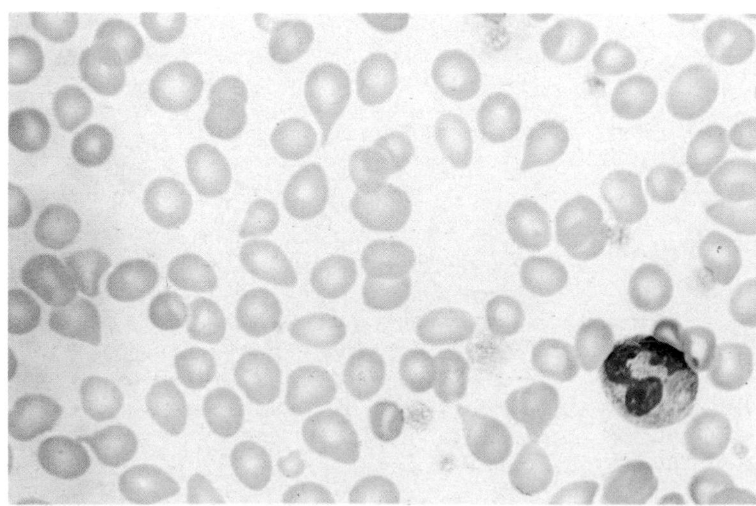

Fig. 9.30 Peripheral blood film in chronic idiopathic myelofibrosis showing anisocytosis and poikilocytosis with prominent tear drop poikilocytes.

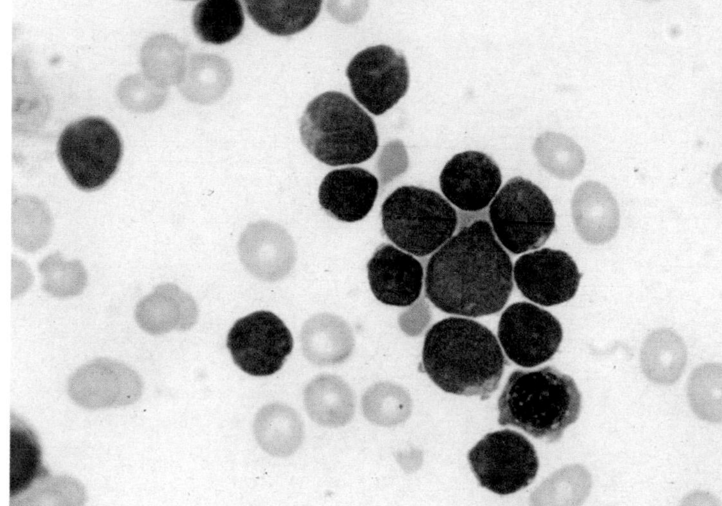

Fig. 9.31 Peripheral blood film in L1 ALL showing lymphoblasts and one NRBC. The lymphoblasts vary in size but are relatively uniform in morphology. The smaller blast cells show some chromatin condensation, which can be a feature of lymphoblasts but not of myeloblasts. This case was shown on immunophenotyping to be of B lineage.

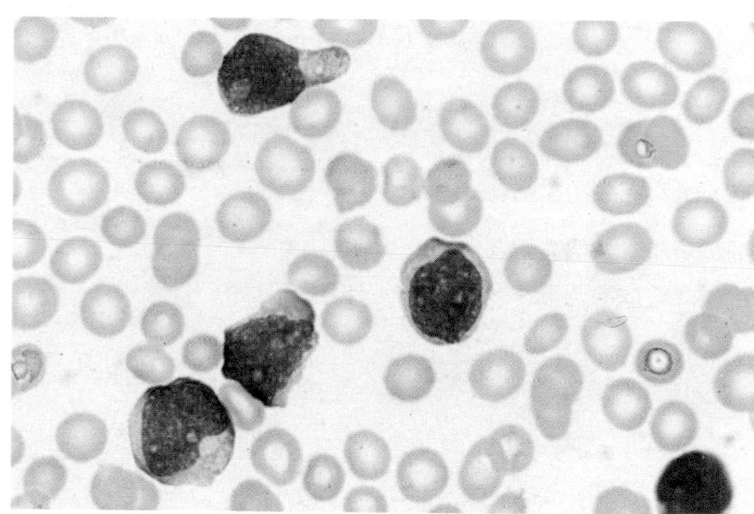

Fig. 9.32 Peripheral blood film in L2 ALL. The blast cells are larger and more pleomorphic than in L1 ALL and in this case have a more diffuse chromatin pattern; one of the blasts has a hand-mirror conformation. This case was shown on immunophenotyping to be of T lineage.

Differential diagnosis

The differential diagnosis is principally with AML and reactive lymphocytosis.

Some cases of ALL have a few azurophilic granules and some cases of AML lack any granules or other light microscopy signs of myeloid differentiation so that reliable differentiation of the two conditions requires further tests. L2 ALL is most readily confused with AML. L1 ALL can usually be distinguished from AML on cytological features. There are usually some quite small blast cells, barely any bigger than a normal lymphocyte, and these cells show some chromatin condensation whereas the blasts of AML are rarely this small and usually have a diffuse chromatin pattern. L3 ALL is so distinctive that a diagnosis based on cytology alone is rarely wrong.

Cases of small cell tumours of childhood with circulating neoplastic cells are sometimes confused with ALL. Immunophenotyping may be necessary to make the distinction.

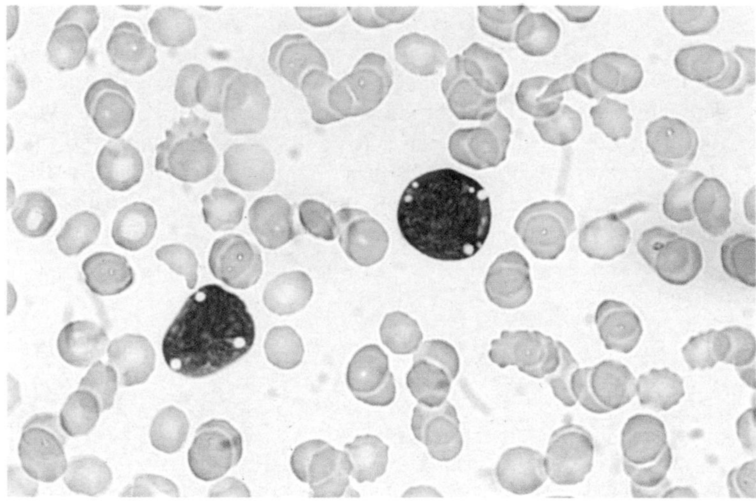

Fig. 9.33 Peripheral blood film in L3 ALL. The blast cells are medium sized with strongly basophilic vacuolated cytoplasm. This case was shown to have a mature B-cell immunophenotype.

In cases of ALL with only small numbers of circulating blasts it is sometimes necessary to do further tests to distinguish ALL from an infection which is causing lymphocytosis with atypical lymphocytes.

In cases with no circulating leukaemic cells the differential diagnosis includes aplastic anaemia and other causes of bone marrow failure. Concern is often expressed as to whether children with severe thrombocytopenia are suffering from ALL. When there are no atypical lymphoid cells and no anaemia this is very unlikely.

Further tests

Bone marrow aspiration and immunophenotyping of either peripheral blood or bone marrow blast cells are essential to confirm the diagnosis of ALL. Cytogenetic analysis to identify prognostically important subgroups is also recommended. Cases of L1 and L2 ALL may be of either B or T lineage. Cases of L3 ALL are almost always of B lineage with the blasts being mature B cells expressing surface membrane immunoglobulin.

Chronic lymphoid leukaemias and lymphomas

Both chronic lymphoid leukaemias and lymphomas are lymphoid neoplasms. By definition, in chronic lymphoid leukaemias there are circulating leukaemic cells whereas lymphomas primarily involve lymph nodes and other tissues. Lymphomas may, however, have a leukaemic phase, either at presentation or with disease progression. The term 'lymphoproliferative disorder' includes both leukaemias and lymphomas. Cytology is very useful in the differential diagnosis of these disorders [49] but it is not always possible to arrive at a definitive diagnosis on the basis of cytological features alone. Diagnosis should be based on clinical features, blood count, cytology and immunophenotype. In some cases histological examination of the bone marrow or lymph nodes is also necessary. Only peripheral blood features will be discussed in any detail here. For further information on immunophenotype and histology the reader is referred elsewhere [33,49–51].

B-LINEAGE LYMPHOPROLIFERATIVE DISORDERS

Chronic lymphocytic leukaemia (CLL)

CLL is a chronic condition characterized by accumulation of mature small B cells with consequent development of lymphadenopathy, hepatomegaly and splenomegaly. In early cases there may be no abnormal physical findings and the diagnosis is made incidentally on a routine blood count. The peripheral blood and bone marrow are always involved.

Blood film and count

The WBC and lymphocyte count range from just above normal to greatly elevated. The Hb and platelet count may be normal or reduced. In the untreated patient, the neutrophil count is rarely reduced. The lymphocytes are similar in size to normal lymphocytes but are more uniform in appearance (Fig. 9.34). The chromatin is usually clumped and nucleoli are small and inconspicuous. Cytoplasm is scanty and weakly basophilic. In some cases there are cytoplasmic crystals (Fig. 9.35) or globular inclusions. Because CLL cells have increased mechanical fragility, there are increased numbers of smear cells. There may be a small number of larger cells with prominent nucleoli resembling the cells of PLL. If there are more than 10% of prolymphocytes or the degree of pleomorphism is greater than usual, the diagnosis of CLL of mixed cell type (CLL/PL) is preferred [50]. Anaemia is usually normocytic and normochromic. If there is complicating autoimmune haemolytic anaemia there are spherocytes and polychromasia.

Differential diagnosis

The differential diagnosis is with other chronic lymphoproliferative disorders, particularly with follicular lymphoma, splenic lymphoma with villous lymphocytes (SLVL), mantle cell lymphoma and the small cell variant of T-lineage PLL. Benign conditions which can be confused with CLL include post-splenectomy lymphocytosis and lymphocytosis induced by acute stress. If the blood film is examined in isolation without reference to the age and clinical features then whooping cough and infectious lymphocytosis can also be confused with CLL.

Further tests

The diagnosis should be confirmed by immunophenotyping which may be supplemented by cytogenetic analysis and trephine biopsy of the bone marrow.

B-lineage prolymphocytic leukaemia (PLL)

B-lineage PLL is characterized clinically by marked splenomegaly with trivial lymphadenopathy. The peripheral blood and bone marrow are always involved. There may be anaemia and other cytopenias. The disease is more rapidly progressive than CLL.

Blood film and count

The WBC is usually greatly elevated. The neoplastic cells are larger than those of CLL and

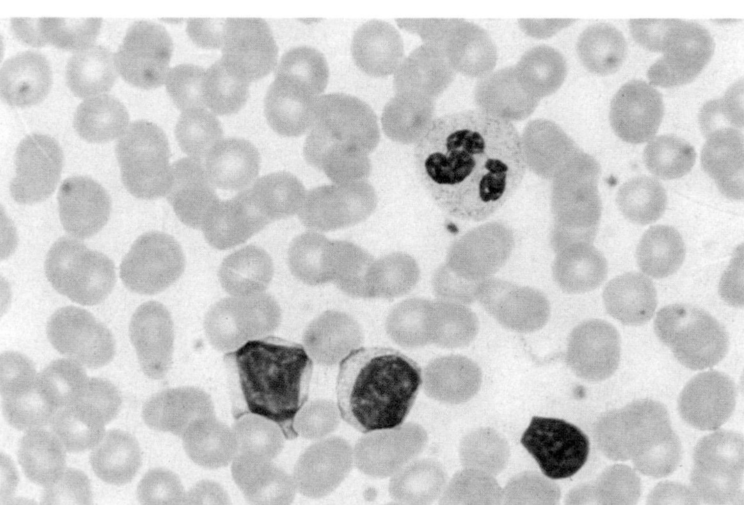

Fig. 9.34 Peripheral blood film in CLL showing a neutrophil, two mature lymphocytes and a smear cell.

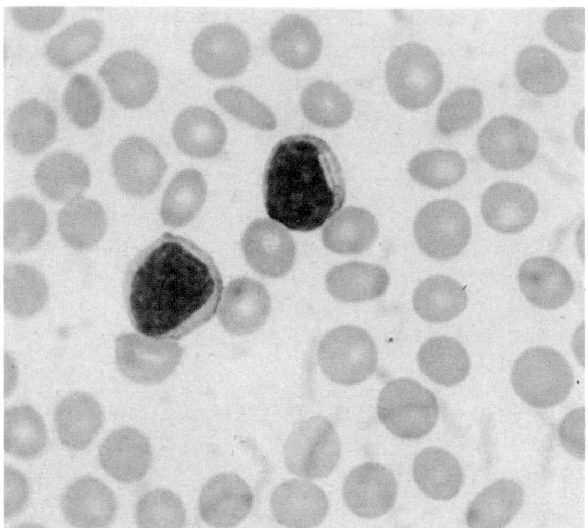

Fig. 9.35 Peripheral blood film in CLL showing two lymphocytes, one of which contains two crystals. Courtesy of Professor D. Catovsky.

show more variation in size. They are predominantly round with round nuclei and weakly basophilic cytoplasm which is more abundant than in CLL (Fig. 9.36). Many cells, particularly the larger ones, have large and prominent nucleoli. There is moderate chromatin condensation which is enhanced around the large nucleolus, giving it a 'vesicular' appearance.

Differential diagnosis

The differential diagnosis is with other chronic lymphoproliferative disorders, particularly with CLL/PL and T-lineage PLL. The best criterion to separate PLL from CLL/PL is that prolymphocytes are at least 55% [52]. In T-lineage PLL, the cells are more irregular in shape, more pleomorphic and often smaller than in B-lineage PLL. Occasionally, the leukaemic phase of large cell lymphoma resembles PLL but generally the degree of pleomorphism is much greater in large cell lymphoma.

Further tests

Immunophenotyping supports a provisional diagnosis of PLL.

Hairy cell leukaemia

Hairy cell leukaemia is a chronic disorder characterized by splenomegaly without lymphadenopathy. Early cases may have no abnormal physical findings and diagnosis may then be made incidentally because of cytopenia.

Blood film and count

The WBC is usually not elevated and hairy cells (Fig. 9.37) are infrequent in the peripheral blood.

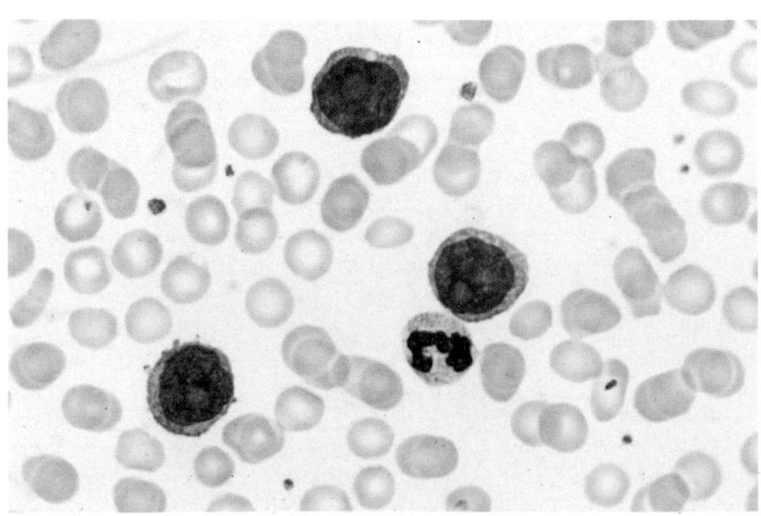

Fig. 9.36 Peripheral blood film in B-lineage PLL showing a neutrophil and three prolymphocytes with characteristic vesicular nucleoli.

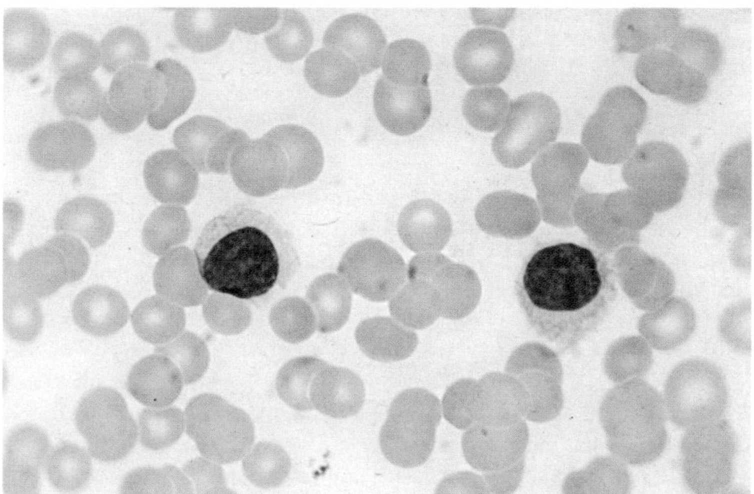

Fig. 9.37 Peripheral blood film in hairy cell leukaemia showing two hairy cells; both have plentiful cytoplasm with irregular margins and in one fine hair-like projections are present.

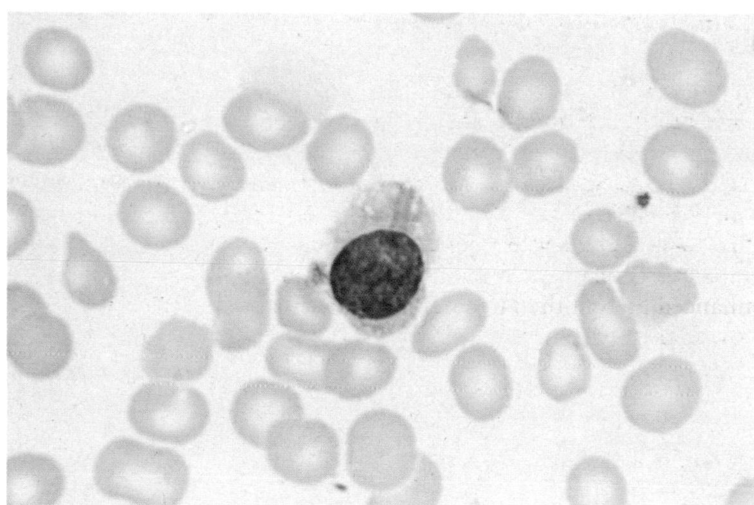

Fig. 9.38 Peripheral blood film in hairy cell leukaemia showing a hairy cell containing a ribosomal–lamellar complex. These structures are more readily observed by ultrastructural examination but can occasionally be identified by light microscopy as two parallel basophilic lines. Courtesy of Professor D. Catovsky.

There is usually normocytic anaemia and marked monocytopenia. In more advanced disease there is also neutropenia and thrombocytopenia. Hairy cells are larger than normal lymphocytes. They have abundant weakly basophilic cytoplasm with irregular 'hairy' margins. Occasionally, there are cytoplasmic inclusions which represent the ribosomal–lamellar complex which has been identified on electron microscopy; on light microscopy these inclusions appear as two indistinct parallel lines (Fig. 9.38). The nucleus may be round, oval, dumbell-shaped or bilobed. It has a bland appearance with little chromatin condensation and sometimes an indistinct nucleolus.

Differential diagnosis

The differential diagnosis is with other lymphoproliferative disorders, particularly with the variant form of hairy cell leukaemia, and with SLVL. Since there may be pancytopenia with very infrequent leukaemic cells, hairy leukaemia can also be confused with aplastic anaemia. The disproportionate reduction of the monocyte count is a useful indicator of the correct diagnosis.

Further tests

The diagnosis is confirmed by immunophenotyping [49], TRAP activity and a highly characteristic trephine biopsy in which neoplastic cells are spaced apart.

Hairy cell leukaemia variant

A variant form of hairy cell leukaemia has been recognized. It has similar clinical features to hairy cell leukaemia but some of the haematological, cytological and immunophenotypic features differ.

Blood film and count

In hairy cell leukaemia variant, the WBC is often elevated and neoplastic cells are numerous. Severe monocytopenia is not a feature. Otherwise haematological features are similar to those of hairy cell leukaemia. The neoplastic cells have similar cytoplasmic characteristics to hairy cells but have a prominent vesicular nucleolus, similar to that of the prolymphocyte (Fig. 9.39).

Differential diagnosis

The differential diagnosis is with hairy cell leukaemia and SLVL. In SLVL the neoplastic cells have less abundant cytoplasm and the nucleolus, if visible, is less prominent than in hairy cell leukaemia variant.

Further tests

Immunophenotype, cytochemistry and a trephine biopsy are useful in confirming the diagnosis. The immunophenotype of the variant form of hairy cell leukaemia differs from that of hairy cell leukaemia and TRAP activity is generally negative. The trephine biopsy usually does not show the spaced cells which are almost invariable in hairy cell leukaemia. SLVL has a similar immunophenotype to hairy cell leukaemia variant so that distinction is mainly on cytological features.

Splenic lymphoma with villous lymphocytes (SLVL)

The clinical features of SLVL are prominent splenomegaly with only minor lymphadenopathy.

Blood film and count

WBC varies from normal to moderately elevated. The blood film (Fig. 9.40) shows variable numbers

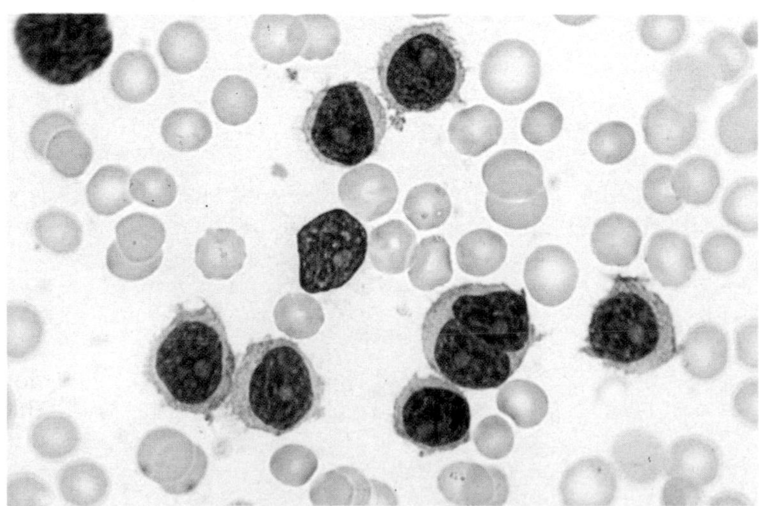

Fig. 9.39 Peripheral blood film in the variant form of hairy cell leukaemia showing cells with the cytoplasmic characteristics of hairy cells but with a prominent nucleolus. There is one binucleate cell. Courtesy of Professor D. Catovsky.

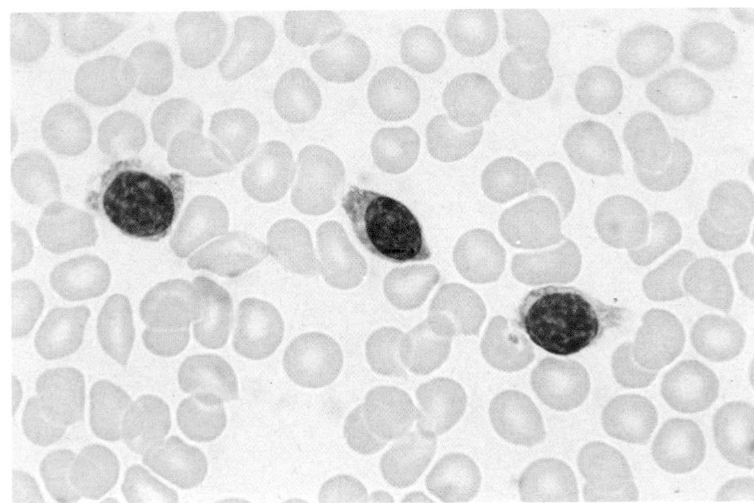

Fig. 9.40 Peripheral blood film in SLVL.

of mature small lymphocytes which are not as uniform in appearance as those of CLL. The nucleus is round with chromatin clumping and sometimes an inconspicuous nucleolus. Cytoplasm is scanty to moderate in amount and weakly to moderately basophilic. Some of the neoplastic cells have irregular or 'villous' margins, often at one pole of the cell. Some neoplastic cells show plasmacytoid differentiation. Some cases show increased rouleaux formation consequent on the presence of a paraprotein.

Differential diagnosis

The differential diagnosis is with CLL and the variant form of hairy cell leukaemia.

Further tests

The immunophenotype is useful in making the distinction from CLL. Analysis of serum immunoglobulins may demonstrate a paraprotein.

Lymphoplasmacytoid lymphoma

Lymphoplasmacytoid lymphoma is a lymphoma in which some cells show differentiation to plasmacytoid lymphocytes and, often, to plasma cells. This is usually a disease of lymph nodes and sometimes of the spleen and other lymphoid organs. A proportion of cases have involvement of the peripheral blood and bone marrow. There is often secretion of a paraprotein, most commonly but not always IgM. Sometimes the paraprotein is a cryoglobulin or shows cold agglutinin activity.

Blood film and count

When the bone marrow is infiltrated, a normocytic normochromic anaemia is common and other cytopenias can also occur. The blood film may show only rouleaux and increased background staining, as a consequence of a paraprotein, or there may be circulating lymphoma cells (Fig. 9.41). In a minority of cases there is red cell agglutination or cryoglobulin deposition. Circulating lymphoma cells resemble small lymphocytes but show some plasmacytoid features such as cytoplasmic basophilia or an eccentric nucleus. A few mature plasma cells may also be present. Sometimes cells have cytoplasmic crystals or globular inclusions.

Differential diagnosis

The differential diagnosis is with CLL. Waldenström's macroglobulinaemia is a variant of lymphoplasmacytoid lymphoma in which large amounts of an IgM paraprotein are secreted with consequent symptoms of hyperviscosity. Chronic

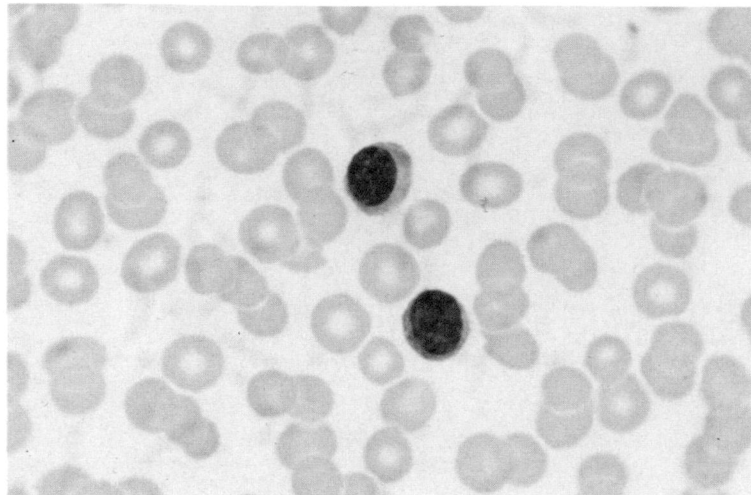

Fig. 9.41 Peripheral blood film in lymphoplasmacytoid lymphoma.

cold haemagglutinin disease is also a variant of lymphoplasmacytoid lymphoma in which the dominant clinical and haematological features are caused by the cold agglutinin activity of the paraprotein. The lymphoma itself is often very low grade and sometimes clinically inapparent.

Further tests

Bone marrow aspiration and trephine biopsy, immunophenotyping and investigations for a serum paraprotein and for urinary Bence-Jönes protein (free monoclonal immunoglobulin light chains) are indicated.

Follicular lymphoma

Centroblastic/centrocytic or follicular lymphoma is mainly a disease of the lymph nodes although in advanced disease the liver and spleen are also involved. Circulating neoplastic cells may be present at diagnosis or a leukaemic phase may develop with disease progression.

Blood film and count

The WBC varies from normal to greatly elevated. The Hb and platelet count may be normal but in advanced disease anaemia and thrombocytopenia can develop. Circulating lymphoma cells may be rare or present in large numbers. Lymphoma cells (Fig. 9.42) are often very small with scanty, almost inapparent, weakly basophilic cytoplasm. Some nuclei show notches or deep narrow clefts. These cytological features are particularly typical of cases with high WBCs. Other cases have larger, more pleomorphic cells, some of which have small but distinct nucleoli. Again there are notches or clefts in a proportion of cells. Smear cells are not a feature.

Differential diagnosis

The differential diagnosis is with CLL and other non-Hodgkin's lymphomas, particularly mantle cell lymphoma.

Further tests

Immunophenotyping is very useful in making the distinction between follicular lymphoma and CLL. The immunophenotypes of follicular lymphoma and mantle cell lymphoma are more similar and when cytological features are insufficient to make a diagnosis lymph node biopsy and cytogenetic analysis may be needed.

Mantle cell lymphoma

Mantle cell lymphoma, also known as diffuse centrocytic lymphoma and lymphoma of intermediate differentiation, is mainly a lymph node

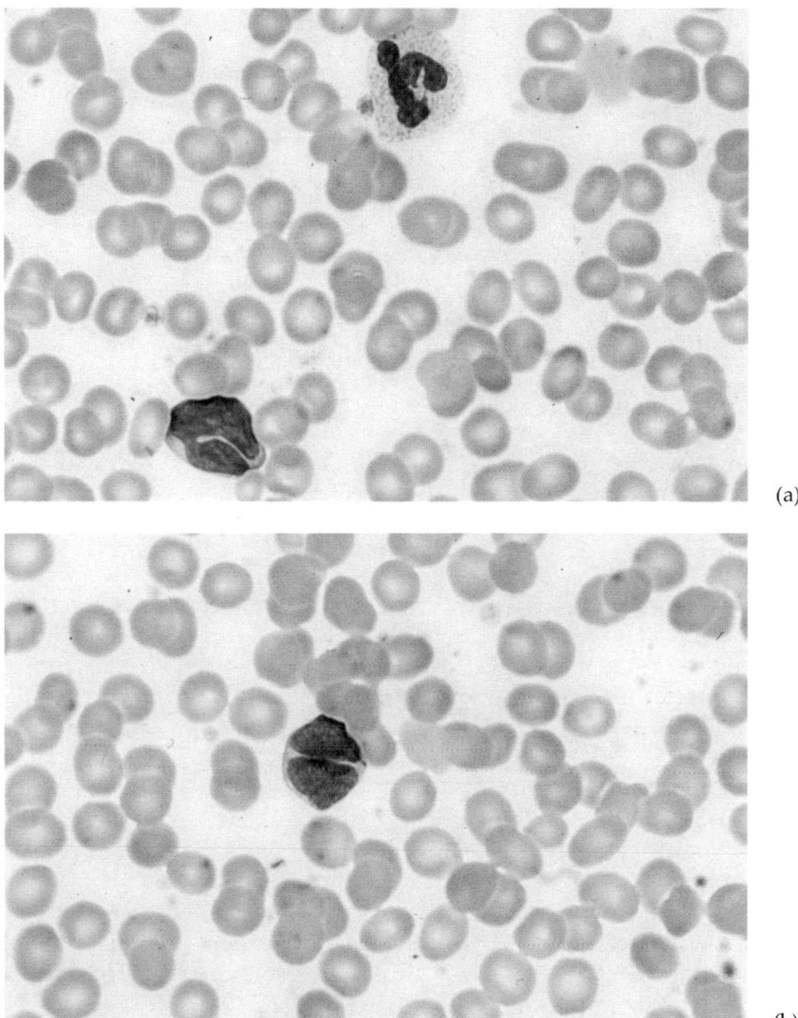

Fig. 9.42 Peripheral blood film in follicular (centroblastic/centrocytic) lymphoma showing: (a) a neutrophil and a cleft lymphocyte; and (b) a cleft lymphocyte.

disease but the peripheral blood is involved in one-fifth to one-quarter of cases.

Blood film and count

Lymphoma cells vary from small to medium in size (Fig. 9.43). Some cases have been confused with CLL but, in general, the cells are more pleomorphic. Cells are variable in shape and nucleocytoplasmic ratio. Some have cleft or irregular nuclei. Chromatin condensation is less than in CLL. Some cells are nucleolated.

Differential diagnosis

The differential diagnosis is with other non-Hodgkin's lymphomas and with CLL and CLL/PL.

Further tests

The immunophenotype is quite distinct from that of CLL and shows subtle differences from that of other non-Hodgkin's lymphomas. In general, cytological and immunophenotypic features are not sufficiently distinctive for a definite diagnosis and either lymph node histology or cytogenetic analysis is needed for confirmation.

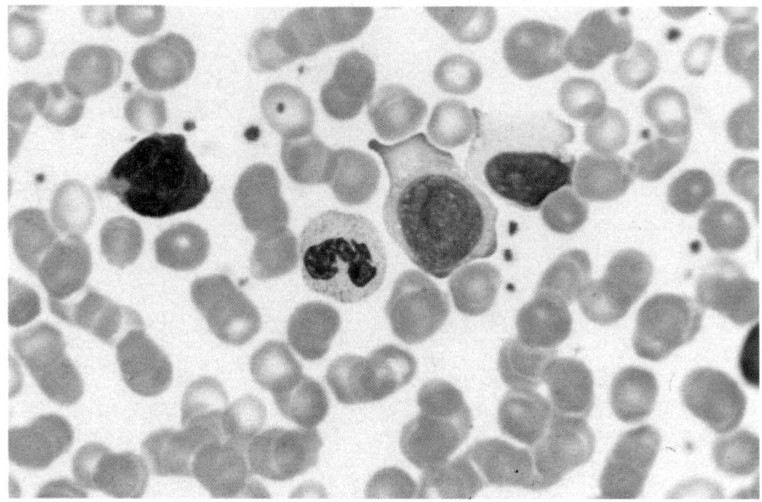

Fig. 9.43 Peripheral blood film of a patient with mantle cell lymphoma showing a neutrophil and three highly pleomorphic lymphocytes. Courtesy of Dr E. Matutes, London.

Other B-lineage lymphomas

Burkitt's lymphoma may involve the peripheral blood. In endemic Burkitt's lymphoma, leukaemia usually occurs only in advanced disease. In non-endemic and AIDS-associated Burkitt's lymphoma peripheral blood involvement is much commoner. When a leukaemic phase occurs, the cells are cytologically identical to those of L3 ALL.

A leukaemic phase is much less common in B-lineage large cell lymphomas than in the low grade lymphoproliferative disorders described above. When it occurs the cells have a diameter about three times that of a red cell (Fig. 9.44). They are usually pleomorphic with abundant moderately basophilic cytoplasm [53]. Nuclei are often lobulated and there may be prominent nucleoli. In some cases the cells resemble monoblasts.

Certain low-grade lymphomas, e.g. mucosa-associated lymphoid tissue (MALT) type lymphoma and monocytoid B-cell lymphoma, rarely have a leukaemic phase although occasional cases have shown peripheral blood dissemination.

Multiple myeloma and plasma cell leukaemia

Multiple myeloma and plasma cell leukaemia are disseminated plasma cell neoplasms. Multiple myeloma is characterized by proliferation of abnormal plasma cells (myeloma cells) in the bone marrow and, in the great majority of patients, secretion of a monoclonal immunoglobulin or immunoglobulin light chain which is referred to as a paraprotein. The monoclonal immunoglobulin is detectable in the serum. The monoclonal light chain, being of low molecular weight, is excreted in the urine where it is referred to as Bence-Jones protein. In multiple myeloma there may be some 'spillover' of neoplastic cells into the peripheral blood.

The term 'plasma cell leukaemia' indicates that neoplastic plasma cells are circulating in the blood. Plasma cell leukaemia may occur *de novo* or as the terminal phase of multiple myeloma. The FAB group [50] have suggested that this term be restricted to a *de novo* presentation in leukaemic phase but others have used it more generally [54]. Plasma cell leukaemia has been arbitrarily defined as an absolute plasma cell count of more than $2 \times 10^9/l$ with the plasma cells also being more than 20% of peripheral blood cells [54]. Plasma cell leukaemia is particularly common in IgD myeloma.

The picture of plasma cell leukaemia can also occur transiently when infection occurs in a patient with multiple myeloma, probably as a consequence of stimulation of plasma cells by interleukin 6 [55].

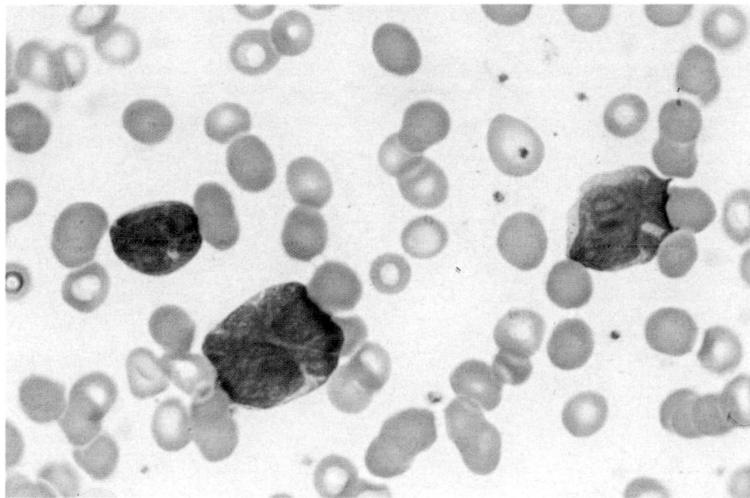

Fig. 9.44 Peripheral blood film of a patient with centroblastic lymphoma showing large pleomorphic lymphoma cells with cleft nuclei.

The most typical clinical features of multiple myeloma are anaemia, bone pain, hypercalcaemia and renal failure.

Blood film and count

The blood film in multiple myeloma usually shows normocytic normochromic anaemia. In the majority of cases in which there is a serum paraprotein there is also increased background staining and increased rouleaux formation. Cases with Bence-Jones protein but no serum paraprotein do not have increased rouleaux or increased background staining so the absence of these features does not exclude the diagnosis. The WBC and platelet count are usually not elevated and may be reduced. There may be occasional NRBC and immature granulocytes. There may also be thrombocytopenia. Circulating myeloma cells may be absent, infrequent or numerous. Circulating myeloma cells may be cytologically normal but often they show abnormalities such as nuclear immaturity (a diffuse chromatin pattern and a nucleolus), high nucleocytoplasmic ratio, reduction of cytoplasmic basophilia and poorly developed Golgi zone, mitotic figures, binuclearity and dissociation of maturation of the nucleus and the cytoplasm.

In plasma cell leukaemia (Fig. 9.45), the neoplastic cells may resemble mature plasma cells or, particularly in the cases with a *de novo* presentation, may be highly abnormal with an immature chromatin pattern, nucleoli and minimal features of plasma cell differentiation.

In some patients with multiple myeloma, the paraprotein is a cryoglobulin or has cold agglutinin activity. In such cases, precipitated cryoglobulin or red cell agglutinates may be noted in blood films.

When paraproteins are cold agglutinins or cryoglobulins they may cause factitious results with automated blood cell counters (see Chapter 4).

Differential diagnosis

In patients with circulating myeloma cells the differential diagnosis is with reactive plasmacytosis. Both conditions may have increased rouleaux formation and background staining but these abnormalities are usually much more striking in multiple myeloma. Neutrophilia, monocytosis, thrombocytosis and reactive changes in neutrophils are often present in patients with reactive plasmacytosis but they are quite uncommon in multiple myeloma. Marked cytological abnormalities are indicative of a neoplastic condition.

The differential diagnosis in cases without circulating plasma cells is with the other causes of

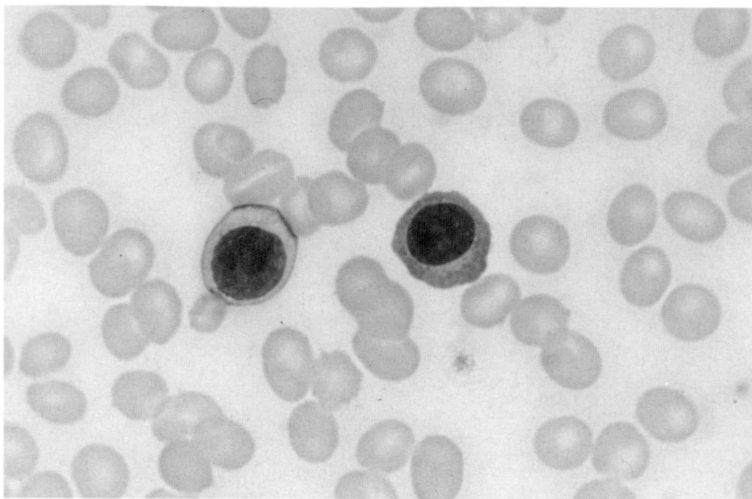

Fig. 9.45 Peripheral blood film of a patient with plasma cell leukaemia showing two neoplastic plasma cells.

normocytic normochromic anaemia (see p. 170), particularly with conditions, such as chronic inflammation or cirrhosis of the liver, in which an increased concentration of plasma proteins leads to increased rouleaux formation.

When the neoplastic cells are cytologically very atypical the differential diagnosis is with non-Hodgkin's lymphoma.

Further tests

The ESR is commonly markedly elevated in multiple myeloma and is often used as a screening test for this condition. However, it should be noted that if there is marked hyperviscosity the ESR may be normal and in cases without a serum paraprotein the ESR may not show much elevation. When multiple myeloma is suspected, tests indicated to confirm the diagnosis are bone marrow aspiration, a radiological survey of the skeleton, serum calcium estimation and investigation for serum and urinary paraproteins. Immunophenotyping is not needed unless there is any reason to doubt that the plasma cells are neoplastic in which case use of anti-κ and anti-λ reagents will demonstrate clonality. Immunophenotyping is also useful when there is doubt as to whether highly abnormal circulating cells are neoplastic or when their lineage is not apparent. The immunophenotype of the terminally differentiated plasma cell differs from that of non-Hodgkin's lymphoma cells.

T-LINEAGE LYMPHOPROLIFERATIVE DISORDERS

T-lineage lymphoproliferative disorders are less common than B-lineage disorders. Precise diagnosis requires immunophenotyping and, sometimes, cytogenetic analysis or histological examination of lymph nodes, skin or other tissues.

T-lineage prolymphocytic leukaemia (T-PLL)

T-lineage PLL is most often a disease of elderly people. Splenomegaly is the commonest clinical feature.

Blood count and film

The WBC is moderately to greatly elevated. T-lineage prolymphocytes (Fig. 9.46) are smaller and more pleomorphic than B-lineage prolymphocytes. Nuclei are irregular or lobulated. Cytoplasm is often scanty and may be moderately basophilic. In some cases cells have protruding cytoplasmic 'blebs'. Nucleoli may be inapparent or prominent but are rarely as large or as prominent as in B-lineage PLL.

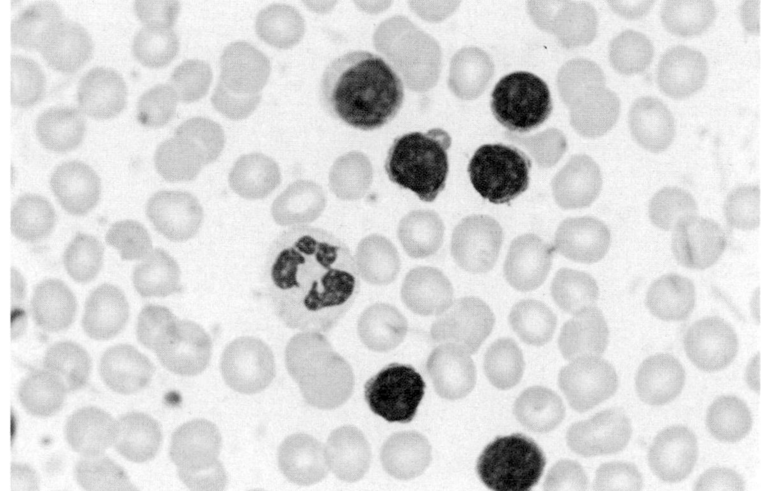

Fig. 9.46 Peripheral blood film of a patient with T-lineage PLL showing lymphocytes with irregular hyperchromatic nuclei, inconspicuous nucleoli and scanty moderately basophilic cytoplasm which in one cell is forming blebs. Only one of the cells resembles those of B-lineage PLL, being larger with a moderate amount of cytoplasm and a more prominent nucleolus.

Differential diagnosis

The differential diagnosis is mainly with B-lineage CLL and PLL.

Further tests

Immunophenotyping is essential to confirm a diagnosis. Cells characteristically express CD7 which is usually negative in other T-lineage lymphoproliferative disorders.

Cutaneous T-cell lymphomas

Mycosis fungoides and Sézary's syndrome are T-cell lymphomas which characteristically infiltrate the skin. The presence of circulating lymphoma cells is essential for the diagnosis of Sézary's syndrome in which there is widespread disease dissemination at diagnosis whereas in mycosis fungoides circulating lymphoma cells are seen only in cases with advanced stage disease. The cytological features do not differ between Sézary's syndrome and mycosis fungoides although they differ greatly between cases.

Blood count and film

The blood count is normal, apart from sometimes showing lymphocytosis. Lymphoma cells, known as Sézary cells, may be predominantly either small (Fig. 9.47) or large (Fig. 9.48) or a case may show a mixture of large and small cells. The most characteristic feature of the Sézary cell is a convoluted or cerebriform nucleus with tightly intertwined nuclear lobes. The cytoplasm is weakly basophilic and may contain a ring of vacuoles which has been likened to rosary beads. In the small Sézary cell, there is scanty cytoplasm and a compact nucleus, the surface of which appears grooved. In large Sézary cells, there is more plentiful cytoplasm and a larger nucleus with more obvious nuclear lobes.

Differential diagnosis

The differential diagnosis is with other lymphomas.

Further tests

Skin biopsy and immunophenotyping are useful in diagnosis. Intraepidermal lymphocyte accumulations (Pautrier's microabscesses) are characteristic. It is sometimes difficult to recognize small Sézary cells by light microscopy. Ultrastructural examination can be useful in such cases since the complex nuclear form is then readily apparent.

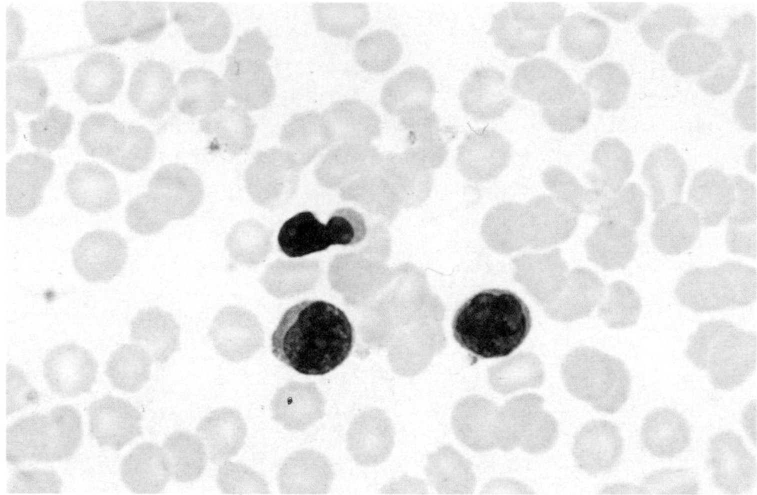

Fig. 9.47 Peripheral blood film of a patient with Sézary's syndrome showing small Sézary cells with hyperchromatic convoluted or cerebriform nuclei.

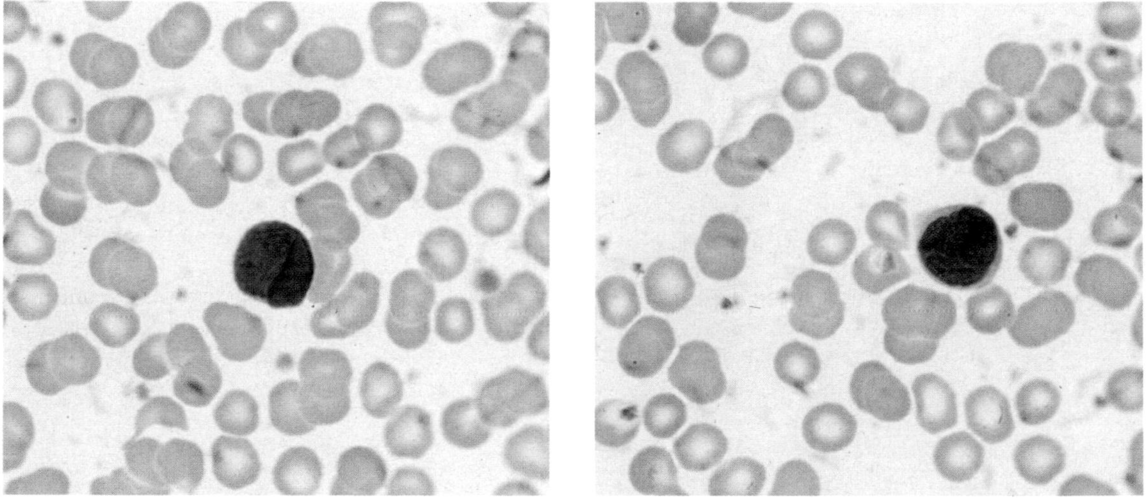

(a) (b)

Fig. 9.48 Peripheral blood film of a patient with Sézary's syndrome showing large Sézary cells.

Adult T-cell leukaemia/lymphoma (ATLL)

ATLL is a disease which develops in a minority of adults who are long-term carriers of the HTLV-I retrovirus. Such carriers mainly live in, or originate from, Japan and the Caribbean but the disease is also found in Taiwan, the Middle-East, Central and West Africa, South America, south-eastern USA and in native Americans in North America. In the majority of cases the disease manifests itself as leukaemia and in a minority as a lymphoma. In those who present with leukaemia there is usually lymphadenopathy and sometimes hepatomegaly and splenomegaly. Skin infiltration and hypercalcaemia are common. Patients with ATLL are also prone to opportunistic infections.

Blood count and film

The WBC is often greatly elevated. Leukaemic cells are generally large and very pleomorphic. Nuclei are often polylobated, their shape resembling a flower or a clover leaf (Fig. 9.49). Some nuclei have condensed chromatin while others have a diffuse chromatin pattern. Some cells are nucleolated. There is a variable amount of cytoplasm which may be basophilic. A minority of cells resemble those of Sézary's syndrome. Some patients have associated eosinophilia. Anaemia and thrombocytopenia may be minimal at diagnosis.

Differential diagnosis

The differential diagnosis is with cutaneous T-cell lymphoma and with other lymphomas of mature T cells. The degree of pleomorphism and the presence of at least a minority of cells with flower-shaped nuclei is useful in the differential diagnosis. The typical acute form of ATLL should also be distinguished from smouldering or chronic ATLL which generally lacks organomegaly, cytopenia and biochemical abnormalities. It also needs to be distinguished from the carrier state for HTLV-I in which there may be small numbers of polyclonal virus-infected atypical lymphocytes in the peripheral blood.

Other tests

Serological tests for HTLV-I are indicated. Immunophenotyping is also useful in the differential diagnosis since CD25 is commonly positive whereas it is usually negative in other leukaemias and lymphomas of phenotypically mature T cells.

Large granular lymphocyte leukaemia

Large granular lymphocyte leukaemia is a heterogeneous group of disorders in which the neoplastic cells have the cytological features of large granular lymphocytes and the immunophenotypic features of either cytotoxic T cells or natural killer cells. The clinical course is variable. Some patients have little organomegaly and a slowly progressive disease, but the course may be complicated by the effects of cytopenia, most often neutropenia. Other patients, particularly those whose cells have the phenotype of natural killer cells, have more typical features of lymphoma and a more rapid clinical course.

Blood count and film

In most cases the leukaemic cells are cytologically very similar to normal large granular lymphocytes (Fig. 9.50) with a small nucleus with condensed chromatin, plentiful weakly basophilic cytoplasm

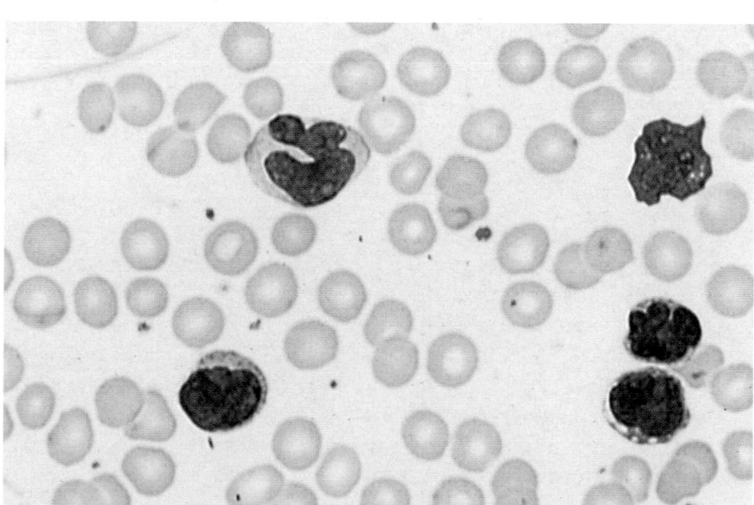

Fig. 9.49 Peripheral blood film of a patient with ATLL showing four pleomorphic lymphocytes and a smear cell; one of the lymphoma cells has a flower-shaped nucleus and two others have convoluted nuclei.

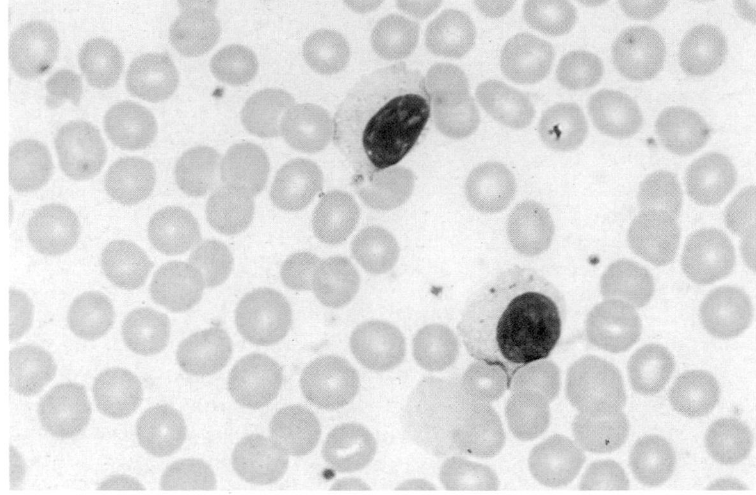

Fig. 9.50 Peripheral blood film of a patient with large granular lymphocyte leukaemia showing two large granular lymphocytes.

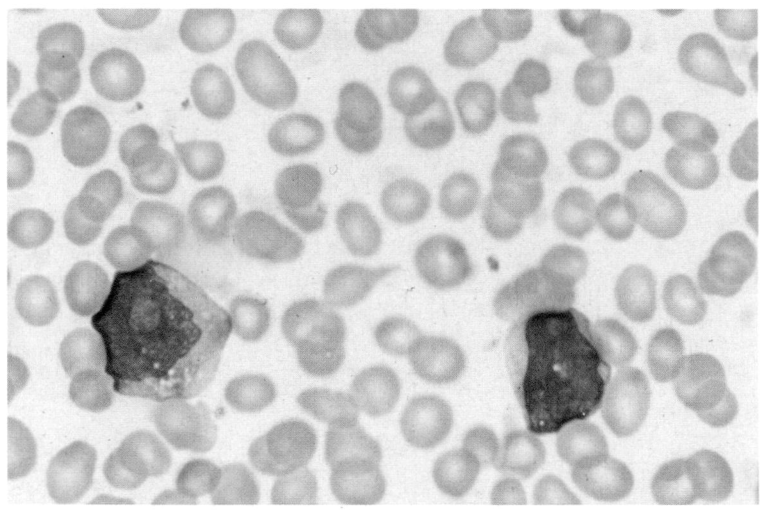

Fig. 9.51 Peripheral blood film of a patient with large cell lymphoma of T lineage showing two large lymphoma cells.

and prominent azurophilic granules in at least some of the cells. Some patients have neutropenia or, less often, anaemia or thrombocytopenia.

Differential diagnosis

The differential diagnosis is with a reactive increase of large granular lymphocytes, e.g., that caused by a chronic viral infection.

Other tests

When the diagnosis is in doubt, immunophenotyping and tests to demonstrate clonality can be of use. Most often the neoplastic cells are CD2-positive, CD3-positive and CD8-positive and show variable expression of natural killer cell markers. CD57 is most often expressed and CD11b, CD16 and CD56 less often. Other cases lack specific T-cell markers such as CD3 but express natural killer markers. A very uniform immunophenotype is suggestive of clonality and therefore of neoplasia. Clonality can be demonstrated in CD3-positive cases by molecular genetic analysis to demonstrate rearrangement of T-cell receptor genes. In CD3-negative cases cytogenetic analysis demonstrates an abnormal clone in some cases.

Other T-cell lymphomas

T-cell lymphomas are less common than B-cell lymphomas and less often have a leukaemic phase.

Blood count and film

Circulating lymphoma cells are often medium sized or large and quite pleomorphic (Fig. 9.51).

Differential diagnosis

T-cell lymphomas cannot be reliably distinguished from certain B-cell lymphomas, particularly mantle cell lymphoma and B-lineage large cell lymphomas. Occasionally, they can also be confused with AML, particularly acute monoblastic leukaemia.

Other tests

Immunophenotyping is indicated and confirms the diagnosis. Cells express T-cell markers but the immunophenotype is often aberrant.

References

1 Lascari AD. *Hematologic Manifestations of Childhood Diseases.* New York: Theme-Stratton, 1984.
2 Manroe BL, Weinberg AG, Rosenfeld CR, Browne R. The neonatal blood count in health and disease. I. Reference values for neutrophilic cells. *J Pediatr* 1979; 95: 89–98.
3 Christensen RD, Rothstein G. Pitfalls in the interpretation of leukocyte counts in newborn infants. *Am J Clin Pathol* 1978; 72: 609–11.
4 Morris CDW, Bird AR, Nell H. The haematological and biochemical changes in severe pulmonary tuberculosis. *Q J Med* 1989; 73: 1151–9.
5 Glasser RM, Walker RI, Herion JC. The significance of hematologic abnormalities in patients with tuberculosis. *Arch Intern Med* 1990; 125: 691–5.
6 Cantow EF, Kostinas JE. Studies on infectious mononucleosis. IV. Changes in the granulocytic series. *Am J Clin Pathol* 1966; 46: 43–7.
7 Habib MA, Babka JC, Burningham RA. Profound granulocytopenia associated with infectious mononucleosis. *Am J Med Sci* 1973; 265: 339–46.
8 Sumaya CV, Ench Y. Epstein–Barr virus infectious mononucleosis in children. I. Clinical and general laboratory findings. *Pediatrics* 1985; 75: 1003–10.
9 Carter JW, Edson RS, Kennedy CC. Infectious mononucleosis in the older patient. *Mayo Clin Proc* 1978; 53: 146–50.
10 Bar RS, Adlard J, Thomas FB. Lymphopenic infectious mononucleosis. *Arch Intern Med* 1975; 135: 334–7.
11 Akashi K, Eizuru Y, Sumiyoshi Y, Minematsu T, Hara S, Harada M, Kituchi M, Niho Y *et al.* Severe infectious mononucleosis-like syndrome and primary human herpesvirus 6 infection in an adult. *N Engl J Med* 1993; 329: 168–71.
12 McDonald JC, MacLean JD, McDade JE. Imported rickettsial disease: clinical and epidemiologic features. *Am J Med* 1988; 85: 799–805.
13 Wilson ME, Brush AD, Meany MC. Murine typhus acquired during short-term urban travel. *Am J Med* 1989; 57: 233–4.
14 McDade JE. Ehrlichiosis — a disease of animals and humans. *J Infect Dis* 1990; 161: 609–17.
15 Chesterman CN. Late adverse effects of streptokinase. *Aust NZ J Med* 1992; 22: 106–8.
16 Cullen MH, Stansfeld AG, Oliver RTD, Lister TA, Malpas JS. Angio-immunoblastic lymphadenopathy: report of ten cases and review of the literature. *Q J Med* 1979; 48: 151–77.
17 Delbarre F, Le Go A, Kahan A. Hyperbasophilic immunoblasts in the circulating blood in chronic inflammatory rheumatic and collagen diseases. *Ann Rheum Dis* 1975; 34: 422–30.
18 Daniele RP, Rowlands DT. Lymphocyte subpopulations in sarcoidosis: correlation with disease activity and duration. *Ann Intern Med* 1976; 85: 593–600.
19 Craig J, Isaacs D. Kawasaki syndrome in a Sydney hospital. *Aust NZ J Med* 1993; 23: 440.
20 Horwitz CA, Henle W, Henle G, Polesky H, Balfour HH, Siem RA, Borken S, Ward PCJ. Heterophile-negative infectious mononucleosis and mononucleosis-like illnesses. *Am J Med* 1977; 63: 947–57.
21 Pol S, Thiers V, Driss F, Devergie A, Berthelot P, Bréchot C. Lack of evidence for a role of HCV in hepatitis-associated aplastic anaemia. *Br J Haematol* 1993; 85: 808–10.
22 Chusid ML, Dale DC, West BC, Wolff SM. The

hypereosinophilic syndrome. *Medicine* 1975; 54: 1–27.
23 Cogan E, Schandené L, Crusiaux A, Cochaux P, Velu T, Goldman M. Clonal proliferation of type 2 helper T cells in a man with the hypereosinophilic syndrome. *N Engl J Med* 1994; 330: 535–8.
24 Spry C. Discussion: Management of the idiopathic hypereosinophilic syndrome. In: Mahmoud AAF, Austen KP, Simon AS, eds. *The Eosinophil in Health and Disease*, New York: Grune & Stratton, 1980: 341.
25 Parker RI. Hematologic aspects of mastocytosis. II. Management of hematologic disorders in association with systemic mast cell disease. *J Invest Dermatol* 1991; 96: 52S–53S.
26 Bain B. Down's syndrome – transient abnormal myelopoiesis and acute leukaemia. *Leuk Lymphoma* 1991; 3: 309–17.
27 Stevens MCG, Darbyshire PJ, Brown SM. Early congenital syphilis and severe haematological disturbance. *Arch Dis Child* 1987; 62: 1073–5.
28 Willoughby MLN. *Paediatric Haematology*. Edinburgh: Churchill Livingstone, 1977.
29 Bennett JM, Catovsky D, Daniel M-T, Flandrin G, Galton DAG, Gralnick H, Sultan C. Proposals for the classification of the acute leukaemias (FAB cooperative group). *Br J Haematol* 1976; 33: 451–9.
30 Bennett JM, Catovsky D, Daniel MT, Flandrin G, Galton DAG, Gralnick H, Sultan C. Proposed revised criteria for the classification of acute myeloid leukaemia. *Ann Intern Med* 1985; 103: 620–5.
31 Bennett JM, Catovsky D, Daniel M-T, Flandrin G, Galton DAG, Gralnick H, Sultan C. Criteria for the diagnosis of acute leukemia of megakaryocyte lineage (M7): a report of the French–American–British Cooperative Group. *Ann Intern Med* 1985; 103: 460–2.
32 Bennett JM, Catovsky D, Daniel M-T, Flandrin G, Galton DAG, Gralnick H, Sultan C. Proposal for the recognition of minimally differentiated acute myeloid leukaemia (AML M0). *Br J Haematol* 1991; 78: 325–9.
33 Bain BJ. *Leukaemia Diagnosis: a Guide to the FAB Classification*. London: Gower, 1990.
34 Soler J, O'Brien M, Tavaras de CJ, San Miguel JF, Kearney L, Goldman JM, Catovsky D. Blast crisis of chronic granulocytic leukemia with mast cell and basophil precursors. *Am J Clin Pathol* 1985; 83: 254–9.
35 Coser P, Quaglino D, de Pasquale A, Colombetti V, Prinoth O. Cytobiological and clinical aspects of tissue mast cell leukaemia. *Br J Haematol* 1980; 45: 5–12.
36 Efrati P, Klajman A, Spitz H. Mast cell leukemia? Malignant mastocytosis with leukemia-like manifestations. *Blood* 1957; 12: 869–82.
37 Parwaresch MR. *The Human Blood Basophil. Morphology, Origin, Kinetics, Function and Pathology*. Berlin: Springer-Verlag, 1976.
38 Bain BJ. Transient leukaemia in newborn infants with Down's syndrome. *Leuk Res* 1994; 18: 723–4.
39 Spiers ASD, Bain BJ, Turner JE. The peripheral blood in chronic granulocytic leukaemia. Study of 50 untreated Philadelphia chromosome-positive cases. *Scand J Haematol* 1977; 18: 25–38.
40 Castro-Malaspina H, Schaison G, Passe S, Pasquier A, Berger R, Bayle-Weisgerber C, Miller D, Seligman M *et al.* Subacute and chronic myelomonocytic leukemia in children (juvenile CML). *Cancer* 1984; 54: 675–86.
41 You W, Weisbrot IM. Chronic neutrophilic leukemia, report of two cases and review of the literature. *Am J Clin Pathol* 1979; 72: 233–242.
42 Kanoh T, Saigo K, Yamagishi M. Neutrophils with ring-shaped nuclei in chronic neutrophilic leukemia. *Am J Clin Pathol* 1986; 86: 748–51.
43 Zoumbos NC, Symeonidis A, Kourakli-Symeonidis A. Chronic neutrophilic leukemia with dysplastic features: a new variant of myelodysplastic syndromes? *Acta Haematol* 1989; 82: 156–60.
44 Srodes CH, Hyde EH, Boggs DR. Autonomous erythropoiesis during erythroblastic crisis of chronic myelocytic leukaemia. *J Clin Invest* 1973; 52: 512–15.
45 Ondreyco SM, Kjeldsberg CR, Fineman RM, Vaninetti S, Kushner JP. Monoblastic transformation in chronic myelogenous leukemia. *Cancer* 1981; 48: 957–63.
46 Rosenthal S, Schwartz JKH, Canellos GP. Basophilic chronic granulocytic leukaemia with hyperhistaminaemia. *Br J Haematol* 1977; 36: 367–72.
47 Marinone G, Rossi G, Verzura P. Eosinophilic blast crisis in a case of chronic myeloid leukaemia. *Br J Haematol* 1983; 55: 251–6.
48 Hogge DE, Misawa S, Schiffer CA, Testa JR. Promyelocytic blast crisis in chronic granulocytic leukaemia with 15;17 translocation. *Leuk Res* 1984; 8: 1019–23.
49 Bain BJ, Catovsky D. The leukaemic phase of non-Hodgkin's lymphoma. *J Clin Pathol* 1994; 48: 189–93.
50 Bennett JM, Catovsky D, Daniel M-T, Flandrin G, Galton DAG, Gralnick H, Sultan C. Proposals for the classification of chronic (mature) B and T lymphoid leukaemias. *J Clin Pathol* 1989; 42: 567–84
51 Bain BJ, Clark D, Lampert IA. *Bone Marrow Pathology*, Oxford: Blackwell Scientific Publications, 1992.
52 Melo JV, Catovsky D, Galton DAG. The relationship between chronic lymphocytic leukaemia and prolymphocytic leukaemia. I. Clinical and laboratory features of 300 patients and characterisation of an

intermediate group. *Br J Haematol* 1986; 63: 377–87.

53 Bain BJ, Matutes E, Robinson D, Lampert IA, Brito-Babapulle V, Morilla R, Catovsky D. Leukaemia as a manifestation of large cell lymphoma. *Br J Haematol* 1991; 77: 301–10.

54 Kyle RA, Maldonado JE, Bayrd ED. Plasma cell leukaemia. Report on 17 cases. *Arch Intern Med* 1974; 133: 813–18.

55 Murayama K, Sawamura M, Tamura K. Transient plasmacytosis with acute infection in myeloma. *Br J Haematol* 1993; 82: 475.

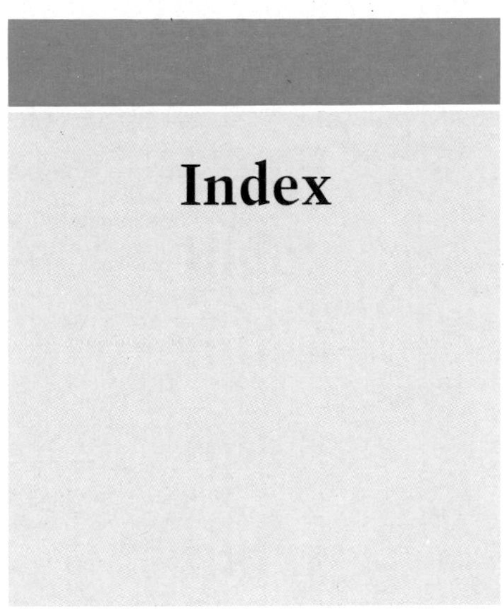

Index

Page numbers in *italic* refer to figures and/or tables